Bariatric Therapy

Elisabeth M. H. Mathus-Vliegen
Jérôme Dargent

Bariatric Therapy

Alliance between Gastroenterologists and Surgeons

Springer

Elisabeth M. H. Mathus-Vliegen
Amsterdam UMC
(University Medical Centres)
Amsterdam
The Netherlands

Jérôme Dargent
Polyclinique Lyon Nord
Lyon
France

ISBN 978-3-319-90073-5 ISBN 978-3-319-90074-2 (eBook)
https://doi.org/10.1007/978-3-319-90074-2

Library of Congress Control Number: 2018945544

Printed on acid-free paper

This Springer imprint is published by the registered company Springer International Publishing AG part of Springer Nature.
The registered company address is: Gewerbestrasse 11, 6330 Cham, Switzerland

Preface

Overweight and obesity are a global epidemic associated with many health consequences and an impressive psychosocial and economic burden. As yet, preventive measures to reverse the global trend have been unproductive and overweight has surpassed the incidence of undernutrition. Therapeutic options are limited. Intensive lifestyle interventions have been able to reduce the cumulative incidence of diabetes over a period of 4–6 years in obese patients with impaired glucose tolerance, but such interventions are difficult to sustain lifelong and thus are usually short-lived. Medical drug treatment is moderately effective and also hampered by a limited duration of prescription. Moreover, the Gaussian curve of the distribution of overweight shifts to the right, signifying that in the category of obesity patients move towards the category of morbid obesity and thus become eligible for bariatric surgery.

Many obesity-associated comorbidities relate to the gastrointestinal tract, and formerly this was the only place where surgeons and gastroenterologist met. Nowadays they should form an alliance, as not only the complications of obesity itself but also the treatment of obesity by endoscopic and surgical bariatric means and possible complications thereof require a close cooperation and mutual understanding. This alliance between the two specialisms is the topic of this book.

Although this book was written in close cooperation, the signature of the gastroenterologist will be visible in Chaps. 1, 2, 4–6 and the signature of the surgeon in Chaps. 3 and 7. These chapters deal with the comorbidities related to the gastrointestinal tract, the endoscopic bariatric treatment, the preoperative screening and perioperative and postoperative guidance and the whole spectrum of surgical options. When postbariatric complications occur, the endoscopic modalities in the early and late postoperative period are discussed at length.

The remaining Chaps. 7–11 were a true challenge and as such cannot be retrieved from the literature: they are the result of weighing the pros and cons. They discuss matters such as when the endoscopist needs the surgeon, when gastroenterologist and surgeons should act as one, and when they are possible opponents. Also, a completely new way of looking at weight loss trajectories is offered.

The detailed discussions should enable gastroenterologists and surgeons to better delineate the options, the responsibilities and knowledge and possibilities of each specialty. The profound conviction that a lot can be gained from a close cooperation lays the foundation of this book and both authors wish the reader as much as pleasure with reading as the authors had with writing. They do hope that it provides the tools for adequate management of the obese patient.

Amsterdam, The Netherlands Elisabeth M. H. Mathus-Vliegen
Lyon, France Jérôme Dargent

Contents

Epidemiology and Comorbidities

1

Contents

Abbreviations

^{1}H-MRS	Proton magnetic resonance spectroscopy
AARP	American Association of Retired Persons
AGE	Advanced glycation end
ALT	Alanine aminotransferase
AMP	Adenosine monophosphate
AMPK	AMP-activated protein kinase
APACHE	Acute Physiology and Chronic Health Evaluation
AST	Aspartate aminotransferase

E. M. H. Mathus-Vliegen, J. Dargent, *Bariatric Therapy*,
https://doi.org/10.1007/978-3-319-90074-2_1

ATBC	Alpha-tocopherol beta-carotene
ATP	Adenosine triphosphate
BEACON	Barrett and Esophageal Adenocarcinoma Consortium
BIA	Body impedance analysis
BMI	Body mass index
COX	Cyclooxygenase
CRC	Colorectal cancer
CRP	C-reactive protein
CT	Computed tomography
CVD	Cardiovascular disease
DEXA	Dual-energy X-ray absorptiometry
EPIC	European Prospective Investigation into Cancer and Nutrition
ERCP	Endoscopic retrograde cholangiopancreaticography
ERK	Extracellular signal-regulated kinase
GI	Gastrointestinal
GORD	Gastro-oesophageal reflux disease
GTT	Glucose tolerance test
H. pylori	*Helicobacter pylori*
HCC	Hepatocellular carcinoma
HDL	High-density lipoprotein
HFCS	High-fructose corn syrup
HMW	High molecular weight
HOMA	Homeostatic model assessment
Hp	*Helicobacter pylori*
HR	Hazard ratio
IGF-1	Insulin-like growth factor-1
IGFBP	Insulin-like growth factor-binding protein
IHTG	Intrahepatic triglyceride content
IL	Interleukin
IR	Insulin resistance
LCD	Low-calorie diet
LDL	Low-density lipoprotein
LMW	Low molecular weight
LOS	Lower oesophageal sphincter
LOSP	Lower oesophageal sphincter pressure
MAPK	Mitogen-activated protein kinase
MCP-1	Monocyte chemoattractant protein-1
MetS	Metabolic syndrome
MMW	Middle molecular weight
MOD	Multi-organ dysfunction
MOF	Multiple organ failure
MR	Magnetic resonance
MRI	Magnetic resonance imaging
mTOR	Mammalian target of rapamycin
MUFA	Mono-unsaturated fatty acid
NAFL	Non-alcoholic fatty liver
NAFLD	Non-alcoholic fatty liver disease

NAS	NAFLD Activity Score
NASH	Non-alcoholic steatohepatitis
NCD-RisC	NCD Risk factor collaboration
NCI	National Cancer Institute
NDDM	non-insulin dependent diabetes mellitus
Nf-κB	Nuclear factor kappa B
NHANES	National Health and Nutrition Examination Survey
NHI	National Institutes of Health
NSAID	Non-steroidal anti-inflammatory drug
OGD	Oesophagogastroduodenoscopy
OR	Odds ratio
PAI	Plasminogen activator inhibitory protein
PCOS	Polycystic ovary syndrome
PI3K	Phosphatidyl inositol 3-kinase
PAR	Peroxisome proliferator-activated receptor
PET	Position emission tomography
PUFA	Polyunsaturated fatty acid
PYY	Polypeptide Y
RR	Relative risk
ROS	Reactive oxygen species
SAT	Subcutaneous adipose tissue
SEER	Surveillance epidemiology and end results
SHBG	Sex hormone binding globuline
SIM	Specialised intestinal metaplasia
SIR	Standardised incidence ratio
SIRS	Systemic inflammatory response syndrome
SRR	Summary relative risk
T2DM	Type 2 diabetes mellitus
TNF-α	Tumour necrosis factor-alpha
TLOSR	Transient lower oesophageal sphincter relaxation
US	Ultrasound
VAT	Visceral adipose tissue
VEGF	Vascular endothelial growth factor
VLCD	Very-low-calorie diet
VLDL	Very-low-density lipoprotein
WHO	World Health Organisation
WHR	Waist-to-hip ratio

1.1 Introduction and Epidemiology

Overweight and obesity have reached epidemic proportions and globally there are now more people who are obese than underweight. This is the case in every region except parts of sub-Saharan Africa and Asia [1]. In 2014 266 million men and 375 million women were obese compared to only 34 million men and 71 million women in 1975 and 58 million men and 126 million women suffered from severe obesity.

In 2016 the Non-Communicable Disease Risk factor Collaboration (NCD-RisC) evaluated 1698 population-based worldwide data sources from 200 countries with more than 19.2 million (9.9 million men and 9.3 million women) participants aged 18 years and older to estimate trends in overweight and obesity from 1975 to 2014 [1]. Over this period the global age-standardised mean Body Mass Index (BMI) in men increased from 21.7 kg/m^2 in 1975 to 24.2 kg/m^2 in 2014, and in women from 22.1 kg/m^2 to 24.4 kg/m^2. The mean increases per decade were 0.63 kg/m^2 for men and 0.59 kg/m^2 for women, signifying an increase in body weight per decade of 1.5 kg. There were large regional differences. The largest increase in men's mean BMI was in high-income English-speaking countries and in women in central Latin America. The prevalence of obesity (BMI ≥30 kg/m^2) increased from 3.2% in 1975 to 10.8% in men and from 6.4% to 14.9% in women (Fig. 1.1). Severe obesity (BMI ≥35 kg/m^2) was present in 2.3% of men and in 5.0% of women and morbid obesity (BMI ≥40 kg/m^2) in 0.64% and 1.6%, respectively. In 2014 more men were obese in 68% of 200 countries and severely obese in 56.5% of countries than underweight. Similar data were 83% and 67.5%, respectively, for women. In 2014 slightly more obese people live in China than in the USA and China moved to the second rank for severe obesity. Notwithstanding this, more than one out of four severely obese men and almost one in five severely obese women in the world live in the USA.

The probability of reaching the global target of halting the rise in obesity by 2025 at the 2010 obesity level is virtually zero. By 2025, the global obesity prevalence will reach 18% in men and surpass 21% in women and severe obesity will surpass 6% in men and 9% in women. If recent trends continue it has been estimated that in 2030 60% of the world's population will be overweight with 3.3 billion people of whom 2.2 billion are overweight and 1.1 billion are obese.

Forty-one million children under the age of five were overweight or obese in 2014 [2, 3]. In Africa, the number of children who are overweight or obese has nearly doubled from 5.4 million in 1990 to 10.6 million in 2014. Nearly half of the children under five who were overweight or obese in 2014 lived in Asia. In European countries the prevalence of overweight and obesity in adults is 50% [4, 5]. Within the range of obesity the segment with a BMI ≥35 kg/m^2 is rapidly growing. In the USA a BMI >35 kg/m^2 is present in 15% of the adult population.

These alarming data signify an enormous burden of well-known obesity-associated diseases such as type 2 diabetes mellitus (T2DM), hypertension, dyslipidaemia, metabolic syndrome, cardiovascular disease, sleep apnoea syndrome and certain cancers. Overweight and obesity are the strongest established risk factor for diabetes which is associated with a 2–3-fold increased risk of mortality [6]. The International Diabetes Federation (IDF) estimated that the cost of caring for diabetes worldwide was at least $673 billion in 2015. The NCD-RisC also estimated the trend in diabetes between 1980 and 2014, without differentiating between type 1 and type 2 diabetes, in 751 studies including almost 4.4 million participants [7]. Global age-standardised diabetes prevalence doubled from 4.3% in 1980 to 9.0% in men and increased by 60% from 5.0% to 7.9% in women. The number of adults with diabetes increased from 108 million in 1980 to 422 million in 2014, a near quadrupling of the number of adults. This impressive increase could be explained for 28.5% due to the rise in prevalence, 39.7% due to population growth and 31.8%

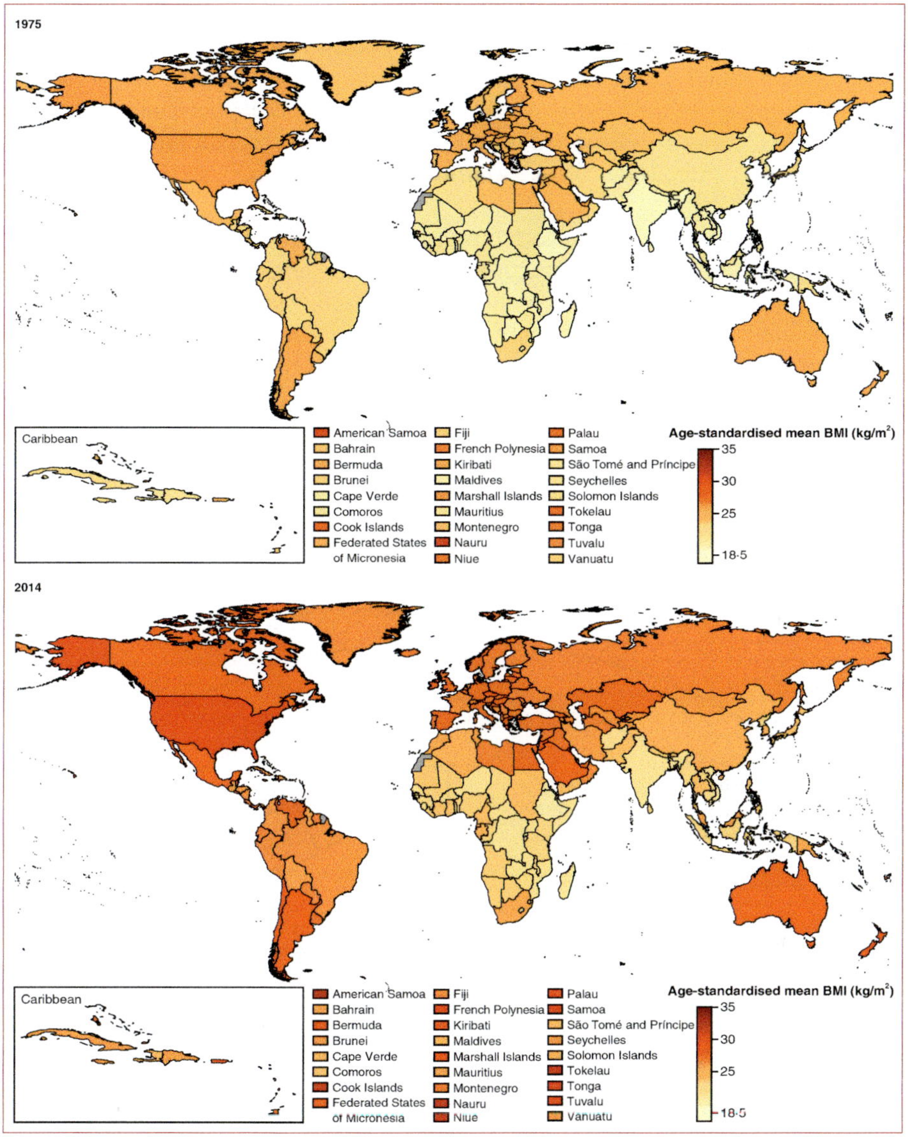

Fig. 1.1 Age-standardised mean BMI in women in 1975 and 2014 worldwide (printed with permission of the editors of the Lancet) [1]

due to the interaction of these two factors. The probability of reaching the goal of halting diabetes at the 2010 level in 2025 is less than 1% in men and is 1% in women. If the trend continues the age-standardised prevalence of diabetes by the year 2025 will be 12.8% in men and 10.4% in women, surpassing a number of 700 million people.

Obesity is an established risk factor for at least ten cancers (oesophagus adenocarcinoma; liver, gallbladder, colorectum and pancreas cancer; kidney cancer; and in males advanced prostate cancer and in females postmenopausal breast cancer and cancer of the endometrium and ovaries) [8]. Besides the already mentioned gastrointestinal (GI) cancers, the GI tract is involved with gastro-oesophageal reflux disease (GORD) with its complications of erosive oesophagitis, Barrett's oesophagus and oesophageal adenocarcinoma, gallstone disease, acute pancreatitis, non-alcoholic fatty liver disease (NAFLD) and colon adenomas.

Apart from these serious comorbidities which may lead to a reduced life expectancy, a range of debilitating conditions such as osteoarthritis, respiratory difficulties, infertility and psychosocial problems, with stigmatisation and discrimination, have a negative impact on the quality of life and result in work absenteeism and disability. Both the life-threatening comorbidities and the impaired quality of life are depicted in the obesity web (Fig. 1.2). Obesity is responsible for 10–13% of deaths. Furthermore, the WHO has emphasized that 44% of T2DM burden, 23% of ischaemic heart disease burden and 7–41% of certain cancer burdens are related to overweight and obesity [2]. In European countries overweight and obesity are

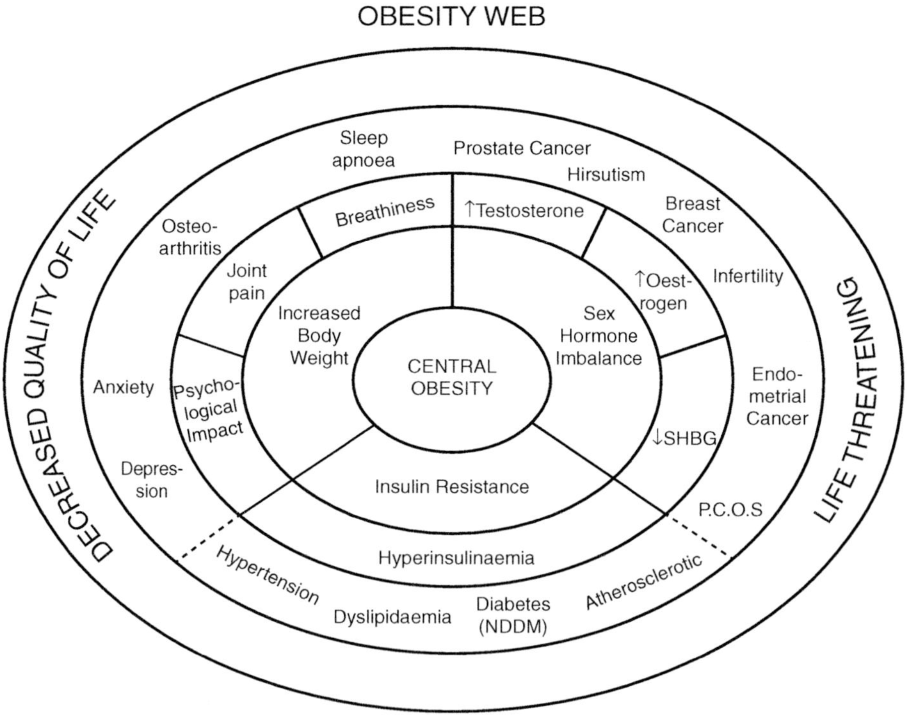

Fig. 1.2 The obesity web illustrates the diverse range of conditions associated with obesity. Furthermore it shows how these conditions are linked in terms of physiological and biochemical mechanisms and how obesity and central obesity may threaten health and cause a decreased quality of life

responsible for 80% of cases of T2DM, 35% of ischaemic heart disease and 55% of hypertension among adults [4].

1.2 Definition and Classification

The term overweight refers to an excess of body weight in relation to height and–in children–age [9]. An excess of body weight may involve water, muscle, osseous and adipose tissue but most overweight people will have an excess of adipose tissue. The terms obesity and adiposity refer specifically to an absolute or a relative excess in body fat mass. This excess fat storage, in addition to the way in which the fat is distributed in the body, places the individual at risk of premature death and many obesity-associated comorbidities. Quantification of the amount of adipose tissue and its distribution is important. For everyday use the body mass index (BMI, calculated by dividing weight in kilogram by height in meters squared, kg/m^2) suffices, which is largely independent of height and, at least in adult Caucasians, correlates closely with the mass of body fat.

The World Health Organisation (WHO) classified people according to their BMI into classes of underweight (BMI <18.5 kg/m^2), normal weight (BMI 18.5–24.9 kg/m^2), overweight or pre-obesity (BMI 25.0–29.9 kg/m^2) and obesity (BMI ≥30 kg/m^2) with obesity class I (BMI 30–34.9 kg/m^2), class II (BMI 35.0–39.9 kg/m^2) and class III (≥40 kg/m^2) (Table 1.1) [10–14]. For Asian countries different BMI categories have been defined as a similar level of BMI in South East Asians is associated with higher risks of comorbidities than in Caucasians [10–14]. The threshold for obesity is 2 kg/m^2 lower (Table 1.1). The term morbid obesity refers to the category of BMI ≥40 kg/m^2.

BMI is known to be an imperfect predictor of metabolic risks [15]. Some individuals with a normal BMI have a metabolic pattern characteristic of those with overweight or obesity. Some with high BMI appear to have a healthy metabolic pattern, the so-called healthy obese, suggesting that the disease risks associated with obesity may not be uniform and that apparently a subgroup of obese patients is resistant to the development of obesity-associated diseases [16]. The meta-analysis by Kramer and colleagues tried to determine the effect of the metabolic status on all-cause mortality and cardiovascular events in adults with data available on the three categories of BMI, all-cause mortality, fatal and non-fatal cardiovascular events and being metabolically healthy or unhealthy defined by the presence of metabolic syndrome components [17, 18]. A total of 61,386 persons in 8 studies, followed over 10 years or more, were included. They concluded that metabolically unhealthy persons, regardless of BMI, were at 2.5–3 times increased risk of death. However, the metabolically healthy obese group was also at risk, although the risk was smaller, 24% higher, thereby casting doubt on the existence of metabolically healthy obesity [17, 18]. Unfortunately, carefully conducted basis scientific studies that tried to determine the beneficial phenotype of obesity were not considered such as studies with euglycaemic insulin clamps and studies with careful measurement of total body, visceral and subcutaneous fat by

Table 1.1 Comparison of cut-offs of BMI, waist circumference and several components of the metabolic syndrome in Western and Asian countries [10–14]

	Western countries	Asian countries[a]
BMI normal weight	18.5–24.9 kg/m^2	18.5–22.9 kg/m^2
BMI overweight	25–29.9 kg/m^2	23.0–27.4 kg/m^2
BMI obesity	≥30 kg/m^2	≥27.5 kg/m^2
BMI obesity class I	30–34.9 kg/m^2	27.5–32.4 kg/m^2
BMI obesity class II	35–39.9 kg/m^2	32.5–37.4 kg/m^2
BMI obesity class III/morbid obesity	≥40 kg/m^2	≥37.5 kg/m^2
BMI obesity super-morbid obesity	≥50 kg/m^2	
Waist circumference, males Overweight Obese	 ≥94 cm ≥102 cm	
Waist circumference, females Overweight Obese	 ≥80 cm ≥88 cm	
Metabolic syndrome		
Waist circumference, males	≥94 cm	≥90 cm
Waist circumference, females	≥80 cm	≥80 cm
Arterial blood pressure	≥130/85 mmHg or treatment for hypertension	≥130/85 mmHg or treatment for hypertension
Fasting glucose	≥5.6 mmol/L or treatment for T2DM	≥5.6 mmol/L or treatment for T2DM
Serum triglycerides	≥1.7 mmol/L or treatment for hyperlipidaemia	≥1.7 mmol/L or treatment for hyperlipidaemia
HLD cholesterol levels, males	<1.03 mmol/L or treatment	<1.03 mmol/L or treatment
HLD cholesterol levels, females	<1.29 mmol/L or treatment	<1.29 mmol/L or treatment

[a]Threshold BMI for obesity in South Asians being 2 kg/m^2 lower and waist being 10 cm smaller

magnetic resonance (MR) imaging (MRI) and those measuring fat in muscle and liver by MR spectroscopy [19, 20]. Moreover, a relatively large fat mass may mask a small muscle mass, a condition known as sarcopenic obesity. The sole use of BMI may thus aggregate different people with differences in nutritional status, disability, disease and mortality risk.

Likewise, the surplus value of the distribution of fat is more and more appreciated [9]. Subcutaneous fat in peripheral parts of the body, also named peripheral, gynoid, femorogluteal or lower body obesity, is physiological and not associated with health hazards. In contrast, increased intra-abdominal and visceral fat, also named central, android, abdominal or upper body obesity, is associated with increased health risks. An estimation of the distribution of adipose tissue can be obtained by body circumference measurements, such as the waist circumference, measured halfway the lower rib cage and the upper crest of the pelvis (in cm), or the waist/hip circumference ratio (WHR), in which the waist circumference is divided by the hip circumference, measured over both femur condyles. As such, a waist circumference of 80–88 cm in females and 94–102 cm in males corresponds with overweight [21]. In patients with a BMI between 25 and 34.9 the measurement of the waist wand waist-to-hip ratio are recommended by current guidelines. Cut-off values to define abdominal obesity and to identify persons at risk are 102 cm for men and 88 cm for women and for the WHR ratio 1.0 in men and 0.85 in women [9, 21]. The WHR is presumably a more specific surrogate for the fat distribution as the WHR is less strongly correlated with BMI as is the waist circumference but mostly the use of the waist circumference has been proposed [9, 21]. In Asians these measures are different: the waist is 10 cm smaller. This has also implications for the definition of the metabolic syndrome, which clusters components predictive for cardiovascular diseases, and which requires the presence of visceral obesity defined by the waist circumference combined with at least two other factors [13]. For Asian populations the new definition for the metabolic syndrome which includes the waist circumference is mentioned in Table 1.1 [11, 12, 14].

Methods to better quantify the absolute amount of adipose tissue and its location are either expensive or only feasible in the context of scientific research [9]. Examples of sometimes readily available methods are ultrasonography, body impedance analysis (BIA), computed tomography (CT), magnetic resonance imaging (MRI) and dual-energy X-ray absorptiometry (DEXA). Magnetic resonance spectroscopy allows the determination of fatty tissues in liver and muscle. Hydrodensitometry and isotope dilution and neutron activation methods are mainly available for scientific purposes and the same holds true for position emission tomography (PET) method to demonstrate brown adipose tissue.

1.3 Pathogenesis of Comorbidities

Treatment of obesity is more than a reduction of excess fat; it is also the treatment of obesity's comorbidities. To better understand the pathogenesis of these comorbidities, both the mechanical load by the excess body mass and the role of the adipose tissue itself should be taken into consideration.

Adipose tissue is no longer considered to be an inert tissue. Brown adipose tissue, being found principally in neonates but also in the neck-scapular region in adults with distinct differences between normal-weight and obese individuals, is mainly involved in the temperature regulation [22–24]. When exposed to cold, for instance 16 °C, the energy expenditure increases by approximately 160 kcal per day and this is likely through brown adipose tissue thermogenesis [23, 24]. White adipose tissue is now considered to constitute an endocrine organ in its own right, being an important mediator of metabolism and inflammation [25, 26] (Fig. 1.3). It secretes adipokines which are divided into *hormone-like adipokines* such as leptin, resistin, adiponectin, visfatin, apelin, vaspin, hepcidin, chemerin, omentin and angiopoietin-like peptide 4, and *inflammatory cytokines*, which include tumour necrosis factor alpha (TNF-α), interleukins such as interleukin-1 (IL-1), IL-6 and IL-10, plasminogen activator protein (PAI) and monocyte chemoattractant protein-1 (MCP-1).

	Effects	Pathways	Involved adipokines and cytokines
White adipose tissue	Metabolism	Energy homeostasis	Leptin, IL-6, IL-1, IL-1Ra
		Adipocyte differentiation	TNF-α, MCP-1, IL-1, IL-1Ra, IL-6
		Insulin sensitivity	IL-1, IL-1Ra, IL-6, TNF-α
	Inflammation	Inflammatory control	IL-1, IL-1Ra, IL-6, IL-8, IL-9, IP-10, TNF-α, MCP-1, PAI, RANTES
		Cardiovascular protection/ Neo-angiogenesis	Adiponectin, IL-1, IL-1Ra, IL-10, VEGF, Leptin, TNF-α
		Vascular inflammation	IL-8, IL-10, MCP-1, RANTES, Resistin

Fig. 1.3 The effects of white adipose tissue on metabolism and inflammation through different pathways with involved adipokines and cytokines [25, 26]. *IL* interleukin, *TNF-α* tumour necrosis factor-alpha, *MCP-1* monocyte chemoattractant protein-1, *PAI* plasminogen activator inhibitory protein, *RANTES* regulated upon activation normal T-cell sequence, *VEGF* vascular endothelial growth factor, *IP-10* interferon-gamma inducible protein 10

These adipokines and cytokines are involved in energy homeostasis, adipocyte differentiation and insulin sensitivity, and thereby have their effect on metabolism. They also exert their influence on inflammation through pathways of inflammatory control, cardiovascular protection, angiogenesis and vascular inflammation. Some hormone-like adipokines and inflammatory cytokines, that are mentioned in a large number of studies, need some more detailed discussion [25, 26].

1.3.1 Hormone-Like Adipokines

Through the hypothalamus *leptin* modulates body weight, food intake and fat stores. High levels of leptin, related to the large fat mass in the obese, do not suppress the appetite because of resistance to the hormone due to leptin receptor signalling defects, downstream blockade in neuronal circuits and defects in leptin transport across the blood-brain barrier. Furthermore, leptin regulates pancreatic islet cell growth, growth hormone levels, immune homeostasis, haematopoiesis, angiogenesis, wound healing, osteogenesis and gastrointestinal function.

Adiponectin has anti-proliferative and anti-atherosclerotic properties and is an antioxidant by decreasing reactive oxygen; it augments endothelial nitrous oxygen production protecting the vasculature by vasodilation and reduced platelet aggregation. Adiponectin concentrations are markedly declined in morbid obesity and a wide array of diseases such as stroke, coronary heart disease, insulin resistance, non-alcoholic fatty liver disease (NAFLD) and steatohepatitis (NASH), and many obesity-related cancers have been associated with decreased adiponectin levels.

	Location	Secretion of	Effects
Local white adipose tissue deposits	Visceral	IL-8, IP-10, MCP-1, RANTES	Local and systemic inflammation
	Muscle	TNF-α, FFA, IL-6	Insulin resistance
	Epicardial	IL-6, IL-1b, TNF-α, MCP-1	Local inflammation and chemotaxis
	Perivascular	IL-1/ IL-1Ra, IL-6, IL-8, IP-10, MCP-1, TNF-α, RANTES	Atherosclerosis and systolic hypertension
	Kidney	Reabsorption of sodium	Increased vascular volume, hypertension

Fig. 1.4 Local effects of white tissue and their secretory products on metabolism and inflammation [25, 26]. *IL* interleukin, *IP-10* interferon-gamma inducible protein 10, *MCP-1* monocyte chemoattractant protein-1, *RANTES* regulated upon activation normal T-cell sequence, *TNF-α* tumour necrosis factor-alpha, *FFA* free fatty acids

1.3.2 Inflammatory Cytokines and Anti-inflammatory Factors

Inflammatory cytokines can be divided into adipocytokines (leptin, resistin, visfatin, adiponectin), interferons (interferon gamma, beta), interleukins (IL-1, IL-5), haematopoietic factors, chemokines (IL-6, IL-10, MCP-1) and growth factors (TNF-α). TNF-α, IL-1 and IL-6 influence growth and immunity, and initiate inflammation, apoptosis and cell division. Anti-inflammatory factors include anti-inflammatory cytokines (IL-4, IL-10, tumour growth factor beta (TGF-β)), receptor antagonists (IL-1Ra), soluble receptors (IL-1RII, sTNFR, sIL-1R) and adipocytokines (adiponectin).

Adding to the complexity is the fact that different fat depots in the body play secrete different sets of adipokines [25, 26] (Fig. 1.4). Whereas visceral adipose tissue can influence both systemic and local inflammatory processes, muscular fat deposits figure more prominently with insulin resistance. Perivascular fat can facilitate the development of atheromas and perirenal fat can contribute to hypertension. In contrast to lean subjects who have normal-sized adipocytes with normal numbers of macrophages with high adiponectin and low leptin levels, obese patients have large adipocytes, more macrophages in their adipose tissue and more apoptotic adipocytes with low adiponectin levels and high leptin levels, promoting atherosclerosis and decreased insulin responsiveness or insulin resistance in liver and muscle.

1.4 Decreased Life Expectancy and Mortality

Most of the curves depicting mortality in relationship to increasing BMI values show a J-shaped or U-shaped configuration with excess mortality at both extremes of BMI values, i.e. underweight defined by a BMI <18.5 and overweight/obesity defined by a BMI ≥ 25 kg/m^2. Reverse causation explains the death at lower BMIs as pre-existent chronic disease and inadequate control for smoking status can distort the true relation between body weight and risk of death. Smoking is associated with a lower BMI and an increased risk of death and pre-existing disease is linked to both decreased weight and increased risk of death. The studies that investigated the cause of death at low BMIs found mainly a higher mortality from non-cancer, non-cardiovascular diseases such as acute or chronic respiratory diseases, infectious disease and injuries or a higher mortality from cardiovascular disease [21, 27–29]. Others have suggested that the higher mortality is a detrimental effect of a low BMI per se.

In the Framingham Heart Study (1948–1990) life expectancy and premature death before 70 years of age were measured in overweight and obese subjects [30]. Because of being overweight, 40-year-old female non-smokers lost 3.3 years and 40-year-old male non-smokers lost 3.1 years of life expectancy and because of obesity the lost years of life were 7.1 and 5.1 years, respectively. Obese women were 115% more likely and obese men 81% more likely to die before age 70. Obese female smokers lost 7.2 years and obese male smokers lost 6.7 years when compared with normal-weight 40-year-old smokers. The survival advantage by non-smoking in the obese was rather small. Obese female smokers lost 13.3 years and obese male smokers lost 13.7 years when compared with normal-weight non-smokers. So, the double burden of obesity and smoking resulted in losing 13–14 years of life expectancy. These data were confirmed in the large Prospective Studies Collaboration publication with a reduced life expectancy by 2–4 years at BMI 30–35 and by 8–10 years at BMI 40–45 [28].

There are not many studies that investigated the effect of both overall and abdominal adiposity. In the European Prospective Investigation into Cancer and Nutrition (EPIC) with a mean follow-up of 9.7 years in 359,387 subjects the lowest mortality was observed at a BMI of 25.3 for men and 24.3 for women and in smokers at a lower BMI of 24.5 for men and 23.9 for women [21]. After adjustment for BMI, relative risks (RR) for death in the highest quintile of waist (≥102.7 cm in males and ≥89.0 cm in females vs., respectively, <86.0 and <70.1 cm) were 2.05 (95% confidence interval 1.80/2.33) for men and 1.78 (1.56/2.04) for women. In the highest quintile of waist-to-hip ratio the relative risks of death were 1.68 (1.53/1.84) for men and 1.51 (1.37/1.60) for women. BMI remained significantly associated with the risk of death in models that included waist and waist/hip ratio. So, both general and abdominal adiposities are associated with an increased risk of death. For a given BMI an increase in waist by 5 cm increased the risk for death with 17% (1.15/1.20) among men and by 13% (1.11/1.15) among women. Similarly, by a given BMI an increase by 0.1 in WHR resulted in an increased death rate of 1.34 (1.28/1.39) for men and 1.24 (1.20/1.29) for women. Alarmingly, the associations of waist and WHR tended to be stronger in the lower BMI category: among men and women of normal weight the relative risks of death in the highest quintile of waist were, respectively, 2.06 (1.32/3.20) and 1.79 (1.39/2.31) and in the highest quintile of WHR, respectively, 1.79 (1.53/2.10) and 1.53 (1.34/1.75), again emphasising the fact that even normal-weight subjects may be at risk when a visceral fat distribution is present.

The Prospective Studies Collaboration publication of 57 studies with almost 900,000 adults gives more details about the effect of stepwise higher BMI values [28]. In both sexes the mortality was lowest at about BMI 22.5–25 kg/m^2. Each 5 kg/m^2 higher BMI was associated with at least 5 mmHg higher systolic blood pressure and about 4 mmHg higher diastolic blood pressure; it was inversely associated with HDL cholesterol (0.16 mmol/L lower in males and 0.14 mmol/L lower in females) and therefore strongly positively related with the ratio of non-HDL to HDL (males 0.85, females 0.54 higher per 5 kg/m^2). Moreover, each 5 kg/m^2 higher BMI was on average associated with about a 30% higher overall mortality (hazard ratio (HR) per 5 kg/m^2 1.29 (1.27/1.32)), a 40% higher vascular mortality (HR 1.41 (1.37/1.45)), a 40% higher ischaemic heart mortality (1.39 (HR 1.34/1.44)) and a 40% higher stroke mortality (HR 1.39 (1.31/1.48)). In the BMI range of 25–50 kg/m^2, BMI was associated with mortality due to heart failure (HR 1.86 (1.55/2.23)) and hypertensive disease (HR 2.03 (1.75/2.36)), but also with mortality due to diabetes (HR 2.16 (1.89/2.46)), renal disease (HR 1.59 (1.27/1.99)), hepatic disease (HR 1.82 (1.59/2.09)), neoplasia (HR 1.10 (1.06/1.15)) and respiratory diseases and lung cancer (HR 1.20 (1.07/1.34)). For several sites of cancer the hazard ratios were different according to age: for deaths at ages 60–89, cancers of the liver (HR 1.47 (1.26/1.71)), kidney (1.23 (1.06//1.43)) and breast (1.15 (1.02/1.31)) were important, and for death at 35–59 years these were cancer of the endometrium (1.38 (1.08/1.77)), prostate (1.13 (1.02/1.24)) and large intestine only in males (1.29 (1.18/1.40)).

The by far largest study published in 2016 by Aune et al. included 230 cohorts with 30.3 million participants and almost 3.8 million deaths [6]. The lowest risk was a BMI of 23–24 in never smokers, 22–23 in healthy never smokers and 20–22 in never smokers with ≥20 years of follow-up. The summary relative risk for all-cause mortality per 5 unit increase in BMI was 1.05 (1.04/1.07) for all participants (228 cohort studies). Due to the large number of participants they could stratify for risk of smoking and several specific causes of early death in the first 1–6 years after inclusion in the study. By doing so they found a summary relative risk per 5 unit increase in BMI of 1.18 (1.15/1.21) for never smokers (53 cohorts), 1.21 (1.18/1.25) for healthy never smokers (26 cohorts) and 1.27 (1.21/1.33) for healthy never smokers with exclusion of early follow-up (11 studies). Their data were at variance with another large study by Flegal et al., a meta-analysis of 97 cohort studies with 2.88 million individuals and more than 270,000 deaths [31]. Flegal et al. found summary hazard ratios of death of 0.94 (0.90/0.97), 0.97 (090/1.04) and 1.34 (1.21/1.47) for BMI categories of 25–30, 30–35 and ≥35, respectively, suggesting a protective effect of overweight on mortality and only severely obese people being at increased risk of mortality. There are two possible explanations to clarify this discrepancy. Flegal et al. defined a normal weight by a wide range of BMI 18.5–24.9 kg/m^2 and used statistical adjustments for smoking and prevalent disease while in the study of Aune et al. stratification for and/or exclusion of smokers and prevalent disease is a more powerful tool but this needs obviously large cohorts [15].

Two other large cohorts were also able to exclude the group of smokers and found data that agreed with the study by Aune et al. The NHI–AARP (National

Institute of Health–American Association of Retired Persons) Diet and Health Study (527,265 participants) found relative risks of death in class I, II and II obesity in non-smoking males of 1.96, 2.46 and 3.82, respectively, and in non-smoking females of 1.99, 2.57 and 3.79, respectively, when compared with a BMI of 23.5–24.9 [32]. In the National Cancer Institute (NCI) Cohort Consortium with 1.46 million white adults, Berrington de Gonzalez et al. excluded patients with smoking and impaired health status [29]. Hazard ratios for death due to overweight were 1.11 (1.07/1.16) for males and 1.13 (1.09/1.16) for females when compared with a BMI 22.5–24.9 as the reference group. In the BMI classes of 30–34.9, 35–39.9 and 40–49.9 hazard ratios of 1.44, 1.88 and 2.51 in women and 1.44, 2.06 and 2.93 for men were reported. Per 5 unit increase in BMI the all-cause mortality HR was 1.31 (1.29/1.33) over the wide BMI range of 25.0–49.9 kg/m^2.

1.4.1 Mortality: All-Cause and Disease-Specific Causes

Obesity is associated with an increase in all-cause mortality and life expectancy is reduced. The impact of obesity on mortality is less in subgroups where competing causes of death are increased such as in elderly and smokers [33]. Flegal et al. combined the data of the three National Health and Nutrition Examination Surveys (NHANES) in the USA and grouped the causes of deaths into three categories: cardiovascular, cancer and all other (non-cardiovascular, non-cancer) [27]. Cancer was further divided into lung cancer; obesity-related cancers such as colon, breast, oesophagus, uterine, kidney, ovarian and pancreas cancer; and other cancers. Obesity was associated with increased all-cause mortality and with increased excess deaths from cardiovascular, coronary heart and non-coronary heart disease (including stroke), from obesity-associated cancers and from the combined presence of diabetes and kidney disease. Overweight was associated with a decreased all-cause mortality with only an increased mortality from diabetes and kidney disease combined, but a decreased mortality from non-cardiovascular, non-cancer disease causes and not associated with cancer and cardiovascular mortality. Similar findings were reported by Berrington de Gonzalez et al. in the NCI Cohort Consortium with overall higher risks for death from cardiovascular disease than for death from cancer [29]. For cardiovascular death these hazard ratios were 1.82 (1.69/1.93) for BMI 30–34.9, 2.63 (2.40/2.88) for BMI 35–39.9 and 3.56 (3.12/4.04) for BMI 40–49.9 kg/m^2. Hazard ratios for cancer death were 1.34 (1.27/1.42), 1.47 (1.34/1.61) and 1.70 (1.48/1.96) in the respective BMI categories. In the European EPIC study significant relative risks were present only for circulatory causes of death in males and females in class I obesity (RR 1.62 (1.38/1.90) and RR 1.31 (1.07/1.61), respectively) and for circulatory cause of death in those with a BMI ≥35 in males and females (RR 2.70 (2.13/3.42) and RR 2.27 (1.78/2.90), respectively), followed by death due to neoplastic disease only in women (RR 1.38 (1.14/1.68)) [21].

1.4.2 Population Attributable Fraction

The population attributable risk of overweight or obesity is an estimate of the percentage of premature death or occurrence of a disease in the cohort that would not have occurred if all persons had been of normal weight at the same age. Excess weight accounted for approximately 7.7% of all premature deaths among men and 11.7% among women [32]. It accounted for 18.1% of premature deaths among non-smoking men and 18.7% among non-smoking women [32].

Cardiovascular mortality accounted for 37% of adult deaths in the USA in 2004 [27]; 13% of total CVD mortality was associated with obesity (BMI >30). Cancer accounted for 24% of total deaths in the USA [27]. Flegal et al. found no to little association of BMI categories to excess all-cancer mortality [27]. When they divided cancers into lung cancer (29% of death of all cancers), obesity-associated cancers (32% of all cancer deaths) and other cancers (40% of cancer deaths) it appeared that obesity was significantly associated with 11% of death from cancers considered to be obesity related. Calle et al. estimated that 4.3% of all cancer deaths in men and 14.3% of all cancer deaths in women were associated with obesity in the large Cancer Prevention Study [8]. The WHO emphasized that 44% of the diabetes burden, 23% of the ischaemic heart disease burden and 7–41% of certain cancer burdens are attributable to overweight and obesity [2]. In Europe about 80% of cases of type 2 diabetes, 35% of ischaemic heart disease and 55% of hypertensive disease among adults are attributable to overweight and obesity [4].

1.4.3 Current Developments

There are currently both negative and positive developments. Oldhansky et al. reported a potential decline in life expectancy in the USA in the twenty-first century [34]. They calculated that the life expectancy at birth would be higher in white men with obesity grade I (BMI >30) by 0.33 years and in white men with obesity grade II (BMI >35) by 0.93 years, if subjects would decrease to a BMI of 24. The years gained would be 0.30 and 0.81 years, respectively, for white females; 0.30 and 1.08 years, respectively, for black males; and 0.21 and 0.73 years, respectively, for black females. But the current negative effect of obesity of 1/3 to 3/4 of a year life shortening could rise to 2–5 years as the prevalence of obesity among adults, and especially among children, is increasing and obese children will carry and express obesity-related risks for more years of their lifetime than previous generations.

On the other hand, a recent analysis in three Danish cohorts (the Copenhagen City Heart study 1976–1978 (n = 13,704) and 1991–1994 (n = 9482), and the Copenhagen General Populations Study 2003–2013 (n = 97,362)) discovered that the BMI associated with the lowest mortality increased from 23.7 in 1976–1978 to 24.6 in 1991–1994 to 27.0 in 2003–2013, thus an increase by 3.3 BMI units over three decades [35]. The corresponding BMIs for cardiovascular disease mortality were 23.2, 24.0 and 26.4 and the BMIs for other mortalities 24.1, 26.8 and 27.8. Analysis of BMI categories against the normal BMI category of 18.5–25 showed decreased risks of all-cause mortality from 1.04 in 1976–1978 and 0.97 in 1991–1994 to 0.86 in the 2003–2013 cohort. The adjusted hazard ratio for all-cause mortality for a BMI of 30 or greater against BMI 18.5–25 changed from 1.31 in 1976–1978 to 1.13 in 1991–1994 and to 0.99 in 2003–2012. The researches provided a potential explanation for the secular trend. They suggested that the improvement of treatment of cardiovascular risk factors or complicating disease has reduced mortality in all weight classes but that these effects may have been greater with subjects at higher BMI levels where hypertension, diabetes and dyslipidaemia place individuals more at risk. Decreased smoking and increased physical activity may also have improved the general health of the population.

In certain circumstances overweight and moderate obesity are not associated with increased mortality, a fact known as the obesity paradox. Especially in the intensive care, the obesity paradox has gained increasing interest: here patients with a BMI between 30 and 40 showed an even lower mortality (relative risk 0.83 (0.74/0.92)) compared with normal-weight subjects, suggesting that increased nutritional reserves are advantageous to survive the intensive care [36].

1.5 Comorbidities in General

Obesity is associated with many comorbidities which relate to weight-bearing influences on bones, joints, ligaments and muscles and respiratory function, to metabolic and hormonal disturbances, cumulating in life-threatening diseases or decreased quality of life as presented in the obesity web (Fig. 1.2). Obesity is a major risk factor for type 2 diabetes mellitus (T2DM) with a 10- to 20-fold increased risk in those with a BMI ≥35 kg/m^2 [33]. It is also associated with hypertension and cardiovascular disease and in men with hypercholesterolaemia and stroke. Obesity is also predictive of diseases that cause serious morbidity such as osteoarthritis and sleep apnoea. The other major disease group associated with BMI is cancer with a dose-response relationship between the risk of cancer and BMI. Obesity is also a key factor for the metabolic syndrome (MetS) characterised by dyslipidaemia, hyperinsulinaemia, diabetes and hypertension (Table 1.1). Guh et al. tried to assess the importance of 20 comorbidities in a meta-analysis comprising 89 relevant studies from Europe, North America, Australia and New Zealand and they included only prospective cohort studies [37]. This meta-analysis was unique to the many previous systematic reviews and meta-analyses because they recognised the fact that (1) most studies used BMI and abdominal obesity defined by waist circumference might be a better predictor of many cardiovascular diseases and T2DM, and (2) many studies found associations defined per unit change in BMI of per cm change in waist while now BMI and waist were categorised by overweight (BMI 25–29.9 kg/m^2 and waist ≥80 cm for females and ≥94 cm for males) and by obesity (BMI ≥30 kg/m^2 and waist ≥88 cm for females and ≥102 cm for males). They found evidence for 18 comorbidities but not for sleep apnoea and dyslipidaemia (Table 1.2).

Statistically significant associations were found for the incidence of T2DM; all cancers except oesophageal (female), prostate and pancreas cancer; all cardiovascular diseases (except congestive heart failure); asthma; gallbladder disease; osteoarthritis and chronic back pain (Table 1.2). Overweight and obesity were very strongly associated with diabetes (RR 3.92 (3.10/4.97) and 12.41 (9.03/17.06)), respectively.

Table 1.2 Meta-analysis of comorbidities related to defined criteria of overweight BMI (BMI 25–29.9 kg/m^2) and obesity BMI (BMI ≥30 kg/m^2) and to overweight waist measures (≥80 cm for females and ≥94 cm for males) and obesity waist measures (≥88 cm for females and ≥102 cm for males) [37]. Relative Risks with 95% Confidence Intervals are given

Comorbidity	No. of studies		RR overweight BMI	RR obese BMI	RR overweight waist	RR obese waist
Breast cancer postmenopausal	14	F	1.08 (1.03/1.14)	1.13 (1.05/1.22)	1.13 (1.01/1.07)	1.30 (1.17/1.44)
Endometrial cancer	10	F	1.53 (1.45/1.61)	3.22 (2.91/3.56)	1.15 (1.02/1.30)	1.42 (0.80/2.49)
Ovarian cancer	9	F	1.18 (1.12/1.23)	1.28 (1.20/1.36)	0.61 (0.35/1.08)	1.35 (0.95/1.93)
Colorectal cancer	12	M	1.51 (1.37/1.67)	1.95 (1.59/2.39)	1.88 (1.47/2.41)	2.93 (2.31/3.73)
		F	1.45 (1.30/1.62)	1.66 (1.52/1.81)	1.25 (0.98/1.59)	1.55 (1.27/1.88)
Oesophageal cancer	1	M	1.13 (1.02/1.26)	1.21 (0.97/1.52)		
		F	1.15 (0.97/1.36)	1.20 (0.95/1.53)		
Kidney cancer	5	M	1.40 (1.31/1.49)	1.82 (1.61/2.05)		
		F	1.82 (1.68/1.98)	2.61 (2.39/2.90)		
Pancreatic cancer	6	M	1.28 (0.94/1.75)	2.29 (1.65/3.15)		
		F	1.24 (0.98/1.56)	1.60 (1.17/2.20)		
Prostate cancer	8	M	1.14 (1.00/1.31)	1.05 (0.85/1.30)		
T2DM	9	M	2.40 (2.12/2.72)	6.74 (5.55/8.19)	2.36 (1.76/3.15)	5.67 (4.46/7.20)
		F	3.92 (3.10/4.97)	12.41 (9.03/17.06)	3.40 (2.42/4.78)	11.1 (8.23/14.96)
Hypertension	4	M	1.28 (1.10/1.50)	1.84 (1.51/2.24)		
		F	1.65 (1.24/2.19)	2.42 (1.59/3.67)	1.38 (1.27/1.51)	1.9 (1.77/2.03)
Stroke	7	M	1.23 (1.13/1.34)	1.51 (1.33/1.72)		
		F	1.15 (1.00/1.32)	1.49 (1.27/1.74)		
CAD	11	M	1.29 (1.18/1.41)	1.72 (1.51/1.96)	1.41 (1.16/1.72)	1.81 (1.45/2.25)
		F	1.80 (1.64/1.98)	3.10 (2.81/3.43)	1.85 (1.41/2.36)	2.68 (2.05/3.53)
Congestive heart failure	4	M	1.31 (0.96/1.79)	1.79 (1.24/2.59)		
		F	1.27 (0.68/2.37)	1.78 (1.07/2.95)		
Asthma	4	M	1.20 (1.08/1.33)	1.43 (1.14/1.79)		
		F	1.25 (1.05/1.49)	1.78 (1.36/2.32)		

(continued)

Table 1.2 (continued)

Comorbidity	No. of studies		RR overweight BMI	RR obese BMI	RR overweight waist	RR obese waist
Chronic back pain	1		1.59 (1.34/1.89)	2.81 (2.27/3.48)		
Osteoarthritis	3	M	2.76 (2.05/3.70)	4.20 (2.76/6.41)		
		F	1.80 (1.75/1.85)	1.96 (1.88/2.04)		
Pulmonary embolism	1		1.94 (1.39/2.64)	3.51 (2.61/4.73)		
Gallbladder disease	4	M	1.09 (0.87/1.37)	1.43 (1.04/1.96)	1.63 (1.42/1.88)	2.51 (2.16/2.91)
		F	1.44 (1.05/1.98)	2.32 (1.17/4.57)		

T2DM type 2 diabetes mellitus, *CAD* coronary artery disease, *RR* relative risk, *F* females, *M* males

1.6 Symptoms and Comorbidities More Specifically Related to the Gastrointestinal Tract

Many of the comorbidities associated with obesity rely to the gastrointestinal tract such as gastro-oesophageal reflux disease (GORD) and its complications, gallbladder stones and pancreatitis, colon polyps and colorectal cancer, liver diseases such as non-alcoholic fatty liver disease (NAFLD) and non-alcoholic steatosis hepatitis (NASH), and gastrointestinal tract cancers. Most of these comorbidities will change favourably by body weight reduction and the way this weight reduction is achieved will not impact them, with GORD presumably being an exception. As GORD and its complications are also the most prevalent diseases, this chapter focuses extensively on GORD and its complications of erosive oesophagitis, Barrett's oesophagus and oesophageal and gastro-oesophageal junction adenocarcinoma. Also, the liver manifestations of obesity with non-alcoholic fatty liver disease (NAFLD) and its progression to non-alcoholic steatohepatitis (NASH) are discussed at length with an eye to increased needs for liver transplantation in the future. The subchapter of gastro-oesophageal tract malignancies will discuss the cancers in a more general perspective as far as these have not been discussed in detail in the preceding paragraphs.

But before discussing the obesity-related gastrointestinal diseases: what is the relationship between GI complaints and BMI?

1.7 Symptoms Related to the Gastrointestinal Tract

The perception of sensations arising from the GI tract may be diminished in obese subjects and thus facilitate overeating. On the other hand, altered food habits, such as skipping meals, binge-eating, periods of excess food intake and periods of food restriction, may induce changes in GI function and thereby produce upper and lower GI symptoms. Two studies investigated gastrointestinal symptoms by validated questionnaires such as the Gastro-Oesophageal Reflux Questionnaire and the Bowel Disease/Symptom Questionnaire in a large cohort [38, 39] (Table 1.3). In the first cohort, consisting of residents of the Olmsted County ($N = 1963$) with 51% females and with at least 53% of subjects ≥50 years of age, the prevalence of overweight was 42.5% [38]. Obesity was present in 23% and severe obesity in 2% of cases. There was a positive relationship between BMI and frequent vomiting, upper abdominal pain, bloating and diarrhoea. The prevalence of frequent lower abdominal pain, nausea and constipation was increased among obese subjects, without a significant association between the BMI and these symptoms. The second cohort was a much younger group of 980 26-year-old subjects (47.9% females) [39]. Comorbidities and use of medication were unlikely to be a confounder given the young age group. The prevalence of overweight was 30% and that of obesity 12%; severe obesity was not present. Overweight was negatively associated with abdominal pain and constipation (odds ratio (OR) 0.4). Diarrhoea (>3 stools/day, loose stools, urgency) was associated with obesity (OR 1.8) as was abdominal pain combined with nausea and vomiting (OR 2.0). IBS and reflux were not associated with obesity and the waist/hip circumference ratio was not associated with GI symptoms. In these two cohorts, no information was available about the presence of GI lesions or diseases. A cross-sectional survey in Australia in adults yielded similar results on diarrhoea (OR 1.4) and abdominal pain (OR 1.3) [40]. However, a study in US subjects recruited for a study on weight loss medication differed from the previously mentioned three studies in a lesser symptomatology of diarrhoea and abdominal pain (OR 1.04 and 1.03, respectively) [41].

In a representative Swedish population 2122 individuals completed the validated abdominal symptom questionnaire on 27 troublesome GI symptoms [42].

Table 1.3 Studies evaluating gastrointestinal symptoms from questionnaires in patients with obesity; only significant associations are presented

Author and year	Number of patients and country	Adjustment in analysis	Associations of obesity with symptoms: odds ratio with 95% confidence interval
Delgado-Aros'04 [38]	1963, USA	Age, gender, alcohol, smoking, psychosomatism	Diarrhoea OR 2.7 (1.1/6.8) Vomiting OR 6.7 (2.7/26.6) Upper abdominal pain OR 3.7 (1.0/13.3)
Talley'04 [39]	980, New Zealand	Gender	Diarrhoea OR 1.81 (1.12/2.91) Vomiting OR 2.04 (1.12/2.90)
Talley'04 [40]	777, Australia	Age, gender, alcohol, smoking, education	Diarrhoea OR 1.41 (1.14/1.74) Upper abdominal pain OR 1.29 (1.03/1.61)
Levy'05 [41]	983, USA	Age, gender	Diarrhoea OR 1.04 (1.02/1.07) Abdominal pain OR 1.03 (1.00/1.05)

These reports could be coupled to findings on upper GI endoscopy in 1001 of these responders. Their mean age was 53.5 years and 51% were women. Overweight was present in 46% and obesity in 16%. There were significant associations between obesity and symptoms such as gastro-oesophageal reflux, vomiting, nocturnal urgency and diarrhoea (OR varying between 2.0 and 3.1) and epigastric or any abdominal pain, irritable bowel symptoms, retching, incomplete rectal evacuation and any stool urgency (OR between 1.58 and 1.63). Gastric ulcer was present in 1.4% of normal-weight, 1.3% of overweight and 5.6% of obese subjects; for duodenal ulcer these figures were 1.9%, 2.0% and 2.5%, respectively. Oesophagitis was present in 9.3 of normal-weight, 16.7 of overweight and 26.5% of obese subjects. When patients with oesophagitis were excluded from the analysis, only vomiting, diarrhoea and incomplete rectal evacuation remained associated with obesity (OR between 1.7 and 4.0) and the association with gastro-oesophageal reflux symptoms disappeared, meaning that gastro-oesophageal symptoms were largely explained by increased upper GI findings by endoscopy. Adjusting for medication did not alter the association between oesophagitis and BMI. A dose-response curve appeared to be present: the higher the BMI, the higher the gastro-oesophageal symptom score.

Dutta et al. compared 101 morbidly obese patients scheduled for Roux-en-Y gastric bypass with age- and sex-matched 101 non-morbidly obese patients and assessed the presence of symptoms of heartburn, regurgitation, dysphagia, nausea, epigastric fullness, postprandial discomfort, belching and bloating [43]. They also performed upper gastrointestinal endoscopy and biopsies in both groups of patients. Morbidly obese patients suffered more from heartburn (32.6% vs. 18.8%, p 0.02) compared with the control group. Endoscopically, the prevalence of a hiatal hernia ≥2 cm was higher (38.6% vs. 13.8%, $p < 0.001$) and the frequency of gastritis identified by endoscopy and histology was higher (23.7% vs. 11.8%, p 0.02) without differences in *Helicobacter pylori* infection. However, data on the use of NSAIDs, aspirin and steroids were not available. This study suggests different mechanisms involved in the development of upper GI symptoms and disorders in morbidly versus non-morbidly obese patients, which may be relevant for the evaluation of patients referred for bariatric surgery. Impaired visceral sensation, likely to be ascribed to a dysfunction of the autonomic nervous system, might explain the asymptomatic presence of endoscopic lesions [44]. The frequent use of proton pump inhibitors (PPIs) may also be an explanation.

As can be seen from Table 1.3, all studies reported a higher risk of diarrhoea and three studies reported increased vomiting and upper abdominal pain. Symptoms may be attributed to the size of the meal ingested leading to rapid gastric distension and vomiting [32]. Also, the rapid delivery of a meal into the small intestine with an increased osmotic load may explain the complaints. Furthermore, the cytokines and adipokines secreted by the adipose tissue may impact the gastrointestinal motility. As functional complaints have been related to an inflammatory insult to the gastrointestinal tract, obesity may therefore increase the risk of functional complaints by the release of pro-inflammatory cytokines [32].

1.8 Comorbid Diseases Related to the Gastrointestinal Tract

Apart from the relevance of being symptomatic or not, the obesity-associated diseases of the gastrointestinal tract are of clinical importance for both gastroenterologists and (bariatric) surgeons.

1.8.1 Oesophagus and Stomach

1.8.1.1 Gastro-Oesophageal Reflux Disease

Gastro-oesophageal reflux disease is a major problem, with a prevalence of 20% in Western countries. Over the last 20 years an increase by 4% per year was noticed in the Western world parallel to the doubling of the prevalence of obesity in that same period [45]. The parallel rise in GORD and obesity suggests a link between the two. A causal association between obesity and GORD-related disorders is suggested by these parallel secular trends, by consistent significant associations and compatible temporal associations and the suggestive dose-response relation found in many studies and associations found even in the normal range of BMI [46, 47].

Putative Causative Mechanisms

Obese patients often complain of gastro-oesophageal reflux with the main symptoms of heartburn and regurgitation. There are many putative mechanisms precipitating gastro-oesophageal reflux in obese subjects that makes the notion of obesity as a cause of GORD biologically plausible [47–49].

Mechanical Mechanisms

1. Increased intra-abdominal pressure (20–40 mmHg) with increased intragastric pressure and abdomino-thoracic pressure gradient over the cardia due to excess subcutaneous and intra-abdominal adipose tissue, which increases with increasing BMI and waist circumference.
2. Defective barrier function of the cardia or so-called incompetence of the cardia: Several mechanisms may lead to a defective barrier function such as stretching of the phrenico-oesophageal membrane that may adversely affect the lower oesophageal sphincter (LOS) by reducing the abdominal length of the sphincter, and an abnormal diaphragmatic pinch-cock and the presence of a hiatal hernia which facilitates gastro-oesophageal reflux by serving as a reservoir of gastric acid and by separating the LOS from the lengthening effect of the right crus of the diaphragm. Obese are more likely than lean subjects to have a hiatal hernia (40% vs. 12.6%) [48].
3. Impaired LOS function: Reflux mainly occurs when the LOS is either fully relaxed or has a resting tone less than 2 mmHg. Diet may have a role in altering the LOS tone, such as a high-fat diet through effects of cholecystokinin on LOS function. The postprandial LOS tone may be lowered by chocolate and coffee by the presence of xanthines, by mint by the presence of carminatives and by alcohol. Another mechanism might be increased transient LOS relaxations

(TLOSRs), with a high incidence of acid exposure during TLOSRs, which can be induced experimentally by gastric distension, use of an intragastric balloon or ingestion of a large meal [50, 51].
4. Dysmotility: Dysmotility of the oesophagus may impair the clearance of acid from the oesophagus; delayed gastric emptying induced by fatty meals or related to disturbances in glucose metabolism may favour reflux of acid material. Changes in hormones involved in gastric emptying, secondary to obesity, such as leptin, ghrelin and polypeptide Y (PYY), may play a role as well.
5. Intake of medication with influence on LOS pressure and tone such as the intake of exogenous oestrogens.

Humoral Mechanisms

The response of the oesophageal mucosa to the gastro-oesophageal refluxed materials is modified by humoral effects arising from the increased visceral fat. These humoral factors also govern the GORD-related complications such as erosive oesophagitis, Barrett's oesophagus and oesophageal adenocarcinoma. Visceral fat secretes pro-inflammatory cytokines like TNF-α, IL-6 and IL-1β. Both IL-6 and TNF-α are overexpressed in oesophagitis and Barrett's oesophagus and may potentially increase the inflammation and hence the malignant transformation [47].

Role of General Adiposity and Visceral Adiposity

There has been a lot of discussion on the role of overweight and whether overweight may influence the tendency for acid reflux in a graded way or whether a threshold value exists above which overweight might be of importance and some authors found no significant correlation between body weight or BMI and abnormal pH measurements [52, 53]. This discussion was fuelled by discrepancies between textbook recommendations and disappointing findings during weight loss in overweight patients [54].

It should, however, be recognised that the ideal study with data on GORD symptoms by validated scale scores, endoscopy to diagnose oesophagitis and presence of a hiatal hernia, manometry and pH measurements in a large number of individuals with both measures of total body fat (BMI) and central fat (waist measures) within a limited time frame does not (yet) exist.

One of the few studies available examined patients referred for GORD symptoms, with negative endoscopy and negative *Helicobacter pylori* (Hp) by manometry and 24-h pH measurements and had data on BMI [49]. This study proved that most but not all of the association between BMI and acid exposure was due to mechanical disturbances as described above. They mimicked their findings by a constricting abdominal belt in healthy volunteers. In a similar study with the new and sensitive technology of intraluminal high-resolution manometry and pH measurements in subjects with intra-abdominal fat and by placing a waist belt, Lee et al. showed that waist belt and intra-abdominal fat caused a partial hiatus hernia and short-segment acid reflux [55].

On the other hand, Anggiansah et al. could only partly confirm the mechanical theory in patients with typical GORD symptoms, assessed by validated questionnaires, by manometry and pH measurements, but in their study data on endoscopy,

H. pylori status and presence of a hiatal hernia were lacking [56]. Oesophageal acid exposure increased with waist and BMI and was also associated with lower LOS pressure (LOSP), reduced abdominal LOS length and peristaltic dysfunction (lower contractile amplitude of the lower oesophagus). BMI correlated negatively with LOSP but not LOS length and waist correlated negatively with both LOS pressure and abdominal length, consistent with the mechanical hypothesis. In multivariate analysis, correction for the manometric findings maintained the significant relation between obesity (BMI and waist) and acid exposure, but also showed an independent effect of oesophageal dysfunction on acid exposure, which is not in agreement with a pure mechanical hypothesis. GORD has been associated with abdominal obesity through increased intra-abdominal pressure, frequent TLOSRs, increased risk of hiatal hernia and oesophageal acid exposure.

In a large cohort study of 728 subjects undergoing oesophagogastroduodenoscopy (OGD) and having visceral (VAT) and subcutaneous adipose tissue (SAT) measurements by computer tomography (CT), 65 (8.9%) had erosive oesophagitis [57]. The patients with erosive oesophagitis were predominantly female. Compared with controls, they had a higher body mass index, metabolic syndrome prevalence, triglyceride levels and blood pressure. On OGD, hiatal hernia was also more prevalent. The mean VAT/SAT ratio was higher in the erosive oesophagitis group than in the non-erosive oesophagitis group (1.30 vs. 0.92). The results of the multivariate logistic regression analysis demonstrated that hiatal hernia, VFA/SFA ratio $\geq$1.165 and high triglyceride level were independent risk factors for erosive oesophagitis. Hiatal hernia was associated with a 12.9 times increased risk of erosive oesophagitis (OR 12.90 (3.57/46.65)). Similarly, a VFA/SFA ratio $\geq$1.165 was a significant risk factor for erosive oesophagitis (OR 2.04 (1.18/3.51)). The severity of the oesophagitis was positively correlated with the VFA/SFA ratio and visceral fat volume. The risk of Los Angeles (LA) oesophagitis types LA-A, LA-B and LA-C/LAC-D increased 1.23-fold, 1.27-fold and 1.56-fold, respectively. So, a VFA/SFA ratio $\geq$1.165 might be a useful indicator for predicting the presence and severity of erosive oesophagitis.

Yet, others performed manometry and/or pH measurements in obese and morbidly obese subjects referred for bariatric surgery and clearly found abnormalities [57, 58]. Comparison of an obese (BMI >30 kg/m^2) with a normal-weight group (BMI <25 kg/m^2) showed a clear dose-response relationship: per unit BMI increase there were 2.76 more acid reflux episodes postprandially and 1.89 more minutes with a pH <4 postprandially [59]. There were 0.8 more episodes of acid reflux per kg weight and 0.85 more acid reflux episodes per cm of waist postprandially. A BMI >30 kg/m^2 was associated with a 2.5-fold increased likelihood of having an abnormal DeMeester score (2.53 (1.18/5.41)). However, when waist circumference was included in the same model, the association between BMI >30 and oesophageal acid exposure became attenuated, indicating that the waist circumference may mediate a large part of the effect of obesity on oesophageal acid exposure. Ayazi et al. examined retrospectively the relationship between BMI, manometry and 24-h pH findings in 1659 symptomatic patients and found that 13% of the variability in the DeMeester composite score of the 24-h pH measurement was explained by variability in BMI [60]. Each unit increase of BMI was associated with an increased proportion of the total oesophageal exposure time at pH <4 of 0.35% and increased postprandial exposure time at pH <4 of 0.48% and an increased composite score by 1.46 points. The association between BMI and oesophageal acid exposure was stronger during supine periods compared with being upright. Also, overweight and obese compared to normal weight subjects had an increased risk of 1.69 (1.32/2.16) and 2.12 (1.623/2.747) of having a defective LOS, without any influence by age or sex. Even in those without a manometrically assessed hiatal hernia the OR was 2.36 (1.93/2.89).

Some have found an increased risk of GORD in obese women, with the suggestion that humoral factors should also be considered as a mechanism relating obesity to reflux. Two studies from the same group in Sweden reported on oestrogens considered as a mechanism relating obesity to reflux [61, 62]. One study showed a significant association between obesity and oesophagitis in women, which was potentiated by the use of oestrogens (oestrogen-only hormone replacement therapy (HRT)) by postmenopausal women. Oestrogen increases the synthesis of nitric oxide, a vasodilator leading to smooth muscle relaxation that can include the LOS. The second larger study found that overweight men and women had a similar increased risk of GORD symptoms. However, obese women compared to men had an increased risk of GORD symptoms, with a highest risk both in premenopausal women and in postmenopausal women using oestrogen replacement therapy. They also found that a weight gain of 3.5 kg/m^2 was associated with a 2.7-fold (2.3/3.2) increased risk for developing new symptoms. Also, the increased rates of GORD in pregnant patients have been attributed to increased sex hormone levels but may in fact be due to an increased transmitted gastric pressure from the enlarged uterus.

A substantial barrier in GORD studies is the imperfect association between GORD symptoms and acid reflux; people with severe symptoms may have little acid damage and patients with severe damage may have little symptoms. Therefore, Nocon et al. studied the relationship between severity of symptoms and BMI in 6215 patients with clinically assessed GORD [63]. A higher BMI was associated with more severe symptoms especially regurgitation, which were twice as likely in women and men, and heartburn being 50% more likely with more frequent reflux symptoms and oesophagitis. Obese women but not men had increased risk for severe oesophagitis compared to women with normal weight (OR 2.5 (1.53/4.12)) probably due to an increased oestrogen activity.

Meta-Analyses and Cohort Studies

Two meta-analyses, which found positive correlation between obesity and GORD, questioned their outcomes because of the significant degree of heterogeneity [64, 65]. Hampel et al. performed a meta-analysis in 2005. Nine studies examined the relationship between GORD, based on validated questionnaires and/or endoscopic findings, and BMI. Six studies showed a statistically significant association and three studies did not. Adjusted odds ratio for GORD symptoms was 1.43 among overweight and 1.94 for obese persons. Erosive oesophagitis was investigated in seven studies and in six studies, the adjusted odds ratio for erosive oesophagitis was 1.76 (1.156/2.677) for a BMI ≥25 kg/m^2. Seven studies examined total calorie intake and dietary fibre, fruits and vegetables and found the effect of BMI on GORD-related disorders to be independent of dietary intake. The second meta-analysis by Corley and Kubo decided to stratify the studies by country of origin [65]. An evaluation of all studies did not demonstrate a consistent association between elevated BMI and GORD. Homogeneous results for seven studies from the USA demonstrated a rising prevalence of GORD with increasing BMI with an OR 1.57 (1.36/1.80) for overweight and an OR 2.15 (1.89/2.45) for obesity. The eight studies from Europe were too heterogeneous and the five studies from outside Europe and the USA were very inconsistent.

A large cohort study in 80,110 subjects revealed gastro-oesophageal reflux symptoms in 11% and tried to correlate BMI and abdominal diameter with gender and ethnicity [66]. They found abdominal diameter to be an independent factor for gastro-oesophageal reflux symptoms in whites without a gender difference and much of the observed association between BMI and gastro-oesophageal reflux symptomatology to be mediated through the abdominal diameter. Abdominal diameter adjusted for BMI increased the risk for symptoms in white (OR 1.85 (1.55/2.21)) but not in black and Asian people. In Caucasian but not in Asian people the abdominal diameter was consistently associated with gastro-oesophageal reflux symptoms. The increased risk with no adjustment for BMI was even greater (OR 2.68 (2.33/3.08)) and also the risk of increasing BMI on symptoms was greater in the white. The attributable fractions among white subjects for a BMI ≥25 versus BMI <25 kg/m^2 and an abdominal diameter of ≥18 cm versus <18 cm were 16.5% and 15.1%, respectively, and among blacks these were 11.9% and 6.5%. In Asians these were not significant.

In the Nurses' Health Study an association between GORD and increasing BMI was found which was not influenced by the WHR [46]. This difference is due to the characteristics of the WHR used: a large waist and a large hip have the same ratio as a small waist and a small hip, whereas in the previous study the absolute abdominal diameter and thus a large abdominal size were measured [66].

What Is the Natural History of GORD?

Longitudinal studies are scarce. The only one available with a large number of subjects is the study by Lee et al. in 3669 subjects who underwent frequent endoscopy during the three periods, separated by 528, 392 and 352 days [67]. At the time points 1.2, 14.9 and 17.9% progressed from non-erosive to erosive oesophagitis whereas 42.5, 37.7 and 34.6% regressed from erosive into non-erosive oesophagitis. Being male (RR 4.31 (3.22/5.75)), being a smoker (RR 1.20 (1.03/1.39)) and having the metabolic syndrome (RR 14.75 (1.29/2.38)) independently increased the likelihood of progression from a non-erosive into an erosive oesophagitis and/or lowered the likelihood of disease regression. Short-term use of acid suppression raises the likelihood of disease regression (RR 0.54 (0.39/0.75)).

1.8.1.2 Barrett's Oesophagus

Although, generally speaking, GORD symptoms are equally distributed over ethnic groups and sexes, oesophagitis, Barrett's oesophagus and oesophageal adenocarcinoma appear to be dominated by white men of Caucasian origin [47]. Men have a twofold higher risk than women and Caucasians have a fivefold higher risk than African-Americans. Barrett's oesophagus is a metaplastic change from the squamous epithelial lining to a specialised columnar epithelial lining, also called specialised intestinal metaplasia (SIM), the key feature of a Barrett's oesophagus and the only known precursor lesion of oesophageal adenocarcinoma. Persons with Barrett's oesophagus have a 30- to 40-fold increased risk of oesophageal adenocarcinoma through the sequence of Barrett's metaplasia → dysplasia → adenocarcinoma but the progression of Barrett's oesophagus to oesophageal adenocarcinoma is low, at a rate of 0.2–3.5% per year. GORD is associated with and probably directly contributes to Barrett's oesophagus. It is not clear whether obesity alone independent of GORD also plays a role. The association between obesity and Barrett is mixed with an increase of Barrett's oesophagus with increasing BMI, increased risk with increasing BMI only in patients with GORD or no association at all with BMI. Abdominal diameter appears to be a risk factor for Barrett independently of BMI and when adjusted for the waist the relationship between BMI and Barrett's oesophagus disappears [47]. However, the most well-known risk factor, i.e. GORD, is not markedly differentially distributed by sex or race. General obesity reflected by the BMI and abdominal obesity reflected by the waist circumference have been consistently associated with the risk of oesophageal adenocarcinoma, but associations between BMI and Barrett's oesophagus have been inconsistent [68]. Abdominal obesity appears to be more consistently related with Barrett's oesophagus. In men no consistent pattern was observed in the association between BMI and Barrett, and in women there was no association present [68]. Barrett cases were more likely to be men, of Caucasian origin, with a longer duration of GORD symptoms, who were more likely to smoke and who were less likely to be infected with *Helicobacter pylori*.

Case-Control Studies and BMI and Waist

A case-control study in veterans showed that, after correction for age and race, a 2.5 times increased risk of Barrett's oesophagus was present both in overweight and obesity and that for each 5 kg increase in body weight or for each 5-point increase in BMI the risk for Barrett was increased by 10% and 35%, respectively [69].

Several studies have demonstrated that obesity may play a role in Barrett's oesophagus beyond the promotion of gastro-oesophageal reflux and that it is the abdominal fat distribution that may play a crucial role in the risk of developing a Barrett's oesophagus independent of BMI.

In a large case-control study in the Kaiser Permanente Northern Carolina population, patients with a Barrett's oesophagus ($n = 320$) were matched to subjects with GORD without a Barrett ($n = 312$) and to population controls ($n = 317$) [70]. There was a general association between Barrett's oesophagus and a larger abdominal circumference (waist >80 vs. <80 cm, OR 2.24 (1.21/4.15)), independent of BMI. The increased risk was only evident at >80 cm, suggesting a possible risk plateau. Also, a dose-response was apparent with increased risks at higher waist circumferences. There was no substantial difference in risk for short-segment versus long-segment Barrett. There was no association between Barrett and BMI. Abdominal waist was also associated with the severity of GORD with increasing risk of severe weekly symptoms (OR 1.86 (1.03/3.38) per 10 cm increased circumference). Adjustment for GORD attenuated the association between Barrett and waist from 2.24 (1.21/4.15) to 1.78 (0.86/3.66), which is to be expected when abdominal obesity → GORD → Barrett. So, waist but not BMI had a modest independent association with Barrett's oesophagus.

Increase in girth may increase the intra-abdominal pressure causing reflux, but may also alter GI motility because of metabolic products from the fat mass, and the plateau effect of the waist circumference may signify that at least a certain albeit modest amount of intra-abdominal fat is necessary.

Jacobson et al. discovered 261 cases of Barrett in 15,861 nurses of the Nurses' Health Study [71]. Only being obese (BMI $\geq$30 kg/m^2), but not being overweight, increased the risk (OR 1.52 (1.02/2.28)) and controlling for frequent GORD symptoms did not alter the observed risks for Barrett, but the association between obesity and Barrett was no longer significant, suggesting that obesity may play a role in Barrett's metaplasia beyond the promotion of GORD. However, waist, WHR and height were not associated with Barrett's oesophagus.

Smith et al. found in a population-based study with 167 cases of Barrett's oesophagus and 261 matched controls that obese people with self-reported symptoms of acid reflux had a markedly higher risk of Barrett (OR 34.4 (6.3/188)) than obese people without reflux (OR 0.7 (0.2/2.4)) or only reflux reporting normal-weight people (OR 9.3 (1.4/62.2)) suggesting that obesity plays a further role in the development of Barrett's oesophagus over and above its role in promoting acid reflux [72].

The strongest available data to date comes from the BEACON consortium with pooled individual participant data from 4 case-control studies including 1102 cases and 1400 controls with also having the possibility to include a sufficient number of females [68]. Waist circumference increased the risk of Barrett's oesophagus both in women and in men, independent of BMI, with a 125% (OR 2.24 (1.08/4.65)) and 275% (OR 3.75 (1.47/9.56)) increased risk for men and women, respectively. There was no association between BMI and risk of Barrett's oesophagus and the association between waist and Barrett strengthened after adjustment for BMI. There was a strong dose-effect association with increased risk by larger waist circumferences whether corrected for gastro-oesophageal reflux symptoms or not. However, the WHR was not associated with a risk in both women and men. Men, particularly of the white race, tend to accumulate more central/visceral fat compared with women. Also the NHANES study showed abdominal obesity to be more common among men and white individuals than among women and other racial/ethnic subgroups [73]. So the greater prevalence of abdominal obesity in men may at least in part explain the observed sex disparities in the incidence of Barrett's oesophagus.

Meta-Analyses

A meta-analysis by Cook et al. tried to solve the issue whether adiposity (BMI) mediates its effect on Barrett's oesophagus independently of GORD [74]. Ten studies were retrieved comparing the BMI of Barrett's and GORD patients and the general population. When comparing Barrett's oesophagus with GORD patients, the pooled estimate was not significant (0.99 (0.97/1.01) per kg/m^2), with no statistically significant point estimates for men and women separately. The pooled estimate comparing Barrett with the general population was statistically significant (1.02 per kg/m^2 (1.01/1.04)) with no difference between males and females. The meta-analysis concluded that increasing BMI did not present an increased risk of Barrett's oesophagus above what would have been expected from GORD alone. The previously mentioned meta-analysis by Hampel et al. suggested that increasing adiposity is a risk factor for the development of Barrett's oesophagus [64]. The meta-analysis by Cook et al. concluded that the increased risk of GORD, caused by increasing BMI, underlies this association [74]. Once GORD occurs there is no additional effect of BMI on its progression to Barrett's oesophagus. Both meta-analysis could not explain the large male-to-female sex ratio of Barrett 's oesophagus and oesophageal adenocarcinoma and the predominance in Caucasians: men are approximately twice as likely as women to develop Barrett's oesophagus and 5–8 times more likely to develop oesophageal adenocarcinoma.

Sometimes, discrepant findings between studies can be explained [75]. The meta-analysis by Cook found a significant association between BMI and Barrett when considering the general population as controls, an effect that disappeared when GORD controls were used [74]. Jacobson's Nurses' Health Study showed that in women the effects of obesity on Barrett are mediated at least in part by mechanisms other than GORD [71]. Whereas in the latter study controls had an endoscopy and did not have a Barrett's oesophagus, in the Cook's meta-analysis controls did not have an endoscopy and were therefore not known as to have a Barrett's oesophagus or not. Also, the different outcomes between studies concerning the importance of the fat distribution can be explained. Corley et al. reported in their case-control study that both waist and WHR were associated with Barrett's oesophagus, independently of the BMI [70]. Jacobson et al. failed to find an association of Barrett with central adiposity defined by increased WHR in women [71]. When using the WHR it should be realised that a large waist and a large hip have the same ratio as a small waist and a small hip. But also when using the waist circumference no association was found. This may be due to the fact that not all adipose tissues behave the same and that it is the metabolically more active visceral adipose tissue (VAT) and not subcutaneous adipose tissue (SAT) that is associated with Barrett's oesophagus.

By measuring the VAT and SAT by computer tomography at the level of the intervertebral disc between L4 and L5, it was found that in women visceral fat constitutes a much smaller fraction of the abdominal fat (and thus the waist circumference) when compared with men [76]. Likewise, 1 cm increase in waist circumference corresponds to a smaller increase in VAT in women. So, BMI is a significant risk factor for Barrett's oesophagus but VAT is an even stronger and independent risk factor [77–79].

The Visceral Fat Pathway

So, apart from general adiposity, the visceral fat accumulation is at least, if not more, important. The humoral role of the visceral fat has attracted great attention.

Overweight and obese men tend to have more centralised fat while women have more fat in their subcutaneous tissue [48, 73, 76–79]. This may explain why measures of fat distribution appear more strongly associated with Barrett's oesophagus than BMI in predominantly male populations, while BMI may be more important in women. Visceral fat is associated with particular metabolic compounds and a different balance of adipose-related hormones including insulin-like growth factor-1 (IGF-1), TNF-α, IL-6 and adipokines (leptin, adiponectin), many of which are linked to carcinogenesis and with processes of healing and injury to gastrointestinal mucosa and have been implicated in the pathogenesis of Barrett's oesophagus [25, 26, 48]. Visceral obesity is also associated with insulin resistance and metabolic syndrome, and this metabolic dysregulation in itself is associated with Barrett's oesophagus and several cancers.

Visceral Fat Measurements

El Serag et al. performed a CT study in 173 Barrett cases, 343 colonoscopy controls and 172 endoscopy controls, who also all underwent an upper endoscopy [79]. As abdominal fat is comprised of two functionally distinct types of fat: visceral adipose tissue (VAT) and subcutaneous adipose tissue (SAT); both fat masses were measured, supposing that on the one hand subcutaneous fat may contribute to the mechanical effect of abdominal fat but is metabolically inert, and on the other visceral fat exerts a mechanical effect on stomach and oesophagus but also secretes multiple pro-inflammatory cytokines and is associated with insulin resistance [79]. Visceral fat but not subcutaneous fat was associated with an increased risk of Barrett's oesophagus; the association was partly explained by the presence of GORD symptoms but was also present in people without symptoms. These important findings point towards humoral mechanisms of obesity-related increased risk of Barrett's oesophagus. Patients with Barrett's were more than twice likely to be in the highest VAT:SAT ratio (OR 2.42 (1.51/3.88)). After adjustment for age, sex, race, *H. pylori* status, smoking, NSAID use and alcohol use, the odds ratio was attenuated, with age and sex being the most attenuating factors. The association was stronger in males (adjusted OR 2.12 (1.15/3.90)) and when a long ≥3 cm Barrett's segment was present (OR 3.42 (1.627/7.01)). With respect to the reported association of Barrett's oesophagus with male gender and Caucasian descent, the analyses were repeated in male Caucasians. The unadjusted association between Barrett's oesophagus and VAT:SAT ratio was similar as in the whole group but now the associations persisted after adjustment for age, NSAIDs, Hp status, smoking and alcohol use (OR 2.27 (1.09/4.72)) as well as after the additional adjustment for GORD and PPI use. VAT and VAT:SAT ratio were associated with both presence and duration of GORD. The fat distribution in male and Caucasian tends to be more abdominal than truncal. Increased obesity may disproportionally increase GORD in white subjects and in males.

Subcutaneous Fat Measurements

Another way to address the fat distribution is to consider a possible protective effect of gluteofemoral (peripherally deposited) fat in oesophagitis and Barrett's oesophagus [80]. Gluteofemoral obesity protects against T2DM and cardiovascular disease and is positively associated with insulin sensitivity and adiponectin levels. Abdominal obesity was measured by waist circumference and gluteofemoral obesity by hip circumference and also the WHR was taken into account. Waist circumference was positively associated with erosive oesophagitis and Barrett's oesophagus, which became stronger after correction for the hip circumference. The hip circumference was negatively associated. It is difficult to explain the protective role of gluteofemoral fat on a mechanistic basis and it has no role in acid reflux. It may be that gluteofemoral obesity may serve as sink for storing fat in a manner that avoids the inflammatory and other humoral effects of the fat, otherwise stored in the visceral compartment.

Metabolic Syndrome

Apart from a more detailed analysis of humoral factors secreted by the visceral fat also the function of visceral fat and its role in the metabolic syndrome (MetS) can be studied as done by Ryan et al. [81]. One hundred and two patients with Barrett's and specialised intestinal metaplasia were investigated. Of these patients, 46% had the metabolic syndrome, 78% were overweight and 6% had central obesity (waist >80 cm for women and >98 cm for men). When comparing long-segment versus short-segment Barrett's oesophagus patients with a long-segment Barrett had more often MetS in 60%, associated with hyperinsulinaemia and elevated levels of IL-6, and central obesity in 92% compared with short-segment Barrett in 23.8% and 62%, respectively. Long-segment Barrett had a 11 cm greater waist circumference. The MetS was associated with elevated C-reactive protein (CRP) and leptin levels and a tendency of decreased adiponectin levels. Both MetS and waist circumference were independent risk factors for long-segment Barrett (OR 4.23 (1.07/18.6) and OR 5.6 (1.01/1.18), respectively), suggesting that MetS and the pro-inflammatory state may induce progression of the length of Barrett's oesophagus.

Secreted Adipokines

Visceral fat, also named the largest endocrine organ in humans, secretes many adipokines, cytokines and chemokines. The role of adipokines, leptin and adiponectin, has been investigated in patients with Barrett's oesophagus and oesophageal adenocarcinoma [25, 26, 48].

Leptin

Leptin has a role in appetite regulation and energy homeostasis and is also known for its effects on angiogenesis, wound healing, tissue repair, fertility, immune function, renal and lung functions, and cancer [26]. Leptin attached to leptin receptors can inhibit apoptosis, and increase proliferation. It is cytoprotective for the GI mucosa but can also induce neoplastic cell proliferation. Leptin is primarily produced by adipocytes but also secreted by chief cells in the gastric mucosa. Leptin receptor expression was seen in the chief and parietal cells of the gastric fundus and in superficial and basal layers of the oesophagus. Leptin levels are high in obesity but do not suppress hunger and appetite by leptin resistance, analogous to the effects of high insulin levels and insulin resistance. Francois et al. hypothesized that leptin of gastric origin may participate in the maintenance of normal (non-inflamed) oesophageal mucosa or the more acid-resistant Barrett's epithelium and examined tissue biopsies for leptin levels and leptin receptors in *H. pylori*-negative persons [82]. Barrett patients had significantly higher fundic leptin levels suggesting that the combination of refluxed acid and high leptin could predispose to mucosal proliferation, which depending on the host context may result in repair of oesophageal inflammation or progression of Barrett's oesophagus. For every twofold increase in fundic leptin the odds of having a Barrett's oesophagus was 3.4 (1.5/7.6) times higher when compared with having a normal oesophagus. Kendall et al. investigated levels of serum leptin in Barrett's oesophagus [83]. Their findings in a pilot study (67 controls; 51 Barrett) were confirmed in a large validation study (306 Barrett, 309 controls). In female controls and female Barrett patients serum leptin levels were 2–3 times higher than in males. Serum leptin levels correlated with BMI both in controls and Barrett patients. In men, serum leptin levels increased with increasing BMI and were higher in Barrett than in controls. The risk of a Barrett's oesophagus was highest in men among those in the highest quartile of serum leptin with a significant threefold increased risk of Barrett (OR 3.3 (1.7/6.6)) and this persisted after further adjustment for symptoms of gastro-oesophageal reflux (OR 2.4 (1.1/5.2)). There was a modest age-adjusted risk of Barrett with increasing BMI in males (BMI ≥30 kg/m^2: 1.7 (1.0/3.1)) but not in females and correction for gastro-oesophageal symptoms attenuated the risk. So, in men a proportion of the effect of obesity in the risk of Barrett was likely thought to be via non-reflux pathways including leptin. In women the risk of Barrett decreased with increased leptin levels and was not related to increasing values of BMI and correction for gastro-oesophageal symptoms attenuated the risk. So, men and women behaved quite differently. In women, the peripheral adipocytes secrete more leptin than the omental adipocytes, whereas in men the leptin secretion is similar at both sites. Women with central obesity would have lower serum leptin levels than peripherally obese women of the same BMI, implying that serum leptin would be negatively associated with central obesity and this would explain the negative association of leptin and Barrett's oesophagus in women. Adiponectin levels were not different between Barrett's and controls.

Adiponectin

Another player might be adiponectin which is secreted by adipose tissue [25, 26, 48, 84, 85]. Specific receptors are found in oesophageal mucosa such as AdipoR1 and R2. Adiponectin is an insulin sensitizer and has cardioprotective and immunomodulating actions. Being an anti-inflammatory agent, adiponectin is involved in the regulation of inflammation and suppresses carcinogenesis: it suppresses growth factors, stimulates apoptosis and suppresses cell proliferation. Adiponectin levels are low in obesity and lower in obese men than in women and low adiponectin levels have been linked to carcinogenesis in colon, gastric, prostate, breast and uterus cancer. Adiponectin has three multimeric forms: low molecular weight (LMW, trimers), middle molecular weight (MMW, hexamers) and high molecular weight (HMW, octadecamers) [84, 85]. These multimeric forms have opposite actions in inflammation: HMW induces the secretion of pro-inflammatory cytokines (IL-6) whereas LMW is anti-inflammatory, suppressing lipopolysaccharide (LPS)-induced release of IL-6 and stimulating the secretion of anti-inflammatory IL-10. In a case-control study Rubenstein et al. compared total adiponectin and different molecular weight adiponectin levels in 112 Barrett patients and in 199 controls [85]. No association of total adiponectin with Barrett's oesophagus was found, but high LMW adiponectin levels and a high LMW/total adiponectin ratio were associated with a decreased risk of Barrett's oesophagus, and the effect was stronger in women than in men. Confounding effects by insulin, glucose and insulin sensitivity were excluded. They hypothesised that normal circulating levels of LMW adiponectin are sufficient to suppress the inflammatory response to GORD and guide the healing of the mucosa towards regeneration of squamous mucosa. LMW suppresses the local expression of IL-6 in the oesophageal mucosa and IL-6 expression has been shown to be increased in Barrett's oesophagus. In the presence of low LMW levels the response to GORD might be directed towards a more exuberant oesophagitis or towards metaplasia in the intestinal epithelium. Unfortunately, IL-6 was not measured and other factors like diet, physical activity and *H. pylori* status were not taken into account.

Both Leptin and Adiponectin

Thompson et al. studied both leptin and adiponectin in men and women in 177 subjects with newly diagnosed Barrett's oesophagus compared with 177 controls [86]. In the whole group both adipokines were predictors of the risk of Barrett's oesophagus independently of each other. In women, those in the highest tertile of BMI and waist had the greatest risk (OR 4.6 (1.9/11.6) and OR 5.1 (2.0/13.0), respectively) for Barrett's metaplasia than those on the lowest tertile. Adjustment for leptin and adiponectin attenuated the risk by 52% and 42%, respectively. In men, those in the highest tertile of WHR were at greatest risk (OR 2.8 (1.3/5.9)) but adjustment for leptin and adiponectin did not attenuate these associations. Taking women and men as a group together, those in the highest tertile of BMI, waist and WHR had increased risks of developing a Barrett's oesophagus (OR 2.3 (1.3/4.1), OR 2.8 (1.6/4.8) and OR 2.4 (1.4/4.2), respectively). Adjustments for both leptin and adiponectin attenuated these with 38%, 17% and 36%, respectively. They concluded that both leptin and adiponectin were significant predictors of Barrett's oesophagus in women and men combined, independent of each other. The associations between adipokine levels and Barrett's risk were the strongest for women. Furthermore, the association between Barrett's risk and obesity was attenuated but not eliminated when adjustments were made for both cytokines by 24–52% in females and by 17–38% in combined male-female models. So, apparently leptin and adiponectin partially account for the relationship between obesity and Barrett's oesophagus.

1.8.1.3 Oesophageal Adenocarcinoma and Gastro-Oesophageal Junction/Gastric Cardia Adenocarcinoma

In the last decades the incidence of oesophageal and gastric adenocarcinoma has increased rapidly with a strong predominance in white Caucasian men, comprising 65% of all cases [48, 87]. Oesophageal adenocarcinoma is fivefold higher in Caucasians than in African-Americans and sixfold higher in men than in women [88]. In some countries the incidence has risen by 500–650% over the last three decades and oesophageal adenocarcinoma now accounts for 50% of all oesophageal cancers in the West [87]. The incidence of oesophageal squamous cell cancer has been stable or is slightly decreasing by 3.6% per year in all ethnic groups and distal gastric cancer is decreasing [48]. Heredity seems to play a role, although the aetiology is mainly non-genetic. Barrett's oesophagus, GORD and obesity are known risk factors and medications that lower the LOS might contribute to the risk through the mechanism of gastro-oesophageal reflux [89]. Polednak et al. used results from published meta-analyses and large cohort studies and reported a steadily increasing impact of obesity on trends in oesophageal adenocarcinoma incidence rates, from 21% in 1976–1980 to approximately 36% in 2001–2004 to 40% in 2007 [90].

Dietary changes with reduced intake of fruits and vegetables with low intake of antioxidants and cereal fibres may contribute; the role of tobacco is probably limited and alcohol consumption is not a risk factor. Heavy alcohol consumption (≥7 drinks/day) was not associated with increased risk of oesophageal and gastric adenocarcinoma in 11 studies and 1800 cases in the BEACON consortium in contrast to the almost ten times increased risk for oesophageal squamous cell carcinoma [91]. Modest consumption (<1 drink per day) had a 37% and 22% decreased risk of oesophageal and gastric cardia carcinoma, respectively. The presence of *H. pylori* with a 50–80% reduced risk was assumed to be related to atrophic gastritis and the use of NSAIDs and selective COX-2 inhibitors, by reducing tumour growth, may be protective. Reasons for this increasing incidence in oesophageal adenocarcinoma include increased obesity rates, with epidemiological evidence linking obesity with up to 40% of cases, increased prevalence of reflux symptoms and Barrett's oesophagus incidence rates and decreasing prevalence of *H. pylori* infection.

Obesity may be an independent risk factor for oesophageal adenocarcinoma by the mechanism of obesity → GORD→ Barrett's oesophagus → adenocarcinoma and it has been postulated that the effects of increased total body fat mass are largely manifested early in the pathogenesis of oesophageal adenocarcinoma, that is, in the development of specialised intestinal metaplasia (SIM), a characteristic feature of Barrett's oesophagus [48]. Later in the pathogenesis, visceral obesity may be more important, by adipokine-induced accelerated rates of cell division and proliferation with progression of Barrett's oesophagus through dysplasia in oesophageal adenocarcinoma. Critically reviewing each of these steps raises many questions [88, 92]. The first question is whether BMI increases the risk of cancer through increasing the chance of GORD. In general the association between both is not very strong and all ethnicities and both sexes commonly have GORD but the risk of cancer is markedly higher in white Caucasian men. Previous studies have demonstrated that both obesity and GORD are independent risk factors. Moreover, patients with GORD treated with PPI should be at lesser risk which is not the case. The second question is whether BMI increases the risk of Barrett's oesophagus independently of GORD; however, BMI on its own is not a strong risk factor for Barrett's oesophagus. The third question is whether BMI in itself increases the risk of progression of a Barrett's oesophagus to adenocarcinoma independently from GORD and again the answer is negative. Both increased total fat mass (mechanic part) and increased abdominal/visceral fat mass (humoral part) may be required for the development of erosive oesophageal damage, the development of Barrett's oesophagus and its malignant progression to oesophageal adenocarcinoma. With all these reflections in mind, one should realise that only 42% of men and 46% of women with oesophageal adenocarcinoma have a history of weekly reflux symptoms and only 22% have previously diagnosed GORD [93]. Moreover, Barrett's oesophagus is only apparent in 31% of patients. Similarly findings for gastric cardia cancer are 29% having a history of reflux symptoms and only 12% having a Barrett [93].

One explanation for the gender and ethnic specificity of oesophageal adenocarcinoma is the fact that for the same BMI, Caucasians and men tend to have more visceral fat [48, 73, 76–80]. Men of all ages and postmenopausal women tend to deposit fat predominantly intra-abdominally whereas premenopausal females tend to deposit fat subcutaneously. This difference may explain the gender and age disparities in incidence and outcome of some cancers such as oesophageal adenocarcinoma.

The negative association between *H. pylori* infection and oesophageal adenocarcinoma may be due to two different factors: (1) the chronic infection by *H. pylori* and the resultant gastric atrophy with diminished acid production, thereby decreasing gastro-oesophageal acid reflux, and (2) the decreased ghrelin secretion by X/A-like endocrine cells in the fundus of the stomach, protecting against obesity by decreasing hunger and appetite, and protecting against GORD by decreasing acid production. Martel et al. investigated both *H. pylori* infection and ghrelin levels and contrary to the original hypothesis they found that high rather than low serum ghrelin levels were associated with protection against oesophageal adenocarcinoma but only among overweight subjects (BMI $\geq$25 kg/m^2) and the lower risk did not change after correction for BMI and *H. pylori* presence (0.18 (0.04/0.78)) and after full correction, including also correction for smoking and education [26, 94]. Also, the strong protective action of *H. pylori* on cancer risk was not modified by ghrelin, and effects of both *H. pylori* and ghrelin were independent. Ghrelin has been shown to stimulate upper GI motility and to accelerate gastric emptying by effects on the vagal nerve and the myenteric plexus, thereby potentially diminishing oesophageal acid exposure and the risk of oesophageal adenocarcinoma, and also possesses profound anti-inflammatory effects with inhibition of TNF-α and inhibition of activation of NF-κB, thus diminishing the consequences of chronic gastric reflux with chronic inflammation and the development of oesophageal adenocarcinoma [26, 94]. For clinical practice it is important to know that obese patients usually have low levels of ghrelin and are therefore presumably less protected.

Meta-Analyses

Several meta-analyses tried to quantify the risk of oesophageal adenocarcinoma and gastric cardia adenocarcinoma. In Hampel's meta-analysis of nine studies there appeared to be a dose-response relationship with an OR of 1.52 at BMI 25–30 kg/m^2 and 2.78 at BMI ≥30 kg/m^2 [64]. Concerning the gastric cardia adenocarcinoma the adjusted OR was 1.68 for BMI ≥25 kg/m^2. Kubo and Corley had similar results in 14 studies [95]. A BMI ≥25 kg/m^2 was associated with an increased oesophageal adenocarcinoma in men (OR 2.2) and women (OR 2.0), and higher BMIs had higher cancer risks both in men and women: the ORs were for men with overweight 1.8 and with obesity 2.4; for females these ORs were, respectively, OR 1.5 and OR 2.1. There was a trend towards a stronger association in men compared with women. Associations with gastric cardia adenocarcinoma were heterogeneous, but after stratification by study location only a weak association (OR 1.5 for male and female and overweight and obese combined) between gastric cardia cancer and BMI was found in studies from the USA and Europe but not in studies from China.

Recent Cohort and Case-Control Studies

An article by Ryan et al. updated the meta-analysis of 2006 by Kubo and Corley with articles between 2005 and 2010 [48]. Twelve articles were retrieved, four from the USA and Canada, six from Europe and two from Australia [96–107]. As can be seen from Table 1.4 risks of oesophageal adenocarcinoma were at least 2.3 times higher and were as high as 5.3, 6.1 and 11.3 times higher compared with the BMI reference values in the different continents. In the study by Corley et al. also the anteroposterior diameter was taken into consideration [97]. The risk of oesophageal adenocarcinoma was 4.67 (1.14/20.11) when the diameter was equal or greater than 25 cm, suggesting that intra-abdominal fat increases the risk independently of BMI. Ryan compared the highest versus the lowest quartile of BMI and found a dose-dependent relationship between BMI and oesophageal adenocarcinoma for males (OR 4.3(2.3/7.9)); for the lower oesophagus the risk was the highest of all reported risks (OR 11.3 (3.5/36.4)); for the gastro-oesophageal junction the risk of adenocarcinoma was 3.4 (1.4/8.7) [100]. In the Netherlands Cohort Study on Diet and Cancer a dose-response curve was found for overweight and obesity in both oesophageal and gastric cardia adenocarcinoma [103]. Each 1 kg/m^2 increment during adulthood increased the risk of adenocarcinoma of the oesophagus by 14% and a weight gain of BMI ≥8 kg/m^2 had a 3.4 times higher risk than those with 0–3.9 kg/m^2 change. In this population 30.2% of oesophageal and 21.8% of gastric adenocarcinoma could be attributed to overweight and obesity. The European Prospective Investigation into Cancer and Nutrition (EPIC) study found that BMI, waist and WHR were all positively associated with oesophageal adenocarcinoma [105]. In an Australian study the risk increased by 46% for every 10 cm increase in waist [106]. Whiteman et al. also investigated morbidly obese subjects with a BMI ≥40 kg/m^2 [107]. Risk increased from OR 1.4 when being overweight to OR 3.3 in subjects with BMI ≥30 and to 7.0 in subjects with a BMI ≥40 kg/m^2. Adjustment for gastro-oesophageal reflux and other factors modestly attenuated this risk. Risk associated with obesity was significantly higher (almost twice as high) for men than for women and for those aged

<50 years (OR 7.5) versus those aged ≥50 years (OR 2.2). Obese people with frequent reflux had significantly higher risks (OR 16.5 (8.9/30.6)) than obese without reflux (OR 2.2 (1.1/4.3)) or normal weight with reflux (OR 5.6 (2.8/11.3)) consistent with a synergistic action between these factors. Risks of combined exposure were threefold higher than expected assuming a synergistic interaction between obesity and reflux. Similar findings were seen for gastro-oesophageal junctional adenocarcinoma but of smaller magnitude. The prevalence of *H. pylori* in this study was 6.3–8.5% and had no impact on the risk estimates. Their data suggested that patients with obesity and frequent reflux symptoms are especially at risk of adenocarcinoma.

Two more recent studies dating back to 2012 are also included in Table 1.4. The pooled analysis of individual participant data by the international Barrett and Esophageal Adenocarcinoma Consortium (BEACON) included 1997 oesophageal adenocarcinomas, 1900 oesophagogastric junction adenocarcinomas and 11,159

Table 1.4 Recent studies investigating the risk of oesophageal adenocarcinoma in obese subjects

Author and year	Design	Country	Cases/ controls	BMI reference	BMI	Results OR (95% CI)
USA and Canada						
Veugelers'06 [96]	CC	Canada	57/102	<25	>30	4.67 (1.27/17.9)
Corley'08 [97]	CC	USA	94/206,974	18.5–24.9	≥30	3.17 (1.43/7.04)
Abnet'08 [98]	Cohort	USA	371/480,475	18.5–<25.0	>35	2.27 (1.44/3.59)
Figueroa'09 [99]	CC	USA	122/695	<25	>30	5.32 (2.75/10.29)
Europe						
Ryan'06 [100]	CC	Ireland	760/893	<22	>30	11.3 (3.5/36.4)
Samanic'06 [101]	Cohort	Sweden	82/362,552	<24.9	>30	2.7 (1.33/5.55)
Reeves'07 [102]	Cohort	UK	150/1.2 × 10^6	22.5–24.9	≥30	2.54 (1.89/3.41)
Merry 07 [103]	Cohort	The Netherlands	293/4452	<24.9	>30	3.96 (2.27/6.88)
Anderson'07 [104]	CC	Ireland	227/260	<25	>28.1	2.69 (1.62/4.46)
Steffen'09 [105]	Cohort	Germany	198/346,554	<20.5	>30	2.8 (1.4/5.9)
Australia						
MacInnis'06 [106]	Cohort	Australia	30/41,295	<25	>30	3.7 (1.1/12.4)
Whiteman'08 [107]	CC	Australia	793/1580	18.5–24.9	>40	6.1 (2.7/13.6)
Most recent studies						
Hoyo'12 [87]	Cohort and CC	USA, EU, Australia	1997/11,159	<25	≥40	4.76 (2.96/7.66)
Doherty'12 [92]	Cohort	USA	253/218,854	18.5- < 25.0	≥35	2.11 (1.09/4.09)

BMI Body mass index, *OR* odds ratio, *95% CI* 95% confidence interval, *CC* case-control, *UK* United Kingdom, *EU* Europe

controls in 12 epidemiological studies (eight North America, three Europe and one Australia) [87]. Compared with BMI <25, a BMI 25–29.9 increased the risk by 54%; a BMI 30–34.9 gave a twofold increased risk (OR 2.39) and a BMI 35–39.9 gave a risk of 2.79. A BMI ≥40 kg/m^2 increased almost fivefold the risk (OR 4.76). For gastro-oesophageal junctional cancer these OR were smaller and were 1.28, 2.08, 2.36 and 3.07, respectively. Analysis testing for synergism or departure from additivity showed a synergism between BMI and GORD symptoms with respect to the oesophageal adenocarcinoma risk. The excess risk attributable to the synergistic interaction of BMI and GORD was 64% versus the non-interaction group. This observation of a synergetic effect of BMI and GORD on the cancer risk supports the idea of at least two pathways: a direct mechanical and an indirect metabolic one.

In the National Institutes of Health–American Association of Retired Persons (NIH-AARP) Diet and Health study 253 cases of oesophageal adenocarcinoma, 191 cases of gastric cardia adenocarcinoma and 125 cases of gastric non-cardia adenocarcinoma were documented [92]. In oesophageal adenocarcinoma weight, BMI, waist, hip and WHR were positively associated with the risk, with an HR between 1.81 and 2.28. For gastric cardia adenocarcinoma BMI and waist displayed an increasing risk of a HR 3.67 and HR 2.22, respectively. No consistent associations were found for gastric non-cardia adenocarcinoma.

1.8.1.4 Gastric Cancer

A meta-analysis studied the relationship between gastric cancer and overweight and obesity and identified ten studies involving 9492 gastric cancers in a population of almost 3.1 million individuals [108]. Overweight (BMI ≥25 kg/m^2) was associated with an increased gastric cancer risk (OR 1.22 (1.06/1.41)) with a small dose-response relationship: overweight (BMI 25–29.9) was associated with a 21% higher gastric cancer risk and obesity with a 36% higher risk. A stratified analysis showed a BMI ≥25 kg/m^2 to be associated with increased risks of gastric cardia cancer (OR 1.55 (1.31/1.84)), with overweight being at excess risk of 40% and obesity being over two times at risk. Overweight non-Asians had a 24% higher gastric cancer risk.

1.8.1.5 Implications for Clinical Practice

What does this imply for the gastroenterologist and for the surgeon? The degree of overweight and the visceral distribution of fat are involved in the aetiology of GORD, and GORD complications. Especially the obese with large waist circumference and severe symptoms of GORD is at risk for GORD complications. For daily practice this means taking a careful history with measurement of weight, height and waist circumference and a diagnostic workup in the presence of symptoms, with not only an endoscopy, sometimes supplied with manometry or 24-h pH measurements, but also an analysis of components of the metabolic syndrome. This is needed to estimate to what extent the obese subject is at risk of GORD complications. This should be followed by adequate treatment of symptoms with emphasis on attempts to lose weight which automatically will also result in a decreased mass of actively secreting visceral fat. Seven studies evaluated the effect of a lifestyle or diet intervention: two studies on very-low-calorie diet (VLCD), one on a low-calorie diet (LCD), one on a low-carb diet and three used combined lifestyle; three of the studies used an intragastric balloon [109]. Disappointingly, three of the studies were negative as to the improvement in GORD. In contrast, Roux-en-Y gastric bypass had a beneficial effect on GORD in all studies, although most of the studies evaluated only symptoms by questionnaires and did not perform 24-h pH measurements, manometry or endoscopy. The studies on restrictive surgery were inconsistent. Moreover, the efficacy of proton pump inhibitors and H_2 receptors antagonists has been reported to be less favourable in obese patients.

One should always bear in mind that symptoms may not be present or may disappear when the oesophagus adapts to the acid exposure by changing into a Barrett's oesophagus. When it comes to bariatric surgery, the intervention with the smallest risk of GORD and GORD complications should be chosen. At present, the discussion will centre around the two possibilities of a gastric sleeve or a gastric bypass. At the one side, procedures that enhance the risk of GORD should be denied to patients having already a Barrett's oesophagus present and thus would favour a gastric bypass over a gastric sleeve. On the other, when severe dysplasia or cancer develops in a Barrett's oesophagus, a gastric sleeve resection may enable the construction of a gastric tube.

1.8.2 Gallbladder and Pancreas

1.8.2.1 Gallbladder

Gallbladder Stones

Obesity is a risk factor for the formation of cholesterol gallstones and exposes patients to increased risk of gallstone-related complications. Rapid weight loss is also a risk factor for gallstone formation in obese patients, making the risks especially high in those who go through prominent cycles of gaining and losing weight [33, 110, 111]. Gallstone disease is one of the most prevalent and costly digestive diseases in Western countries with a prevalence of 10–15% in adults [112]. According to the third National Health and Nutrition Examination Survey (NHANES III) about 6.3 million of men and 14.2 million of women aged 20–74 in the USA might suffer from gallbladder disease [113].

Depending on the chemical composition, gallstones are often classified as pure cholesterol, pure pigment and mixed stones. In developed countries, cholesterol gallstones account for about 75% of stones [114–117]. For cholesterol gallstones, the textbooks always mention the 5F's which are still valid: at risk are Females, Fat people, Fair (in this context meaning prosperous) subjects, Fertile women and 40–50 years of age, with endogenous oestrogens, oral oestrogens and contraceptives being involved, as well as conditions leading to gallbladder stasis. Ethnics and genetics also play a role: the Pima Indians of Arizona display the highest prevalence rate of cholesterol gallstones in the world (about 80% in women by age 25–30), together with a high prevalence of both obesity and type 2 diabetes mellitus, thus combining the most provoking factors [118].

Obesity as such is associated with a higher risk of gallbladder stones linearly increasing over the BMI range compared with a BMI of 22 kg/m^2 with a factor of 1.7 at a BMI of 25, a factor of 3.7–6.0 at a BMI 30–35 and of 7.4 at a BMI >45 kg/m^2 [119, 120]. In males, risks are lower and more related to the central/visceral distribution of adipose tissue. In the Health Professional Study focusing on men, being 40–55 years of age at inclusion and followed for up to 10 years, a 2.5-fold increased risk of developing gallstones was found [121]. Besides obesity per se, the metabolic syndrome has a marked influence on cholesterol gallstones in men [122]. Many obesity-associated factors contribute to the risk of gallstone formation such as the diet, physical inactivity, metabolic syndrome, dyslipidaemia, insulin resistance and gallbladder stasis [110, 116, 117, 123]. Also, the treatment may contribute to the risks: the rapid weight loss as seen with very low calorie diets and with bariatric surgery, i.e., >1.5 kg/week, but also treatment with orlistat, a lipase inhibitor [124, 125]. The risks increase with weight cycling: with greater risks the greater the weight fluctuations and the greater its frequency of occurrence [33, 110, 111].

Gallstones and Complications

Increased BMI is also a risk factor for symptomatic gallstone disease and other complications of gallstone disease such as acute cholecystitis, choledocholithiasis, cholestatic jaundice, acute cholangitis and acute pancreatitis [124, 126]. In women, 30–55 years of age at inclusion in the Nurses' Health Study and followed for up to 18 years, increasing BMI was associated with a threefold increased risk of gallstones [120]. A dramatic increase was observed in the incidence of symptomatic gallstones with a need of cholecystectomy, or newly diagnosed symptomatic gallstones. The incidence of symptomatic gallstones increased from approximately 0.25% per year of follow-up in women with a BMI <24 kg/m^2 to more than 2% per year of follow-up in women with a BMI above 45 kg/m^2.

The presence of gallstones in the gallbladder is associated with the increased prevalence of gallbladder cancer [127]. Overall, the estimated prevalence of gallbladder cancer is 0.5–3%. Gallbladder cancer has a high grade of malignancy and is diagnosed late: it is a rare but often lethal complication of gallstones.

Pathophysiology of Gallstone Formation in Obesity

Central to the formation of gallbladder stones in obesity are the following:

1. Increased cholesterol synthesis and secretion by the liver [114–117]: The amount of cholesterol synthesised by the liver is linearly related to body fat (i.e. about 20 mg of additional cholesterol is synthesised daily for each kg of extra body fat). Because of insulin resistance, hyperinsulinaemia and dyslipidaemia, the liver secretes more cholesterol in the bile with an increased propensity to cholesterol-rich stones.

2. Supersaturated bile: Supersaturated bile is characterised by excess cholesterol relative to bile salts and phospholipids allowing solid cholesterol monohydrate crystals to aggregate and grow in the gallbladder [116, 128]. Gallbladder bile was supersaturated with cholesterol in all obese patients [129]. Also, increased cholesterol pronucleating factors such as gallbladder mucin and biliary calcium were present [129, 130].
3. Gallbladder-emptying disturbances: Reduced gallbladder emptying and gallbladder stasis are often a feature of obese subjects [131]. It might be related to their eating pattern with a prolonged period of fasting because of skipping breakfast and might act as a contributing factor for the aggregation of solid cholesterol crystals and stone growth. Mathus-Vliegen et al. showed that obese subjects with the largest fasting gallbladders had the largest residual and least emptying gallbladders and scored the highest in every aspect of body size, composition and fat distribution, and also had the highest insulin levels [132]. Body weight and fasting insulin levels explained 35.2% of the variance in fasting volume, lean body mass and insulin explained 28.1% of the residual volume and waist circumference explained 23.6% of the ejection volume.
4. Rapid and substantial weight loss after a very-low-calorie diet or bariatric surgery, secondary to enhanced mobilisation of cholesterol and thereby increased biliary cholesterol secretion: Also, secondarily a decreased hepatic bile acid pool and reduced hepatic secretion of biliary bile salts may play a role [111, 116, 117, 130, 133, 134]. Orlistat, reducing the fat absorption by 30% by lipase inhibition, might impair gallbladder emptying, thus further predisposing weight-losing obese subjects to gallstone formation [125]. One month of lipase inhibition by orlistat significantly impaired gallbladder motility, which persisted to some extent after 1 year. Therefore, obese subjects with diabetes or hyperlipidaemia, who are more at risk of gallstones, should be followed carefully.

Solid conglomerates of cholesterol monohydrate crystals, mucin gel, calcium bilirubinate and proteins accumulate and are deposited in the gallbladder to form gallstones. Obesity is also likely to act on and to potentiate lithogenic mechanisms by several associated conditions. These include the metabolic syndrome, insulin resistance, diabetes mellitus, autonomic neuropathy, gallbladder stasis, hypertriglyceridaemia, low HDL-cholesterol levels, sedentary lifestyle and the Western high-calorie, high-fat and refined sugar diet [110, 135]. The metabolic syndrome combines a visceral fat distribution with hypertriglyceridaemia, low HDL-cholesterol levels, impaired fasting glucose levels and hypertension and the central feature is insulin resistance and hyperinsulinaemia. These metabolic syndrome criteria have either isolated or combined effects on the process of cholesterol gallstone formation as shown in a cross-sectional study from China [136]. A number of 7570 subjects including 918 gallstone patients were investigated as to the different components of the metabolic syndrome during a physical check-up. Gallstone prevalence increased with the number of the criteria of the metabolic syndrome being present, from a prevalence of about 5% without any criteria to about 25% when all five criteria were present. This appeared to increase the risk of gallstone disease by four times in both men and women.

1.8.2.2 Pancreas

Acute Pancreatitis

Gallstones (45%) and alcohol (35%) are the most common aetiologies for acute pancreatitis [137]. Other factors are metabolic derangements such as hypertriglyceridaemia (1–4%) and hypercalcaemia (1.5%), drugs (1.3–1.4%), genetic mutations, trauma (blunt or penetrating trauma or post-ERCP (endoscopic retrograde cholangiopancreaticography)), smoking and infections. The aetiology is different according to gender, age and country: in men acute pancreatitis occurs at ages 30–45 due to alcohol, and in females at ages 50–70 due to gallstone disease. In the UK and Germany gallstones prevail as a causal factor whereas in Italy, the USA and Australia one of the major causes is alcohol [138]. The annual incidence ranges from 4.9 to 35 per 100,000 and acute pancreatitis was the leading gastrointestinal cause of hospitalisation in the USA in 2012 [139]. There is an increase in the incidence of acute pancreatitis in the past 40 years, probably due to a greater prevalence of risk factors such as increased alcohol consumption, obesity and diabetes.

Whatever the cause, exposure to toxins, including alcohol and medication; elevated serum triglycerides or calcium levels; overdistension, obstruction and increased permeability of the pancreatic duct; or ischaemia, trauma and viral infections, the final common pathway to clinical pancreatitis involves activation of pancreatic enzymes with autodigestion of the gland and peripancreatic tissues [137, 138, 140–147]. Normally, autodigestion of the pancreas is prevented by storing the proteases (trypsinogen, chymotrypsinogen, proelastase, phospholipase A) in a precursor form and by the synthesis of protease inhibitors. Pancreatitis occurs when premature activation of these enzymes occurs and the balance between activated proteases and protease inhibitors is disrupted. Premature activation and intracellular release of intrinsic enzymes lead to pancreatic acinar cell injury and, when released into the interstitium, to autodigestion of the organ with devastating effects on its function [138]. The activated pancreatic enzymes subsequently enter the bloodstream, resulting in elevated amylase and lipase blood levels, and leak into the peripancreatic tissue producing characteristic fat necrosis and exudation. The local injury is amplified through the induction of a systemic inflammatory response syndrome (SIRS), mediated by the generation and release of cytokines and the recruitment of aggressive inflammatory cells [137, 138, 143–145]. The gut hypothesis of multiple-organ failure (MOF) supposes that failure of the intestinal barrier function and increased intestinal permeability allow macromolecules, bacteria, endotoxins and antigens to pass into the portal circulation, and thus enter into the tissues of mesenteric nodes, liver, spleen and pancreas. This evasion elicits an inflammatory response by stimulating the macrophages and circulating neutrophil granulocytes and by inflammatory cytokines (interleukin-1 (IL-1), IL-2, IL-6 and TNF-α) [144]. These inflammatory mediators may exacerbate the systemic inflammatory response associated with this process, worsening the overall clinical severity of the pancreatitis and contributing to complications of organ failure and nosocomial infections. The importance of preventing bacterial gut translocation is further stressed since almost 40% of severe acute pancreatitis cases develop infectious complications such as infected necrosis, pancreatic phlegmons and peripancreatic fluid collections [137, 138]. The organisms responsible for the majority of pancreatic infections are typically those found to colonise the gastrointestinal tract.

The severity of acute pancreatitis forms a continuum from a relatively mild, self-limiting illness in 80–85%, which usually resolves spontaneously within days, to a moderately severe disease with transient organ failure and/or local and systemic complication that resolve within 48 h to a fulminant, rapidly progressive and severe disease with persistent organ failure and development of local and systemic complications in 15–20%. The mortality is between 5% and 15% [137, 148]. An Italian study in 1005 patients reported a mortality of 5%, with a low mortality of 1.5% in mild acute pancreatitis and 17% in severe pancreatitis [149]. A systematic review on acute pancreatitis reported an overall mortality of 5%, with a mortality of 3% in interstitial pancreatitis with acute oedema and inflammation of the pancreas and 17% in necrotising pancreatitis with inflammation and pancreatic and peripancreatic necrosis [150]. In patients with necrotising pancreatitis the mortality may be as high as 12% in sterile necrosis, 30% with infected necrosis and 47% with multi-organ dysfunction. Early death is often linked to systemic inflammatory response syndrome (SIRS) and multi-organ dysfunction (MOD); late death is more often associated with infected pancreas necrosis, sepsis and its complications [137, 148, 150–152].

Monitoring the severity of acute pancreatitis by biochemical, radiological and multifactorial scales of several prognostic factors is relevant but none has proven to be perfect and the most ideal prognostic system is still undetermined. Some scores take 48 h to complete such as the Ranson and Imrie/Glasgow scores where for example in the Ranson score five parameters need to be judged at entry and another six after 48 h [153]. Mortality increased with an increasing score and severe pancreatitis was defined by a Ranson score ≥3 with a mortality of 11–15% whereas a score of ≥6 was associated with a 40% mortality and a score of ≥7 with 100% mortality. Although already in 1999 a meta-analysis found the Ranson score to be a poor predictor of severity, it is still widely used [154]. Probably the most widely studied severity scoring system in acute pancreatitis is the APACHE-II score with 12 physiologic measures; a score of ≥8 is associated with a mortality of 11–18% and therefore it is taken as an indication of severe pancreatitis [148, 150]. New severity scores including obesity such as the APACHE-O have been proposed [155]. One point was added for a BMI of 25–30 and two points were added for a BMI >30 kg/m^2.

Meta-Analyses

Four meta-analyses have studied the relationship between obesity and the risk of acute pancreatitis, the severity and its complication [156–159]. No general accepted definitions of acute pancreatitis were proposed until September 1992, when the so-called Atlanta criteria were launched which were revised in 2012 [150, 160]. All four meta-analyses used the Atlanta criteria and the aetiology was mainly biliary (about 60%) followed by alcohol (about 17%). None of the meta-analysis took into account the distribution of fat and also could not adjust for gallbladder and other obesity-associated diseases.

Martinez et al. updated their 2004 meta-analysis in 2006. Obesity was defined by a BMI $\geq$30 kg/m^2 [156, 157]. The meta-analysis involved 739 patients. Severe acute pancreatitis, defined by the Atlanta criteria, was 2.9 times more frequent in obese subjects (OR 2.9 (1.8/4.6)). They were also more at risk for systemic complications such as respiratory failure, renal failure and shock (OR 2.3 (1.4/3.8)) and for local complications (OR 3.8 (2.4/6.6)) such as severe necrosis and pancreatic infection with a twice as great risk of mortality (OR 2.1 (1.0/4.8)). This meta-analysis could not answer the question if the relationship between obesity and gallstones is associated with the relationship between obesity and acute pancreatitis.

Hong et al. retrieved 14 studies: five studies evaluated BMI as a risk factor (N = 1571) and nine evaluated obesity as a prognostic marker for acute pancreatitis (N = 1365) [158]. Although the heterogeneity was high, obese patients when compared with normal-weight subjects had a 34% increased risk of acute pancreatitis. There was an increased risk of severe acute pancreatitis (summary relative risk (SRR) 1.82 (1.44/2.30)), an increased risk of systemic (SRR 1.71 (1.147/2.50)) and local complications (SSR 2.32 (1.79/3.00)) and an increased mortality (2.21 (1.28/3.83)), all without significant heterogeneity.

Wang et al. decided to study the impact of overweight besides that of obesity [159]. In eight studies including 939 patients the risks of severe pancreatitis (OR 2.48 (1.34/4.60)), local complications (OR 2.58 (1.20/5.57)) and mortality (OR 3.81 (1.22/11.83)) but not for systemic complications were increased in overweight patients. The poor prognosis for obese patients was again confirmed: in seven studies involving 786 obese patients obesity was associated with severe acute pancreatitis (OR 3.36 (2.35/4.81)). Complications were studied in four studies (n = 567). Both local (OR 6.23 (3.90/9.94)) and systemic (OR 2.95 (1.85/4.69)) complications were increased in the obese. The seven studies that looked at mortality (n = 889) found obesity to be related with significant mortality (OR 3.31 (1.96/5.60)). So, not only obesity but also overweight are additional prognostic factors of severity, local complications and mortality in acute pancreatitis.

Why Are the Obese at Risk of Acute Pancreatitis and Local and Systemic Complications?

Obesity is associated with several factors associated with the development of acute pancreatitis, such as gallstones, use of alcohol, smoking and high serum levels of triglycerides. There are two theories explaining the initiation of pancreatitis in gallstones: either obstruction at the ampulla due to an impacted stone or oedema as a result of the passage of a stone or reflux of bile into the pancreatic duct during transient obstruction by a stone at the ampulla [137, 141, 148]. Alcohol may increase the synthesis of digestive and lysosomal enzymes responsible for the development of acute pancreatitis by the pancreatic acini, making them oversensitive to the action of cholecystokinin [161, 162]. Smoking is an independent risk factor but the mechanism remains unclear [163]. Hypertriglyceridaemia occurs in the setting of obesity, diabetes and use of medications such as β-blockers, but the pathogenesis of pancreatitis in this condition is unexplained.

Besides the obese having several factors predisposing them to acute pancreatitis, there are obesity-related peculiarities that make them at risk for an adverse outcome [156–158]. Patients with obesity have a large visceral fat mass and increased accumulations of peripancreatic fat. The risk of infection is associated with the amount of pancreatic necrosis. They also have hyperinsulinaemia and thereby changes in their microcirculation which are predisposing to ischaemia. The excess visceral adipose tissue contributes to and accelerates the inflammatory cascade as adipose tissue is an important source of pro-inflammatory cytokines. The inflammatory condition of obesity may thus enhance the systemic inflammatory response syndrome (SIRS) and multi-organ dysfunction (MOD) in acute pancreatitis. Obese have a restricted movement of chest wall and diaphragm and a reduced inspiratory capacity, leading to hypoxia and respiratory failure. The ischaemia and hypoxia result in deficient tissue oxygenation, which may aggravate the consequences of the excessive inflammatory response with multi-organ failure and death [156–158].

Pancreatic Cancer

There is a strong role for obesity and diabetes in the risk of pancreatic cancer. At least ten prospective trials have reported an elevated risk of pancreatic cancer when those with a BMI ≥30 kg/m^2 were compared with those with a normal weight (BMI <25 kg/m^2). The risks varied from 1.2 to 3.0 [164]. A meta-analysis of 14 studies showed a 19% increased risk when comparing a BMI of 30 with that of BMI 22 (RR 1.19 (1.10/1.29)) [165].

The problem of the association between pancreatic cancer and type 2 diabetes is the obvious reverse causality: patients may develop type 2 diabetes as a result of their disease. Also, type 2 diabetes is often present in overweight and obese people and correction for the presence of overweight is lacking in most of the studies. A meta-analysis of 20 studies by Everhart et al. estimated that long-standing diabetes, for more than 5 years, increased the risk of pancreatic cancer twofold (RR 2.0 (1.2/3.2)) [166]. A more recent meta-analysis of 50 studies by Huxley et al. found a slightly weaker association compared with non-diabetics; the risk was 50% higher both when diabetes existed for 5–9 or 10 years and longer (RR 1.5 (1.3/1.8) and RR 1.5 (1.2/2.0), respectively) [167].

Four studies examined the role of elevated glucose levels in the risk of pancreatic cancer [168–171]. Two studies, the Chicago Heart Association Detection Project and the Whitehall study, looked at glucoses after a glucose tolerance test (GTT) and found a 2.4 times (especially in men) and a 4 times increased risk of pancreatic cancer, respectively, in those with elevated versus normal post-GTT glucose levels [168, 169]. The Korean Cancer Prevention Study followed patients with diabetes for 10 years and found a 70% increased risk of pancreas cancer [170]. In the Alpha Tocopherol Beta Carotene (ATBC) study a twofold increase in risk was observed for those with glucose ≥7 versus <7 mmol/L and a similarly increased risk in those with insulin in the highest versus the lowest quartile [171]. So there were statistically significant dose-response associations between glucose levels and pancreatic cancer. Apart from insulin there may be a role for insulin-like growth factor-1 (IGF-1) and oxidative stress.

The role of the diet composition with respect to carbohydrates, glucose and glycaemic index is debated. The relationship between carbohydrate intake, glycaemic index and glycaemic load and pancreatic cancer is inconsistent [164]. The role of added sugar, refined sugar and fructose has been examined in different studies showing a 2- to 3-fold increased risk with added sugar, a 2-fold increased risk with the intake of refined sugar and a 2.3-fold increased risk for ≥2 sweetened soda servings per day and a non-significant risk for fructose from high-fructose syrup [172–175].

1.8.2.3 Implications for Clinical Practice

As obese patients are at risk of gallstone development and of severe pancreatitis and cholangitis when duct obstruction occurs, all measures should be taken to diminish at least the risks. Besides a gradual weight loss when they attempt to lose weight, they should be advised to have a normal three-meal eating pattern without skipping breakfast and without having long periods of fasting. Advices of not drinking alcohol and not smoking should be given. When weight losses exceed the limit of safe weight loss of <1.5 kg/week, ursodeoxycholic acid should be recommended. As a preventive measure attention to the fat content of the diet should be given, which should at least contain 10 g of fats (which is often not the case with very-low-calorie diets). The prophylactic use of 600 mg ursochol for 6 months following gastric bypass has been shown to reduce the incidence of gallstones to 2% in the treatment group compared to 32% in the placebo group [176]. Six months' daily intake resulted in prolonged absence of gallstone formation as at 24 months the differences were still present [177]. This is important as gallstone formation is correlated with the rate of weight loss and bile cholesterol normalises when the weight stabilises, usually after 24 months, and stones may disappear spontaneously. More importantly, the effectiveness of ursodeoxycholic acid prophylaxis has been confirmed by a meta-analysis [178].

1.8.3 Rectocolon

Colorectal cancer is, after lung cancer, breast cancer in women and prostate cancer in men, the fourth most incident cancer and the third leading cause of cancer-related death [179, 180]. The cumulative lifetime risk of developing colorectal cancer in the general population is 5%. As there is a distinct precursor in the form of an adenoma with the well-known adenoma-carcinoma sequence, a screening programme for colon cancer either by examination of stools or by sigmoidoscopy or colonoscopy, with removal of adenomas when present, has been instituted in many countries and has come to fruition with a favourable cost-benefit balance. The adenoma carcinoma sequence is a multistep, multipath and multifocal process with progression of normal mucosa to small polyps and later larger ones that change from advanced adenomas with advanced histology to invasive cancer. The advanced adenomas, defined by size ≥1 cm, villous component and/or high-grade dysplasia, are adenomas that more likely progress to colorectal cancer.

Known risk factors for colorectal cancer (CRC) are the presence of colon polyps, age, menopausal status, family history of CRC, genetic alterations such as in familial adenomatous polyposis (FAP) and the Lynch syndrome, and inflammatory bowel disease [179]. The rapid rise of colon cancer in several populations previously considered at low risk for colon cancer, the incidence changes in migrant populations and the 20-fold difference in incidence between high- and low-risk areas suggest environmental factors as aetiological agents [181]. Obesity has been proposed as a risk factor for CRC and more for colon than for rectum cancer and the association is weaker for women than for men. The risk is increased in younger and premenopausal women compared to older and postmenopausal women. In Europe 11% of the CRC cases are attributed to overweight and obesity [180]. Other factors like the distribution of adipose tissue, oestrogen levels, physical activity and diet also influence the risk of colorectal cancer. Dietary factors include the consumption of red meat and processed meat, low consumption of fruits and vegetables, low-fibre diet and foods low in calcium and folate.

1.8.3.1 Colorectal Adenoma

Obesity doubles the risk of development of colon adenomas and weight gain is also associated with an increased risk [179]. The risk appears higher in men than in women. The obesity risk is increased further by the abdominal, visceral distribution of fat which is reflected in an increased waist circumference or in increased visceral adipose tissue (VAT) as measured by computer tomography (CT) at the level of L4–L5. For instance, patients with adenomas had on average 1.5 times the VAT area compared with subjects without adenomas and increased VAT area was also associated with the number, size and aggressive histology of adenomas and advanced adenomas [164, 181]. VAT was not associated with recurrence of adenomas, suggesting that visceral adiposity promotes growth rather than increasing the occurrence.

Patients with diabetes are also at increased risk for colon adenoma, especially those who are obese [164]. In the Nurses' Health Study an increased risk for adenomas was found (RR 1.63) in the highest quartile of C-peptide levels when controlling for BMI and exercise [164]. In the Veteran Study, advanced adenomas were found in 2903 older and male veteran patients [182]. Obese patients had a greater prevalence of advanced adenomas when compared with overweight and normal-weight patients (28% vs. 23% and 24%). The risk of advanced adenoma by obesity was 1.01 (1.0/1.02) and there was a corresponding 1% increase in the frequency of finding an advanced adenoma per unit increase of BMI above 30. The findings were controlled for NSAID use, statin use, age and family history of CRC without changing the association. Controlling for NSAID use is important as they block cyclooxygenase (COX) enzymes and nuclear factor-kappa B (NF-κB) and thus prevent angiogenesis and have a pro-apoptotic effect on colonocytes. Statins in rodents have been shown to reduce the CRC risk by 47%.

In a case-control study 2244 age- and sex-matched Korean subjects (1122 with and 1122 without adenomas) underwent an abdominal CT with measurement of visceral adipose tissue (VAT) and subcutaneous adipose tissue (SAT), colonoscopy, and were also investigated for the 5 different components of the metabolic syndrome (MetS) adapted for use in Asian populations and for insulin resistance by the HOMA-IR index [183]. The prevalence of smoking, hypertension and MetS and a family history of CRC were higher in the adenoma group than in the normal control group. In addition BMI, SAT and VAT areas, waist circumference, insulin and triglycerides were higher and HDL cholesterol levels lower in the adenoma group. Mean HOMA was also higher in the adenoma group. In univariate analysis the presence of the MetS (OR 1.55 (1.27/1.90)) appeared to be a risk factor and when analysing the five components of the MetS after correction for NSAID aspirin and positive family history, increased waist (OR 1.66 (1.38/1.99)) and elevated triglycerides (OR 1.53 (1.25/1.89)) were found to be the most prominent MetS components that were significantly associated with colon adenoma. These two factors of the MS were considered to be closely related to visceral obesity but they were lost in the multivariate analysis when also VAT was included, meaning that VAT more sensitively predicts the presence of colorectal adenoma. In multivariate analysis VAT was independently associated with the risk of colorectal adenoma (OR 3.09 (2.19/4.36) for the highest quintile versus the lowest quintile) and there appeared to be a dose-dependent relationship: for a 10 cm^2 increase in VAT area the risk of colorectal adenoma increased by 9%. VAT but not SAT was found to be related to the number of polyps, maximum polyp size and advanced adenoma.

Two recent studies urged the need to look at the colon in patients with non-alcoholic fatty liver disease (NAFLD) [184, 185]. Hwang et al. investigated 2917 participants by colonoscopy, ultrasound and liver tests; they found a prevalence of 41.5% of NAFLD in patients with adenomatous polyps and of 30.2% in the control group [184]. Wong et al. recruited subjects of 40–70 years referred for colonoscopic screening from two study cohorts: one cohort from the community, who had their liver fat estimated by proton magnetic resonance spectroscopy (^{1}H-MRS), and the other cohort from patients with biopsy-proven NAFLD [185]. Patients with NAFLD had a higher prevalence of adenomas (34.7% vs. 21.5%) and advanced adenomas (18.6% vs. 5.5%) than healthy controls. Moreover, 46.4% of adenomas in NAFLD and 44.7% of the advanced adenomas were right-sided lesions. In the group of biopsy-proven NAFLD, patients with inflammation, i.e. patients with non-alcoholic steatohepatitis (NASH), had a higher adenoma rate (51.0% vs. 25.6%) and advanced adenoma (34.7% vs. 14%) than non-NASH NAFLD patients. After adjustment, NASH was associated with an about five times higher risk of adenoma (OR 4.89 (2.04/11.7)) and advanced adenoma (OR 5.34 (1.92/14.84)) rate compared with simple steatosis. Patients with simple steatosis were similar to control subjects in adenoma and advanced adenoma rates. So, NASH was associated with a high prevalence of adenomas and advanced adenomas and these were mainly located in the right colon, needing a total colonoscopy procedure. NAFLD patients are characterised by a profound insulin resistance, with high insulin and IGF-1 levels and low adiponectin levels, and a pro-inflammatory state [185].

Meta-Analyses

A significant increased risk of colorectal polyps was found in patients with obesity and with abdominal obesity. Lee et al. included 25 studies in their meta-analysis and found a pooled odds ratio for obesity and abdominal obesity of 1.43 (1.23/1.67) in 22 studies and 1.42 (1.30/1.56) in 12 studies, respectively [186]. In a subgroup meta-analysis the risk was present for both men and women, for Asian and non-Asian countries and for distal and total colorectum, and the risk was highest for advanced polyps (OR 2.16 (1.49/3.14)). Also a dose-response relationship was present with risks increasing from 1.19 in the lowest category of BMI to 1.40 in the middle and 1.69 in the highest BMI category. They suggested that the strong positive association of abdominal adiposity with large and advanced polyps supported the hypothesis of the role of hyperinsulinaemia, in which insulin and insulin-like growth factor-1 (IGF-1) are the molecules mediating the progression of small to advanced polyps. The growth and progression by the effects of insulin and IGF-1 seem stronger in advanced than in less advanced polyps. In an extensive and comprehensive review Bardou et al. summarised their findings on four meta-analysis on colorectal adenoma [180, 186–189] (Table 1.5). All meta-analyses showed a small but significant association with similar trends over sexes, races, countries, site in the colon other than rectum, etc. The most recent meta-analysis by Okabayashi found a dose relationship with BMI 25–30 of 1.21 and BMI ≥30 of 1.32 when compared with a BMI <25 kg/m^2 [188]. Ben et al. looked at the dose-response per 5 unit increase in the BMI (Table 1.5) [188, 189].

1.8.3.2 Colorectal Carcinoma

Several large studies and also different meta-analyses have found a consistent positive association of obesity defined as a BMI ≥30 kg/m^2 and colon cancer in men and women. Bardou et al. summarised the findings of 5 meta-analyses and found a moderately increased risk of 1.5–2-fold (Table 1.6) [37, 180, 190–193]. The association was weaker for women than for men. This was also true for the waist circumference and the WHR. Most studies showed that the associations of waist circumference and WHR with colon cancer were stronger than for BMI and the associations remained when they corrected for BMI but attenuated when they corrected for waist circumference and WHR, indicating the strongest influence of abdominal obesity [191]. Most of the studies report a lower but significant association of rectum cancer with BMI in males; in females this association is inconsistent and also the relationship of rectum cancer with waist and WHR is unclear or absent (Table 1.6).

There seems also to be an ethnic difference as findings of the USA and Europe are in the same direction and with a somewhat higher risk estimate in the USA concerning the relation between obesity and colon cancer or CRC whereas in Asian countries mainly obese males seem to be affected by colon cancer (Table 1.6). Many of the studies did not take into consideration the effect modification by age and menopausal status which may explain the inconsistent or weak findings among women. The menopausal status was addressed by the Canadian Breast Screening Study which found a weak and insignificant association with

Table 1.5 Published meta-analyses on colorectal adenoma (CRA) with only mentioning of risk ratios that were statistically significant

Author and year	No. of studies/ search period	Reported analysis	Outcomes	Risk ratios (95% CI)
Lee'11 [186]	25 studies/1964–June 2010	Lower class BMI ≥25 and ≥23 in Asians Moderate-class BMI ≥30 and ≥25 in Asians	Men	1.39 (1.10/1.76)
			Women	1.37 (1.08/1.73)
			Asian countries	1.88 (1.30/2.71)
			Western countries	1.30 (1.11/1.52)
			Waist	1.42 (1.30/1.56)
			Site distal CR	1.46 (1.46/1.72)
			Site total CR	1.45 (1.17/1.78)
			Large/advanced	2.16 (2.16/3.14)
			Small/ non-advanced	1.51 (1.15/1.99)
Hong'12 [187]	21 studies/up to October 2011	Dose-response per 10 cm increase in waist and 0.1 unit increase in WHR	Waist	1.39 (1.24/1.56)
			WHR	1.22 (1.10/1.36)
			Men waist	1.38 (1.11/1.70)
			Women waist	1.24 (1.00/1.56)
			Men WHR	1.34 (1.14/1.58)
			Asian waist	1.38 (1.17/1.56)
			Non-Asian waist	1.39 (1.20/1.61)
			Non-Asian WHR	1.26 (1.11/1.43)
Okabayashi'12 [188]	23 studies/1980–August 2011	BMI 25–30 and ≥30 vs. BMI <25	BMI risk CRA	1.24 (1.16/1.33)
			Western countries	1.18 (1.04/1.34)
			Asian countries	1.35 (1.27/1.44)
Ben'12 [189]	36 studies/up to July 2011	Dose-response per 5 unit increase in BMI	BMI risk CRA	1.19 (1.13/1.26)
			Men	1.15 (1.05/1.26)
			Women	1.08 (1.02/1.14)
			White	1.12 (1.04/1.21)
			USA	1.18 (1.09/1.26)
			Europe	1.16 (1.06/1.27)
			Asia	1.29 (1.11/1.51)
			<10 mm	1.53 (1.18/1.98)
			≥10 mm	1.49 (1.16/1.91)
			Non-advanced	1.36 (1.17/1.58)
			Advanced	1.70 (1.12/2.58)

BMI Body mass index; *WHR* waist/hip ratio; CI confidence interval; CR colorectal

obesity (BMI ≥30 kg/m^2) in the entire cohort (HR 1.08 NS) [194]. Obesity was associated with an approximately twofold risk (HR 1.88 (1.24/2.86)) in women who were premenopausal at inclusion and no altered risk was present among postmenopausal women (with a trend of a small to moderately decreased risk (HR 0.92) for colon cancer). Similar results were found in three older studies with a twofold increased risk in Swedish obese subjects below age 55, in female Seventh Day Adventists, and in obese women in the Nurses' Health Study who were between 34 and 59 at entrance [195–197]. These findings are surprising given that the menopause is associated with a redistribution of fat towards the abdomen [181]. Age is a bias here, as Swedish obese subjects older than 55 years and nurses older than 65 years did not have a higher CRC risk [196, 197]. So, the association

Table 1.6 Published meta-analyses on colorectal cancer (CRC) with only mentioning of risk ratios that were statistically significant

Author and year	No. of studies/ search period	Reported analysis	Outcomes	Risk ratios (95% CI)
Dai'07 [190]	15 studies/up to January 2007	BMI ≥30	Men colon cancer	1.71 (1.33/2.19)
			Men rectal cancer	1.75 (1.17/2.62)
			Men CRC	1.37 (1.21/1.56)
			Waist men colon	1.68 (1.36/2.08)
			Waist women colon	1.48 (1.19/1.84)
			WHR men colon	1.91 (1.46/2.49)
			WHR women colon	1.49 (1.23/1.81)
			WHR men rectum	1.93 (1.19/3.13)
Larsson'07 [191]	31 studies/1966–April 2007	Per 5 unit increase in BMI, per 10 cm increase in waist and per 0.1 unit increase in WHR	Men colon	1.30 (1.25/1.35)
			Women colon	1.12 (1.07/1.18)
			Men rectum	1.12 (1.09/1.16)
			Waist men colon	1.33 (1.19/1.49)
			Waist women colon	1.16 (1.09/1.23)
			Waist men rectum	1.12 (1.03/1.22)
			WHR men colon	1.43 (1.19/1.71)
			WHR women colon	1.20 (1.08/1.33)
			USA men colon	1.39 (1.31/1.48)
			USA women colon	1.17 (1.08/1.25)
			EU men colon	1.27 (1.22/1.32)
			EU women colon	1.04 (1.02/1.07)
			Asia men colon	1.16 (1.05/1.28)
Moghaddam'07 [192]	31 studies/up to April 2007	BMI ≥30	Men CRC	1.46 (1.36/1.56)
			Women CRC	1.15 (1.06/1.24)
Guh'09 [37][a]	12 studies/up to January 2007	BMI ≥30	Men CRC	1.95 (1.59/2.39)
			Women CRC	1.66 (1.52/1.81)
			USA men CRC	1.86 (1.40/2.46)
			USA women CRC	1.47 (1.30/1.66)
			EU men CRC	2.00 (1.40/2.87)
			EU women CRC	1.74 (1.68/1.81)
			Waist men CRC	2.93 (2.31/3.73)
			Waist women CRC	1.55 (1.27/1.88)
Harriss'09 [193]	28 studies/1966–December 2007	Per 5 unit increase in BMI	Men colon	1.24 (1.20/1.28)
			Women colon	1.09 (1.04/1.14)
			Men rectum	1.09 (1.06/1.12)
			USA men colon	1.35 (1.21/1.50)
			USA women colon	1.13 (1.06/1.19)
			EU + A men colon	1.21 (1.18/1.24)
			EU + A women colon	1.04 (1.00/1.07)
			Asian men colon	1.32 (1.20/1.46)

BMI Body mass index, *WHR* waist/hip ratio, *EU* Europe, *EU + A* Europe + Australia; *CI* confidence interval

[a]Data given as incidence risk ratio

between obesity and CRC in premenopausal women may be as strong and as consistent as that in men.

Apart from age and menopausal status physical activity is a confounding factor [181]. A meta-analysis of the association between CRC and physical activity by

Samad et al. could demonstrate a similar decrease in colon cancer (not rectal cancer) risk by increased physical activity both in men and women [198]. Slattery showed that 12–14% of colon cancers can be attributed to lack of involvement in vigorous exercise [199]. Two meta-analysis by the same authors found a decreased risk of colorectal adenoma (OR 0.84 (0.77/0.92)) and colorectal carcinoma (OR 0.76 (0.71/0.82)) with increased physical activity [200, 201]. Adjustment for a confounding factor such as diet (increased red meat and processed meat, low folate and low fibre consumption) did not change the association. Physical inactivity also increases the risk of dying after the diagnosis of colon cancer.

Meta-Analyses

Three of the five meta-analyses as shown in Table 1.6 compared categories of BMI $\geq$30 kg/m^2 with normal-weight categories. Three of these meta-analyses have also estimated the strength of the association between obesity and CRC and the dose-response relationship: in the meta-analysis of Moghaddam et al. the risk of developing CRC increased by 7% per 2 unit (kg/m^2) increase in BMI and with 4% for each 2 cm increase in waist [192]. In the meta-analysis of Larsson et al. each 5 unit increase in BMI increased the risk by 30% in males and by 12% in females; for each 10 cm increase in waist circumference the risk increased by 33% in men and by 16% in women and for each 0.1 unit increase in WHR the risk increased by 43% in men and by 20% in women [191]. Similarly, Harriss et al. found an increased risk of colon cancer by 24% in males and 9% in females by each 5 kg/m^2 increase in BMI, but only a 9% increased risk in males and no increased risk in females for rectal cancer [193].

1.8.3.3 Pathophysiology of Obesity in Relation to Adenoma and Carcinoma

High BMI, physical inactivity and visceral adiposity are consistent risk factors for colon adenoma and colon cancer [164]. Also patients with type 2 diabetes and metabolic syndrome are at risk. They all have a common feature: hyperinsulinaemia which is a consistent marker of increased colon cancer risk. Also, altered levels of adipokines seem to be of importance. Other biological factors such as bile acids and gut microbiota are still under investigation.

In the pathophysiology of adenoma and carcinoma the role of the visceral fat is predominant by itself or indirectly which is in contrast to gastro-oesophageal reflux disease where also mechanical factors play a role. Colon cancer in men is positively associated with BMI and central adiposity whereas in women these associations are weak or non-existing. Such relationships of rectal cancer are either not investigated and thus unknown, or weak and restricted to men. Visceral fat deposition, reflected in waist circumference measurements or visceral adipose tissue (VAT) measurement by CT, is associated with insulin resistance and higher circulating insulin levels. Especially, hyperinsulinaemia is the critical factor [164, 180, 181]. BMI is strongly correlated with plasma insulin levels. Increased insulin lowers blood levels of insulin-like growth factor-binding proteins (IGFBP-1 and IGFBP-2), resulting in more free and bioactive insulin and IGF-1, which is associated with the risk of CRC in men and women. IGF-1 has a role in the control of normal growth, maintenance of tissue homeostasis, altering the balance between proliferation and apoptosis, and differentiation, angiogenesis, cell migration, cell adhesion and wound healing. IGF-1 is a procarcinogen that stimulates cell growth and decreases apoptosis. Serum C-peptide is a surrogate test for insulin secretion and many studies found a relation between the highest levels of C-peptide and colon cancer [164, 180, 181]. In the Physicians' Health Study, men with a C-peptide in the highest versus the lowest quintile had a 2.7 times higher risk for CRC after adjustment for BMI and exercise [202]. After controlling for the components of the MetS the risk rose to 3.4. In the Nurses' Health Study both an increased risk of adenomas (RR 1.63) and an increased risk of colorectal carcinoma (RR 1.73) were found in the highest quartile of C-peptide versus the lowest quartile after adjustment for BMI and exercise [203]. Patients with acromegaly have an increased risk of colon cancer because of elevated IGF-1 from excessive growth hormone secretion.

The stronger associations in men may be explained by a more prevalent abdominal obesity. As women tend to accumulate lesser VAT than men with weight gain, this may be an explanation for the gender differences between the risk of cancer and obesity, apart from the role of gonadal hormones. Endogenous oestrogens may be protective and are associated with a lower risk of CRC by inhibiting proliferation and increasing apoptosis [194, 197]. Adipose tissue is the only tissue that expresses oestrogen aromatase and is therefore a primary source of oestrogens by conversion of androgens into oestrogens both in men and women. So, in postmenopausal women extraglandular endogenous oestrogen may counteract the deleterious effects of insulin and IGF-1 and may result in a reduced risk of CRC, which is rather surprising as postmenopausal women behave like men and are more likely to store their fat intra-abdominally [194]. Postmenopausal hormone use has been associated with decreased risk of colon or colorectal cancer in 7 of the 14 studies by Calle et al. [8, 181]. In premenopausal women obesity increases insulin and the contribution of adipose oestrogens is relatively unimportant when compared to that derived from the ovaries [164, 194, 197]. The balance between insulin and IGF-1 and the oestrogens is towards the adverse effects of insulin, thus having a net effect of increasing the risk of CRC. Moreover, adiposity is inversely correlated with testosterone in men but positively associated in women [191]. Androgen deprivation increases adiposity and insulin resistance in men. An obesity-induced reduction of testosterone would be another reason for a higher CRC risk in men.

Physical activity increases insulin sensitivity and reduces plasma insulin levels. It reduced the risk of CRC by 25–50% in physically active individuals [179, 198, 200, 201]. The protection by increased physical activity, related to improved insulin sensitivity, is stronger for colon cancer and absent for rectum cancer [164, 180, 181]. This suggests that colon cancer is more related to insulin resistance and hyperinsulinaemia than rectum cancer. A diet high in refined sugars and low in dietary fibre, linked to colon cancer, also causes hyperinsulinaemia [181].

Metabolic Syndrome

Type 2 diabetes has a 1.43 times increased risk of colon carcinoma and there appears also to be an increased risk for colon adenoma, especially in those who are obese. Hyperglycaemia is associated with increased risk of colon carcinoma. Also, the presence of the metabolic syndrome increases the risk of colon carcinoma [164, 180]. One study investigated the risk of CRC with increasing number of components of the MetS and found a significantly increased risk of 2.40 and of 2.57 for two and three component versus none [204]. The study by Hu et al. in Taiwan did the same for colorectal adenoma and found a significantly increased risk of 1.61, 2.57 and 3.23 for 3, 4 and 5 components, respectively, of the MetS [205]. Kang et al. [183] measured VAT, SAT and metabolic syndrome components adapted for use in Asian people. In univariate analysis the presence of the MetS (OR 1.55 (1.27/1.90)) is a risk factor and, when analysing the five components of the MS after correction for NSAID, aspirin and positive family history, increased waist and elevated triglycerides were found to be significantly associated with colon adenoma. These two factors of the MetS were lost in the multivariate analysis when also VAT was included. Apparently, VAT predicts more sensitively the presence of colorectal adenoma. VAT has been identified as a risk factor for colorectal adenoma (risk 1.6) and for colorectal cancer with risks varying between 1.9 and 4.0, either independently or via VAT-secreted adipokines [180]. VAT is associated with colorectal adenoma independently of BMI.

Visceral Fat and Adipokines

Omental and subcutaneous fat are metabolically different [206]. The glucose uptake in general, insulin-stimulated glucose uptake and depressed insulin-induced glucose uptake by steroid blockade were greater in omental fat. Also, liposuction of a substantial amount of subcutaneous fat (a mean of 6.3 kg in subjects with normal glucose tolerance and 8.9 kg in type 2 diabetes patients) did not change insulin sensitivity in liver, muscle and adipose tissue; did not change blood levels of glucose, insulin or lipids; and did not result in changes in inflammatory mediators [207]. However, in a pilot study, omentectomy, i.e. removal of visceral fat, together with gastric banding resulted in 2–3 times greater improvements in oral glucose tolerance, insulin sensitivity and fasting plasma glucose and insulin with no differences in blood lipids and these improvements were statistically independent of the loss in body mass index [208].

The relationship between adiposity and insulin sensitivity can be summarised as follows: weight gain increases visceral adipose tissue past a threshold and then the patient passes into a phase of insulin resistance in which the VAT area correlates with C-peptide, insulin and leptin [209].

Insulin is the best established biochemical mediator between obesity and colon cancer. Obesity is also associated with high leptin and low adiponectin levels and both high leptin and low adiponectin levels are related to increased risks of colorectal carcinoma.

Both leptin and adiponectin have an influence on intracellular signal pathways such as the phosphatidylinositol 3-kinase/Akt (PI3K/Akt), mitogen-activated protein kinase (MAPK) and extracellular signal-regulated kinase (ERK), which play an important role in colon carcinogenesis [210]. Leptin is secreted by white adipose tissues and leptin receptors are present in colon tissue. It activates the signal transduction pathways such as Jack kinase, mTOR, AMP-activated protein kinase

(AMPK), ERK and MAPK [180, 209, 210]. High leptin levels are associated with increased colorectal cancer risk and also with more aggressive tumours; it does not initiate tumours but is involved in tumour growth.

Adiponectin is an insulin-sensitising hormone with two known receptors, ADIPOR1 expressed in skeletal muscle and ADIPOR2 expressed in the liver. Also, adiponectin and its receptors are expressed in colonic tissue and adiponectin is inversely associated with colorectal cancer risk [180, 209, 210]. Compared with males in the lowest quintile, men in the highest quintile had a 58% lower risk of colorectal cancer [211]. Two meta-analyses found an inverse association of adiponectin and CRC [212, 213]. One meta-analysis of 13 studies found that per 1 μg/mL higher adiponectin the risk of CRC decreased by 2% [212]. In mice, adiponectin suppresses colonic epithelium proliferation by inhibition of the mTOR pathway and stimulation of the AMP-activated protein kinase pathway, under the condition of a high-fat diet but not a basal diet [84, 214]. A high-fat diet might be able to affect the expression of molecules which link metabolism, inflammation and cancer [214]. Adiponectin counteracts leptin and decreases the PI3K/Akt signal pathway activated by leptin [210, 215]. Adiponectin also modulates genes involved in inflammation and can inhibit inflammatory pathways such as IL-6 and TNF.

1.8.3.4 Implications for Clinical Practice

Current guidelines recommend CRC screening in adults aged 50–70 years. However, it has been demonstrated that males with abdominal obesity and metabolic syndrome might benefit from screening starting at 45 years of age. In the study by Wong et al. males and females aged 40–50 years with biopsy-proven NAFLD, and even more so when inflammation, i.e. NASH, was present, had a higher prevalence of adenomas and advanced adenomas compared with controls, which were in 45% of cases right-sided [184, 185]. The clinical implication might be screening by total colonoscopy at an earlier age than indicated by the guidelines. At least gastroenterologist should be aware of the association.

Apart from being at risk for colorectal cancer while being obese the question is whether obesity influences the outcome after surgery. The outcome might also be related to lifestyle factors associated with obesity such as decreased physical activity and indeed physical inactivity increases the risk of dying after the diagnosis of colon cancer [181]. As to the short-term outcomes for CRC Bardou et al. reviewed the literature on surgery [180]. They retrieved 20 published observational studies and found indications of a significantly longer hospital stay, an increased complication rate, more wound infection and significantly more blood loss. A meta-analysis of 8 studies and a narrative review of 33 studies showed increased conversion rates, operating times and postoperative morbidity [216, 217]. Obesity might be associated with a decreased overall survival in patients with CRC independently of MetS [180].

Bardou et al. also reviewed the response to chemotherapy [180]. Visceral fat and its metabolic hormones promote angiogenesis and thus might predict a less well response to vascular endothelial growth factor (VEGF)-targeted therapy (bevacizumab). They summarised the available literature as follows. When comparing bevacizumab-based regimen with chemotherapy, obese patients with high BMI and more visceral fat had no response to the former and did well on the latter. High visceral fat was independently associated with time to progress, response and overall survival. These results were confirmed in a study that showed that responders had lower visceral adipose tissue than non-responders. Also in the CAIRO and CAIRO2 studies a high BMI predicted a better survival in the chemotherapy group but not in combined chemotherapy + targeted treatment.

So, to reduce the risk of colorectal cancer, obese patients should lose weight, be more active physically and eat a more healthy food with less meat and more fruits, vegetables, fibre, calcium and folic acid. Although bariatric surgery has resolved or improved many comorbidities and also reduced the mortality risk, there is still some debate about potentially adverse effects. Hull and Lagergren cautioned against the assumption that bariatric surgery will lead to a decreased future incidence rate of CRC [218]. They studied a large cohort of 15,095 patients after bariatric surgery and both restrictive and malabsorptive interventions were included [219]. They found an increased standardised incidence ratio (SIR) of 2.0 (1.48/2.64) for colorectal cancer 10 years after surgery whereas the comparator obese group of 62,016 subjects who had never undergone surgery had a stabile SIR of 1.26 (1.14/1.40). Several factors have to be taken into account: the effect of residual excess weight and a tendency to gain weight postoperatively, but also less desirable consequences of certain operations such as higher intraluminal bile concentrations and changes in microbiota after a gastric bypass, but also the general recommendation to increase the dietary protein postoperatively.

1.8.4 Liver

Non-alcoholic fatty liver disease (NAFLD) encompasses the entire spectrum of fatty liver disease from simple non-alcoholic fatty liver (NAFL) on the one hand to the more complicated non-alcoholic steatohepatitis (NASH), with eventually liver fibrosis/cirrhosis, and hepatocellular carcinoma (HCC) on the other [220, 221]. The natural course and the different stages of the disease with frequencies of evolution are depicted in Fig. 1.5 [222].

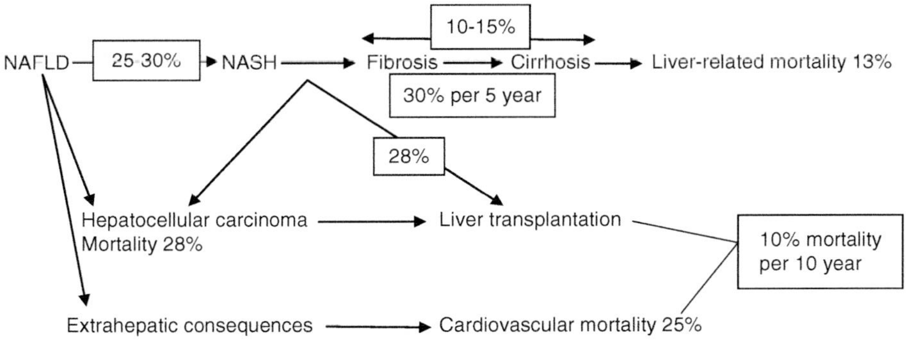

Fig. 1.5 The NAFLD spectrum with rates of prevalence, changeover and mortality

1.8.4.1 Non-alcoholic Fatty Liver Disease

NAFLD is characterised by excessive hepatic fat accumulation, associated with insulin resistance, and is defined by the presence of steatosis in >5% of hepatocytes according to histological analysis, or by a proton density fat fraction, a rough estimation of the volume fraction of fatty material in the liver, >5.6% assessed by proton magnetic resonance spectroscopy (^{1}HMRS) or quantitative fat/water-selective magnetic resonance imaging (MRI) [221].

The diagnosis of NAFLD requires (1) the exclusion of chronic liver diseases associated with fat accumulation such as viral hepatitis, Wilson's disease, lipodystrophy and abetalipoproteinaemia, systemic diseases or certain lipogenic drugs such as amiodarone, corticosteroids and antiretroviral medications and (2) hepatic fat accumulation in the absence of significant alcohol use in the last 2 years, defined as >21 drinks per week in men and >14 drinks per week in women, or a daily alcohol consumption ≥30 g for men and ≥20 g for women [220, 221]. There are also data to suggest that hypothyroidism, hypogonadism, hypopituitarism, sleep apnoea and PCOS, common comorbidities of obesity, further drive NAFLD prevalence and severity independent of obesity [220, 221].

In NAFL simple steatosis is present with an absent to low risk of progression to cirrhosis. The diagnosis of NASH requires the joint presence of steatosis and inflammation with hepatocyte ballooning and lobular inflammation. They may be at risk of progressive disease. The NAFLD Activity Score (NAS) scoring system is a composite score to quantify features of steatohepatitis and to assess treatment response in NASH clinical trials [223]. It is composed of steatosis (0–3), lobular inflammation (0–3) and hepatocyte ballooning (0–2) grades and ranges from 0 to 8. Fibrosis in NASH is staged separately on a scale from 0 to 4 with stages 3–4 considered advanced fibrosis.

NAFLD is tightly associated with insulin resistance, not only in the liver, but also in muscle and adipose tissues, and thus with metabolic risk factors and components of the metabolic syndrome (MetS) and may be considered as the hepatic manifestation of the MetS. The clinical burden of NAFLD being closely related to obesity and other metabolic syndrome risk factors is expected to grow with the bourgeoning epidemics of obesity and diabetes. Moreover, NASH is assumed to be the underlying cause in 30–75% of cryptogenic cirrhosis [224]. NASH-related cirrhosis is the most rapidly rising indication for liver transplantation and by the year 2020 may be the leading cause of liver transplantation.

Patients with NAFLD are mostly asymptomatic and when symptoms are present patients complain of fatigue, malaise and right upper quadrant discomfort. Incidence data are sparse and both incidence and prevalence data of NAFLD vary according to the assessment methods used such as histology, ultrasound, liver aminotransferases or proton magnetic resonance spectroscopy (^{1}H-MRS) or magnetic resonance imaging (MRI). The incidence of NAFLD is 31 and 86 cases per 1000 person-years based on elevated liver enzymes and/or on ultrasound (US), and 34 per 1000 person-years by ^{1}H-MRS, but is also reported as low as 29 cases per 100,000 person-years in a study from the UK [220, 221]. Sherif et al. reviewed the epidemiological data and found a worldwide prevalence of NAFLD between 4 and 46% with a reported

3–5% prevalence of NASH [225]. For Western countries these data are for NAFLD and NASH, 20–40% and 2–3%, respectively. In the USA prevalences of 27–34% and 3–5%, and in Canada 7% and 3%, have been reported for NAFLD and NASH, respectively. So, one can state that in the general population a median prevalence of NAFLDF of 20% is estimated with only a prevalence of NASH between 3% and 5%; the prevalence of NASH-related cirrhosis is not known. They also reviewed the NHANES studies in the USA and found an increased prevalence according to the NHANES study from 5.5% in 1988 to 11% in 2008 and an increased proportion of NAFLD among chronic liver disease from 47% in 1998 to 75% in 2008, attributable to a rise in the prevalence of obesity, insulin resistance and significantly altered dietary habits [222, 225]. Indeed, when considering obese patients and patients with the metabolic syndrome or type 2 diabetes, prevalence was high: the prevalence in obese patients, especially with hyperlipidaemia, is 60–85%, and in diabetic patients it is 30–50%. From the NHANES, the Dallas and the San Antonio study, Sherif et al. also found US Hispanics to be the most disproportionally affected ethnic group with African-American being the least affected, presumably explained by genetic disparities [225].

NAFLD increases with age and is more prevalent in men. Somewhat alarming are the findings in healthy and non-obese young living liver donors, who were reported to have a prevalence of NAFLD varying from 17.9% in Japan to 34% in the USA [225].

The natural course of NAFLD has been studied in two meta-analyses by Vernon et al. and Musso et al. [226, 227]. They show that a minority will progress from simple fatty liver to NASH and also that only NASH is associated with an increased risk of progressive liver disease. In the spectrum of NAFLD only one-third will develop NASH and NASH is the only disease in the NAFLD spectrum that is associated with progression to cirrhosis (9–20% over 5–10 years) and HCC [228]. In a meta-analysis of three population-based and four community-based studies with a follow-up between 7.3 and 24 years, the overall mortality was 57% higher in NAFLD compared with the normal population with a 2.16 times increased cardiovascular mortality but not an increased extrahepatic malignancy mortality [227]. Looking at all deaths 13% of all deaths were related to liver, 28% related to malignancy and 25% of all cases related to ischaemic heart disease. Patients with NASH and a fibrosis score of 3–4 had a 3.3 times higher overall and disease-related mortality. When patients with NASH were compared with patients with NAFL they had an 18% higher mortality, but the liver-related mortality was 5.7 times higher.

A number of factors have been mentioned as potentially leading to the progression of the fatty liver disease such as obesity, type 2 diabetes mellitus (T2DM), age, degree of inflammation, alanine aminotransferase (ALT), aspartate aminotransferase (AST)/ALT ratio, triglycerides, C-peptide, insulin resistance, female sex and hypertension [229]. Also findings at biopsy are important as the degree of inflammation is the strongest and independent predictor of fibrosis progression [230]. Two studies from Sweden demonstrated that the stage of fibrosis was the only independent histological feature on liver biopsy associated with long-term overall mortality and disease-specific mortality [231, 232].

As earlier mentioned, coronary heart disease is the primary cause of morbidity and mortality in patients with NAFLD [233]. There is a strong association between NAFLD and risk of coronary heart disease and cardiac complications such as left ventricle dysfunction, heart valve disease and atrial fibrillation. NAFLD is associated with the metabolic syndrome and therefore with multiple cardiac risk factors such as abdominal obesity, hyperglycaemia, insulin resistance, atherogenic dyslipidaemia, hypertension, ectopic fat accumulation and an altered adipocyte-related hormonal and cytokine profile which results in the development of a pro-inflammatory and pro-atherogenic milieu.

Recent studies have challenged the dogma that NAFL is not progressive. Singh et al. studied the progression of the disease in a meta-analysis of six studies in 133 NAFLD patients and of seven studies in 116 NASH patients [234]. The pooled data from six studies with 133 patients with simple steatosis with over 2146 person-years of follow-up showed that 52 (39.1%) patients developed progressive fibrosis and 70 (52.6%) remained stable while 11 patients (8.3%) had improvement of fibrosis. Accordingly, the fibrosis progression rate in patients with simple steatosis and absence of fibrosis at baseline was 0.07 stages, translating into 1 stage of fibrosis progression over 14.3 years. The pooled data of 116 NASH patients found that 40 patients (34.5%) developed progressive fibrosis, 45 (38.8%) remained stable and 31 (26.7%) showed improvement in fibrosis. The annual fibrosis progression rate in NASH without baseline fibrosis was 0.14 stages, translating into 1 stage of progression over an average of 7.1 years. Predictors associated with progression of fibrosis in NASH appeared to be age, inflammation at index biopsy, hypertension and a baseline low AST/ALT ratio. The long-term outcome related to histology was reported by Matteoni in 132 patients over 8 years [235]. Cirrhosis developed in 21–28% of patients with NASH compared to 3% in non-NASH with a liver-related mortality of 11% versus 2%. They updated their cohort with 18.5 years of follow-up and found increased liver-related mortality of 18% in the NASH and 3% in the non-NASH groups [236].

In the Million Women Study with 1.3 million women the admission rates and death rates for liver cirrhosis in a 6-year follow-up period were investigated [237]. Compared with the reference group with a BMI of 22.5–24.9 kg/m^2, those with a BMI of 25–27.4 had a non-significant 5% higher risk and with a BMI of 27.5–29.9 a non-significant 11% higher risk of liver cirrhosis. However, those with a BMI 30–34.9 had a 49% higher risk (RR 1.49 (1.33/1.68)) and those with a BMI 35–39.9 a 77% higher risk (RR 1.77 (1.49/2.10)) and per 5 units of increased BMI the risk of cirrhosis increased by 24% (RR 1.24 (1.19/1.38)). The relative risk did not change according to the amount of alcohol consumed but the absolute risk did. The absolute risk of liver cirrhosis per 1000 women over a period of 5 years was 2.7 (2.1/3.4) and 5.0 (3.8/6.6) in women who reported drinking 150 g or more per week (18 units) with a BMI of 22.5–25.0 and BMI ≥30 kg/m^2, respectively. Also, Hart et al. showed that being overweight or obese and drinking 15 or more units each week had a synergistic effect which amplified the insult to the liver and greatly increased the risk of liver-related morbidity and mortality [238].

Hamaguchi et al. examined the relationship between the metabolic syndrome and NAFLD diagnosed by ultrasound in 4401 Japanese men and women drinking 20 g or less of ethanol each day [239]. On ultrasound at the start, a fatty liver was identified in 18% with a 2.5-fold higher incidence in men than women. Patients with a fatty liver were more likely to be obese and to have the metabolic syndrome. Those who were free of NAFLD diagnosis at the start developed NAFLD in the 1-year interval period in 14% of males and 5% of women; they gained only little body weight, 1.7 and 1.3 kg, respectively. The most important finding was that the presence of the metabolic syndrome carried a 4–11 times higher risk for future NAFLD. Fourteen percent of males and 25% of females showed regression to normal of their initially fatty livers; they lost 2.5 kg and 2.3 kg, respectively, and had less components of the metabolic syndrome. Hamaguchi et al. thus provided strong support for the central role of insulin resistance in the pathophysiology of NAFLD and also showed that weight gain and metabolic syndrome are risk factors for NAFLD. More importantly, NAFLD may be reversible if obesity and certain aspects of the metabolic syndrome are managed effectively, even without normalisation of body weight. In a study from Italy with 304 patients by Marchesini et al., the presence of the metabolic syndrome conferred a higher risk of NASH (OR 3.2 (1.2/8.9)) and a higher risk for advanced fibrosis (OR 3.5 (1.1/11.2)) [240].

1.8.4.2 Hepatocellular Carcinoma

Patients with NASH are also at risk for the development of hepatocellular carcinoma (HCC) and the increased risk for HCC is likely to be limited to those with advanced fibrosis and cirrhosis. Advanced fibrosis remains a strong risk factor for HCC with cumulative incidence rates reported between 2.4 and 12.8% [222]. The recent Surveillance Epidemiology and End Results (SEER) study compared a total of 4929 HCC cases and 14,937 controls without HCC over the years 2004–2009 [241]. Of the HCC cases, 54.9% were related to hepatitis C, 16.4% to alcoholic liver disease, 14.1% to NAFLD and 9.5% to hepatitis B. Across the 6-year period the number of NAFLD-HCC showed a 9% annual increase. NAFLD-HCC patients were older, had shorter survival time, more heart disease and were more likely to die from their primary liver cancer. In multivariate analysis, NAFLD increased the risk of HCC by a factor of 2.6 (OR 2.62 (2.28/3.00)) and increased the 1-year mortality by 21% (OR 1.21 (1.01/1.45)).

Hassan et al. from the MD Anderson Cancer Centre performed a case-control study to evaluate the association between obesity and HCC and they tried to correct for confounding factors such as hepatitis B and C, diabetes, a family history of cancer, smoking and alcohol consumption [242]. Obesity, but not overweight, in early adulthood (in the mid-20–mid-40 years of age) was a significant risk factor for HCC in the total population (OR 2.6 (1.4/4.4)), both in men (OR 2.3 (1.2/4.4)) and in women (OR 3.6 (1.5/8.9)). For each 1 kg/m^2 increase in BMI in early adulthood, hepatocellular carcinoma occurred 3.9 months earlier in life. Obesity had no influence on HCC outcome. Obesity and virus infections had a synergistic interaction, suggesting that obesity, in addition to its own direct effects, may exacerbate the effect of chronic hepatitis. For example, the population attributable risk percentages were 21% for diabetes, 10% for early adulthood obesity and 11% for the combination. So, 42% of cases of hepatocellular cancer could be explained by obesity and diabetes.

In 2010 the American Diabetes Association and the American Cancer Society concluded that T2DM was convincingly associated with increased risk of cancers such as colorectal, pancreas, liver, breast, endometrial and bladder cancer [243]. Tsilidis et al. in their umbrella review confirmed the robust associations for some of these cancers but not for others [244].

The incidence of HCC has tripled in the USA in the last decades. Due to the falling incidence because of prevention and adequate treatment of viral hepatitis, the increase is consequent to the rising prevalence of obesity and T2DM, the two major risk factors for NAFLD.

Sex and ethnic-specific studies suggested that not adiposity in general but specific fat depots in viscera and liver might be more relevant. In the Multiethnic Cohort Study, overweight was associated with a 50% increased risk (HR 1.50 (1.16/1.95)) and obesity with a 82% increased risk (HR 1.82 (1.31/2.52)) of HCC with an increased risk per 5 kg/m^2 increase in BMI of 1.26 (1.26 (1.12/1.42)) in males and no increased risks in women [245]. There were also ethnic differences with BMI $\geq$30 kg/m^2 and the increased risk per 5 kg/m^2 increase in BMI being strongly associated with HCC with the greatest risk in Japanese, followed by Latinos, whites and native Hawaiians but not in black men. Detailed adiposity measurements showed that Asians and Latinos were likely to accumulate more and blacks less fat in the abdominal visceral compartment, suggesting that studying the association between obesity and HCC should move beyond BMI and should use a measure for fat-specific depots. Similarly, the European Prospective Investigation into Cancer and Nutrition (EPIC) study showed that WHR had the strongest association with HCC and also that in multivariate analysis the association of BMI with HCC disappeared whereas that of WHR remained [246]. A Japanese study determined the visceral fat mass quantitatively by CT and found that visceral fat was an independent risk factor for (recurrent) HCC in patients with suspected NASH [247].

Pathophysiology of Obesity in Relation to NAFLD

The pathophysiology of non-alcoholic fatty liver disease has been discussed in a number of recent review articles and is summarised below [228, 248–251].

The fundamental derangement in NAFLD is insulin resistance. Insulin resistance is also the pathogenic denominator of the metabolic syndrome which includes type 2 diabetes mellitus, essential hypertension, hypertriglyceridaemia, low circulating levels of HDL cholesterol and (visceral) obesity (Table 1.1). Steatosis of the liver may therefore be considered the hepatic manifestation of the metabolic syndrome and is closely associated with diabetes, obesity and hyperlipidaemia. In healthy subjects insulin, secreted by the pancreas and entering the portal circulation, stimulates glycogen synthesis, lipogenesis and lipoprotein synthesis and suppresses gluconeogenesis and glycogenolysis. Insulin resistance may present as whole-body insulin resistance as shown by a 50% reduction in glucose disposal, but also at the tissue level of the hepatocyte, adipocyte and skeletal muscle. Hepatic insulin resistance is characterised by a reduced suppression of endogenous glucose production via gluconeogenesis and reduced VLDL secretion because of an altered apolipoprotein B synthesis, which normally exports lipids from the liver in a complex of apolipoprotein B, lipids and phospholipids. Insulin resistance in the adipocyte promotes lipolysis and increased free fatty acid flux to the liver, and in skeletal muscle it impairs glucose uptake and disposal. Hyperinsulinaemia is a consequence of target cells, such as liver, adipose tissue and skeletal muscle being resistant to normal concentrations of insulin. As insulin stimulates lipogenic enzymes and portal insulin levels are high, the de novo lipogenesis in the liver is increased, contributing to hepatic fat accumulation. Apart from the increased fatty acid influx from adipocyte lipolysis, the increased de novo lipogenesis and the impaired fatty acid hepatic efflux due to reduced synthesis of apolipoprotein B or reduced secretion of VLDL, excess free fatty acids that can be stored in the liver as triglycerides may come from a reduced hepatic fatty acid oxidation as a result of hyperinsulinaemia and from excess dietary consumption of fat or carbohydrates in the condition of excess caloric intake.

A study by Donelli et al. has demonstrated that in obese NAFLD patients 59% of triglycerides arose from non-esterified fatty acids, 26% from de novo lipogenesis and 15% from the diet [252]. Nielsen et al. found that in lean individuals 5% of the portal vein free fatty acids originated from visceral fat in contrast to a 20% in obese patients [253]. Free fatty acids and their metabolites are highly toxic to the liver and in this way the storage of fatty acids in triglycerides as lipid droplets in the liver has a protective role. Simple steatosis patients with non-alcoholic fatty liver (NAFL) thus may be considered as good fat storers [228]. However, when excessive fatty acids cannot be converted into triglycerides and when excessive fatty acids overload the mitochondrial capacity for fatty acid oxidation, good fat storers may change into bad fat storers [228].

Progression of NAFLD to NASH is assumed to occur by two or multiple hits. Some, however, do not support the continuum of NAFLD → NASH→ advanced fibrosis → cirrhosis, but consider NAFL and NASH as discrete entities rather than two points on a spectrum, supported by the fact that progression from pure fatty liver to NASH is very rare [228]. The two-hit hypothesis in the progression of NAFLD put forward by Day and James in 1998 has been replaced by the multiple-hit model [228]. The first hit consists of insulin resistance with a resultant hyperinsulinaemia causing an impaired inhibition of adipose tissue lipolysis, an increased efflux of free fatty acids from the adipose tissue to the liver and increased hepatic de novo lipogenesis resulting in a simple fatty liver. Due to the hepatic fat infiltration, the liver may become vulnerable to a series of hits. These hits consist of oxidative injury and stress from reactive oxygen species (ROS), leading to lipid peroxidation, impaired mitochondrial and peroxisome oxidation of fatty acids, endoplasmatic reticulum stress, dysregulated hepatic apoptosis and activation of profibrinogenic cytokines and of hepatic stellate cells, all together resulting in inflammation (steatohepatitis) and fibrosis. Also, the release of adipokines, cytokines and chemokines plays a role: adipokines such as leptin, adiponectin and resistin; acylation-stimulating protein; TNF-α; and IL-6 are associated with insulin resistance and IL

1, TGF-β, VEGF, angiotensinogen and angiotensin II are inflammatory mediators (Figs. 1.3 and 1.4). Furthermore, low levels of adiponectin may predispose patients to the progressive form of NAFLD or NASH. Adiponectin is produced by omental fat and levels are low in diabetes and metabolic syndrome.

A high-calorie diet, excess (saturated) fats, refined carbohydrates, sugar-sweetened beverages, a high fructose intake and a Western diet have all been associated with weight gain and obesity, and more recently with NAFLD [220, 221]. Apart from the role of the diet as a source of excess energy and excess fat, the role of carbohydrates and especially simple carbohydrates such as fructose, sucrose, glucose and high-fructose corn syrup (HFCS) should be discussed. Carbohydrates can stimulate lipogenesis via carbohydrate response element-binding proteins, converting excess glucose to fatty acids. Fructose, present in HFCS, fruit juices and sucrose (glucose:fructose 1:1), has attracted much attention especially in the USA, where fat was substituted by carbohydrates during the low-fat lobby and sweetened soda contained fair amounts of HFCS. In the USA, HFCS is the most common consumed sugar.

Several properties make fructose a particularly lipogenic carbohydrate [254]. The liver is exposed to much higher fructose concentrations as compared to other tissues because fructose is absorbed from the intestine and delivered to the liver via the portal vein. In contrast, long-chain fatty acids are absorbed from the intestine as chylomicron particles and enter the systemic circulation via the lymphatic system and the thoracic duct and thus expose liver and peripheral tissue to a similar degree. Furthermore, fructose absorption and metabolism are insulin independent in contrast to glucose absorption. After absorption, carbohydrates are metabolised to acetyl CoA and activate lipogenic transcriptional factors in the liver stimulating every step in the de-novo lipogenesis that converts acetyl CoA into triglycerides [254]. Fructose phosphorylation into fructose-1-phosphate requires ATP, thereby decreasing ATP levels. Decreased ATP levels in the liver may also be the result of decreased mitochondrial ATP production because of the inhibition of β-oxidation by malonyl CoA. The depletion of ATP leads to uric acid production which may promote lipogenesis through the generation of mitochondrial oxidative stress. The suppression of mitochondrial lipid oxidation results in increased production of reactive oxygen species which augment steatosis through insulin-independent pathways [254]. Fructose increases protein levels of enzymes involved in de-novo lipogenesis during its conversion into triglycerides. Fructose promotes stress in the endoplasmatic reticulum resulting in upregulation of de-novo lipogenesis. So, in summary, fructose supports lipogenesis in the presence of insulin resistance and contributes further to insulin resistance.

Fructose has also been implicated in the progression to fibrosis. The major risk factor for development of NAFLD is excess calorie intake mainly derived from high-fat foods and increased intake of sugar-sweetened beverages [220, 221]. Overconsumption of refined sugar is a risk factor for the development of obesity, diabetes and NAFLD and in countries with high intakes of HFCS diabetes is 20% higher compared to countries that do not use HFCS. Chung et al. performed a meta-analysis of 21 intervention studies on the effects of sucrose, fructose, HFCS and glucose on NAFLD [255]. They found a low level of evidence that a hypercaloric fructose diet (supplemented by pure fructose) increased liver fat and AST in healthy men when compared with the consumption of a weight-maintenance diet. In addition, hypercaloric fructose and glucose had similar effect on liver fat and liver enzymes in healthy adults. There was insufficient evidence to draw a conclusion on the effects of HFCS or sucrose on NAFLD. The apparent association between indexes of liver health and fructose of sucrose intake appeared to be confounded by excessive energy intake and they concluded that the available evidence is not sufficiently robust to draw conclusions regarding the effect of fructose, HFCS or sucrose consumption on NAFLD [221, 255].

The importance of the location of the ectopic fat, i.e. liver versus visceral fat, was demonstrated in a study that used sophisticated methods for total fat and visceral adipose tissue (VAT) measurements (by dual-energy X-ray absorptiometry (DEXA) and MRI), intrahepatic triglyceride content (IHTG by proton magnetic resonance spectroscopy) and kinetic studies (hyperinsulinaemic euglycaemic clamp and VLDL-triglyceride kinetic studies) [256]. Subjects matched for VAT were dissimilar in IHTG, and subjects matched for IHTG differed in VAT. Subjects with higher IHTG content and matched on VAT had 41%, 13% and 36% lower insulin sensitivity in liver, adipose tissue and muscle, respectively, whereas VLDL-triglyceride secretion from mainly non-systemic fatty acids was almost double. Patients with high IHTG had twofold greater insulin and 50% lower adiponectin levels. No differences were found in insulin sensitivity and VLDL secretion when subjects with different VAT masses but matched for IHTG levels were examined. So, the relationship between VAT and metabolic disease is because of the relationship between VAT and IHTG and therefore the level of intrahepatic triglycerides is a better marker of metabolic derangements than visceral adiposity.

Pathophysiology of Obesity in Relation to Hepatocellular Carcinoma

Many studies have supported a key role of obesity in the risk of hepatocellular carcinoma and accumulating evidence exists that type 2 diabetes mellitus (T2DM) predisposes to a number of cancers [243, 244]. As mentioned above, both obesity and diabetes may contribute to NAFLD and the contribution of NAFLD to the prevalence of HCC has been reported repeatedly. Moreover, inactivity and excess food intake link obesity and NAFLD.

There are both systemic and local factors that contribute to the HCC risk and that may explain the association of obesity, T2DM and metabolic syndrome with HCC and the predominant presence of HCC in males [251]. *Systemic* factors contributing to the HCC risk are hyperinsulinaemia, obesity-related hypoxia, systemic inflammation, systemic effects of cytokines and adipokines, systemic immune dysregulation and systemic effects of the microbiome. High levels of insulin promote cell survival and cell proliferation and the binding of insulin at the insulin receptor activates mitogenic and anti-apoptotic pathways intracellularly. Insulin also suppresses the production of insulin-like growth factor-1-binding proteins which cannot bind sufficiently IGF-1 and cannot inhibit its mitogenic, anti-apoptotic and proangiogenic action [251].

Hypoxia of adipose tissue contributes to insulin resistance and to elevated pro-inflammatory adipokines and cytokines, increased levels of leptin involved in initiation and progression of HCC, and decreased levels of adiponectin that delays hepatocarcinogenesis and antagonises the oncogenic effect of leptin. Also macrophages accumulating in adipose tissue secrete inflammatory cytokines such as TNF-α, IL 6, IL-1β, nitric oxide, leukotrienes and chemokines that attract fibroblasts and other inflammatory cells. Persistent inflammation and persistent reactive oxygen species generation promote DNA damage and HCC [251].

Local factors in the liver contributing to the HCC risk are similar as described in adipose tissue and similar to the progression of NASH with liver cell damage, inflammatory infiltrates, pro-inflammatory signalling and insulin resistance, generation of reactive oxygen species that interfere with endoplasmatic reticulum and mitochondrial function, and release of TNF-α and IL-6, which promote proliferation and malignant progression [251].

1.8.4.3 Implications for Clinical Practice

In NAFLD/NASH, strategies should point to metabolic conditions such as obesity, diabetes and metabolic syndrome that favour progressive fibrosis. However, prevention is the key and advices to change the food consumption and increase physical exercise should be given to all patients. Related to potential mechanisms of hepatotoxicity are foods high in energy density with large portion sizes, high in fat and saturated fat, high in refined carbohydrate, high-fructose corn syrup (HFCS) and caramel colouring (cola soft drinks rich in advanced glycation end products that can promote insulin resistance and inflammation), low in fibre, low in antioxidants, high in red meat, high in industrially produced trans fatty acids, and promoting free fatty acid overload in the liver and local inflammation [220, 221, 223, 249, 251, 257–259].

Advices derived from this knowledge are a reduced calorie diet, reduction in saturated fatty acids along with an increase in MUFA and ω-3 PUFA, consumption of low glycaemic index carbohydrates, a reduced consumption of simple sugars especially in sweetened beverages, a higher intake of fruit and vegetables and a higher intake of fibre. Also adherence to a Mediterranean diet may be useful but scientific evidence to recommend specific diets is currently lacking [251, 257, 258].

Regular exercise reduces the risk of T2DM, insulin resistance, hypertension, dyslipidaemia, impaired fasting glucose and metabolic syndrome, all of which are factors involved in the pathogenesis of NAFLD. Exercise also has immunostimulatory effects, reduces systemic inflammation and decreases the activity of the mTOR system, thereby reducing HCC risk. Physical activity should be at least 30 min of moderate-intensity physical activity on most, and preferably all days of the week, or vigorous-intensity physical activity ≥ 3 times a week for ≥ 20 min each time.

What is the evidence for these lifestyle interventions by diet and physical exercise and how much weight should be lost? Promrat et al. randomised 21 patients with NASH to an intervention group which received a diet between 1000 and 1500 kcal/day with 25% of total energy from fat and ten patients to the control group, which received basal nutrition education [260]. The goal was a 7–10% weight reduction and the primary endpoint was improvement in NAFLD activity score (NAS) after 48 weeks. The intervention group lost 9.3% of total bodyweight versus 0.2% in the control arm with a significantly higher proportion of histological improvement in 72% versus 30%, respectively. Those with ≥7% weight loss showed improvements in steatosis, lobular inflammation and NAFLD activity score, but a weight loss of at least 10% was required to improve fibrosis and portal hypertension. Evidence for the substantial effects of moderate weight losses followed in larger studies. Villar-Gomez et al. evaluated 293 patients with biopsy-proven NASH after 52 weeks of lifestyle intervention consisting of a low-fat calorie-reduced diet (750 kcal less per day) and walking 200 min/week [261]. Paired biopsies were present in 261 patients. Among the entire cohort a weight loss was obtained of 4.6 kg, NASH resolution occurred in 25%, NAS reduction in 47% and fibrosis regression in 19%. The degree of weight loss was independently associated with improvements in all NASH-related histology features. Those who obtained a weight loss ≥5% (30% of subjects) had NASH resolution in 58%, a 2-point reduction in NAS score in 82%. Of those who achieved a ≥10% weight reduction (11% of subjects), 90% experienced a resolution of NASH and 100% a reduction in NASH and 45% a regression of fibrosis. Harrison et al. had similar findings: a ≥5% weight loss resulted in a significant improvement of insulin sensitivity and steatosis and those with a ≥9% weight loss improved in steatosis, inflammation and hepatocyte ballooning and NAS [262].

So all studies agreed that a minimum of 9–10% weight loss is needed to achieve NASH improvement and fibrosis regression.

Keating et al. reviewed 16 studies on exercise in a meta-analysis [263]. There was a significant pooled effect size for the comparison between exercise therapy and controls, even in the absence of significant weight loss. A recent systematic review of 23 studies on lifestyle interventions showed that diet or physical activity consistently reduced liver fat and improved glucose control and insulin sensitivity [264].

Important in this context is the rate of weight loss. Weight loss should be moderate and gradual (<1.6 kg/week) as a rapid reduction in body weight may decrease hepatic fat content but can induce hepatic inflammation and exacerbate NASH and thus worsening of liver disease. Ketosis may be deleterious for patients with NAFLD. Data on the upper limit of weight loss came from a study by Andersen et al. who provided a 400 kcal formula diet to 41 morbidly obese subjects [265]. They showed improvement of steatosis and improvement in liver biochemistry but 24% developed slight portal inflammation and portal fibrosis but none of the patients who lost less than 1.6 kg/week developed fibrosis.

Another important point for clinical practice is the recognition that all components of the metabolic syndrome correlate with liver fat content, independently of BMI. So, the presence of the metabolic syndrome in any given patient should lead to an evaluation of the risk of NAFLD, and vice versa the presence of NAFLD should lead to an assessment of all components of the metabolic syndrome [220]. Patients with steatosis or steatosis with non-specific inflammation are on the one end of the spectrum and are not candidates for pharmacological treatment that specifically targets the liver condition [230]. On the other end are patients with the progressive form of NAFLD (i.e. NASH), particularly when associated with advanced fibrosis. At-risk patients (age > 50 years, type 2 diabetes mellitus or metabolic syndrome) should be identified because of its prognostic implications. Treatment for the prevention of liver-related comorbidities should be focused on patients with NASH and particularly those with a fibrosis stage ≥2 [220]. For the many therapeutic options and the many medications in phase II and III studies the reader is referred to superb and very recent overviews and meta-analysis [223, 230, 249, 259, 266, 267] and the two recent guidelines from the USA in 2012 [220] and from Europe in 2016 [221].

1.8.5 Gastrointestinal Cancers

Mechanisms explaining the association between obesity and gastrointestinal cancers include hormonal effects of adipose tissue, insulin resistance, inflammation, effects on predisposing conditions such as GORD, Barrett's oesophagus, gallbladder disease, colorectal adenomas and effects through the immune system [48]. In obesity, endogenous hormones such as sex steroids, insulin and IGF-1 are increased and are important in the control of growth, differentiation and metabolism of cells [268]. Patients with diabetes type 2, which often accompanies overweight and obesity, have increased rates of cancer [243, 244]. Obesity is a state of low-grade chronic systemic inflammation characterised by pro-inflammatory cytokines produced by adipocytes and chronic inflammation is an important factor in the initiation and promotion of cancer cells. Obesity is also associated with enhanced oxidative stress by local ischaemia and through the inflammatory process. The World Cancer Research Fund and the American Institute for Cancer Research estimated in 2007 that a large percentage of cancers are attributable to obesity: 28% of gallbladder cancers, 35% of pancreatic, 16% of colorectal, 17% of breast and 49% of endometrial cancers, and 28% of kidney and 35% of oesophageal cancers [269]. Calle et al. estimated that in the USA obesity is responsible for up to 14% and 20% of all cancer deaths in males and females, respectively, signifying that 90,000 annual deaths are avoidable if BMI was kept below 25 [8]. In Europe, it is estimated that 36,000 cancer cases could be avoided by halving the prevalence of overweight and obesity [270].

Several large cohort studies and meta-analyses have examined cancer incidence and cancer mortality for all obesity-related cancers.

1.8.5.1 Cohort Studies

A large cohort study by Calle et al. followed more than 900,000 US adults free of cancer at enrolment in 1982 in the Cancer Prevention Study II, with an average age at that time of 57 years, over 16 years [8]. Death due to cancer was related to the BMI measured between 1982 and 1988. Of the 900,053 included persons 57,145 died (6.3%) of whom 16,962 (30%, one-third) being non-smokers. A BMI above the reference BMI (18.5–24.9 kg/m^2) was associated with cancer of the oesophagus, colon and rectum, liver, gallbladder, pancreas and kidney; the same was true for death due to non-Hodgkin's lymphoma and multiple myeloma. Significant trends for an association with higher BMI were present for gastric and prostate cancer in men and breast, uterus, cervix and ovary cancer in women. An inverse association was observed between BMI and lung cancer in male and females.

The highest relative death rate was for uterine cancer in females with a BMI $\geq$40 kg/m^2 with a RR 6.25; in males the highest relative death rate was for liver cancer (RR 4.52). There was, however, no clear documentation of presence or absence of liver disease in affected individuals. Also, no information about impaired glucose tolerance or NAFLD was present. At a BMI $\geq$40 kg/m^2 the cancer death rates were 52% higher in men and 62% higher in women when compared with normal-weight subjects and went even up to 88% in non-smoking women with a BMI $\geq$40 kg/m^2. The risks according to the BMI classes for gastrointestinal cancer are visible in Table 1.7 and in Fig. 1.6 for males and Fig. 1.7 for females. The population attributable fraction of death of all cancers varied between 4.2% in the population of men and 14.2% among male non-smokers and in women between 14.3% and 19.8%. So the avoidable proportion of cancers was as high as 14% for males and 20% for females, signifying that 90,000 cancer deaths could have been avoided when BMI had remained 25.0 throughout life [8].

The critics concerning this landmark study touched upon the fact that comparison was made with weight 16 years ago and the people could have gained 1–2 units BMI over the 16-year period of the study and 10% of people have an increased BMI by 5 units over less than 10 years. This was addressed in the Northern Sweden Health and Disease Cohort (1985–2003) which consisted of 35,362 women and 33,424 men with weights and heights measured and repeated at 10-year intervals [271]. After 10 years of follow-up >70% preserved their initial BMI classification in the quartiles; on average women gained about 1.8 BMI units and men about 1.4 BMI units and the annual increase in BMI was 0.1 BMI units among men and 0.06 BMI units among women. Obese women had a 36% higher cancer incidence than normal-weight women while overweight women had a risk largely similar to that of normal-weight women [271]. Obese women had a 2.0 times higher risk of colorectal cancer and 2.25 times higher risk of colon cancer. In men there was no association of BMI with total cancer risk. Obese men were 1.77 times at risk of developing colon cancer. In women up to 7% of cancer were attributable to overweight and obesity, with a larger attribution on endometrium (30%), ovarian (22%), colon (20%) and colorectal (16%) which could have been avoided by keeping BMI in the normal range [271].

A cohort study by Reeves et al. and a meta-analysis by Reneman et al. investigated the effect of an increase in BMI by 5 or 10 BMI units [102, 272]. Reeves et al. investigated 1.2 million women in the Million Women breast cancer screening study, with an age of 55.9 years at recruitment and recruited over the years 1996–2001 [102]. The reference BMI group had a BMI 22.5–24.9 kg/m^2 and the trend in risk per 10 units BMI was taken as this was equivalent to the difference in median

Table 1.7 Relative risks (with 95% confidence intervals in brackets) for cancer death according to BMI classes of overweight (BMI 25–29.9), class I (BMI 30–34.9), class II (BMI 35–39.9) and class III of obesity (BMI ≥40 kg/m²) [8]

	BMI 25–29.9	BMI 30–34.9	BMI 35–39.9	BMI ≥40	*p* for trend
Males *N* = 404,576					
All cancers	0.97 (0.94/0.99)	1.09 (1.05/1.14)	1.23 (1.11/1.34)	1.52 (1.13/2.05)	0.001
Oesophagus	1.15 (0.99/1.32)	1.28 (1.00/1.63)	1.63 (0.95/2.80)		0.008
Stomach	1.01 (0.88/1.16)	1.20 (0.94/1.52)	1.94 (1.21/3.13)		0.03
Colorectal	1.20 (1.12/1.30)	1.47 (1.30/1.66)	1.84 (1.39/2.41)		<0.001
Liver	1.13 (0.94/1.34)	1.90 (1.46/2.47)	4.52 (2.94/6.54)		<0.001
Gallbladder	1.34 (0.97/1.84)	1.76 (1.06/2.94)			0.02
Pancreas	1.13 (1.03/1.25)	1.41 (1.19/1.66)	1.49 (0.99/2.22)		<0.001
Non-smoking males *N* = 107,030					
All cancers	1.11 (1.05/1.18)	1.38 (1.24/1.52)	1.31 (1.01/1.70)		<0.001
Oesophagus	1.76 (1.08/2.86)	1.91 (0.92/3.96)			0.04
Pancreas	1.24 (1.01/1.54)	1.34 (0.92/1.95)	2.61 (1.27/5.35)		0.005
Females *N* = 495,477					
All cancers	1.08 (1.05/1.11)	1.23 (1.18/1.29)	1.32 (1.20/1.44)	1.62 (1.40/1.87)	<0.001
Oesophagus	1.20 (0.86/1.66)	1.39 (0.86/2.25)			NS
Stomach	0.89 (0.72/1.09)	1.30 (0.97/1.74)	1.08 (0.61/1.89)		NS
Colorectal	1.10 (1.01/1.19)	1.33 (1.17/1.51)	1.36 (1.06/1.74)	1.46 (0.94/2.24)	<0.001
Liver	1.02 (0.80/1.31)	1.40 (0.97/2.00)	1.68 (0.93/3.05)		0.04
Gallbladder	1.12 (0.86/1.47)	2.13 (1.56/2.90)			<0.001
Pancreas	1.11 (1.00/1.24)	1.28 (1.07/1.52)	1.41 (1.01/1.99)	2.76 (1.74/4.36)	<0.001
Non-smoking females *N* = 276,564					
All cancers	1.14 (1.09/1.18)	1.33 (1.25/1.41)	1.40 (1.25/1.58)	1.88 (1.56/2.27)	<0.001
Oesophagus	1.49 (0.85/2.59)	2.64 (1.36/5.12)			0.004

BMI among obese women and the reference category. They found that an increased BMI was associated with increased risk of cancer for 10 of the 17 examined cancer types. More specifically, the risk of adenocarcinoma of the oesophagus was 2.38 times higher per 10 kg/m² increase in BMI, followed by CRC in premenopausal women (1.61 (1.05/2.48)) and pancreatic cancer (1.24 (1.03/1.48)) (Table 1.8). Postmenopausal women were not at increased risk (0.99 (0.88/1.12)), a finding strengthened by findings by Terry et al. who also showed different risks in premenopausal obese (RR 1.88 (1.24/2.86)) and postmenopausal obese (0.73 (0.48/1.10)) women [194, 197].

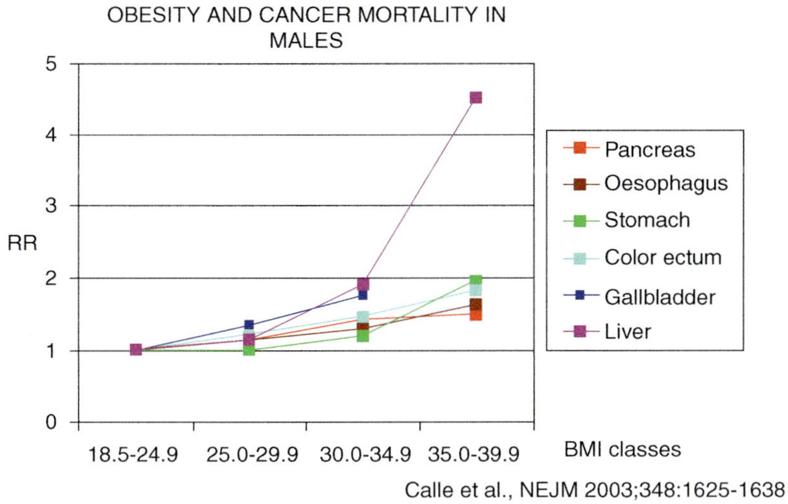

Fig. 1.6 The risks according to the BMI classes for gastrointestinal cancer for males

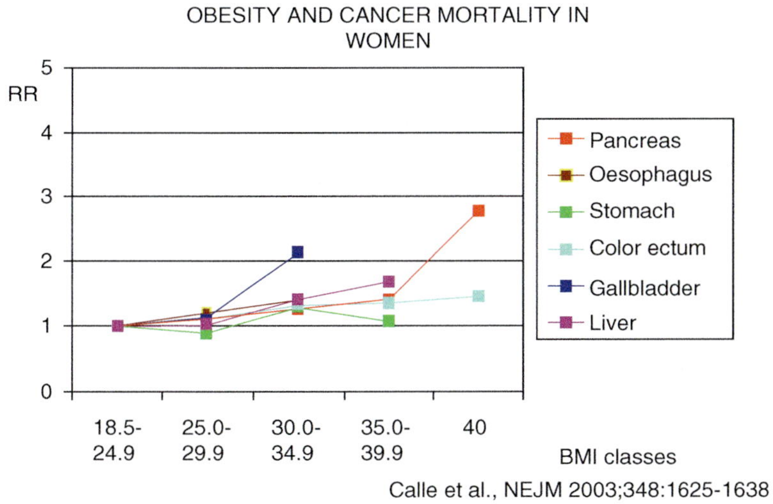

Fig. 1.7 The risks according to the BMI classes for gastrointestinal cancer for females

1.8.5.2 Meta-Analyses

Bergstrom et al. examined the prevalence of six cancer sites (colon, endometrium, prostate, kidney, gallbladder and postmenopausal breast cancer) and the proportion of these six cancers attributable to overweight (BMI 25–29.9 kg/m^2) and obesity (BMI $\geq$30 kg/m^2) in the European union [270]. Overweight (BMI >25 kg/m^2) was slightly more prevalent in southern countries (61% for men and 52% for women) compared with the northern countries (59% for men and 47% for women). Obesity was more prevalent in women and overweight more in men. Excess body weight

Table 1.8 Relative risk (with 95% confidence interval) associated with a 5 kg/m² increase in BMI or a 10 kg/m² increase in BMI in the Million Women Cohort Study [102, 272]

Cancer type	RR per 5 kg/m² males	*p*-Value	RR per 5 kg/m² females	*p*-Value	RR per 10 kg/m² females
Oesophagus adenocarcinoma	1.52 (1.33/1.74)	<0.001	1.51 (1.31/1.74)	<0.001	2.38 (1.59/3.56)
Colon cancer	1.24 (1.20/1.28)	<0.001	1.09 (1.05/1.13)	<0.001	1.00 (0.92/1.08)
Liver cancer	1.24 (0.95/1.62)	NS	1.07 (0.55/2.08)	NS	
Rectum cancer	1.09 (1.06/1.12)	<0.001	1.02 (1.00/1.05)	NS	1.00 (0.92/1.08)
Gallbladder cancer	1.09 (0.99/1.21)	NS	1.59 (1.02/2.47)	0.04	
Pancreas cancer	1.07 (0.93/1.23)	NS	1.12 (1.02/1.22)	0.01	1.24 (1.03/1.48)
Stomach cancer	0.97 (0.88/1.06)	NS	1.04 (0.90/1.20))	NS	0.90 (0.72/1.13)
Oesophagus squamous cell cancer	0.71 (0.60/0.85)	<0.001	0.57 (0.47/0.69)	<0.001	0.26 (0.18/0.38)
All cancers					1.12 (1.09/1.14)

accounted for 5% of all cancers in Europe, 3% for men and 6% for women, corresponding to 27,000 cases in males and 45,000 cases in females. So, more than 70,000 of the 3.5 million new cases of cancer each year in the European union are attributable to overweight (34,800 cases) and to obesity (37,000). This is likely to be an underestimation as only six cancers, for which there is existing evidence to suggest a link between obesity and cancer, were examined in Bergstrom's study. The attributable proportion varied by gender and country: for males the attributable proportion varied between 2.1% for Greece and 4.9% for Germany, and for women between 3.9% for Denmark and 8.8% for Spain.

Of the 19 studies related to colon cancer six were used in the meta-analysis. Per unit increase in BMI the risk increased by 3% (RR 1.03 (1.02/1.04)). Overweight attributed to a 15% increase and obesity to a 33% increase in risk. The average proportion attributable to excess body weight was 11% with a number of 11,000 new cases per year. For gallbladder cancer, six epidemiological studies were found with conflicting data. Only two studies could be used and assessed a risk of 1.06 (1.00/1.12)) per unit BMI increase. Overweight attributed to a 34% and obesity to a 78% increase in risk. Twenty-four percent of gallbladder cancers could be attributed to excess body weight amounting to 6000 new cases/year. The highest attributable proportions were found for endometrium (39%), kidney (25% in both sexes) and gallbladder (25% in men and 24% in women). More important is the absolute number of cases and then the highest attributable number of cases were attributable to colon cancer (21,500 annual cases) followed by endometrium (14,000 cases) and breast (12,800). In Europe, an estimated 36,000 cases could have been avoided by halving the prevalence of overweight and obesity.

In a meta-analysis of 221 data sets by Reneman et al., the incidence of 20 most common cancers were studied per 5 unit increase in BMI, corresponding to a 15 kg weight gain in males and 13 kg in females with an average BMI at baseline of 23 kg/m² [272] (Table 1.8). In men, a 5-point increase in BMI was strongly associated with an increased risk of oesophageal adenocarcinoma and colon cancer, and in women with gallbladder and oesophageal adenocarcinoma. Weaker positive associations (RR < 1.20) were discovered between increased BMI and rectal cancer in men and pancreas and colon cancer in women. The associations for colon cancer were stronger in men than in women. The associations did not differ in studies from Europe, North America and Australia and the Asia Pacific group.

Guh et al. considered overweight and obesity not only as defined by BMI criteria, but also as defined by waist circumference in their meta-analysis [37]. As can be seen in Table 1.2, relative risks in men were higher for colorectal cancer and gallbladder cancer when overweight waist and obese waist were compared by their respective BMIs. For women this was not the case as far as colorectal cancer was concerned.

1.8.5.3 Implications for Clinical Practice

It is evident that keeping the body weight at a level below BMI 25 kg/m^2 can reduce substantially the burden of cancer and also that weight stability, even when it is in the overweight range, is preferable over weight gain. An at least 50% greater risk was only observed in people with a BMI ≥35 kg/m^2. In males with a BMI 30–34.9 kg/m^2 the RR for cancer death was greater than 50% in liver, gallbladder and non-Hodgkin's lymphoma; in women this was true for cancer of the gallbladder, breast, uterus and kidneys. Evidence for a reduction in cancer risk by attempts of weight loss by lifestyle measures is lacking. The only available evidence in a prospective, controlled trial comes from the Swedish Obesity Subjects (SOS) study [273]. The SOS study involved 2010 obese subjects who underwent gastric bypass in 13%, gastric banding in 19% and vertical banded gastroplasty in 68%. They were compared with 2037 contemporaneously matched obese controls who received usual care. Over 10 years there was a significantly different mean weight reduction of 19.9 kg in the bariatric group versus a weight gain of 1.3 kg in controls. The risk of incident cancers was reduced by 33% in the whole group (HR 0.67 (0.53/0.85)) but there was clearly a gender-treatment interaction: in women the incidence was significantly lower (HR 0.58 (0.44/0.77)) but there was no effect of surgery in men. With respect to the above-mentioned attributable fractions by overweight and obesity and the impressive reduction when excess weight was halved or wiped out, the adage remains: prevention is the key!

References

1. NCD (Non-Communicable Disease) Risk Factor Collaboration (NCD-RisC). Trends in adult body-mass index in 200 countries from 1975 to 2014: a pooled analysis of 1698 population-based measurement studies with 19·2 million participants. Lancet. 2016;387:1377–96.
2. WHO: fact sheetno.311; updated June 2016. www.who.int/mediacentre/factsheets/fs311/en/. Accessed May 2017.
3. WHO: fact sheet no 311; updated June 2016. www.who.int/dg/speeches/2016/obesity-diabetes-disaster/en/. Accessed May 2017.

4. Frühbeck G, Toplak H, Woodward E, Yumuk V, Maislos M, Oppert J-M. Obesity: the gateway to ill health—an EASO position statement on a rising public health, clinical and scientific challenge in Europe. Obes Facts. 2013;6:117–20.
5. Fried M, Yumuk V, Oppert J-M, Scopinaro N, Torres AJ, Weiner R, et al. Interdisciplinary European guidelines on metabolic and bariatric surgery. Obes Facts. 2013;6:449–68.
6. Aune D, Sen A, Prasad M, Norat T, Janszky I, Tonstad S, et al. BMI and all cause mortality: systematic review and non-linear dose-response meta-analysis of 230 cohort studies with 3.74 million deaths among 30.3 million participants. BMJ. 2016;353:i2156.
7. NCD (Non-Communicable Disease) Risk Factor Collaboration (NCD-RisC). Worldwide trends in diabetes since 1980: a pooled analysis of 751 population-based studies with 4·4 million participants. Lancet. 2016;387:1513–30.
8. Calle EE, Rodriguez C, Walker-Thurmond K, Thun MJ. Overweight, obesity, and mortality from cancer in a prospectively studied cohort of U.S. adults. N Engl J Med. 2003;348:1625–38.
9. Mathus-Vliegen EMH, Romijn JA, Belachew M, Greve JW. Morbid obesity. Gastrointestinal aspects/surgical aspects. In: van Lanschot JJB, Gouma DJ, Jansen PLM, Jones EA, Pinedo HM, Schouten WR, et al. (eds). Integrated medical and surgical gastroenterology. Houten, The Netherlands; Bohn Stafleu Van Loghum, 2004: 124-145.
10. WHO Expert Consultation. Appropriate body-mass index for Asian populations and its implications for policy and intervention strategies. Lancet. 2004;363:157–63.
11. Chandalia M, Lin P, Seenivasan T, Livingston EH, Snell PG, Grundy SM, Abate N. Insulin resistance and body fat distribution in south Asian men compared to Caucasian men. PLoS One. 2007;2:e812.
12. Chitturi S, Farrell GC, Hashimoto E, Saibara T, Lau GKK, Sollano JD, et al. Non-alcoholic fatty liver disease in the Asia–Pacific region: definitions and overview of proposed guidelines. J Gastroenterol Hepatol. 2007;22:778–87.
13. Alberti KG, Zimmet P, Shaw J. Metabolic syndrome—a new worldwide definition. A consensus statement from the international diabetes federation. Diabet Med. 2006;23:469–80.
14. Tan C-E, Ma S, Wai D, Chew S-K, Tai E-S. Can we apply the National Cholesterol Education Program Adult Treatment Panel definition of the metabolic syndrome to Asians? Diabetes Care. 2004;27:1182–6.
15. Heymsfield SB, Cefalu WT. Does body mass index adequately convey a patient's mortality risk? JAMA. 2013;309:87–8.
16. Wildman RP, Muntner P, Reynolds K, McGinn AP, Rajpathak S, Wylie-Rosett J, et al. The obese without cardiometabolic risk factor clustering and the normal weight with cardiometabolic risk factor clustering. Arch Intern Med. 2008;168:1617–24.
17. Kramer CK, Zinman B, Retnakaran R. Are metabolically healthy overweight and obesity benign conditions? Ann Intern Med. 2013;159:758–69.
18. Hill JO, Wyatt HR. The myth of healthy obesity. Ann Intern Med. 2013;159:789–90.
19. Ferrannini E, Natali A, Bell P, Cavallo-Perin P, Lalic N, Mingrone G. Insulin resistance and hypersecretion in obesity. J Clin Invest. 1997;100:1166–73.
20. Stefan N, Kantartzis K, Machann J, Schick F, Thamer C, Rittig K, et al. Identification and characterisation of metabolically benign obesity in humans. Arch Intern Med. 2008;168:1609–16.
21. Pischon T, Boeing H, Hoffmann K, Bergmann M, Schulze MB, Overvad K, et al. General and abdominal adiposity and risk of death in Europe. N Engl J Med. 2008;359:2105–20.
22. Virtanen KA, Lidell ME, Orava J, Heglind M, Westergren R, Tiemi T, et al. Functional brown adipose tissue in healthy adults. N Engl J Med. 2009;360:1518–25.
23. Blondin DP, Labbe SM, Tingelstad HC, Noll C, Kunach M, Phoenix S, et al. Increased brown adipose tissue oxidative capacity in cold-acclimated humans. J Clin Endocrinol Metab. 2014;99(3):E438–46.
24. Van der Lans AA, Hoeks J, Brans B, Vijgen GH, Visser MG, Vosselman MJ, et al. Cold acclimation recruits human brown fat and increases nonshivering thermogenesis. J Clin Investig. 2013;123:3395–403.
25. Juge-Aubry CE, Henrichot E, Meier CA. Adipose tissue a regulator of inflammation. Best Pract Res Clin Endocrinol Metab. 2005;19:547–66.

26. Wozniak SE, Gee LL, Wachtel MS, Frezza EE. Adipose tissue: the new endocrine organ? A review article. Dig Dis Sci. 2009;54:1847–56.
27. Flegal KM, Graubard BI, Williamson DF, Gail MH. Cause-specific excess deaths associated with underweight, overweight, and obesity. JAMA. 2007;298:2028–37.
28. Prospective Studies Collaboration. Body mass index and cause-specific mortality in 900 000 adults: collaborative analyses of 57 prospective studies. Lancet. 2009;373:1083–96.
29. Berrington de Gonzalez A, Hartge P, Cerhan JR, Flint AJ, Hannan L, MacInnis RJ, et al. Body-mass index and mortality among 1.46 million white adults. N Engl J Med. 2010; 363:2211–9.
30. Peeters A, Barendregt JJ, Willekens F, Mackenbach JP, Al Mamun A, Bonneux L. Obesity in adulthood and its consequences for life expectancy: a life-table analysis. Ann Intern Med. 2003;138:24–32.
31. Flegal K, Kit BK, Orpana H, Graubard BI. Association of all-cause mortality with overweight and obesity using standard body mass index categories. JAMA. 2013;309:71–82.
32. Adams KF, Schatzkin A, Harris TB, Kipnis V, Mouw T, Ballard-Barbash R, et al. Overweight, obesity, and mortality in a large prospective cohort of persons 50 to 71 years old. N Engl J Med. 2006;355:763–78.
33. Moayyedi P. The epidemiology of obesity and gastrointestinal and other disease: an overview. Dig Dis Sci. 2008;53:2293–9.
34. Oldhansky SJ, Passaro DJ, Hershow RC, Layden J, Carnes BA, Brody J, et al. A potential decline in life expectancy in the United Sates in the twenty-first century. N Engl J Med. 2005;352:1138–45.
35. Afzal S, Tybjaerg-Hansen A, Jensen GB, Nordestgaard BG. Change in body mass index associated with lowest mortality in Denmark, 1976–2013. JAMA. 2016;315:1989–96.
36. Akinussi ME, Pineda LA, El-Sohl AA. Effect of obesity on intensive care morbidity and mortality: a meta-analysis. Crit Care Med. 2008;36:151–8.
37. Guh DP, Zhang W, Bansback N, Amarsi Z, Birmingham L, Anis AH. The incidence of co-morbidities related to obesity and overweight: a systematic review and meta-analysis. BMC Public Health. 2006;9:88.
38. Delgado-Aros S, Locke GR III, Camilleri M, Talley NJ, Fett S, Zinsmeister AR, et al. Obesity is associated with increased risk of gastrointestinal symptoms: a population-based study. Am J Gastroenterol. 2004;99:1801–6.
39. Talley NJ, Howel S, Poulton R. Obesity and chronic gastrointestinal symptoms in young adults: a birth cohort study. Am J Gastroenterol. 2004;99:1807–14.
40. Talley NJ, Quan C, Jones MP, Horowitz M. Association of upper and lower gastrointestinal tract symptoms with body mass index in an Australian cohort. Neurogastroenterol Motil. 2004;16:413–9.
41. Levy RL, Linde JA, Feld KA, Crowell MD, Jeffery RW. The association of gastrointestinal symptoms with weight, diet, and exercise in weight-loss program participants. Clin Gastroenterol Hepatol. 2005;3:992–6.
42. Aro P, Ronkainen J, Talley NJ, Storskrubb T, Bolling-Sternevald E, Agreus L. Body mass index and chronic unexplained gastrointestinal symptoms: an adult endoscopic population based study. Gut. 2005;54:1377–83.
43. Dutta SK, Arora M, Kireet A, Bashandy H, Gandsas A. Upper gastrointestinal symptoms and associated disorders in morbidly obese patients: a prospective study. Dig Dis Sci. 2009;54:1243–6.
44. Carabotti M, Avallone M, Cereatti F, Paganini A, Greco F, Scirocco A, et al. Usefulness of upper gastrointestinal symptoms as a driver to prescribe gastroscopy in obese patients candidate to bariatric surgery. A prospective study. Obes Surg. 2016;26:1075–80.
45. El-Serag HB. Time trends of gastroesophageal reflux disease: a systematic review. Clin Gastroenterol Hepatol. 2007;5:17–26.
46. Jacobson BC, Somers SC, Fuchs CS, Kelly CP, Camargo CA Jr. Body-mass index and symptoms of gastroesophageal reflux in women. N Engl J Med. 2006;354:2340–8.
47. El-Serag H. Role of obesity in GORD-related disorders. Gut. 2008;57:281–4.

48. Ryan AM, Duong M, Healy L, Ryan SA, Parekh N, Reynolds JV, et al. Obesity, metabolic syndrome and esophageal adenocarcinoma: epidemiology, etiology and new targets. Cancer Epidemiol. 2011;356:309–19.
49. Derakhshan MH, Robertson EV, Fletcher J, Jones G-R, Lee YY, Wirz AA, et al. Mechanisms of association between BMI and dysfunction of the gastro-oesophageal barrier in patients with normal endoscopy. Gut. 2012;61:337–43.
50. Hirsch DP, Mathus-Vliegen EM, Holloway RH, Fakry N, D'Amato M, Boeckxstaens GE. Role of CCK(A) receptors in postprandial lower esophageal sphincter function in morbidly obese subjects. Dig Dis Sci. 2002;47:2531–7.
51. Hirsch DP, Mathus-Vliegen EM, Dagli U, Tytgat GN, Boeckxstaens GE. Effect of prolonged gastric distension on lower esophageal sphincter function and gastroesophageal reflux. Am J Gastroenterol. 2003;98:1696–704.
52. Lundell L, Ruth M, Sandbergh N, Bove-Nielsen M. Does massive obesity promote abnormal gastroesophageal reflux? Dig Dis Sci. 1995;40:1632–5.
53. Lagergren J, Bergström R, Nyren O. No relation between body mass and gastro-oesophageal reflux symptoms in a Swedish population based study. Gut. 2000;47:26–9.
54. Kjellin A, Ramel S, Rossner S, Thor K. Gastroesophageal reflux in obese patients is not reduced by weight loss. Scand J Gastroenterol. 1996;31:1047–51.
55. Lee YY, Wirz AA, Whiting JGH, Robertson EV, Smith D, Weir A, et al. Waist belt and central obesity cause partial hiatus hernia and short-segment acid reflux in asymptomatic volunteers. Gut. 2014;63:1053–60.
56. Anggiansah R, Sweis R, Anggiansah A, Wong T, Cooper D, Fox M. The effects of obesity on oesophageal function, acid exposure and the symptoms of gastro-oesophageal reflux disease. Aliment Pharmacol Ther. 2013;37:555–63.
57. Ze EY, Kim BJ, Kang H, Kim JG. Abdominal visceral to subcutaneous adipose tissue ratio is associated with increased risk of erosive esophagitis. Dig Dis Sci. 2017;62:1265–71.
58. Fisher BL, Pennathur A, Mutnick JLM, Little AG. Obesity correlates with gastroesophageal reflux. Dig Dis Sci. 1999;44:2290–4.
59. El-Serag HB, Ergun GA, Pandolfino J, Fitzgerald S, Tran T, Kramer JR. Obesity increases oesophageal acid exposure. Gut. 2007;56:749–55.
60. Ayazi S, Hagen JA, Chan LS, DeMeester SR, Lin MW, Ayazi A, et al. Obesity and gastroesophageal reflux: quantifying the association between body mass index, esophageal acid exposure, and lower esophageal sphincter status in a large series of patients with reflux symptoms. J Gastrointest Surg. 2009;13:1440–7.
61. Nilsson M, Lundegardh G, Carling L, Ye W, Lagergren J. Body mass and reflux oesophagitis: an oestrogen-dependent association? Scand J Gastroenterol. 2002;37:626–30.
62. Nilsson M, Johnsen R, Ye W, Hveem K, Lagergren J. Obesity and estrogen as risk factors for gastroesophageal reflux symptoms. JAMA. 2003;290:66–72.
63. Nocon M, Labenz J, Jaspersen D, Meyer-Sabellek W, Stolte M, Lind T, et al. Association of body mass index with heartburn, regurgitation and esophagitis: results of the progression of Gastroesophageal reflux disease study. J Gastroenterol Hepatol. 2007;22:1728–31.
64. Hampel H, Abraham NS, El-Serag HB. Meta-analysis: obesity and the risk for gastroesophageal reflux disease and its complications. Ann Intern Med. 2005;143:199–211.
65. Corley DA, Kubo A. Body mass index and gastroesophageal reflux disease: a systematic review and meta-analysis. Am J Gastroenterol. 2006;108:2619–28.
66. Corley DA, Kubo A, Zhao W. Abdominal obesity, ethnicity and gastro-oesophageal reflux symptoms. Gut. 2007;56:756–62.
67. Lee Y-C, Yen AM, Tai JJ, Chang SH, Lin JT, Chiu HM, et al. The effect of metabolic risk factors on the natural course of gastro-oesophageal reflux disease. Gut. 2009;58:174–81.
68. Kubo A, Cook MB, Shaheen NJ, Vaughan TL, Whiteman DC, Murray L, et al. Sex-specific associations between body mass index, waist circumference and the risk of Barrett's oesophagus: a pooled analysis from the international BEACON consortium. Gut. 2013;62:1684–91.

69. Stein DJ, El-Serag HB, Kuczynski J, Kramer JR, Sampliner RE. The association of body mass index with Barrett's esophagus. Aliment Pharmacol Ther. 2005;22:1005–10.
70. Corley DA, Kubo A, Levin TR, Block G, Habel L, Zhao W, et al. Abdominal obesity and body mass index as risk factors for Barrett's esophagus. Gastroenterology. 2007;133:34–41.
71. Jacobson BC, Chan AT, Giovannucci EL, Fuchs CS. Body mass index and Barrett's oesophagus in women. Gut. 2009;58:1460–6.
72. Smith KJ, O'Brien SM, Smithers BM, Gotley DC, Webb PM, Green AC, et al. Interaction among smoking, obesity, and symptoms of acid reflux in Barrett's esophagus. Cancer Epidemiol Prev. 2005;14:2481–6.
73. Ford ES, Li C, Zhao G, Tsai J. Trends in obesity and abdominal obesity among adults in the United States from 1999–2008. Int J Obes. 2012;7:e48528.
74. Cook MB, Greenwood DC, Hardie LJ, Wild CP, Forman D. A systematic review and meta-analysis of the risk of increasing adiposity on Barrett's esophagus. Am J Gastroenterol. 2008;103:292–300.
75. Abrams JA. Obesity and Barrett's oesophagus: more than just reflux. Gut. 2009;58:1437–8.
76. Pou KM, Massaro JM, Hoffmann U, Lieb K, Vasan RS, O'Donnell CJ, et al. Patterns of abdominal fat distribution: the Framingham heart study. Diabetes Care. 2009;32:481–5.
77. El-Serag HB, Graham DY, Satia JA, Rabeneck L. Obesity is an independent risk factor for GERD symptoms and erosive gastritis. Am J Gastroenterol. 2005;100:1243–50.
78. Akiyama T, Yoneda M, Imamori M, Iida H, Endo H, Hosono K, et al. Visceral obesity and the risk of Barrett's oesophagus in Japanese patients with non-alcoholic liver disease. BMC Gastroenterol. 2009;9:56.
79. El-Serag HB, Hashmi A, Garcia J, Richardson P, Alsarraj A, Fitzgerald S, et al. Visceral abdominal obesity measured by CT scan is associated with an increased risk of Barrett's oesophagus: a case-control study. Gut. 2014;63:220–9.
80. Rubenstein JH, Morgenstern H, Chey WD, Murray J, Scheiman JM, Schoenfeld P, et al. Protective role of gluteofemoral obesity in erosive oesophagitis and Barrett's oesophagus. Gut. 2014;63:230–5.
81. Ryan AM, Healy LA, Power DG, Byrne M, Murphy S, Byrne PJ, et al. Barrett oesophagus. Prevalence of central adiposity, metabolic syndrome, and a proinflammatory state. Ann Surg. 2008;247:909–15.
82. Francois F, Roper J, Goodman AJ, Pei Z, Ghumman M, Mourad M, et al. The association of gastric leptin with oesophageal inflammation and metaplasia. Gut. 2008;57:16–24.
83. Kendall BJ, Macdonald GA, Hayward NK, Prins JB, Brown I, Walker N, et al. Leptin and the risk of Barrett's oesophagus. Gut. 2008;57:448–54.
84. Tilg H, Kaser A. Adiponectin and JNK: metabolic inflammatory pathways affecting gastrointestinal carcinogenesis. Gut. 2009;58:1576–7.
85. Rubenstein JH, Kao JY, Madanick RD, Zhang M, Spacek MB, Donovan JL, et al. Association of adiponectin multimers with Barrett's oesophagus. Gut. 2009;58:1583–9.
86. Thompson OM, Beresford SAA, Kirk EA, Bronner MP, Vaughan TL. Serum leptin and adiponectin levels and risk of Barrett's esophagus and intestinal metaplasia of the gastroesophageal junction. Obesity. 2010;18:2204–11.
87. Hoyo C, Cook MB, Kamangar F, Freedman ND, Whiteman DC, Bernstein L, et al. Body mass index in relation to oesophageal and oesophagogastric junction adenocarcinomas: a pooled analysis from the International BEACON Consortium. Int J Epidemiol. 2012;41:1706–18.
88. Corley DA. Obesity and the rising incidence of oesophageal and gastric adenocarcinoma: what is the link? Gut. 2007;56:1493–4.
89. Lagergren J. Adenocarcinoma of oesophagus: what exactly is the size of the problem and who is at risk? Gut. 2005;54(Suppl I):i1–5.
90. Polednak AP. Estimating the number of US incident cancers attributable to obesity and the impact on temporal trends in incidence rates for obesity-related cancers. Cancer Detect Prev. 2008;32:190–9.

91. Freedman ND, Murray LJ, Kamangar F, Abnet CC, Cook MB, Nyren O, et al. Alcohol intake and risk of oesophageal adenocarcinoma: a pooled analysis from the BEACON consortium. Gut. 2011;60:1029–37.
92. O'Doherty MG, Freedman ND, Hollenbeck AR, Schatzkin A, Abnet CC. A prospective cohort study of obesity and risk of oesophageal and gastric adenocarcinoma in the NIH-AARP Diet and Health Study. Gut. 2012;61:1261–8.
93. Robertson EV, Derakhshan MH, Wirz AA, Lee YY, Seenan JP, Ballantyne SA, et al. Central obesity in asymptomatic volunteers is associated with increased intrasphincteric acid reflux and lengthening of the cardiac mucosa. Gastroenterology. 2013;145:730–9.
94. Martel de C, Haggerty TD, Corley DA, Vogelman JH, Orentreich N, Parsonnet J. Serum ghrelin levels and risk of subsequent adenocarcinoma of the esophagus. Am J Gastroenterol. 2007;102:1166–72.
95. Kubo A, Corley DA. Body mass index and adenocarcinomas of the esophagus or gastric cardia: a systematic review and meta-analysis. Cancer Epidemiol Biomark Prev. 2006;15:872–8.
96. Veugelers PJ, Porter GA, Guernsey DL, Casson AC. Obesity and lifestyle risk factors for gastroesophageal reflux disease, Barrett esophagus ad esophageal adenocarcinoma. Dis Esophagus. 2006;19:321–8.
97. Corley DA, Kubo A, Zhao W. Abdominal obesity and the risk of esophageal and gastric cardia carcinoma. Cancer Epidemiol Biomark Prev. 2008;17:352–8.
98. Abnet CC, Freedman ND, Hollenbeck AR, Fraumeni JF Jr, Leitzmann M, Schatzkin A. A prospective study of BMI and risk of oesophageal and gastric adenocarcinoma. Eur J Cancer. 2008;44:465–71.
99. Figueroa JD, Terry MB, Gammon MD, Vaughan TL, Risch HA, Zhang FF, et al. Cigarette smoking, body mass index, gastro-esophageal reflux disease and non-steroidal anti-inflammatory drug use and risk of subtypes of esophageal and gastric cancers by P53 expression. Cancer Causes Control. 2009;20:361–8.
100. Ryan AM, Rowley SP, Fitzgerald AP, Ravi N, Reynolds JV. Adenocarcinoma of the oesophagus and gastric cardia: male preponderance in association with obesity. Eur J Cancer. 2006;42:1151–8.
101. Samanic C, Chow WH, Gridley G, Jarvholm B, Fraumeni JF Jr. Relation of body mass index to cancer risk in 362,552 Swedish men. Cancer Causes Control. 2006;17:901–9.
102. Reeves CK, Pirie K, Beral V, Green J, Spencer E, Bull D. Cancer incidence and mortality in relation to body mass index in the Million Women Study: cohort study. BMJ. 2007;335:1134.
103. Merry AH, Schouten LJ, Goldbohm RA, van den Brandt PA. Body mass index, height and risk of adenocarcinoma of the oesophagus and gastric cardia: a prospective cohort study. Gut. 2007;56:1503–11.
104. Anderson LA, Watson RG, Murphy SJ, Johnston BT, Comber H, McGuigan J, et al. Risk factors for Barrett's oesophagus and oesophageal adenocarcinoma: results from the FINBAR study. World J Gastroenterol. 2007;13:1585–94.
105. Steffen A, Schultze MB, Pischon T, Dietrich T, Molina E, Chirlaque MD, et al. Anthropometry and esophageal cancer risk in European prospective investigation into cancer and nutrition. Cancer Epidemiol Biomark Prev. 2009;18:2079–89.
106. MacInnis RJ, English DR, Hopper JL, Giles GG. Body size and composition and the risk of gastric and esophageal adenocarcinoma. Int J Cancer. 2006;118:2628–31.
107. Whiteman DC, Sadeghi S, Pandeya N, Smithers BM, Gotley DC, Bain CJ, et al. Combined effects of obesity, acid reflux and smoking on the risk of adenocarcinomas of the oesophagus. Gut. 2009;57:173–80.
108. Yang P, Zhou Y, Chen B, Wan H-W, Jia G-Q, Bai H-L, et al. Overweight, obesity and gastric cancer risk: results from a meta-analysis of cohort studies. Eur J Cancer. 2009;45:2867–73.
109. Groot de NL, Burgerhart JS, van de Meeberg PC, de Vries DR, Smout AJPM, Siersema PD. Systematic review: the effects of conservative and surgical treatment for obesity on gastro-oesophageal reflux disease. Aliment Pharmacol Ther. 2009;30:1091–102.
110. Bonfrate L, Wang DQ-H, Garruti G, Portincasa P. Obesity and the risk and prognosis of gallstone disease and pancreatitis. Best Pract Res Clin Gastroenterol. 2014;28:623–35.

111. Tsai CJ, Leitzmann MF, Willett WC, Giovannucci EL. Weight cycling and risk of gallstone in men. Arch Intern Med. 2006;166:2369–74.
112. Shaffer EA. Gallstone disease: epidemiology of gallbladder stone disease. Best Pract Res Clin Gastroenterol. 2006;20:981–96.
113. Everhart JE, Khare M, Hill M, Maurer KR. Prevalence and ethnic differences in gallbladder disease in the United States. Gastroenterology. 1999;117:632–9.
114. Carey MC. Pathogenesis of gallstones. Am J Surg. 1993;165:410–9.
115. Beckingham IJ. Gallstone disease. BMJ. 2001;322:91–4.
116. Portincasa P, Moschetta A, Palasciano G. Cholesterol gallstone disease. Lancet. 2006;368:230–9.
117. Portincasa P, Wang DQ. Intestinal absorption, hepatic synthesis, and biliary secretion of cholesterol: where are we for cholesterol gallstone formation? Hepatology. 2012;55:1313–6.
118. Sampliner RE, Bennett PH, Comess LJ, Rose FA, Burch TA. Gallbladder disease in Pima Indians. Demonstration of high prevalence and early onset by cholecystography. N Engl J Med. 1970;283:1358–64.
119. Maclure KM, Hayes KC, Colditz GA, Stampfer MJ, Speizer FE, Willett WC. Weight, diet, and the risk of symptomatic gallstones in middle-aged women. N Engl J Med. 1989;321:563–9.
120. Stampfer MJ, Maclure KM, Colditz GA, Manson JE, Willett WC. Risk of symptomatic gallstones in women with severe obesity. Am J Clin Nutr. 1992;55:652–8.
121. Sahi T, Paffenbarger RS Jr, Hsieh CC, Lee IM. Body mass index, cigarette smoking, and other characteristics as predictors of self-reported, physician-diagnosed gallbladder disease in male college alumni. Am J Epidemiol. 1998;147:644–51.
122. Tsai CJ, Leitzmann MF, Willett WC, Giovannucci EL. Prospective study of abdominal adiposity and gallstone disease in US men. Am J Clin Nutr. 2004;80:38–44.
123. Mendez-Sanchez N, Chavez-Tapia NC, Motola-Kuba D, Sanchez-Lara K, Ponciano-Rodriguez G, Baptitsa H, et al. Metabolic syndrome as a risk factor for gallstone disease. World J Gastroenterol. 2005;11:1653–7.
124. Johansson K, Sundstrom J, Marcus C, Hemmingsson E, Neovius M. Risk of symptomatic gallstones and cholecystectomy after a very-low-calorie diet or low-calorie diet in a commercial weight loss program: 1-year matched cohort study. Int J Obes. 2014;38:279–84.
125. Mathus-Vliegen EM, van Ierland-van Leeuwen ML, Terpstra A. Lipase inhibition by orlistat: effects on gall-bladder kinetics and cholecystokinin release in obesity. Aliment Pharmacol Ther. 2004;19:601–11.
126. Stender S, Nordestgaard BG, Tybjaerg-Hansen A. Elevated body mass index as a causal gallstone disease: a Mendelian randomization study. Hepatology. 2013;58:2133–41.
127. Misra S, Chaturvedi A, Misra NC, Sharma ID. Carcinoma of the gallbladder. Lancet Oncol. 2003;4:167–76.
128. Mabee TM, Meyer P, DenBesten L, Mason EE. The mechanism of increased gallstone formation in obese human subjects. Surgery. 1976;79:460–8.
129. Freeman JB, Meyer PD, Printen KJ, Mason EE, DenBesten L. Analysis of gallbladder bile in morbid obesity. Am J Surg. 1975;129:163–6.
130. Shiffman ML, Sugerman HJ, Kellum JM, Moore EW. Changes in gallbladder bile composition following gallstone formation and weight reduction. Gastroenterology. 1992;103:214–21.
131. Portincasa P, Di Ciaula A, Palmieri V, Van Berge-Henegouwen GP, Palasciano G. Effects of cholestyramine on gallbladder and gastric emptying in obese and lean subjects. Eur J Clin Investig. 1995;25:746–53.
132. Mathus-Vliegen EM, van Ierland-van Leeuwen ML, Terpstra A. Determinants of gallbladder kinetics in obesity. Dig Dis Sci. 2004;49:9–16.
133. Weinsier RL, Ullmann DO. Gallstone formation and weight loss. Obes Res. 1993;1:51–6.
134. Erlinger S. Gallstones in obesity and weight loss. Eur J Gastroenterol Hepatol. 2000;12:1347–52.
135. Diehl AK. Cholelithiasis and the insulin resistance syndrome. Hepatology. 2000;31:528–30.

136. Chen LY, Qiao QH, Zhang SC, Chen YH, Chao GQ, Fang LZ. Metabolic syndrome and gallstone disease. World J Gastroenterol. 2012;18:4215–20.
137. Forsmark CE, Baillie J. AGA Institute clinical practice and economics committee, AGA Institute governing board. AGA Institute technical review on acute pancreatitis. Gastroenterology. 2007;132:2022–44.
138. Mathus-Vliegen EMH. Facts and fallacies of diets in gastroenterology. Institute Danone. 2010. ISBN 2-930151-28-5.
139. Peery AF, Dellon ES, Lund J, Crockett SD, McGowan CE, Bulsiewicz WJ, et al. Burden of gastrointestinal disease in the United States: 2012 update. Gastroenterology. 2012;143:1179.
140. Niederau C, Nierdeau M, Luthen R, Strohmeyer G, Ferrell LD, Grendel JH. Pancreatic exocrine secretion in acute experimental pancreatitis. Gastroenterology. 1990;99:1120–7.
141. Lerch MM, Saluja AK, Rünzi M, Dawra R, Saluja M, Steer ML. Pancreatic duct obstruction triggers acute necrotizing pancreatitis in the opossum. Gastroenterology. 1993;104:853.
142. Rattner DW. Experimental models of acute pancreatitis and their relevance to human disease. Scand J Gastroenterol. 1996;219(suppl):6.
143. Steer ML. Pathogenesis of acute pancreatitis. Digestion. 1997;58(suppl 1):46.
144. Kingsnorth A. Role of cytokines and their inhibitors in acute pancreatitis. Gut. 1997;40(1):1–4.
145. Purohit V, Russo D, Salin M, Brown R. Mechanisms of alcoholic pancreatitis, introduction and summary of the symposium. Pancreas. 2003;27:281–5.
146. Russell MK. Acute pancreatitis: a review of pathophysiology and nutrition management. Nutr Clin Pract. 2004;19:16–24.
147. Kingsnorth A, O'Reilly D. Acute pancreatitis. BMJ. 2006;332:1072–6.
148. Banks PA, Freeman ML. Practice Parameters Committee of the American College of Gastroenterology. Practice guidelines in acute pancreatitis. Am J Gastroenterol. 2006;101:2379.
149. Cavallini G, Frulloni L, Bassi C, Gabbrielli A, Castoldi L, Costamagna G, et al. Prospective multicentre survey on acute pancreatitis in Italy (ProInf-AISP): results on 1005 patients. Dig Liver Dis. 2004;36:205.
150. Bradley EL 3rd. A clinically based classification system for acute pancreatitis. Summary of the international symposium on acute pancreatitis. Arch Surg. 1993;128:586.
151. Gloor B, Müller CA, Worni M, Martignoni ME, Uhl W, Büchler MW. Late mortality in patients with severe acute pancreatitis. Br J Surg. 2001;88:975.
152. Mutinga M, Rosenbluth A, Tenner SM, Odze RR, Sica GT, Banks PA. Does mortality occur early or late in acute pancreatitis? Int J Pancreatol. 2000;28:91.
153. Ranson JH, Rifkind KM, Roses DF, Fink SD, Eng K, Spencer FC. Prognostic signs and the role of operative management in acute pancreatitis. Surg Gynecol Obstet. 1974;139:69.
154. De Bernardinis M, Violi V, Roncoroni L, Boselli AS, Giunta A, Peracchia A. Discriminant power and information content of Ranson's prognostic signs in acute pancreatitis: a meta-analytic study. Crit Care Med. 1999;27:2272.
155. Johnson CD, Toh SK, Campbell MJ. Combination of APACHE-II score and an obesity score (APACHE-O) for the prediction of severe acute pancreatitis. Pancreatology. 2004;4:1.
156. Martinez J, Sanchez-Paya J, Palazon JM, Suazo-Barahona J, Robles-Diaz G, Perez-Mateo M. Is obesity a risk factor in acute pancreatitis? A meta-analysis. Pancreatology. 2004;4:42–8.
157. Martinez J, Johnson CD, Sánchez-Payá J, de Madaria E, Robles-Díaz G, Pérez-Mateo M. Obesity is a definitive risk factor of severity and mortality in acute pancreatitis: an updated meta-analysis. Pancreatology. 2006;6:206.
158. Hong S, Qiwen B, Ying J, Wei A, Chaoyang T. Body mass index and the risk and prognosis of acute pancreatitis: a meta-analysis. Eur J Gastroenterol Hepatol. 2011;23:1136–43.
159. Wang S-Q, Li S-J, Feng Q-X, Feng X-Y, Xu L, Zhao Q-C. Overweight is an additional prognostic factor in acute pancreatitis: a meta-analysis. Pancreatology. 2011;11:92–8.
160. Banks PA, Bollen TI, Dervenis C, Gooszen HG, Johnson CD, Sarr MG, et al. Classification of acute pancreatitis—2012: revision of the Atlanta classification and definitions by international consensus. Gut. 2013;62:102.
161. Apte MV, Wilson JS, McCaughan GW, Korsten MA, Haber PS, Norton ID, et al. Ethanol-induced alterations in messenger RNA levels correlate with glandular content of pancreatic enzymes. J Lab Clin Med. 1995;125:634.

162. Tiscornia OM, Celener D, Perec CJ, De Lehmann ES, Cresta M, Dreiling DA. Physiopathogenic basis of alcoholic pancreatitis: the effects of elevated cholinergic tone and increased "pancreon" ecbolic response to CCK-PZ. Mt Sinai J Med. 1983;50:369.
163. Majumder S, Gierisch JM, Bastian LA. The association of smoking and acute pancreatitis: a systematic review and meta-analysis. Pancreas. 2015;44:540.
164. Giovannucci E, Michaud D. The role of obesity and related metabolic disturbances in cancers of the colon, prostate, and pancreas. Gastroenterology. 2007;132:2208–25.
165. Berrington de Gonzalez A, Sweetland S, Spencer E. A meta-analysis of obesity and the risk of pancreatic cancer. Br J Cancer. 2003;89:519–23.
166. Everhart J, Wright D. Diabetes mellitus as a risk factor for pancreatic cancer. A meta-analysis. JAMA. 1995;273:1605–9.
167. Huxley R, Ansary-Moghaddam A, Berrington de Gonzalez A, Barzi F, Woodward M. Type-II diabetes and pancreatic cancer: a meta-analysis of 36 studies. Br J Cancer. 2005;92:2076–83.
168. Gapstur SM, Gann PH, Lowe W, Liu K, Colangelo L, Dyer A. Abnormal glucose metabolism and pancreatic cancer mortality. JAMA. 2000;283:2552–8.
169. Batty GD, Shipley MJ, Marmot M, Smith GD. Diabetes status and post-load plasma glucose concentrations in relation to site-specific cancer mortality: findings from the original Whitehall study. Cancer Causes Control. 2004;15:873–81.
170. Jee SH, Ohrr H, Sull JW, Yun JE, Ji M, Samet JM. Fasting serum glucose levels and cancer risk in Korean men and women. JAMA. 2005;293:194–202.
171. Stolzenberg-Solomon RZ, Graubard BI, Chari S, Limburg P, Taylor PR, Virtamo J, et al. Insulin, glucose, insulin resistance, and pancreatic cancer in male smokers. JAMA. 2005;294:2872–8.
172. Lyon JL, Slattery ML, Mahoney AW, Robison LM. Dietary intake as a risk factor for cancer of the exocrine pancreas. Cancer Epidemiol Biomark Prev. 1993;2:513–8.
173. Baghurts PA, McMichael AJ, Slavotinek AH, Baghurst KI, Boyle P, Walker AM. A caseconrol study of diet and cancer of the pancreas. Am J Epidemiol. 1991;134:167–79.
174. Schernhammer ES, Hu FB, Giovannucci E, Michaud DS, Colditz GA, Stampfer MJ, et al. Sugar-sweetened soft drink consumption and risk of pancreatic cancer in two prospective cohorts. Cancer Epidemiol Biomark Prev. 2005;14:2098–105.
175. Larsson SC, Bergkvist L, Wolk A. Consumption of sugar and sugar-sweetened foods and the risk of pancreatic cancer in a prospective study. Am J Clin Nutr. 2006;84:1171–6.
176. Sugerman HJ, Brewer WH, Shiffman ML, Brolin RE, Fobi MA, Linner JH, et al. A multicenter, placebo-controlled, randomized, double-blind, prospective trial of prophylactic ursodiol for the prevention of gallstone formation following gastric-bypass-induced rapid weight loss. Am J Surg. 1995;169:91–6.
177. Miller K, Hell E, Lang B, Lengauer E. Gallstone formation prophylaxis after gastric restrictive procedures for weight loss: a randomized double-blind placebo-controlled trial. Ann Surg. 2003;238:697–702.
178. Uy MC, Talingdan-Te MC, Espinosa WZ, Daez ML, Ong JP. Ursodeoxycholic acid in the prevention of gallstone formation after bariatric surgery: a meta-analysis. Obes Surg. 2008 Dec;18(12):1532 8.
179. El-Sherag HB. Obesity and disease of the esophagus and colon. Gastroenterol Clin N Am. 2005;34:63–82.
180. Bardou M, Basrkun AN, Martel M. Obesity and colorectal cancer. Gut. 2013;62:933–47.
181. Frezza EE, Wachtel MS, Chiriva-Internati M. Influence of obesity on the risk of developing colon cancer. Gut. 2005;55:285–91.
182. Siddiqui A, Sahdala HNP, Nazario HE, Mahgoub A, Patel M, Cipher D, et al. Obesity is associated with an increased prevalence of advanced adenomatous polyps in a male veteran population. Dig Dis Sci. 2009;54:1560–4.
183. Kang HW, Kim D, Kim HJ, Kim CH, Kim YS, Park MJ, et al. Visceral obesity and insulin resistance as risk factors for colorectal adenoma: a cross-sectional, case-control study. Am J Gastroenterol. 2010;105:178–87.
184. Hwang ST, Cho YK, Park JH, Kim HJ, Park DI, Sohn CI, et al. Relationship of non-alcoholic fatty liver disease to colorectal adenomatous polyps. J Gastroenterol Hepatol. 2010;25:562–7.

185. Wong VW-S, Wong GL-H, Tsang SW-C, Fan T, Chu WC-W, Woo J, et al. High prevalence of colorectal neoplasm in patients with non-alcoholic steatohepatitis. Gut. 2011;60:829–36.
186. Lee YJ, Myung S-K, Cho BL, Park B-J, Park JH, Ju W, et al. Adiposity and the risk of colorectal adenomatous polyps: a meta-analysis. Cancer Causes Control. 2011;22:1021–35.
187. Hong S, Cai Q, Chen D, Zhu W, Huang W, Li Z. Abdominal obnesity and the risk of colorectal adenoma: a meta-analysis of observational studies. Eur J Cancer Prev. 2012;21:523–31.
188. Okabayashi K, Ashrafian H, Hasegawa H, Yoo JH, Patel VM, Harling L, et al. Body mass index category as a risk factor for colorectal adenoma: a systematic review and meta-analysis. Am J Gastroenterol. 2012;107:1175–85.
189. Ben Q, An W, Jiang Y, Zhan X, Du Y, Cai QC, et al. Body mass index increases risk for colorectal adenomas based on meta-analysis. Gastroenterology. 2012;142:762–72.
190. Dai Z, Xu YC, Niu L. Obesity and colorectal cancer risk: a meta-analysis of cohort studies. World J Gastroenterol. 2007;13:4199–206.
191. Larsson SC, Wolk A. Obesity and colon and rectal cancer risk: a meta-analysis of prospective studies. Am J Clin Nutr. 2007;86:556–65.
192. Moghaddam AA, Woodward M, Huxley R. Obesity and risk of colorectal cancer: a meta-analysis of 31 studies with 70,000 events. Cancer Epidemiol Biomark Prev. 2007;16:2533–47.
193. Harriss DJ, Atkinson G, George K, Cable NT, Reilly T, Haboubi N, et al. Lifestyle factors and colorectal cancer risk (1): systematic review and meta-analysis of associations with body mass index. Color Dis. 2009;11:547–63.
194. Terry PD, Miller AB, Rohan TE. Obesity and colorectal cancer risk in women. Gut. 2002;51:191–4.
195. Phillips R, Snowdon D. Dietary relationships with fatal colorectal cancer among seventh-day adventists. J Natl Cancer Inst. 1985;74:307–17.
196. Martinez M, Giovannucci E, Spiegelman D, Hunter DJ, Willett WC, Colditz GA. Leisure-time physical activity, body size, and colon cancer in women. J Natl Cancer Inst. 1997;89:948–55.
197. Terry P, Giovannucci E, Bergkvist L, Holmberg L, Wolk A. Body weight and colorectal cancer risk in a cohort of Swedish women: relation varies by age and cancer site. Br J Cancer. 2001;85:346–9.
198. Samad AKA, Taylor RS, Marshall T, Chapman MA. A meta-analysis of the association of physical activity with reduced risk of colorectal cancer. Color Dis. 2005;7:204–13.
199. Slattery ML. Physical activity and colorectal cancer. Sports Med. 2004;34:239–52.
200. Wolin KY, Yan Y, Colditz GA. Physical activity and risk of colon adenoma: a meta-analysis. Br J Cancer. 2011;104:882–5.
201. Wolin KY, Yan Y, Colditz GA, Lee IM. Physical activity and colon cancer prevention: a meta-analysis. Br J Cancer. 2009;100:611–6.
202. Ma J, Giovannucci E, Pollak M, Leavitt A, Tao Y, Gaziano JM, et al. A prospective study of plasma C-peptide and colorectal cancer risk in men. J Natl Cancer Inst. 2004;96:546–53.
203. Wei EK, Ma J, Pollak MN, Rifai N, Fuchs CS, Hankinson SE, et al. A prospective study of C-peptide, insulin-like growth factor-1, insulin-like growth factor binding protein-1, and the risk of colorectal cancer in women. Cancer Epidemiol Biomark Prev. 2005;14:850–5.
204. Stocks T, Lukanova A, Johansson M, Rinaldi S, Palmqvist R, Hallmans G, et al. Components of the metabolic syndrome and colorectal cancer risks: a prospective study. In J Obes (Lod). 2008;32:304–14.
205. Hu NC, Chen JD, Lin YM, Chang JY, Chen YH. Stepwise relationship between components of metabolic syndrome and risk of colorectal adenoma in a Taiwanese population receiving screening colonoscopy. J Formos Med Assoc. 2011;10:100–8.
206. Lundgren M, Buren J, Ruge T, Myrnäs T, Eriksson JW. Glucocorticoids down-regulate glucose uptake capacity and insulin signaling proteins in omental but not subcutaneous human adipocytes. J Clin Endocrinol Metab. 2004;89:2989–97.
207. Klein S, Fontana L, Young VL, Coggan AR, Kilo C, Patterson BW, et al. Absence of an effect of liposuction on insulin action and risk factors for coronary heart disease. New Engl J Med. 2004;350:2549–57.

208. Thörne A, Lönnqvist F, Apelman J, Hellers G, Arner P. A pilot study of long-term effects of a novel obesity treatment: omentectomy in connection with adjustable gastric banding. Int J Obes. 2002;26:193–9.
209. Freedland ES. The role of a critical visceral adipose tissue threshold (CVATT) in metabolic syndrome: implications for controlling dietary carbohydrates: a review. Nutr Metab. 2004;1:12.
210. Huang X-F. Adiponectin and signal pathways in obesity-induced colon cancer. Gut. 2009;58:1169–70.
211. Kaklamani VG, Wisinski KB, Sadim M, Gulden C, Do A, Offit K, et al. Variants of the adiponectin (ADIPOQ) and adiponectin receptor 1 (ADIPOR1) genes and colorectal cancer risk. JAMA. 2008;300:1523–31.
212. Xu XT, Xu Q, Tong JL, Zhu MM, Huang ML, Ran ZH, et al. Meta-analysis: circulating adiponectin levels and risk of colorectal cancer and adenoma. J Dig Dis. 2011;12:234–44.
213. An W, Bai Y, Deng SX, Gao J, Ben QW, Cai QC, et al. Adiponectin levels in patients with colorectal cancer and adenoma: a meta-analysis. Eur J Cancer Prev. 2012;21:126–33.
214. Fujisawa T, Endo H, Tomimoto A, Sugiyama M, Takahashi H, Saito S, et al. Adiponectin suppresses colorectal carcinogenesis under the high-fat diet condition. Gut. 2008;57:1531–8.
215. Eraslan E, Turkay C, Koktener A, Koca C, Uz B, Bavbek N. Association of visceral fat accumulation and adiponectin levels with colorectal neoplasia. Dig Dis Sci. 2009;54:862–8.
216. Zhou Y, Wu L, Li X, Wu X, Li B. Outcome of laparoscopic colorectal surgery in obese and nonobese patients: a meta-analysis. Surg Endosc. 2012;26:783–9.
217. Makino T, Shukla PJ, Rubino F, Milsom JW. The impact of obesity on perioperative outcomes after laparoscopic colorectal resection. Ann Surg. 2012;255:228–36.
218. Hull M, Lagergren J. Obesity and colorectal cancer. Gut. 2014;63:205.
219. Derogar M, Hull MA, Kant P, Östlund M, Lu Y, Lagergren J. Increased risk of colorectal cancer after obesity surgery. Ann Surg. 2013;258(6):983–8. https://doi.org/10.1097/SLA.0b013e318288463a.
220. Chalasani N, Younossi Z, Lavine JE, Diehl AM, Brunt EM, Cusi K, et al. The diagnosis and management of non-alcoholic fatty liver disease: practice guideline by the American Gastroenterological Association, American Association for the Study of Liver Disease, and American College of Gastroenterology. Gastroenterology. 2012;142:1592–609.
221. EASL–EASD–EASO Clinical Practice Guidelines for the management of non-alcoholic fatty liver disease. European Association for the Study of the Liver (EASL), European Association for the Study of Diabetes (EASD) and European Association for the Study of Obesity (EASO). J Hepatol. 2016;64:1388–402.
222. Goh GB-B, McCullough AJ. Natural history of nonalcoholic fatty liver disease. Dig Dis Sci. 2016;61:1226–33.
223. Corey KE, Rinella ME. Medical and surgical treatment options for non-alcoholic steatohepatitis. Dig Dis Sci. 2016;61:1387–97.
224. Anstee QM, McPherson S, Day CP. Uncertainty pages. How big a problem is non-alcoholic fatty liver disease? BMJ. 2011;343:d3897.
225. Sherif ZA, Saeed A, Ghavimi S, Nouraie S-M, Laiyemo AO, Brim H, et al. Global epidemiology of nonalcoholic fatty liver disease and perspectives on US minority populations. Dig Dis Sci. 2016;61:1214–25.
226. Vernon G, Baranova A, Younossi ZM. Systematic review: the epidemiology and natural history of non-alcoholic fatty liver disease and non-alcoholic steatohepatitis in adults. Aliment Pharmacol Ther. 2011;34:274–85.
227. Musso G, Gambino R, Cassader M, Pagano G. Meta-analysis: natural history of non-alcoholic fatty liver disease (NAFLD) and diagnostic accuracy of non-invasive tests for liver disease severity. Ann Med. 2011;43:617–49.
228. Yilmaz Y. Review article: is non-alcoholic fatty liver disease a spectrum or are steatosis and non-alcoholic steatohepatitis distinct conditions? Aliment Pharmacol Ther. 2012;36:815–23.
229. Strengel JZ, Harrison SA. Nonalcoholic steatohepatitis: clinical presentation, diagnosis, and treatment. Gastroenterol Hepatol. 2006;6:440–7.

230. Ratziu V. Novel pharmacotherapy options for NASH. Dig Dis Sci. 2016;61:1398–405.
231. Ekstedt M, Hagstrom H, Nasr P, Fredrikson M, Stål P, Kechagias S, et al. Fibrosis stage is the strongest predictor for disease-specific mortality in NAFLS after up to 33 years of follow-up. Hepatology. 2015;61:1547–54.
232. Angulo P, Kleiner DE, Dam-Larsen S, Adams LA, Bjornsson ES, Charatcharoenwitthaya P, et al. Liver fibrosis, but no other histologic features, is associated with long-term outcomes of patients with non-alcoholic fatty liver disease. Gastroenterology. 2015;149:389–97.
233. Mantovani A, Ballestri S, Lonardo A, Targher G. Cardiovascular disease and myocardial abnormalities in nonalcoholic fatty liver disease. Dig Dis Sci. 2016;61:1246–67.
234. Singh S, Allen AM, Wang Z, Prokop LJ, Murad MH, Loomba R. Fibrosis progression in non-alcoholic fatty liver vs non-alcoholic steatohepatitis: a systematic review and meta-analysis of paired-biopsy studies. Clin Gastroenterol Hepatol. 2015;13:643–54.
235. Matteoni CA, Younossi ZM, Gramlich T, Prokop LJ, Murad MH, Loomba R. Nonalcoholic fatty liver disease: a spectrum of clinical and pathological severity. Gastroenterology. 1999;116:1413–9.
236. Rafiq N, Bai C, Fang Y, Srishord M, McCullough A, Gramlich T, et al. Long-term follow-up of patients with nonalcoholic fatty liver. Clin Gastroenterol Hepatol. 2009;7:234–8.
237. Liu B, Balkwill A, Reeves G, Beral V, on behalf of the Million Women Study Coordinators. Body mass index and risk of liver cirrhosis in middle aged UK women: a prospective study. BMJ. 2010;340:c912.
238. Hart CL, Batty GD, Morrison DS, Mitchell RJ, Smith GD. Obesity, overweight and liver disease in the Midspan prospective cohort studies. Int J Obes. 2010;34:1051–9.
239. Hamaguchi M, Kojima T, Takeda N, Nakagawa T, Taniguchi H, Fujii K, et al. The metabolic syndrome as a predictor of nonalcoholic fatty liver disease. Ann Intern Med. 2005;143:722–8.
240. Marchesini G, Bugianesi E, Forlaini G, Cerrelli F, Lenzi M, Manini R, et al. Nonalcoholic fatty liver, steatohepatitis, and the metabolic syndrome. Hepatology. 2003;37:917–23.
241. Younossi ZM, Otgonsuren M, Henry L, Venkatesan C, Mishra A, Erario M, et al. Association of Nonalcoholic Fatty Liver Disease (NAFLD) with Hepatocellular Carcinoma (HCC) in the United States from 2004 to 2009. Hepatology. 2015;62:1723–30.
242. Hassan MM, Abdel-Wahab R, Kaseb A, Shalaby A, Phan AT, El-Serag H, et al. Obesity early in adulthood increases risk but does not affect outcomes of hepatocellular carcinoma. Gastroenterologia. 2015;149:119–29.
243. Giovannucci E, Harlan DM, Archer MC, Bergenstal RM, Gapstur SM, Habel LA, et al. Diabetes and cancer: a consensus report. Diabetes Care. 2010;33:1674–85.
244. Tsilidis KK, Kasimis JC, Lopez DS, Ntzani EE, Ioannidis JP. Type 2 diabetes and cancer: umbrella review of meta-analysis of observational studies. BMJ. 2015;350:g7607.
245. Setiawan VW, Lim U, Lipworth L, Lu SC, Shepherd J, Ernst T, et al. Sex and ethnic differences in the association of obesity with risk of hepatocellular carcinoma. Clin Gastroenterol Hepatol. 2016;14:309–16.
246. Schlesinger S, Aleksandrova K, Pischon T, Fedirko V, Jenab M, Trepo E, et al. Abdominal obesity, weight gain during adulthood and risk of live rand biliary tract cancer in a European cohort. Int J Cancer. 2013;132:645–57.
247. Ohki T, Tateishi R, Shiina S, Goto E, Sato T, Nakagawa H, et al. Visceral fat accumulation is an independent risk factor for hepatocellular carcinoma recurrence after curative treatment in patients with suspected NASH. Gut. 2009;58:839–44.
248. Parekhi S, Anania FA. Abnormal lipid and glucose metabolism in obesity: implications for non-alcoholic fatty liver disease. Gastroenterology. 2007;132:2191–207.
249. Kopec KL, Burns D. Nonalcoholic fatty liver disease: a review of the spectrum of disease, diagnosis, and therapy. Nutr Clin Pract. 2011;26:565–76.
250. Sattar N, Forrest E, Preiss D. Non-alcoholic fatty liver disease. BMJ. 2014;349:g4596.
251. Reeves HL, Zaki MYW, Day CP. Hepatocellular carcinoma in obesity, type 2 diabetes, and NAFLD. Dig Dis Sci. 2016;61:1234–45.
252. Donelly KL, Smith CI, Schwarzenberg SJ, Jessurun J, Boldt MD, Parks EJ. Sources of fatty acids stored in live rand secreted via lipoproteins in nonalcoholic fatty liver disease. J Clin Invest. 2005;115:1343–51.

253. Nielsen S, Guo Z, Johnson CM, Hensrud DD, Jensen MD. Splanchnic lipolysis in human obesity. J Clin Invest. 2004;113:1582–8.
254. Softic S, Cohen DE, Kahn CR. Role of dietary fructose and hepatic de novo Lipogenesis in fatty liver disease. Dig Dis Sci. 2016;61:1282–93.
255. Chung M, Ma J, Patel K, Berger S, Lau J, Lichtenstein AH. Fructose, high-fructose corn syrup, sucrose, and non-alcoholic fatty liver disease or indexes of liver health: a systematic review and meta-analysis. Am J Clin Nutr. 2014;100:833–49.
256. Fabbrini E, Magkos F, Mohammed BS, Pietka T, Abumrad NA, Patterson BW, et al. Intrahepatic fat, not visceral fat, is linked with metabolic complications of obesity. PNAS. 2009;106:15430–5.
257. Leclercq IA, Horsmans Y. Nonalcoholic fatty liver disease: the potential role of nutritional management. Curr Opin Clin Nutr Metab Care. 2008;11:766–73.
258. Zelber-Sagi S, Ratziu V, Oren R. Nutrition and physical activity in NAFLD: an overview of the epidemiological evidence. World J Gastroenterol. 2011;17:3377–89.
259. Hannah WN Jr, Harrison SA. Lifestyle and dietary interventions in the management of non-alcoholic fatty liver disease. Dig Dis Sci. 2016;61:1365–74.
260. Promrat K, Kleiner DE, Niemeier HM, Jackvony E, Kearns M, Wands JR, et al. Randomized controlled trial testing the effects of weight loss on nonalcoholic steatohepatitis. Hepatology. 2010;51:121–9.
261. Villar-Gomez E, Martinez-Perez Y, Calzadilla-Bertot L, Torres-Gonzalez A, Gra-Oramas B, Gonzalez-Fabian L, et al. Weight loss through lifestyle modification significantly reduced features of non-alcoholic hepatitis. Gastroenterology. 2015;149:367–78.
262. Harrison SA, Fecht W, Brunnt EM, Neuschwander-Tetri BA. Orlistat for overweight subjects with non-alcoholic steatohepatitis: a randomised prospective trial. Hepatology. 2009;49:80–6.
263. Keating SE, Hackett DA, George J, Johnson NA. Exercise and non-alcoholic fatty liver disease: a systematic review and meta-analysis. J Hepatol. 2012;57:157–66.
264. Thoma C, Day CP, Trenell MI. Lifestyle inteventions for the treatment of non-alcoholic fatty liver disease in adults: a systematic review. J Hepatol. 2012;56:255–66.
265. Andersen T, Gluud C, Franzmann MB, Christoffersen P. Hepatic effects of dietary weight loss in morbidly obese subjects. J Hepatol. 1991;12:224–9.
266. Musso G, Cassader M, Rosina F, Gambino R. Impact of current treatments on liver disease, glucose metabolism and cardiovascular risk in non-alcoholic fatty liver disease (NAFLD): a systematic review and meta-analysis of randomised trials. Diabetologia. 2012;55:885–904.
267. Younossi ZM, Reyes MJ, Mishra A, Mehta R, Henry L. Systematic review with meta-analysis: non-alcoholic steatohepatitis—a case for personalised treatment based on pathogenic targets. Aliment Pharmacol Ther. 2014;39:3–14.
268. McMillan DC, Sattar N, Lean M, McArdle CS. Obesity and cancer. BMJ. 2006;333:1109–11.
269. World Cancer Research Fund/American Institute for Cancer Research. Food, nutrition, physical activity and the prevention of cancer: a global perspective. Washington DC: AICR; 2007.
270. Bergstrom A, Pisani P, Tenet V, Wolk A, Adami HO. Overweight as an avoidable cause of cancer in Europe. Int J Cancer. 2001;91:421–30.
271. Lukanova A, Björ O, Kaaks R, Lenner P, Lindahl B, Hallmans G, et al. Body mass index and cancer: results from the Northern Sweden Health and Disease Cohort. Int J Cancer. 2005. https://doi.org/10.1002/ijc.21354.
272. Renehan AG, Tyson M, Egger M, Heller RF, Zwahlen M. Body-mass index and incidence of cancer: a systematic review and meta-analysis of prospective observational studies. Lancet. 2008;371:569–78.
273. Sjöström L, Gummesson A, Sjöström CD, Narbro K, Peltonen M, Wedel H, et al. Effects of bariatric surgery on cancer incidence in obese patients in Sweden (Swedish Obese Subjects Study): a prospective, controlled intervention trial. Lancer Oncol. 2009;10:653–62.

Current Endoscopic/Laparoscopic Bariatric Procedures

2

Contents

Abbreviations

ABS	Adjustable balloon system
ACC	American College of Cardiology
ACE	Articulating circular endoscopic
AE	Adverse event
AHA	American Heart Association
ANGPTL	Angiopoietin-like protein
ASGE	American Society for Gastrointestinal Endoscopy
ASMBS	American Society for Metabolic and Bariatric Surgery
ATIIP	Adjustable totally implanted intragastric prosthesis
BED	Binge-eating disorder
BIB	BioEnterics Intragastric Balloon
BMI	Body mass index

E. M. H. Mathus-Vliegen, J. Dargent, *Bariatric Therapy*,
https://doi.org/10.1007/978-3-319-90074-2_2

BTA	Botulinum toxin A
CA	Completers' analysis
CCK	Cholecystokinin
CI	Confidence interval
CLGES	Closed-loop gastric electrical stimulation
CRP	C-reactive protein
DEXA	Dual-energy X-ray absorptiometry
DJBL	Duodenojejunal bypass liner
DJBS	Duodenojejunal bypass sleeve
DMR	Duodenal mucosal resurfacing
EBMIL	Excess BMI loss
EBMT	Endoscopic bariatric and metabolic therapy
EBT	Endoscopic bariatric therapy
EDNOS	Eating disorders not otherwise specified
EMA	European Medicines Agency
ESG	Endoscopic sleeve gastroplasty
EVG	Endoluminal vertical gastroplasty
EWL	Excess weight loss
FDA	Food and Drugs Administration
FGF	Fibroblast growth factor
GEGB	Garren-Edwards gastric bubble
GI	GastroIntestinal
GIP	Gastric inhibitory peptide or glucose-dependent insulinotropic polypeptide
GJBS	Gastroduodenojejunal bypass sleeve
GLP-1	Glucagon-like peptide-1
H. pylori	*Helicobacter pylori*
HbA1c	Glycated haemoglobin
HDL	High density lipoprotein
HIV	Human immunodeficiency virus
HTG	High triglycerides
ICU	Intensive care unit
IFN-γ	Interferon-γ
IGB	Intragastric balloon
IL	Interleukin
IMAS	Incisionless magnetic anastomotic systems
IOP	Incisionless operating platform
ITT	Intention-to-treat
IU	International unit
LA(S)GB	Laparoscopic adjustable (silicone) gastric banding
LDL	Low-density lipoprotein
LS	Long segment
MAO	Monoamine oxidase
MCP-1	Monocyte chemoattractant protein-1
mITT	Modified intention-to-treat

mL	Millilitre
NAFLD	Non-alcoholic fatty liver disease
NICE	National Institute for Health and Clinical Excellence
NIH	National Institute of Health
NTG	Normal Triglycerides
OSAS	Obstructive sleep apnoea syndrome
PEG	Percutaneous endoscopic gastrostomy
PIVI	Preservation and Incorporation of Valuable endoscopic Innovations
POSE	Primary obesity surgery endolumenal
PP	Pancreatic polypeptide
PP	Per-protocol
PPI	Proton pump inhibitor
PYY	Peptide YY
RCT	Randomised controlled trial
RYGB	Roux-en-Y gastric bypass
SAB	Semistationary antral balloon
SAE	Serious adverse event
SAGES	Society of American Gastrointestinal and Endoscopic Surgeons
SG	Sleeve gastrectomy
SGB	Silimed gastric balloon
SMC	Standard medical care
SS	Short segment
T2DM	Type 2 diabetes mellitus
TAPES	Transmural antero-posterior endoscopic suture
TBWL	Total body weight loss
TERIS	Transoral endoscopic restrictive implant system
TGF-1	Transforming growth factor-1
TGVR	Transoral gastric volume reduction
TNF-α	Tumour necrosis factor-α
TOGa	Transoral gastroplasty
TOS	The Obesity Society
TPS	Transpyloric shuttle
VBloc	Vagal blocking
WHO	World Health Organization

2.1 Introduction

Obesity is a chronic, lifelong, multifactorial and genetically related, life-threatening disease of excessive fat storage, which in addition to how the fat is distributed places the individual at risk of premature death and obesity-associated diseases. As discussed in Chap. 1 almost every organ system is affected by obesity, and the gastrointestinal tract is involved as well. This is the first reason why gastroenterologists should take care of the obese patient and the desired weight loss together with drug therapy will, apart from the allusion in Chap. 1, be discussed more in detail in this chapter. In the second place, the gastrointestinal tract is involved in the regulation of the energy balance and many treatments will concentrate on the digestive tract and the gut-brain axis. Side effect of medication and endoscopic bariatric surgery comes here into play, which is discussed in this chapter. The third reason is the burgeoning interest in bariatric surgery. There is still a debate whether a gastroenterologist should be part of the multidisciplinary team and whether he/she should take part in the preoperative screening. This will be discussed in Chap. 4. The widespread use of bariatric surgery and the increasing number of patients being operated also means that a significant proportion of these patients will suffer from surgical complications that may be solved by minimally invasive endoscopic techniques. These have to be distinguished in early complications, discussed in Chap. 5, or midterm and late complications, discussed in Chap. 6.

Authoritative institutions such as the National Heart, Lung and Blood Institutes (National Institute of Health, NIH), the World Health Organization (WHO), the National Institute for Health and Clinical Excellence (NICE) and the American Heart Association, the American College of Cardiology and The Obesity Society (AHA/ACC/TOS) have documented that weight loss reduces many of the risk factors for increased death and obesity-related diseases [1–4]. Improvements after weight loss have been noticed for type 2 diabetes mellitus (T2DM), hypertension, dyslipidaemia, metabolic syndrome, osteoarthritis, cancer and sleep apnoea. As far as non-alcoholic fatty liver disease (NAFLD) is concerned outcomes are variable and there is insufficient evidence for an effect on major depression [5]. The initial goal of weight loss is to reduce body weight by approximately 5–10% from baseline. A reasonable timeline for a 10% reduction in body weight is 6 months. Although this weight loss may appear insignificant, it is associated with a fall in systolic blood pressure of 10 mmHg and in diastolic blood pressure of 20 mmHg [1]. Dyslipidaemia is corrected by a decrease of 10% in total cholesterol, 15% in LDL cholesterol and 30% in triglycerides and an increase of 8% in HDL cholesterol. A 5–10% weight loss is associated with improved glycaemic control and a weight loss of 15–20% is able to reverse the elevated mortality risk of diabetes and to cure diabetes. Ovarian function and quality of life are improved by a 5% weight loss. Resolution of sleep apnoea usually needs a greater weight loss of 15–20%. After 6 months of effective weight loss, treatment efforts to maintain the weight loss over a period of at least 1–2 years but preferentially lifelong should be instituted [1, 2].

Treatment algorithms are typically staged, with the first step consisting of intensive lifestyle intervention; the second step consists of drug treatment, and the final step involves surgery [1–4]. However, as obese patients may suffer from many comorbidities, one of the first actions should be to screen the medication list. Medications commonly prescribed for hypertension (β-blockers), diabetes (sulphonylurea derivatives, insulin), depression (paroxetine, amitriptyline), epilepsy (almost all anti-epileptic drugs), rheumatoid arthritis (corticosteroids) and psychiatric illnesses (neuroleptic drugs) may promote weight gain. For most of these disease, a weight neutral of weight-reducing alternative exists [5].

Based on evidence-based guidelines, the first approach should consist of lifestyle modification: a combination of an energy-restricted diet, physical exercise and behaviour modification [1–4]. With intensive lifestyle treatment, a majority of obese participants in clinical trials lose 7–10% of their initial weight at 1 year [6]. Also, many lifestyle intervention trials in obese people with impaired glucose tolerance show a moderate weight loss between 3% and 5% and an impressive reduction in the transition of impaired glucose tolerance into frank diabetes by 40–55% [7, 8]. However, results from these trials are far better than those attained in everyday clinical practice, where studies using low-intensity counselling have not demonstrated clinically meaningful weight losses [9, 10]. Energy restriction can be a fixed amount of daily energy intake, usually 1200–1500 kcal for women and 1500–1800 kcal for men, but many studies used a 500–750 kcal deficit or a 30% energy deficit, subtracted from the calculated daily energy intake or needs. There has been a lot of discussion whether macronutrient composition has an important contribution in the adherence to a diet and subsequent weight loss. Low-carbohydrate and low-glycaemic diets and the Mediterranean diet have a central role in this discussion [10]. Albeit this is not the place to discuss all dietary options and referral to a dedicated dietician with interest in the problem of obesity is highly appropriate, patients prefer the low-carb diets as they lose a lot of (water) weight in the beginning and they can check their compliance with the diet every day with keto sticks, indicating the presence of ketones in the urine, and do not have to wait for weeks to see an effect on the scales. The legendary study by Sacks et al. in 2009 is illustrative in this regard [11]. They randomly assigned 811 overweight adults to four diets with different macronutrient compositions and offered the participants also group and individual instructional sessions for 2 years. Satiety, hunger ratings, satisfaction with the diet and attendance at group sessions were similar for all diets as were the weight losses. Attendance at the sessions, however, was the only finding that was strongly associated with weight loss (0.2 kg per session attended) [11]. Regular contact with a multidisciplinary team has been shown to be critical in maximising patient outcomes. The American Heart Association, the American College of Cardiology and The Obesity Society (AHA/ACC/TOS) Task Force reviewed all clinical studies related to lifestyle interventions and concluded that a face-to-face contact of 16 times per year on average was a major determinant of body weight loss outcomes and included this recommendation in their guideline [4]. A systematic review of multicomponent weight management programmes (diet, exercise and behaviour therapy) in overweight and obese adults included 12 randomised controlled trials. Weight changes were small, a significant weight loss of 10–15% was rarely achieved and weight regain was common in those studies that measured it [12]. It is known that weight loss that is based on caloric restriction through dieting results in significant increase in appetite with an increase in orexigenic gut hormones such as ghrelin and a decrease in anorexigenic gut hormones such polypeptide YY (PYY) [13]. This suggests that the high rate of relapse among obese patients after restrictive diets has a strong physiological basis [10, 13].

The components of behaviour modification include self-monitoring, stimulus control, slowing the rate of eating, social support, cognitive restructuring, problem solving and relapse prevention. Exercise has many benefits: it improves cardiorespiratory fitness, enhances weight loss, preserves lean muscle tissue during weight loss and is an important tool for weight maintenance which resulted in a recommendation of ≥150 min per week of moderate intensity in the AHA/ACC/TOS guideline [4]. More exercise is needed for weight loss maintenance: 200–300 min per week of moderate-intensity exercise [4].

When motivated patients have seriously attempted but failed to achieve weight loss, pharmacotherapy with approved medication may be recommended. To get approval, current efficacy benchmarks for weight loss relative to placebo are a mean weight loss ≥5% more than that of the placebo group or the proportion of drug-treated participants who lose ≥5% of initial weight is ≥35% and approximately double the proportion who lose ≥5% in the placebo group at 1 year [14]. Drugs should always be embedded in an intensive lifestyle programme. Pharmacotherapy is indicated in subjects with a body mass index (BMI) ≥30 kg/m^2 or a BMI ≥27 kg/m^2 in the presence of obesity-associated comorbidity [5]. Guidelines on the pharmacological management of obesity were published by the Endocrine Society in 2015 [5]. The Endocrine Society, the European Society of Endocrinology and The Obesity Society recommend in their guideline that if a patient's response to a weight loss medication is deemed effective (weight loss ≥5% of body weight at 3 months) and safe, the medication may be continued [5]. If deemed ineffective (weight loss <5% at 3 months) or if there are safety or tolerability issues, they recommend that the medication be discontinued and alternative medications or referral for alternative treatment approaches be considered. The available drugs approved by the Food and Drugs Administration (FDA) are mentioned in Table 2.1, orlistat being approved in 1999 by the Food and Drug Administration (FDA) for indefinite treatment of obesity [5]. In Europe, the European Medicines Agency (EMA) only approved orlistat. Gastroenterologist should be aware that orlistat acts on the digestive system by inhibiting gastric and pancreatic lipase, thereby interfering with the fat absorption. This results in a 30% fat malabsorption with complaints of oily spotting, flatulence with discharge, faecal urgency, oily evacuation, increased defecation and faecal incontinence. These complaints may be decreased by co-administration of fibre-containing supplements. In addition to promoting malabsorption of fat calories, the medication reinforces avoidance of high-fat (energy-dense) foods. These adverse effects may cause patients who do not reduce their fat intake to discontinue therapy. Despite its FDA approval for lifelong intake, fewer than 10% of patients take orlistat three times 120 mg daily for at least 1 year and less than 2% take the medication for 2 years [15, 16]. Yanovski and Yanovski systematically reviewed the literature on long-term drug treatment for obesity up to September 2013 [14]. When prescribed with lifestyle interventions, these drugs produce additional weight loss relative to placebo ranging from approximately 3% of initial weight for orlistat and lorcaserin to 9% for top-dose (15/92 mg) phentermine/topiramate–extended release at 1 year. The proportion of patients achieving clinically meaningful weight loss of ≥5% ranges from 37% to 47% for lorcaserin, 35% to 73% for orlistat and 67% to 70% for top-dose phentermine/topiramate–extended release [14]. All these three medications

Table 2.1 Drugs approved by the FDA for use in the USA; in Europe only orlistat is approved by the EMA

Drug name	Class of drugs/dosage	Advantages	Disadvantages
Phentermine	Noradrenergic, 30 mg OD[a]	Inexpensive Greater weight loss[b]	Side effect profile No long-term data[c]
Phentermine/ topiramate	Noradrenergic/GABA modulator, 7.5/46 mg OD[a] Start 3.75/46 mg, escalating to maximally 15/92 mg	Robust weight loss[b] Long-term data[c]	Expensive Teratogen
Lorcaserin	5HT2c receptor agonist, 10 mg BDD, start with 10 mg OD[a]	Side effect profile Long-term data[c]	Expensive
Orlistat by prescription	Pancreatic and gastric lipase inhibitor 120 mg TDD[a]	Nonsystemic Long-term data[c]	Less weight loss[b] Side effect profile
Orlistat over-the-counter	Pancreatic and gastric lipase inhibitor 60 mg TDD[a]	Inexpensive	Less weight loss[b] Side effect profile
Naltrexone/ bupropion	Opioid antagonist/ dopamine and norepinephrine reuptake inhibitor 8/90 mg 2 tablets BDD[a], start with 8/90 mg 1 tablet BDD[a]	Greater weight loss[b] Food addiction Long-term data[c]	Side effect profile Moderately expensive
Liraglutide	3 mg OD[a], start with 0.6 mg	Side effect profile Long-term data[c]	Expensive Injectable

[a]*OD* once daily; *BDD* twice daily; *TDD* thrice daily
[b]Less weight loss 2–3%; greater weight loss >3–5%; robust weight loss >5%
[c]Long term is 1–2 years; the noradrenergic drugs available in the USA were already in the market before the current efficacy benchmarks for weight loss relative to placebo were issued and they are thus only approved for short term, a 12-week use

produce greater improvements in many cardiometabolic risk factors than placebo. However, less than 2% of people who qualify for pharmacological therapy receive it, mainly because of assumed limited effectiveness and high costs [17].

A surgical approach is restricted to very obese subjects (BMI ≥40 kg/m^2 or BMI ≥35 kg/m^2 with obesity-associated comorbidity). Yet, only approximately 1% of eligible individuals with morbid obesity in the USA receive bariatric surgery [18]. Barriers often mentioned are concern both of patients and referring physicians about the risk of surgical complications and mortality, the fear of reoperations, the perceived invasiveness and irreversible nature of the intervention, limited access and difficulty in obtaining insurance and financing treatment [18–21]. The limited capacity of the healthcare system and the inability of surgeons to meet the grand demand are factors that come into play when more than the current 1% of eligible patients will apply for surgery in the near future.

Notwithstanding these treatment options, there is an intermediate group of patients who do not respond to medical therapy but are not or not yet surgical candidates. Some patients refuse surgery because of its invasiveness and fear of complications. For this group, an endoscopic treatment might look attractive [22]. The same holds true for severely obese patients with a BMI ≥40 kg/m^2, being poor surgical candidates for elective surgery such as hip replacement or organ transplantation, and for patients with a BMI ≥50 kg/m^2 being bariatric surgical candidates, as a bridge to surgery, in whom the achievement of a moderate preoperative weight loss might reduce anaesthesia risks and surgical complications and might allow to better visualise the operative field. So, endoscopic therapy, often labelled endoscopic bariatric therapy (EBT), or more recently endoscopic bariatric and metabolic therapy (EBMT), has a role to play in the treatment of obesity either as an alternative or as an adjunct to medical treatment. This has been discussed at length in many recent superb overviews [23–35]. New therapies have to be more effective and durable than lifestyle interventions alone, less invasive and risky than bariatric surgery, and easily performed at lower costs, thereby allowing improved access and application to a larger segment of the population with moderate obesity. They should be a viable and safe alternative for patients who have been unsuccessful at weight loss with diet and exercise, and should be appropriate for patients who are not suitable for, or are unwilling to undergo, a more invasive surgical procedure [34]. Emerging endoscopic bariatric therapies potentially meet these criteria [35].

The different endoscopic modalities may vary in mechanisms of action: by space occupation, delayed gastric emptying, gastric restriction and decreased distensibility, impaired gastric accommodation, stimulation of antroduodenal receptors, or duodenal exclusion and malabsorption. Vagal signalling to the hypothalamus and hormonal influences may play a role as well. Only treatments will be discussed that are covered in peer-reviewed articles. Figure 2.1 graphically summarises the different endoscopic bariatric modalities. One should realise that these developments are very costly and several companies went bankrupt. Except for intragastric balloons, duodenojejunal bypass liner and aspiration therapy, most of the other endoscopic tools are still investigational or under further development or refinement. Most of the endoscopic modalities are not reimbursed. The FDA approval process represents another challenge that any new device must navigate before becoming available for patients outside of clinical trials. To give an example: the ReShape Duo balloon applied for approval since its starting in 2007 and received it only in 2015 [36].

2.2 Endoscopic Bariatric and Metabolic Therapies

Roughly, the endoscopic bariatric and metabolic interventions can be separated into

1. Early intervention in obese patients (BMI ≥30 kg/m^2) to provide weight loss.

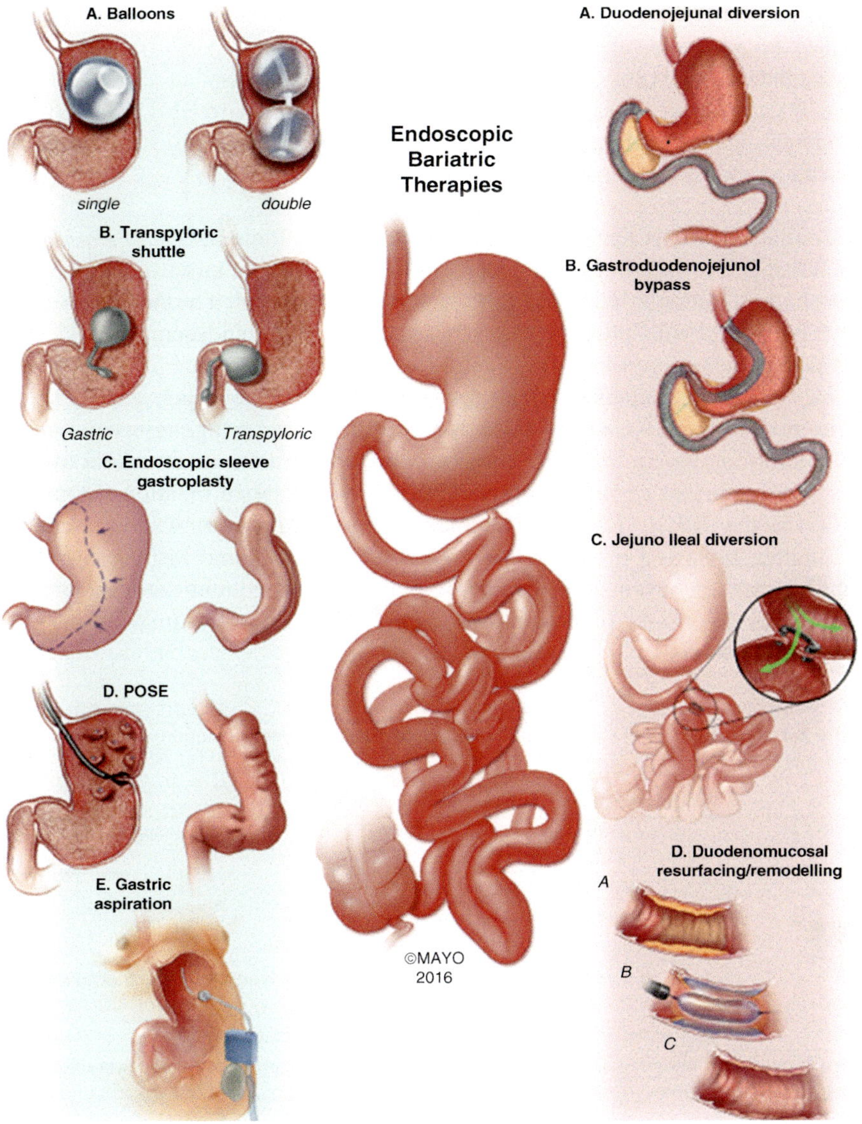

Fig. 2.1 Overview of currently used and approved endoscopic devices and devices that are under development or that apply for FDA approval. Devices are divided into those that work in the stomach (left-hand side) or those that affect the duodenum and small intestine (right-hand side) [35]. Reprinted from Gastroenterology 2017; 152: 716–729, Abu Dayyeh BK, Edmundowicz S, Thompson CC. Clinical practice update: expert review on endoscopic bariatric therapies with permission from Elsevier

2. Primary intervention in subjects eligible for surgery but who refuse surgery or have no access to surgery.
3. Secondary intervention as a bridge to elective surgery in those with BMI ≥ 40 kg/m^2 or as a bridge to bariatric surgery in those with BMI ≥ 50 kg/m^2.
4. Metabolic intervention, primarily addressing comorbid diseases such as diabetes with a modest effect on weight [37].

Contraindications have to be taken into account (Table 2.2) [22, 38, 39]. They can be related to weight loss in general or to the procedure more specifically. Each endoscopic treatment will have its own contraindications. The American Society for Gastrointestinal Endoscopy (ASGE) and the American Society for Metabolic and Bariatric Surgery (ASMBS) Task Force wrote a white paper in 2011 on endoscopic bariatric therapies in which they reviewed the requirements of such procedures as to weight loss, safety, efficacy, durability, reversibility, repeatability, costs and alteration of anatomy [39]. They recommended minimum threshold of weight loss and definitions of successful weight loss for the above-mentioned categories. In 2015, the ASGE Bariatric Endoscopy Task Force and ASGE Technology Committee reviewed the endoscopic bariatric therapies and in that same year a joint task force convened by the ASGE and the ASMBS published the thresholds in a Preservation and Incorporation of Valuable endoscopic Innovations (PIVI) document [39–41].

Table 2.2 General weight loss and more procedure-specific contraindications for endoscopic bariatric treatment [38, 54]

	Endocrine or metabolic cause of obesity
General	Severe underlying disease or ASA ≥ III (renal or hepatic insufficiency, cardiovascular disease)
	Alcoholism or drug abuse
	(Desire of) pregnancy, lactating
	Not co-operative at endoscopy
	Lack of motivation or compliance, (inadequately treated) psychiatric disease, bulimia
	Malignancy in previous 5 years (except skin cancer)
Procedure specific	Oesophageal disorders (oesophagitis grade C or D, severe candida infection, varices, dysmotility, stenosis, webs, scleroderma, Zenker's diverticulum)
	Gastric disorders (peptic ulcer, hiatal hernia >3 cm, angiodysplasia, gastric varices, gastric dysmotility, gastroparesis)
	Severe coagulopathy or need of anticoagulants
	Use of NSAIDs, aspirin, corticosteroids, or immunosuppressants
	Inflammatory disease (Crohn's disease, active *Helicobacter pylori*)
	Previous abdominal or bariatric surgery
	Unwillingness to take PPIs
	Scuba diving and travel in unpressurised airplane cabins, as well as living at high altitudes: specific for gas-filled balloons [38]
	Allergy to the material in the system
	Serotonin syndrome or the use of drugs known to affect levels of serotonin in the body (if methylene blue is used in the balloon)

The PIVI criteria were as follows [41]:

- EBT intended as a primary obesity intervention in Class II/III obese individuals (body mass index (BMI) >35 kg/m^2) should achieve a mean minimum threshold of 25% excess weight loss (% EWL) measured at 12 months. Primary obesity interventions are stand-alone interventions in combination with lifestyle modification and/or behavioural therapy to induce weight loss and improvement in obesity-associated medical comorbidities.
- In addition to the above-mentioned absolute threshold of weight loss, the mean % EWL difference between a "primary" EBT and control group should be a minimum of 15% EWL and be statistically significant.
- Five percent of the total body weight loss (5% TBWL) should represent the absolute minimum threshold for any non-primary EBT (e.g. early intervention, bridge to surgery or metabolic therapy). Bridge-to-surgery obesity intervention is an intervention to promote weight loss, specifically to reduce the risk from a subsequent intervention, including bariatric and non-bariatric surgery, such as orthopaedic, cardiovascular and organ-transplant surgeries. Patients with a BMI >50 kg/m^2 present greater technical challenges and surgical risk than less obese, healthier patients; therefore, EBTs used for this indication should perform well in higher BMI groups.
- The risk associated with EBT should equate to a ≤5% incidence of serious adverse events.
- If a low-risk EBT proves to have a significant impact on one or more obesity-related comorbidities, the threshold for intervention may extend to Class I obese individuals (BMI 30–35 kg/m^2).

ASGE Bariatric Endoscopy Task Force and ASGE Technology Committee reviewed the different EBTs against these PIVI criteria and found an adequate number of studies for a meta-analysis on the Orbera intragastric balloon (IGB) and the EndoBarrier DuodenoJejunal Bypass Sleeve (DJBS), which are discussed in the respective subchapters [41]. Newer IGB had insufficient studies for an analysis such as the ReShape Duo IGB (two studies), the Spatz3 IGB (three studies), the Silimed IGB (three studies) and the Heliosphere IGB (five studies). Also the aspiration therapy and endoscopic gastroplasty techniques had insufficient data to be included in a meta-analysis.

The American Society for Metabolic and Bariatric Surgery (ASMBS), the Society of American Gastrointestinal and Endoscopic Surgeons (SAGES) and, more recently, the American Society for Gastrointestinal Endoscopy (ASGE) and the ASMBS more specifically in the context of intragastric balloons have written position statements focused on these new procedures which are incorporated throughout this manuscript [42–46].

A very recent manuscript by Abu Dayyeh et al. had the intention to update the gastroenterologist on EBTs and to provide practice advices on how to implement them in clinical practice [35]. These Best Practice Advices are reiterated here literally because they are formulated very clear and succinct. The following advices are given:

Best Practice Advice 1	EBTs should be considered in patients with obesity who have been unsuccessful in losing or maintaining weight loss with lifestyle interventions.
Best Practice Advice 2	EBTs can be used in patients with severe obesity as a bridge to traditional bariatric surgery. They can also be used as a bridge to allow unrelated interventions that are unable to be performed because of weight limits (i.e. orthopaedic surgery, organ transplantation).
Best Practice Advice 3	Clinicians should use EBTs as part of a structured weight loss programme that includes dietary intervention, exercise therapy and behaviour modification, in both the active weight loss phase and the long-term maintenance phase.
Best Practice Advice 4	Clinicians should screen all potential EBT candidates with a comprehensive evaluation for medical conditions, comorbidities, and psychosocial or behavioural patterns that contribute to their condition before enrolling patients in a weight loss programme that includes EBTs.
Best Practice Advice 5	Clinicians incorporating EBTs into their clinical practice should follow up patients prospectively to capture the impact of the EBT programme on weight and weight-related comorbidities, and all related adverse outcomes. Poor responders should be identified and offered a detailed evaluation and alternative therapy.
Best Practice Advice 6	Clinicians embarking on incorporating EBTs into their clinical practice should have a comprehensive knowledge of the indications, contraindications, risks, benefits and outcomes of individual EBTs, as well as a practical knowledge of the risks and benefits of alternative therapies for obesity.
Best Practice Advice 7	Institutions should establish specific guidelines that are applied consistently across disciplines for granting privileges in EBTs that reflect the necessary knowledge and technical skill a clinician must achieve before being granted privileges to perform these procedures [35].

As will be discussed in Chap. 4, these advices will be easier to follow when a gastroenterologist is part of an obesity group or a bariatric team, because some of the mentioned tasks can be delegated to team members who are more experienced in certain tasks such as mentioned in Best Practice Advices three and four. Fanelli and Andrew noted that workforce readiness poses another inhibitor to adoption of EBTs, because who will do all the work [29]? Surgeons, who are experts in weight loss interventions of the present, will need to develop robust endoscopic expertise to provide these technologies in a safe and effective manner. Gastroenterologists, who are experts in endoscopic techniques, are often not involved in multidisciplinary weight loss programmes but may need to develop these relationships to responsibly care for the obese. Therefore, Fanelli and Andrew cautiously suggest that "the surgical endoscopist may very well be best positioned to aid patients in this new age of obesity intervention". However, not every country allows surgeons to perform endoscopy, certainly not in the Netherlands because of endoscopic quality measures and required volume of (emergency) endoscopies.

2.3 Gastric Endoscopic Bariatric and Metabolic Therapies

Gastric EBMTs include non-invasive devices that essentially leave the normal anatomy intact and are reversible such as space-occupying devices in the stomach (intragastric balloons) or a device that removes a portion of the calories consumed after a meal (aspiration therapy), and more invasive devices that alter the gastric anatomy to reduce gastric volume and accommodation and to delay gastric emptying (suturing and stapling). Other treatments are presented at the end of the subchapter on gastric EBMTs as they are unproven, not further developed since the last publication, or have an unknown status at this moment.

2.3.1 Non-invasive Endoscopic Bariatric and Metabolic Therapies

2.3.1.1 Intragastric Balloon Treatment

Intragastric balloons have been used for over 35 years. Although being available for three decades, intragastric balloon treatment (IGB) is not covered by the existing evidence-based guidelines. This is partly the result of ineffective and hazardous balloons in the 1980s such as the FDA-approved Garren-Edwards Gastric Bubble (GEGB, American Edwards Laboratories, Santa Ana, CA, USA) [22]. The Garren Edwards Bubble is a 220 mL IGB made from polyurethane in the shape of a cylinder and filled with air. It had a central hollow channel to permit fluid passing down and to permit an easier free movement in the stomach. However, the GEGB had sharp ridges at the place where parts were sealed together. It was approved for use in the USA by the FDA in 1985, but was removed from commercial use in 1988 due to serious complications and lack of effective weight loss [36, 47]. Deflations occurred in 31% which needed surgical interventions in 2.3%. Gastric ulcers were seen in 26% and the balloon was not tolerated in 7% [48].

With the concerns of the design, construction and integrity of previous balloons in mind, experts participating in the workshop "Obesity and the gastric balloon" formulated the fundamental requirements for an optimal balloon design in 1987 [47]. Intragastric balloons should be smooth, seamless and constructed of long-lasting material with a low ulcerogenic and obstructive potential. They should have a radiopaque marker to allow appropriate follow-up in case of deflation. There was uncertainty about the ideal shape, fill volume and fill medium, but yet a preference was expressed to have the ability to be adjusted to a variety of sizes and be filled with fluid rather than air. None of the existing balloons conformed to these requirements (Table 2.3) and this resulted in the withdrawal of balloons from the American market [22]. Many years of research finally resulted in the development of a balloon (BioEnterics Intragastric Balloon, BIB™, currently named the Orbera balloon) that fulfilled the specified requirements. Over the last 15 years the balloon market is booming (Table 2.4) with the availability of many intragastric balloons around the world [22]. Only very recently three balloons are approved by the FDA for 6-month therapy for patients with a BMI 30–40 kg/m^2 with the requirement of supportive treatment for a total of 12 months: the Orbera balloon (formerly the BioEnterics Intragastric Balloon or BIB) since 2015, the ReShape Duo balloon with the requirement of the presence of ≥1 comorbidity besides the BMI values since 2015 and the Obalon balloon since 2016.

Table 2.3 Intragastric balloons removed from the market [22]

Balloon and country	Shape	Content and fill medium
Air filled		
Garren-Edwards (USA)	Cylindrical	200–220 mL Air
Wilson-Cook (USA)	Pear	300 mL Air, connected with fill tube to the nose
Ballobes (DK)	Oval	450–500 mL Air
Fluid filled		
Dow Corning (CAN)	Disc-like	200 mL Air + 200 mL Saline
Willmen (G)	Disc-like	275–400 mL Methylcellulose
Taylor (UK)	Pear	500–550 mL Water

USA United Stated of America, *DK* Denmark, *Can* Canada, *G* Germany, *UK* United Kingdom

Table 2.4 Intragastric balloon available at present [22]

Balloon and country	Shape	Content and fill medium
Fluid filled		
Orbera intragastric balloon (IGB, formerly BIB) (USA)	Spherical	400–800 mL Saline +10 mL MB
Semistationary antral balloon (SAB) (Br)	Oval	150–180 mL Saline, 30 cm duodenal stem at caudal end with 7 g metallic counterweight
Silimed gastric balloon (SGB) (Br)	Spherical	650 mL Saline + MB, introduced alongside endoscope with snare
Spatz Adjustable Balloon System (ABS) (USA)	Spherical	400–600 mL Saline + MB, adjustable by (re)fill tube, migration-preventing anchor
MedSill (Russia)	Spherical	400–700 mL Saline + MB
ReShape Duo (USA)	Spherical	900 mL Saline in two separate balloons, connected with each other; 375 mL per balloon for patients <1.64 m (64.5 in.) in stature
Fluid and air filled		
Endball (F)	Spherical	300 mL Saline and 300 mL Air, mounted on tip of endoscope
Air filled		
Heliosphere Bag (F)	Spherical	Double-bag polymer balloon covered with a silicone envelope, 650–750 mL Air
Adjustable totally implantable intragastric prosthesis/ Endogast (ATIIP) (F)	Oval	300 mL Air, adjustable by port
Orally ingested balloons		
Air filled		
Ullrorex (USA)	Spherical	300 mL Carbon dioxide
Obalon (USA)	Spherical	300 mL Gas mixture
Fluid filled		
Elipse (USA)	Spherical	550 mL Saline

USA United Stated of America, *DK* Denmark, *Can* Canada, *G* Germany, *UK* United Kingdom, *Br* Brasil, *F* France, *MB* Methylene Blue

Intragastric balloons are endoscopically placed or swallowed, endoscopically removed or excreted rectally after planned degradation, air or saline filled, single or dual, spherical or oval, adjustable or nonadjustable, silicone or polymer balloons that are resistant to breakdown by gastric secretions (Table 2.4, Fig. 2.1) [22]. Some balloons have anti-migration characteristics.

Single Ballloons

Orbera Balloon (Formerly Bioenterics Intragastric Balloon (BIB); Apollo Endosurgery, Austin, TX, USA)

The Orbera balloon (formerly the BioEnterics Intragastric balloon (BIB)) is the most commonly used balloon. It is a spherical large-volume (500–750 mL) silicone balloon, usually filled with 500 mL saline (Table 2.4, Fig. 2.2a). Some prefer to add 10 mL of methylene blue (10 mg/mL), which is systemically absorbed from the gastrointestinal tract and excreted by the kidneys. It acts as an indicator of balloon deflation as it colours the urine green. Methylene blue is an inhibitor of monoamine oxidase (MAO) and may thus potentiate other MAO inhibitors [49]. More dangerous with even a fatality is the serotonin syndrome that may develop when drugs affecting serotonin such as serotoninergic antidepressants are used [49–51]. The syndrome is well known in cardiology where methylene blue is administered intravenously during cardiac surgery, but also cases after systemic absorption without intravenous administration are described [49–51].

Prior to positioning, an endoscopy has to be performed to rule out abnormalities that preclude insertion (Table 2.2) [52]. After removal of the endoscope the placement assembly, that consists of a sheath with the collapsed balloon and a balloon fill tube, is inserted up to 10 cm beyond the distance from incisor teeth to the gastro-oesophageal junction. Then the endoscope is reinserted into the stomach, to observe the balloon-filling and -releasing steps. With a syringe, attached to the balloon fill tube, the balloon is filled with the recommended initial volume of 500 mL saline. After filling the balloon, gentle suction by withdrawing the plunger of the syringe creates a vacuum that seals the valve. The balloon is released by a short pull at the fill tube upon which fill tube and empty placement assembly are removed [52]. The balloon should be

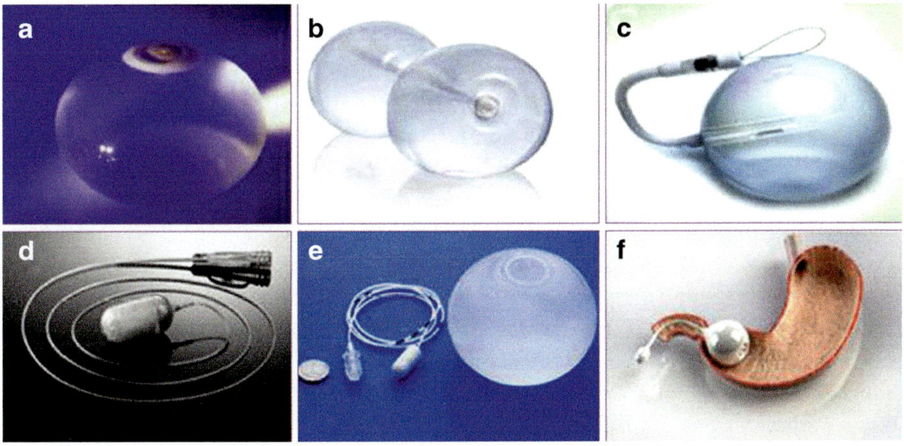

Fig. 2.2 Intragastric endoscopic balloon devices: (**a**) Orbera balloon; (**b**) ReShape Duo balloon; (**c**) Spatz adjustable balloon system; (**d**) Obalon swallowable balloon; (**e**) Elipse swallowable balloon; (**f**) transpyloric shuttle [66]. Reprinted from Clin Endosc 2017; 50: 42–66, Bazerbachi F, Vargas Valls EJ, Abu Dayyeh BK. Recent clinical results of endoscopic bariatric therapies as an obesity intervention (Open Access Article)

removed after a maximum of 6 months because beyond this period there is a higher risk of spontaneous balloon deflation. In case of balloon removal, a needle aspirator is available to puncture the balloon and to remove as much fluid as possible by suction before grasping the balloon with a snare or a two- or three-pronged grasper [52]. The endoscope and the grasped balloon are gently removed. Because of a risk of aspiration of solid food materials coated on top of the balloon, an important advice to patients is to only take clear liquids the day before balloon removal [52].

After insertion, nausea, vomiting, abdominal cramps and acid reflux are to be expected for 72 h and require aggressive treatment with anti-emetics, antispasmodics, analgesics, suppositories or acid suppressants [52]. Instructions for a 72-h post-insertion liquid diet have to be provided. Thereafter, antacids or acid-suppressing drugs are given upon request. However, most of the treating physicians prescribe proton pump inhibitors (PPIs) during the whole period of balloon treatment.

Most of the studies with the Orbera balloons were done in the era when they were named BIB. To avoid confusion, the name BIB has been replaced by the current name Orbera or the general abbreviation intragastric balloon (IGB) is used.

Efficacy and Safety

To assess efficacy and safety of the Orbera balloon three systematic reviews and one meta-analysis are available [53–56]. A Cochrane review included many studies with older balloon designs that were withdrawn from the market because of unsafety [53]. This review concluded that despite the evidence for some additional benefit of the intragastric balloon in the loss of weight, its costs should be considered against a programme of eating and behavioural modification. Two reviews and one meta-analysis discussed newly designed balloons, mainly the Orbera balloon [54–56]. Imaz et al. pooled 15 articles (3608 patients) to estimate Orbera effectiveness [56]. The estimates for weight lost at balloon removal after 6 months were 14.7 kg, 12.2% total body weight loss (TBWL), and 5.7 kg/m^2 (BMI units) or 32.1% excess weight loss (EWL). A meta-analysis of two randomised controlled trials (RCTs) which compared balloon with placebo – one in favour of the balloon and one showing no difference – estimated that patients with balloon group lost more weight than the placebo group; differences in weight loss were 6.7 kg, 1.5% TBWL, 3.2 kg/m^2 or 17.6% EWL [52, 57]. The two systematic reviews included a third RCT which showed no difference but which did not have efficacy evaluation as a primary aim [58]. Safety was assessed in 13 articles with 3442 patients on early balloon removal and 12 studies with 3429 patients on complications [56]. Early balloon removal occurred in 4.2% of cases. Nearly half of the early removals were voluntary in 1.8%, followed by abdominal pain in 0.9% and obstruction of the digestive tract in 0.6%. An overall complication rate was not given because each patient could suffer from more complications [56]. Early deflation occurred in 0.1%, gastric ulceration in 0.1%, gastric perforation in 0.2% and gastrointestinal (GI) tract obstruction in 0.6%. There were two deaths from gastric perforation, both in patients with prior gastric surgery [56]. The two systematic reviews found gastric perforations in a total of nine patients, five of whom had previous gastric surgery, an absolute contraindication for balloon positioning (Table 2.2) [54, 55]. The most feared complications are oesophageal and gastric perforation and small-bowel obstruction due to deflated balloons. Recently, Abou Hussein et al. reported three gastric perforations, two with the Spatz balloon and one with the Orbera balloon that were treated minimally invasive with combined endoscopy and laparoscopy [59]. They reviewed the literature and found 18 cases since 2003, three of them being lethal and six occurring after gastric surgery. One case of cardiac arrest after BIB placement has been described, which was thought to be secondary to vagal nerve activation caused by stretching of the gastric wall [60]. Oesophagitis has been analysed by Rossi et al. who reported oesophagitis to be present at insertion in 15% and slightly increasing up to 18% with IGB treatment [61]. Therefore, an advice to use PPIs was given. Mathus-Vliegen et al. performed pH measurements and manometry in balloon-treated patients who did not receive PPIs [62, 63]. They studied in a double-blind study two times a 13-week consecutive period. Group 1 had first a sham placement followed by verum balloon and group 2 had twice a verum balloon. The Orbera balloon was filled with 500 mL saline. Impaired lower oesophageal sphincter (LOS) function and increased gastro-oesophageal reflux were observed in one-quarter of the untreated obese subjects [63]. In group 1, weight loss ameliorated manometry and pH values, but subsequent balloon positioning tended to counteract these beneficial changes. In group 2 patients with balloon treatment from the start, the adverse effects on manometry and pH measurements by the first balloon seemed to wear off with prolonged balloon treatment [62, 63]. They ascribed the increased gastro-oesophageal reflux and oesophagitis to increased rates of LOS relaxations by the presence of a balloon with a potential involvement of cholecystokinin A receptors in their triggering [64, 65].

The ASGE Bariatric Endoscopy Task Force systematic review and meta-analysis assessed the ASGE PIVI thresholds for the Orbera balloon [41]. They reviewed the literature published between January 1988 and December 2014 and found 82 manuscripts for Orbera intragastric balloons. Three RCTs reported the % EWL over a sham or control group at balloon removal, and 17 studies reported % EWL at 12 months, which is 6 months after balloon removal. Fifty-five studies reported the percentage of total body weight loss (% TBWL) at 6 months, three reported % TBWL at 12 months, and two reported % TBWL at 36 months. Sixty-eight studies were used to calculate adverse events and early removal rates.

Based on a meta-analysis of 17 studies including 1638 patients, the % EWL with the Orbera IGB at 12 months was 25.4 and TBWL was 11.3%; this finding was associated with a high degree of heterogeneity. Three RCTs compared % EWL in patients who received the Orbera IGB (n = 131) with a sham or control group (n = 95). The mean difference in % EWL in patients who received the Orbera IGB over controls was 26.9% (95% CI, 15.6–38.2; $P < 0.001$); also this finding was associated with a high degree of heterogeneity. So, the Orbera balloon fulfilled the PIVI criteria for primary treatment of Class II/III obese individuals (BMI >35 kg/m^2) [41]. As to the criteria for non-primary/bridge therapy, the pooled % TBWL after Orbera implantation was 12.3% at 3 months, 13.2% at 6 months and 11.3% at 12 months after implantation [41]. Another criterion for the Orbera balloon to be used as non-primary obesity therapy is the need to perform sufficiently well in patients with a BMI >40 kg/m^2. A metaregression of the efficacy of the Orbera balloon over a wide range of BMIs showed its efficacy over the whole range and also in high-BMI subjects, thereby fulfilling both criteria for non-primary therapy [41]. A manual review of 68 studies rated the adverse events after placement of the Orbera balloon (Fig. 2.3). Because of accommodation of the stomach to the balloon, abdominal distension and pain, or nausea were frequent side effects, occurring in 33.7% and 29%, respectively. Gastro-oesophageal reflux disease was noticed in 18.3% and erosions in 12.0% of subjects. Early balloon removal occurred in 7.5% [41]. However, early and more aggressive use of proton pump inhibitors, antispasmodic drugs and anti-emetics in the peri- and post-procedural period may allow for a higher rate of balloon conservation [66]. Serious side effects such as balloon migration and gastric perforation were rare, with an incidence of 1.4% and 0.1%, respectively. Four out of eight (50%) gastric perforations occurred in patients who had undergone previous gastric surgeries, a from-the-outset well-known absolute contraindication (Table 2.2). Small-bowel obstruction occurred in 0.3%. Four deaths (0.08%) associated with the Orbera IGB were related to gastric perforation or pulmonary aspiration [41]. So, besides conforming to the criteria for the use as primary and non-primary treatment, the Orbera balloon also fulfilled the safety criteria.

Unfortunately, the committee did not consider the impact on one or more obesity-related comorbidities despite the fact that the safety risk of Orbera was below the threshold value of 5%. So no verdict was given upon the extension to use the Orbera balloon in class I obese individuals (BMI 30–35 kg/m²).

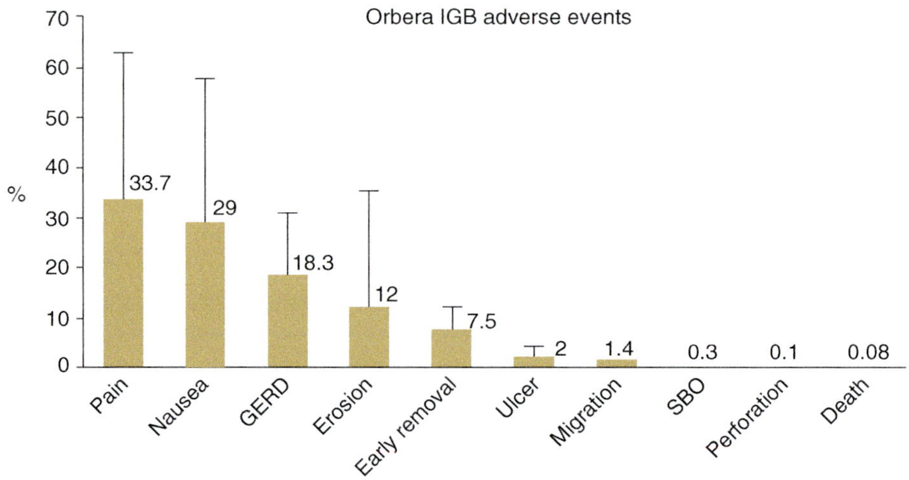

Fig. 2.3 Adverse events with the Orbera balloon as retrieved by a manual review of 68 studies [41]. Reprinted from Gastrointest Endosc 2015; 82: 425–438, ASGE Bariatric Endoscopy Task Force and ASGE Technology Committee. Abu Dayyeh BK, Kumar N, Edmundowicz SA, Jonnalagadda S, Larsen M, Sullivan S, et al. ASGE Bariatric Endoscopy Task Force systematic review and meta-analysis assessing the ASGE PIVI thresholds for adopting endoscopic bariatric therapies with permission from Elsevier

However, class I obese subjects were included in the approval of the FDA, who approved the Orbera balloon for primary treatment of obesity (BMI 30–40 kg/m^2) in August 2015, thereby, however, excluding the use as non-primary therapy for those with a BMI >40 kg/m^2, making this an off-label use of the device [67]. Also, the FDA did not approve the device for use in successive implantations.

The pivotal US trial for Orbera, a "Randomized, Multicentre Study to Evaluate the Safety and Effectiveness of the BIB IGB System as an Adjunct to a Behavioural Modification Program, in Comparison with a Behavioural Modification Program Alone in the Weight Management of Obese Subjects", known as IB-005, included 225 patients (BMI 30–40 kg/m^2) in a multicentre, prospective, randomised, non-blinded trial [68]. All participants were engaged in a 12-month behavioural modification programme, while 125 patients were randomly assigned to also have the Orbera placed for the first 6 months. At 6 months, weight loss was −3.3% of total body weight (−3.2 kg) in the lifestyle modification arm versus −10.2% (−9.9 kg) in the balloon plus lifestyle intervention arm ($P < 0.001$); at 9 months (3 months after balloon removal), weight loss was −3.4% (−3.2 kg) versus −9.1% (−8.8 kg, $P \leq 0.001$); and at 12 months, −3.1% (−2.9 kg) versus −7.6% (−7.4 kg, $P \leq 0.001$). There were two co-primary endpoints: the achievement of a ≥25% EWL and the achievement of at least 15% EWL over the mean of the control group. Both primary endpoints were achieved. IGB-treated subjects had a mean % EWL of 26.5% where the target was 25% EWL and the lifestyle-treated subjects 9.7%, and 45.6% (36.7–54.8, $P < 0.001$) of IGB-treated subjects achieved at least 15% EWL over the mean of the control group. A ≥10% total body weight loss at the time of device removal (6 months) was obtained by 46% of the IGB and 12% of the control group ($P < 0.001$). At 9 months, 3 months after balloon removal, 41% of IGB and 14% of the control group ($P < 0.001$), and at 12 months, 6 months after device removal, 32% of IGB subjects and 16% of the control group achieved ≥10% total body weight loss ($P = 0.003$). The majority of balloon subjects experienced adverse events of nausea (86.9%), vomiting (75.6%) and abdominal pain (57.5%). The balloon removal rate in 30 (18.8%) was fairly high; eight had their device removed before 6 months because of an adverse event, seven for miscellaneous reasons and 15 on subject request [68]. The rate of serious adverse events (SAEs) in the Orbera US pivotal trial was 10% ($n = 16$), with the vast majority due to hospital admissions for nausea, vomiting, abdominal pain or early device removal, anticipated as a result of the gastric accommodation to the balloon. This is twice as high as the PIVI threshold of ≤5% SAEs [41]. There were no ulcerations and no balloon deflations. Other SAEs included one case of gastric outlet obstruction with diffuse gastritis, one case of gastric perforation with sepsis, one case of aspiration pneumonia, two cases of mucosal oesophageal tears (managed endoscopically) and one case of laryngospasm. All SAEs resolved without sequelae, and there was no mortality. Baseline predictors of % TBWL loss at 12 months revealed to be the % TBWL at 3 months [68]. There were no significant improvements in comorbidities at 9 months compared with the lifestyle group. So, the FDA trial affirmed the results of the PIVI threshold criteria and allowed the Orbera for use as primary treatment in adults with a BMI of 30–40 kg/m^2 for the duration of 6 months [68]. The FDA requires a comprehensive 12-month weight management programme to be employed with Orbera placement.

Predictors of Weight Loss

Several studies investigated factors predicting a greater weight loss, and apart from the already mentioned % TBWL at 3 months the weight loss in the first month, initial BMI, female gender, adherence to the dietary programme, allocation to balloon treatment and guess, correctly or not, of having a balloon in the double-blind studies, and changes in gastric emptying induced by the balloon predicted a greater weight loss [52, 68–70]. There was no influence of balloon fill volume or balloon location [52]. The influence of fill volume was again studied in a very recent meta-analysis of 44 studies, including 5549 patients [71]. A meta-regression showed no statistically significant association between filling volume and % TBWL at 6 months. When the BMI was investigated in BMI strata, only BMI 40–50 kg/m^2 demonstrated a small significant correlation between fill volume and weight loss. There was a statistically significant, but clinically irrelevant, increase of 0.5% TBWL per 100 mL balloon fill volume ($P = 0.03$). The authors explained the lack of fill volume effect by their observation of the relationship between change in size and change in volume; the diameter of a 400 mL balloon is 9.14 cm, while a 700 mL balloon is only 20% wider at 11.0 cm [71]. Yet, they found an important effect of balloon volume <600 mL versus higher volumes and therefore recommended a 600 mL fill volume; the rate of oesophagitis of 2.4% and the rate of migration of 0.5% were both less with balloons >600 mL versus 9.4% and 2.3%, respectively, with balloons <600 mL [71].

Binge-eating is not always a contraindication but at least it is a predictor of poor results [72].

Improvement of Comorbidities

Weight loss with the BIB resulted in improvement of metabolic abnormalities in serum levels of glucose, insulin, LDL cholesterol, total cholesterol and triglycerides [52]. Other studies demonstrated improvement in liver dysfunction and liver steatosis, insulin sensitivity, diabetes and serum HbA1c, metabolic syndrome, fertility, plasma total antioxidant capacity and obstructive sleep apnoea syndrome and a significant improvement of the quality of life [52, 58, 73–79]. In one centre in Spain, 714 consecutive patients treated with an Orbera IGB in 2005–2007 had a mean BMI loss of 6.5 kg/m^2 after 6 months [80]. The overall complication rate was 4.1%. Comorbidities were resolved in 64 (40%) of the 162 patients with one or more diagnosed comorbidities before start of the treatment [80]. Genco et al. demonstrated in 2515 Italian patients with a BMI of 44.8 kg/m^2 an % EWL of 33.9% or a BMI decrease of 4.9 kg/m^2 with only 0.08% failed balloon insertions [81]. Preoperative comorbidities were present in 56.4% of patients and these resolved in 44.3% of cases and improved in a further 44.8%. Resolution or improvement occurred in 87.2% of the 488 patients suffering from diabetes, in 93.7% in patients with hypertension, 100% in patients with respiratory disorders and 87% in patients with osteoarthritis. Dyslipidaemia resolved or improved in 51.9% [81].

Course of Body Weight and Prevalence of Comorbidities After Balloon Removal
One of the major drawbacks is the limited duration of therapy for only 6 months and weight regain after balloon removal. In the meta-analysis by Imaz et al. two studies provided data on maintenance of weight loss after 1 year of treatment [56]. The 143 patients included in these studies lost a mean of 15.9 kg at balloon removal; 133 patients were followed 1 year after balloon removal and had recovered 6.3 kg, representing 39.6% of the weight lost at removal. Hervé et al. detailed that still 56% had ≥20% EWL at 1 year and Mathus-Vliegen and Tytgat reported that 47% of patients still had ≥10% weight loss 1 year after removal of the balloons after a 1-year active balloon treatment episode, suggesting that some proportion of the weight loss can be maintained for 24 months [52, 82].

Dastis et al. followed a cohort of 100 patients who had received an IGB for 6 months over a period of 2.5 years without a structural weight maintenance programme after balloon removal [83]. Ninety-eight patients completed final follow-up at a mean of 4.8 years. With the IGB they lost 12.6 kg or 38.3% EWL and 63 had a ≥10% body weight loss. After 1 and 2 years of follow-up they had regained 4.2 kg and 2.3 kg or 37% of the lost weight, and ≥10% weight loss was present in 57% and 38%, respectively. After a mean of 4.8 years, 28% had lost ≥10% weight at final follow-up, 35 patients had undergone bariatric surgery and 34 had no significant weight change from baseline. Kotzampassi et al. followed 474 patients after a 6-month balloon positioning [84]. Average BMI before therapy was 43.7 kg/m^2. Success was defined as ≥20% EWL; 83% attained this successful weight loss with an average loss of 23.9 kg and a BMI loss of 8.3 kg/m^2. Out of 395 successful subjects 53%, 27% and 23% maintained a ≥20% EWL after 12, 24 and 60 months, respectively. After 5 years, an % EWL of 17% and a TBWL of 9 kg were observed [84].

The ORBERA pivotal study showed a 7.6% TBWL 26 weeks after balloon removal (12 months after balloon placement) and the AGSE meta-analysis a 11.7% TBWL 18 months after IGB placement [41, 68]. A review to assess the kinetics of weight loss during and after Orbera balloon therapy and the timing of serious adverse events included seven studies that reported weight losses at 3 and 6 months, with two studies reporting body weights monthly [85]. In seven studies, the average weight loss after 3 and 6 months of Orbera balloon therapy was 12.9 kg and 16.0 kg, respectively, indicating that 80% of the weight loss achieved in 6 months of Orbera balloon therapy occurs within the first 3 months. Two studies (253 patients) reported the timing of adverse events related to malfunction and leaking of the Orbera balloon. In one study 49 of the 51 balloons leaked beyond the recommended removal date of 6 months, whereas two occurred before that date [86]. Only two caused a partial large-bowel obstruction and were removed, once by using colonoscopy and once by laparoscopy. The other study reported 15 balloons that leaked: seven occurred in the first 4 months of Orbera balloon therapy, whereas eight occurred after 4 months of therapy [87]. All balloons passed per vias naturales. Nine studies with 547 patients reported weight losses 6 and 12 months after removal and demonstrated a sustained weight loss of 95% and 52%, respectively, of the weight lost during IGB treatment [85]. Similarly, 3 cohorts with 572 patients reported weight losses at 12 months after balloon removal and 43–68% of the weight loss was sustained [84, 88, 89].

Besides the weight loss obtained and maintained thereafter, the effects on obesity-associated comorbidity and its sustainment are even more important.

Crea et al. followed 143 patients for 1 year after balloon removal [88]. They had lost 6.6 BMI points, 14.1% of total body weight and 29.3% of excess weight at balloon removal. After 12 months these figures were 4.2 kg/m², 11.2% TBWL and 26.1% EWL. The prevalence of diabetes, hypercholesterolaemia, hypertriglyceridaemia and hypertension decreased during balloon treatment from 32.6%, 33.4%, 37.7% and 44.9% to 20.9%, 16.7%, 14.5% and 30.4%, respectively, but increased very modestly in the balloon-free year to 21.3%, 18.9%, 17.4% and 34.8%, respectively (Fig. 2.4). The metabolic syndrome kept on declining from 34.8% to 14.5% over the 1.5 years, and the 11.6% maintenance of at least 10% body weight loss was associated with these improvements which agrees with the guideline advices, mentioned before, of obtaining and maintaining a 10% body weight loss [1, 5, 88]. A 3-year follow-up of 261 overweight patients with a BMI of 27–30 kg/m² (mean 28.6 kg/m²) with at least one comorbidity, which could be evaluated from the original group of 349 subjects treated in a multicentre European study, showed that the reported excess weight loss of 55.6% at 6 months was fairly good maintained with a 29.1% EWL at 3 years [90]. Mean %BMI loss was 11.5% and 6.1% at 6 months and 3-year follow-up, respectively. Forty (15%) patients had post-IGB surgery; 172 (66%) patients followed a dietician's plan after removal of the intragastric balloon. The rate of hypertension decreased from 29% at the start to 16% after 3 years, diabetes from 15 to 10%, hyperlipidaemia from 32 to 21% and osteoarthritis from 25 to 13% at 3 years [90]. Even

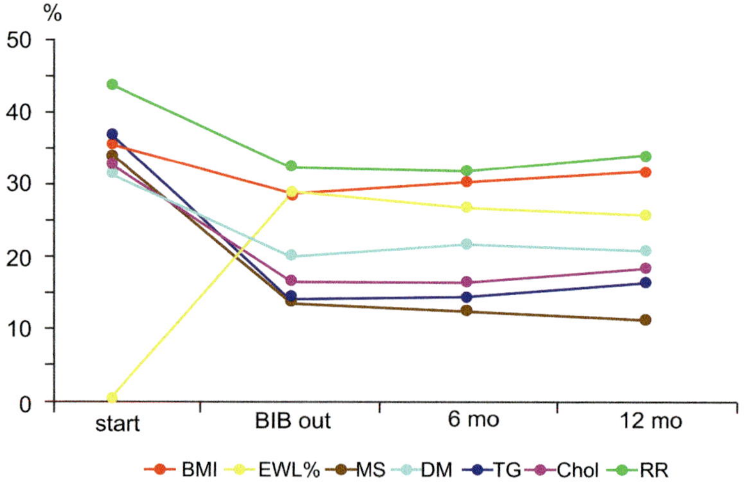

Fig. 2.4 Results obtained 1 year after balloon removal and persistence of effects on body weight and obesity-associated comorbidities [88]. *BMI* body mass index, *EWL* excess weight loss, *MS* metabolic syndrome, *DM* type 2 diabetes mellitus, *TG* hypertriglyceridaemia, *Chol* hypercholesterolaemia, *RR* hypertension

more impressive and clinically very relevant are their 6-year follow-up data of 83 patients who asked for a second or even third or fourth balloon [91]. The "weight cycling" or "yo-yo dieting", a pattern of alternating phases of dieting and relapse, has been the subject of several studies suggesting that increased risks of morbidity and mortality may be associated with fluctuations in weight, although contested by others [92–96]. It is certainly a matter of public concern. Despite their "weight cycling" or "yo-yo dieting", the percentage of comorbidities that resolved or improved at follow-up was 73% for diabetes, 65% for hypertension and 89% for the obstructive sleep apnoea syndrome (OSAS) [91]. No worsened comorbidities were present after 6 years. A significant difference was recorded in the presence of comorbidities at baseline (80% of the patients) and follow-up after 72 months (30%; $P = 0.02$). So, as the authors stated: "Yo-yo dieting may be better than not dieting at all" [91].

Special Subgroups

Special subgroups are important to consider as the FDA approved the Orbera IGB for subjects with a BMI between 30 and 40 kg/m^2 and the PIVI review indicated that the Orbera IGB met both the criteria for primary as well as non-primary treatment [41, 67]. This subgroup analysis is also important as it gives information on patients, usually excluded from studies because of contraindications.

Super-Obese (BMI ≥50 kg/m^2) and Super-Super-Obese (BMI ≥60 kg/m^2) Subjects

Laparoscopic surgery in extremely obese patients is technically complex due to technical limitations of instrument length and reduced ability to reach the angle of His [97]. Large fatty omental tissue is often an obstacle in visualising the stomach and technical difficulties are due to markedly thickened abdominal walls hindering fine laparoscopic movements and control of laparoscopic instruments. Huge ponderous fatty livers are not well retracted by laparoscopic retractors and may result in poor exposure and increased susceptibility to injury. It is honest to say that some surgeons consider such statements exaggerated. The IGB may be used to bridge the time until surgery and to reduce the surgical complications as has been shown by modest proportions of preoperative weight boss (10–20% EWL or 5% weight loss) [98, 99]. Patients with a BMI >60 kg/m^2 obtained a 20–30% EWL with a preoperative balloon [100]. Busetto et al. performed a case-control study (N = 43/43) and showed a lower conversion rate, shorter operative time and hospital stay, and a lower rate of band-related and port-related complications after laparoscopic gastric banding after a preoperative 26.1% EWL in balloon-treated patients [101]. In the first phase of weight loss a preferential reduction of visceral fat and a reduction of liver volume are seen, explaining these beneficial results. Frutos et al. showed a 31.8% reduction in liver volume after 6 weeks of IGB therapy [102]. The reduction in liver volume facilitated subsequent laparoscopic gastric bypass [102]. The metabolic effects of 6 months of Orbera balloon placement and a 1000–1200 kcal diet were examined in detail in a prospective trial including 130 patients (average BMI 43.1 kg/m^2) [76]. Premature balloon removal was required in ten patients due to intolerance, abdominal pain or vomiting. The average weight loss of 13.1 kg was associated with a decrease of hyperglycaemia from 50% to 12%, and hypertriglyceridaemia from 58% to 19%. In patients with a decrease in BMI of greater than 3.5 kg/m^2 a significant and important decrease in the prevalence of severe hepatic steatosis from 52% to 4% was observed [76]. A larger study in 60 consecutive super-super-obese subjects with an average BMI of 66.5 kg/m^2 studied the utility of a balloon as a bridge to gastric bypass [103]. The balloon was placed in 23 patients and remained for a mean of 155 days, while 37 patients went to surgery without prior balloon therapy. The balloon group achieved BMI loss of 5.5 kg/m^2 at the time of the gastric bypass. This resulted in a 55-min shorter operation time and in fewer major adverse events (defined as conversion to laparotomy, ICU stay longer than 2 days and total hospital stay longer 2 weeks): two events versus thirteen events in patients who did not have balloon placement [103]. The effect of BIB on obstructive sleep apnoea has been specifically studied because it poses challenges to the anaesthesiologist during the perioperative period and a nearly complete resolution of sleep apnoea was reported in 17 very obese men (BMI 55.8 kg/m^2) [104]. Spyropoulos et al. treated 26 high-risk super-super-obese patients with a BMI of 65.3 kg/m^2 and at least three comorbidities, who were refused for surgery [105]. One death was related to cardiac arrest after aspiration related to the positioning of the balloon. They lost 22.4% excess weight after 6 months and improved their diabetes and hypertension in 81% and 83%, respectively. From the group of 25 patients 20 became fit enough for bariatric surgery and underwent their operation the day after balloon removal [105]. A systematic review by Yorke et al. which captured studies that reflected the use of IGB only for bariatric specific weight loss, showed a 15.7 kg, 5.9 kg/m^2 and 36.2% EWL before surgery but did not comment on outcomes of subsequent surgery [106].

Coffin et al. disagreed with the salutary influence of balloon-induced weight loss on subsequent bariatric surgery [107]. They performed a prospective randomised multicentre study to compare the impact of a preoperative 6-month intragastric balloon treatment with standard medical care (SMC) in super-obese patients before undergoing laparoscopic gastric bypass [107]. The primary endpoint was the proportion of patients requiring a stay at the intensive care for >24 h and secondary endpoints were weight change, operation time, duration of hospital stay and perioperative complications. The authors calculated a need of randomisation of 314 patients (157 in each group). Due to insufficient enrolment the study had to be interrupted after the inclusion of only 115 patients (BMI 54.3 kg/m^2), of whom 55 had a balloon placement. The proportion of patients who stayed in ICU >24 h was similar in both groups, mean operation time was similar and both groups had a similar hospitalisation stay. At 6 months before the operation, the weight loss in BMI units was significantly greater in the IGB group (2.8 kg/m^2) than in the SMC group (0.4 kg/m^2), and the weight loss occurred mainly in the first 3 months. However, in the end, already at 6 months post-operatively the weight loss was not different anymore. Three severe complications occurred during IGB removal. Five patients had one or more surgical complications, all in the IGB group. Although conclusions may be not well founded because of insufficient numbers, the authors concluded that it is true that IGB insertion before gastric bypass induced weight loss but it did not improve the perioperative outcomes or affect post-operative weight loss.

Some surgeons also warn against balloon therapy prior to surgery. Jones et al. reported a complicated case with stenosis on the second post-operative day after a sleeve gastrectomy, in whom balloon dilation to 18 mm failed to relieve the stenosis and necessitated stent therapy on day 4 [108]. This super-obese patient was treated preoperatively with an intragastric balloon and because the authors had observed that intragastric balloons induced a thickening of the stomach their policy was to wait for an interval of minimally 2 weeks after balloon removal to allow the stomach tissues to decrease in thickness before the operation. This patient refused to wait and therefore the balloon was removed under the same anaesthesia as needed for the sleeve gastrectomy. The first firing with the green staple cartridge failed to close the stomach wall. The procedure was completed using hand-sewn sutures, with a midline laparotomy. They believe that failure of the staple line results from the excessive thickness of the antral stomach where most surgeons would use a green cartridge to initiate the sleeve [108]. The thickness of the stomach wall in this area corresponded to the lower end of the greater curvature of the stomach where the intragastric balloon was seen at endoscopy [108]. Although surgeons often express their fears of either a thickened or a decompensated gastric wall after balloon therapy, a search in the literature did not result in any report on this matter. Two studies examined the removal of balloons in the same setting as surgery [109, 110]. De Goederen–van der Mey et al. removed the balloon at the operation room and proceeded thereafter with a gastric band positioning by laparoscopy without difficulties [109]. Khan et al. investigated 40 consecutive super-super-obese subjects with a BMI 69.3 kg/m^2 which decreased to 62.3 kg/m^2 after 6-month balloon therapy [110]. In an attempt to reduce the number of interventions for these high-risk patients, they decided to offer simultaneous single-stage balloon removal and laparoscopic sleeve gastrectomy to all super-super-obese patients. The only contraindication to proceeding to surgery was the presence of active gastric ulceration. Simultaneous balloon removal and sleeve gastrectomy were achieved in 39 cases; one patient refused surgery. There was no operative mortality, there were no leaks and their new policy appeared safe [110].

IGB as a First Step Towards Bariatric Surgery

The potential role of the IGBs as a psychological bridge to surgery is a matter of debate [73, 89]. Angrisani et al. reported the almost total regain of excess weight 1 year after Orbera balloon removal in patients who had refused any other kind of treatment [89]. On the contrary, IGB therapy facilitated the acceptance of bariatric surgery in 32% of 140 patients who had initially refused surgery but accepted balloon therapy [73]. Bariatric surgery was most frequent in the group that had successfully lost weight with the IGB but then started to regain weight (64%). It was mixed in the group (33%) who had not lost weight and very low (7%) in those who had maintained a successful weight loss during follow-up [73]. Also, Genco et al. demonstrated that in a group of 83 patients who refused surgery and who were offered active guidance with repeat balloon positioning when indicated, 18 patients (22%) requested bariatric surgery after a mean interval of 47.7 months (range 12–72) [91]. They underwent laparoscopic gastric banding (2), laparoscopic gastric bypass (6) and laparoscopic sleeve gastrectomy (10).

Testing of Patient's Eligibility for a Restrictive Surgical Operation: The "BIB Test"

Another potential use is to predict how well a patient will respond to a purely restrictive bariatric procedure; those that lose a significant amount of weight with the Orbera balloon (BioEnterics Intragastric Balloon (BIB), therefore the usual term "BIB test") would, in theory, respond better to surgical procedures that involve gastric volume reduction instead of intestinal bypass [111]. Some surgeons use the balloon as a predictive instrument to single out subjects who would not benefit from gastric restrictive surgery (sweet eaters, snackers, grazers, compulsive eaters and binge-eaters). A BIB test is positive when >10 kg weight is lost with the Orbera balloon. Loffredo et al. tested whether patients with a positive BIB test appeared eligible for a restrictive procedure or when the BIB test is negative a malabsorption procedure had to be considered [87]. Indeed, following a previously positive BIB procedure a significant further weight loss for more than 6 months after laparoscopic gastric banding (LAGB) was reported. De Goederen-van der Meij et al. tested this prospectively in 40 patients who underwent Orbera IGB therapy for 6 months followed by laparoscopic adjustable gastric banding [109]. Successful treatments were defined as ≥10% baseline weight loss with the balloon and a further weight loss of ≥15% with surgery. They found that the BIB test had a mixed predictive value for further weight loss with gastric banding (positive and negative predictive values of 56% and 73%, respectively). The final weight loss was higher in patients with successful versus unsuccessful IGB therapy (12.4 vs. 9.0 kg/m^2 at 18 months, respectively, $P < 0.05$). Genco et al. divided 1357 patients in a successful IGB group A (≥25% EWL, $n = 699$) and in a less successful IGB group B (<25% EWL, $n = 658$) [112]. During subsequent surgery there were significant differences between group A and B: group B had longer mean operation time, more complications, more often difficult anatomy, more perioperative bleedings, more conversion and lengthier hospital stay. After 1, 3 and 5 years the differences in BMI and % EWL observed at the time of balloon removal persisted, and patients with good results after intragastric balloon treatment gain an advantage in terms of BMI and % EWL in the short and medium terms [112].

Consecutive Balloons

The restricted duration of therapy, i.e. 6 months, the main limitation of the treatment, might be overcome by successive balloons. Dumonceau et al. studied 118 patients treated with an IGB in a prospective non-randomised study over a period of 5 years [113]. Nineteen patients (16%) asked for a repeat IGB to prolong their first treatment ($n = 8$) or after a balloon-free interval of 16.4 months ($n = 11$) in which they regained 13.6 kg on average. The repeat balloon fill was 100 mL greater than the initial fill. Compared with subjects with a single treatment ($n = 99$), those with repeat treatment ($n = 19$) had greater weight loss in kilograms at 1 year (12.0 kg vs. 6.0 kg) and in excess weight loss (40.9% vs. 20.8% EWL; $P < 0.008$), but the difference became less than 2 kg starting at 3 years and the effect of a second balloon placement dissipated by the third year of follow-up [113]. They lost less weight with the second balloon (9.0 kg vs. 14.6 kg, or 18.2% EWL vs. 49.3% EWL) when compared with the first balloon, and had a trend towards more complications.

Dumonceau et al. found this strategy of repeating balloon therapy disappointing, as 3 years after removal of the first balloon weight loss curves and proportions of subjects with ≥10% baseline weight loss were almost identical for subjects treated with a single or repeat balloon [113]. Lopez-Nava et al. studied 714 patients who underwent IGB placement: 112 had a second IGB placement after an interval of 1 month [80]. A second balloon could be positioned without difficulties and after a second balloon patients continued to lose weight though not at the same rate as with the first balloon, an average BMI loss of 2.5 kg/m^2 with the second balloon in addition to BMI loss of 6.5 kg/m^2 with the first balloon. Genco et al. randomised patients to two groups: IGB for 6 months followed by diet therapy for 7 months (group A, $n = 50$) and IGB for 6 months followed by a second balloon after 1 month, for again 6 months (group B, $n = 50$) [114]. The 1-month period between the two balloons was to allow the stomach to restore to pre-IGB placement conditions and to reset the normal motility of the stomach before repeating therapy to provide further weight loss. In that intermediate month, both groups gained 0.9 BMI units in weight. After removal of the first balloon weight loss parameters were not different: % EWL 43.5 and 45.2 and BMI 34.2 and 34.8 kg/m^2, respectively, for group A and group B [114]. At the end of the13-month study, weight loss parameters were significantly more beneficial in patients who underwent consecutive balloons in group B: BMI 30.9 kg/m^2 and % EWL 51.9% versus 35.9 kg/m^2 and 25.1% in group A [114]. A second balloon achieved good results with continuing weight loss. A similar investigation by the same group was done in 50 patients with eating disorders not otherwise specified (EDNOS) [115]. At the end of 6-month balloon treatment, the BMI in both groups decreased with 8 kg/m^2. The eating scores did not differ at the outset and decreased to a similar extent in groups A and B. At the end of 13 months BMI was significantly more reduced in group B by 11.9 kg/m^2 versus 7.5 kg/m^2 in group A [115]. Also, the consecutive balloon positioning in group B significantly reduced scores for grazing, emotional eating, after-dinner grazing and sweet eating when compared with group A. Two consecutive balloons demonstrated significant advantage over a single procedure in terms of influencing EDNOS [115]. One of the longest term studies was performed in the Netherlands in 2005 [52]. Forty-three patients were enrolled in 2-year study. Patients in group 1 had an Orbera balloon placed for an initial 3 months followed by replacement at 3-month intervals for three more occurrences (12 months total and four balloons). Group 2 had an initial sham procedure followed by balloon placement every 3 months for three occurrences (12 months total and three balloons). Both groups were subsequently followed up for a second year to assess weight loss maintenance. Although more than 40% of patients achieved greater than 20% total body weight loss in group 1 (four balloons) at 1 year, this was similar to group 2 (three balloons). At 2 years, 60% of the weight loss was maintained [52]. The IGB does seem to have a legacy effect for up to a year with some persistent weight loss (perhaps due to changed dietary habits and behaviour), so repeated therapy may become the most common paradigm for this device to maintain a long-term effect.

A very long-term study with follow-up of 6 years was published by Genco et al. [91]. Eighty-three patients with a BMI >40 kg/m^2, good candidates for surgery but refusing it, were enrolled in a clinical treatment protocol allowing multiple intragastric balloon placements. The protocol was such that a second balloon was placed when the patients had regained ≥50% of the weight loss achieved with the previous balloon. After the first balloon removal, patients were encouraged to maintain the weight by physical exercise, diet and, if needed, psychological support. A dietician was involved who gave a specific low-calorie diet to all. With their first balloon patients decreased in weight from a BMI of 43.7 to a BMI of 35.9 kg/m^2. Every patient asked for a second balloon placement after a mean of 12 months (range 1–55); 18 patients (22%) had a third device placed and 1 (1.2%) patient had a fourth device placed. Although they initially refused surgery, after a mean interval of 47.7 months (range 12–72), 18 patients (22%) requested and underwent bariatric surgery. Only three patients were lost to follow-up (4.1%). After the first balloon treatment, their BMI went up from 35.9 kg/m^2 to 37.9 kg/m^2, and at the end of second IGB treatment, mean BMI was again down to 34.8 kg/m^2. At 76-month follow-up, mean BMI was 37.6 kg/m^2. Apart from the earlier mentioned significant improvement in comorbidity despite this weight cycling or yo-yo dieting, they also experienced a far better quality of life [91]. Obesity is a chronic disease and the authors showed that physicians must be prepared to provide long-term guidance and treatment and the authors must be congratulated for doing so. It would have been nice to have a cost-benefit analysis of such an approach.

Miscellaneous Indications

There are some subgroups that should have been excluded based on the exclusion criteria but were examined to justify these criteria.

(a) Eating disorders: Apart from the above-mentioned study in eating disorders by Genco et al. [91], Puglisi et al. investigated the effect of treatment in patients presenting with binge-eating disorders (BED) [72]. The degree of BMI reduction was significantly less in BED patients (3.3 vs. 5.7 kg/m^2), the BED group requested more often early balloon removal and complications and failure were statistically higher than in the non-BED group, suggesting that the presence of binge-eating disorder is a negative predictive factor for treatment success.

(b) Depressed patients: Often, depressed patients are excluded from pharmaceutical trials and sometimes also do not pass the psychological screening before bariatric surgery. Many antidepressants are associated with weight gain [5]. Therefore, the study by Deliopoupou et al. was urgently needed [116]. A hundred consecutive female patients, characterised as depressed (65 patients) or non-depressed (35 patients) using the Beck Depression Inventory score, were treated with Orbera balloons. The weight loss was similar between groups (39.3% EWL in depressed patients vs. 36.1% EWL in non-depressed patients) and the Beck Depression Inventory score improved from 20.3 to 7.9 during balloon therapy. Resolution of depression occurred in 70.8% of the depressed patients, with a decrease in the prevalence of severe depression (from 27.7% to 1.5%), so demonstrating significant mental health benefits and refuting the customary exclusion of depressed patients.

(c) Overweight subjects (BMI 27–30 kg/m^2) with at least one comorbidity: A retrospective study in 261 subjects showed a decrease in BMI from 28.6 to 25.4 kg/m^2 after 6 months, which after 3 years was still lower than at the start (BMI 27.0 kg/m^2) [90]. Psychological disorders decreased from 54 to 13% at 6 months. The proportions of patients with diabetes, hypertension, dyslipidaemia and osteoarthritis were all reduced to one-third and one-half. The finding that many patients maintained the weight loss achieved by the 6-month balloon treatment in the medium term (3 years) suggests that intragastric balloon therapy can be used, in combination with other treatments, as part of a strategy for preventing the progression of overweight to obesity. It may well be that disordered alimentary behaviours and comorbidities are not as deeply rooted in overweight patients as in obese patients and that these may have greater potential for reversal.

Combined Treatments

Though sibutramine (a centrally acting serotonin-norepinephrine reuptake inhibitor) has been withdrawn from the market due to increased risk for cardiovascular events, the addition of sibutramine has been shown to augment the weight loss effects of IGB, providing a rationale for additive benefits of pharmacotherapy in conjunction with IGBs [117, 118]. Dargent et al. investigated the four-quadrant injection of hyaluronic acid, an absorbable filling agent similar to collagen, which is genetically bioengineered, non-allergenic and currently widely used in cosmetic surgery, at the gastro-oesophageal junction as an adjunct treatment before or after balloon placement and compared this with a balloon-only group [119]. A combined treatment was significantly more effective than single-balloon treatment (at 18 months a BMI loss of 2.8 BMI units vs. 1 BMI units, $P < 0.05$). The treatment that started with hyaluronic acid was inferior to the two groups that started with balloons (balloon-only group or balloon followed by hyaluronic acid after 6 months). Injection of hyaluronic acid after an intragastric balloon, which seemed to be the preferential order, was hampered by food stasis on top of the balloon and at the gastro-oesophageal junction and resulted in a liver abscess in one patient. Dargent et al. did not recommend to add hyaluronic acid to the treatment with balloons [119].

Comparison with Surgery

Orbera balloons have been compared with controls, receiving either no therapy or sham treatment or some form of lifestyle intervention with a diet, exercise, behavioural therapy or a combination of these. It might be interesting to see how they perform when comparing with surgery. There are two retrospective studies comparing IGBs with sleeve gastrectomy and one prospective study [120–122]. Peker et al. compared prospectively 1 year of IGBs (so two connected periods of 6-month balloon treatment, $n = 16$) with 1 year of laparoscopic adjustable gastric banding (LAGB, $n = 16$) [120]. Although the % EWL (39.3% vs. 32.3%) and % excess BMI loss (% EBMIL) (47.1% vs. 36.3%) after the first 6 months were more encouraging in the IGB patients compared with LAGB patients, it was not statistically significant. But at the 12-month period, when the IGB treatment is completed, the % EWL (57%) and % EBMIL (70%) were significantly higher in favour of the IGB group ($P = 0.023$, and $P = 0.011$, respectively). They reported no complications in either group over the 12-month treatment period [120]. The authors suggested that two consecutive IGB applications may be offered to obese patients who do not feel ready for surgery. After 18 months, when the continuous effect of LAGB on food intake restriction continued and the IGB group did not have any restricting device, the % EWL and % EBMIL parameters were similar for LAGB and IGB [120]. So, consecutive IGB applications are feasible and apparently more efficient for weight loss, at least in their hands, in comparison to the LAGB at the 12-month period.

The two retrospective studies compared sleeve gastrectomy with IGB. Milone et al. compared their own 20 patients with a sleeve gastrectomy (SG) in the USA with 57 patients as a historical group who had their balloons placed in Germany and Italy [121]. There were no complications for patients undergoing the SG. For patients undergoing IGB, four patients (7%) had the balloon removed due to intolerance. Body weight loss was significantly better for the sleeve group with 45.5 versus 22.3 kg, 35% versus 24% EWL and change in BMI with 16 versus 8 BMI units. Weight loss decreased comorbidities in 90% of patients after both procedures. Milone et al. suggested that sleeve gastrectomy may be a superior procedure compared with IGB as a first stage for super-obesity [121]. In their clinic, treatment for super-obese subjects ≥60 kg/m^2 consists of an initial sleeve gastrectomy, followed 6–12 months later by a definitive biliopancreatic diversion with duodenal switch, and this study did not change their practice. Genco et al. compared data from their own department and performed a case-control study with two IGB cases for one sleeve gastrectomy case [122]. Mortality, intra- and post-operative complications in SG group, and complications during endoscopy and in the 6 months thereafter in IGB group were absent. BMI at baseline was 54.1 kg/m^2 and 54.8 kg/m^2 in IGB and SG patients, respectively (NS). At 6-month follow-up, mean BMI was 46.2 kg/m^2 and 45.3 kg/m^2 in the BIB and SG patients, respectively (NS). After 12 months, IGB patients were 6 months without a balloon and had to comply with a strict diet regimen and regained weight, while SG patients continued to lose weight. Despite this, at 12-month follow-up, the mean BMI was still not significantly different with 48.1 kg/m^2 and 43.1 kg/m^2 in BIB and SG groups [122]. So, BMI values were not different and also there were no significant differences between the groups as far as comorbidities are considered. Both groups had a similar failure rate: 2/40 SG and 4/80 IGB patients did not achieve a weight loss ≥10% TBWL. In contrast to Milone, Genco et al. concluded that laparoscopic sleeve gastrectomy and intragastric balloon are both valid options for producing weight loss as a first-step procedure in super-obese subjects [122].

Other Intragastric Balloon Types

Spatz Adjustable Balloon System (ABS) (Spatz FGIA Inc., Great Neck, NY, USA)

The Spatz Adjustable Balloon System (ABS) is a spherical silicone balloon filled with 400–800 mL saline with an anchor to prevent migration and a filling tube

(Table 2.4, Fig. 2.2c). One of its key advantages is the ability to adjust the balloon volume, tailoring it to the tolerance of the patient with a decrease in volume in case of intolerance, and to the weight loss with an increase in volume in case of regain of appetite or halting of weight loss. For placement the sheath containing the balloon is fixed with a releasable rubber tape on the tip of the endoscope which ruptures upon balloon inflation. Also removal is by endoscopy. The balloon is adjustable by extracting outwards the fill tube by endoscopy. It is allowed to stay for 12 months. Weight losses are comparable to or slightly better than with the Orbera balloon, although RCTs are missing. In a case-control study, twice as many Orbera IGB subjects who received two balloons to cover the 12-month period were compared with subjects having the ABS for 12 months [123]. At the end of the study weight loss parameters were similar (EWL 55.6% vs. 56.7%, respectively, for Orbera and Spatz balloons). Complications were more frequent in the ABS group in 7 out of 40 (14.5%) of whom 6 needed balloon removal [123]. These complications consisted of migration (4), anchor system rupture (1), deflation (1) and an asymptomatic ulcer (1). In the Orbera IGB there were two complications of intolerance (2/80, 2.5%) [123]. The two open studies which reported on 91 subjects showed a 45.0–48.8% EWL at 52 weeks [124, 125]. Adjustments for intolerance were needed in 17.6% and for weight gain or stabilisation in 67%. Intolerance and physical problems were encountered in 10 (11%) and balloon- or tube-related problems in 11 (12.1%) patients; a total of 5 (5.5%) needed surgery. These previous generations of Spatz adjustable balloons had significant weight losses of up to 20% TBWL over 12 months, but had complications related to the design of the device. The Spatz 3 is the most recent generation of the balloon, which overcomes many of the shortcomings of the previous designs. It is currently being used in a pivotal multicentre randomised trial in the USA to support its regulatory approval in the country.

Silimed Gastric Balloon (SGB) (Silimed, Rio de Janeiro, Brazil)

This spherical silicone balloon is advanced by scope traction, rolled up inside a thin silicone sheath, anchored to the top of the endoscope with a snare. It is filled with saline 650 mL, contrast dye 20 mL and methylene blue 10 mL (Table 2.4). For removal the balloon is punctured by a specially developed catheter containing the needle and used also to empty the balloon. The balloon is grasped by a polypectomy snare and pulled and held in an overtube and withdrawn as an entire system. Carvalho et al. performed 2 studies in a total of 71 patients [126, 127]. Weight losses were 8–10 kg or 3.1–3.9 BMI points. Thirteen patients (18.3%) did not tolerate the balloon and there were four deflated balloons (5.6%).

MedSil Intragastric Balloon (MedSil, Moscow, Russia)

The MedSil Intragastric balloon is very similar to the Orbera balloon with a similar introduction sheath and filled with saline between 400 and 700 mL (Table 2.4). A small study with 22 patients reported an 18.4 kg and 5.5 BMI units weight loss, the % EWL was 26.3% and the % EBMI loss was 26.3% [128]. Fasting glucose did not change but HbA1c was significantly reduced. The authors also measured a whole battery of adipokines and found decrease in leptin levels and no change in levels of adiponectin, angiopoietin-like protein 3 (ANGPTL-3), angiopoietin-like protein 4 (ANGPTL-4) and fibroblast growth factor 19 (FGF19). Fibroblast growth factor 21 (FGF21) decreased significantly after 6 months. Ghrelin was significantly increased after 3 and 6 months. They measured the body composition by DEXA after 6 months and found a decrease in fat mass of 11.3 kg but also a fairly high decrease in fat-free mass of 5.3 kg [128]. There were no complications at placement or removal of the balloon and no complications during balloon stay except from transient gastrointestinal complaints in the beginning.

Intragastric Balloon Types with Unknown Status

Some intragastric balloons are under reconstruction or reconsideration or did not provide further studies, so their status was considered as unknown. Attempts at contacting the companies were fruitless.

Heliosphere Bag (Helioscopie Medical Implants Company, Vienne, France)

The Heliosphere Bag consists of a double-bag polymer balloon covered with a silicone envelop which is inflated with 840–960 cm^3 of air which gives the final volume of 650–700 cm^3 of air as air is compressed (Table 2.4). Two RCTs compared the Heliosphere Bag with the Orbera IGB and both studies showed a better tolerance of the Heliosphere Bag due to differences in balloon weight (500–800 g for the Orbera IGB filled with fluid, 30 g for the Heliosphere Bag) [129, 130]. Weight loss was similar for both balloon types. However, one of the studies was stopped prematurely for safety reasons [129]. A non-randomised study compared Heliosphere Bag in 13 patients (BMI 45.0 kg/m^2) with the Orbera balloon in 19 patients (BMI 45.6 kg/m^2) who failed after 6 months of medical and dietary weight loss therapy [131]. The Orbera balloon was more effective, with weight loss of 19.0 kg versus 13.0 kg with the Heliosphere Bag (38% EWL vs. 21% EWL, $P = 0.01$). One patient with the Orbera balloon required removal for persistent nausea and vomiting at 1 month. One patient died (3.1%) of cardiac arrest due to aspiration at day 13 after Orbera balloon placement. In the largest published study, which included 82 consecutive patients with a median follow-up of 182 days, 70% of patients with the Heliosphere Bag achieved more than 10% body weight loss [132].

Six studies with reports on 189 Heliosphere Bag-treated patients showed a system failure at positioning in 7.4%, a high rate of spontaneous deflation in 11.1% and a difficult extraction of the balloon in 35.4% with difficulties to pass the cardia and upper oesophageal sphincter because of the large size, rigidity and low pliability that needed surgery in two and rigid oesophagoscopy in three [129, 130, 132–135]. The balloon was discontinued because of high system failure at positioning, high rate of spontaneous deflation and difficult extraction. Upon contact with the company, the company mentioned a new balloon product, distributed ad promoted in 52 countries, without further providing details or scientific studies.

Semistationary Antral Balloon (SAB) (JP Industria Farmaceutica S.A., Ribeirao Preto, Sao Paulo, Brazil)

This is a pear-shaped silicone balloon with a conical pole oriented to the pylorus and here fixed to a 30 cm silicone duodenal stem and a 7 g counterweight at the tip designed for anchoring the balloon in the antrum (Table 2.4). The balloon is filled with 150–180 mL saline. The mechanism of action is somewhat different from the other balloons and hypothesised to act through intermittent occlusion of the pyloric opening, prolonged gastric emptying and stimulation of the antroduodenal satiety receptors. Twenty-six patients received the device for 4 months and lost 6.5 kg [136]. In four the balloons deflated spontaneously, were expelled rectally in two and retrieved endoscopically in the stomach in one and once it had to be removed surgically. The design looks very similar to the transpyloric shuttle discussed later.

Adjustable Totally Implanted Intragastric Prosthesis ATIIP–Endogast (Districlass Medical S.A., France)

The ATIIP-Endogast balloon is an air-filled balloon of polyurethane material, filled with 210-330 mL of air and by a percutaneous endoscopic gastrostomy procedure, followed by a surgical procedure for the placement of subcutaneous stainless steel chamber that is connected with the balloon, avoids its dislocation and enables adjustment of balloon volume by accessing the chamber by needle puncture similar as being done with the adjustable gastric band in LAGB procedures (Table 2.4). Besides the contraindications mentioned in Table 2.2, the contraindications for gastrostomy placement are operative. The mechanism of action is different; it is positioned proximally in the gastric fundus-corpus area. This proximal gastric positioning is aimed at affecting various control processes such as gastric accommodation, electrical activity and neurohormonal mechanisms to enhance satiety. The only publication dates back to 2007. A multicentre study in 57 patients showed a good tolerance without vomiting [137]. The main complications were early local infection related to PEG placement in seven (12.2%), one with a severe subcutaneous infection which required removal of the prosthesis, and late port erosions in three (5.2%). A symptomatic pneumoperitoneum occurred in three, treated conservatively. Weight losses were 7.4 BMI points (22.3% EWL) at 3 months in 40 patients and 12.2 BMI points (39.2% EWL) at 12 months in 20 patients.

Dual Balloons

The ReShape Duo Balloon (ReShape Medical, San Clemente, CA, USA)

The Integrated Dual Balloon System or ReShape Duo balloon consists of two silicone spheres attached to each other (Table 2.4, Fig. 2.2b). The system is inserted over a guidewire introduced by endoscopy. They are separately filled with saline and independently sealed. The ReShape Duo is designed to maximise space occupation in the stomach and is filled with an evenly distributed volume of 900 mL of saline, 450 mL in each balloon, with the advice to fill with less saline (375 mL) in females less than 1.64 m (64.5 in.) in height. The proximal balloon sits high in the fundus which might contribute to early satiety. The dual balloon design provides significant protection against deflation-related complications. If one balloon deflates the second balloon will maintain the device in the stomach. Another hypothesis is that because the shape of the dual balloon is better adapted to the gastric silhouette, impaction should be avoided and tolerability be improved. The first prospective trial of the ReShape Duo included 30 patients in a 2:1 randomisation ratio at three centres (21 ReShape Duo vs. 9 controls) [138]. Both groups received diet and exercise counselling. Four of the 21 ReShape Duo patients were admitted for nausea, and two patients were found to have gastritis at the time of balloon removal. Percentage of excess weight loss (% EWL) at device removal (6 months) was 32% in the treatment group compared with 18% in the controls. After 48 weeks, almost 6 months after balloon removal, 30% of the ReShape Duo patients remained at 25% EWL versus 25% of the control patients [138]. Lopez-Nava et al. performed a similar study in Spain in 60 patients with a BMI of 38.8 kg/m^2 [139]. After 6 months, a decrease in BMI with 6.1 units, in total weight of 16.6 kg, and a 15.4% TBWL and 47.1% EWL were obtained without any difference in weight loss between different grades of obesity, age or sex. Morbidly obese patients demonstrated a greater total body weight loss, and women and less obese subjects obtained higher excess weight losses. There was one early removal for patient intolerance, one early deflation without migration and one gastric perforation. Fourteen patients had small, clinically insignificant ulcers or erosions noted at the time of removal but the study was conducted with the first design device, before modification of the balloon [139].

The pivotal study in the USA, the REDUCE study ("A Prospective, Randomized Multicentre Study to Evaluate the Safety and Efficacy of the ReShape Duo Intragastric Balloon System in Obese Subjects"), included a total of 326 patients, randomly assigned to a treatment (n = 187) or sham endoscopy group (n = 139) [140]. Both groups were followed up for an additional 6 months after balloon removal to determine weight loss maintenance. The sham group was given the option of device placement during this second 6-month follow-up period. The primary endpoints in this study were the achievement of at least 25% EWL by the treatment group and a significant difference in % EWL versus diet and lifestyle modification. Both of these primary endpoints were met, as the treatment group achieved a significantly higher % EWL of 25.1% and the sham group 11.3%. The % TBWL was 7.6% in the balloon and 3.6% in the sham group. The mean % EWL dropped to18.8% 24 weeks after balloon removal. Statistically significant improvements of comorbid conditions were also seen in the intervention group, including decreases in HbA1c, systolic blood pressure and serum lipids which persisted in the additional 6 months after removal. There was a 15% rate of early removal for device intolerance including nausea and abdominal pain [140]. Although 6% of patients experienced a deflation, there were no balloon migrations due to the presence of two independent balloons. An initial frequent finding was gastric ulceration, which was observed in 39.6% of balloon patients, even in the presence of mandatory PPI therapy. In only one patient this was clinically relevant because of a bleeding ulcer at the gastro-oesophageal junction requiring transfusion. After modifications in the balloon design the ulcer frequency declined to 10.3% and ulcer size diminished from 1.6 to 0.8 cm. Severe adverse events, apart from the bleeding ulcer, were one oesophageal mucosal tear treated with clips, one oesophageal perforation treated conservatively with antibiotics, and one post-retrieval aspiration pneumonitis. The device placement was successful in 99.4% and the retrieval of the balloon in 100% with short procedure times [140]. The ReShape Duo is FDA – approved for adults with BMI of 30–40 kg/m^2 and one or more obesity-related comorbidities and for the duration of 6 months [141].

Orally Ingested Intragastric Balloons

In the search for minimally invasive placement and removal of intragastric balloons there was an intensive search for balloons that could be ingested orally without the need of endoscopy. Endoscopy and conscious sedation or anaesthesia used for placement and removal can lead to adverse events in an overweight or obese individual and significantly add to the cost. Moreover, endoscopic removal of balloons can be unsafe and patients incur risks of aspiration pneumonitis or mechanical damage of the stomach or oesophagus. Finally, endoscopic balloons that have not been removed from individuals who were lost to follow-up have been reported to migrate into the intestines and to cause bowel obstruction. Even though the available balloons can be inserted under fluoroscopy, they still need an endoscopy for removal and the challenge here is to also eliminate the removal endoscopy. One potential concern regarding a swallowed balloon is the absence of a screening endoscopy prior to balloon placement and the lack of ascertainment of mucosal damage by the balloon upon balloon removal. Therefore, the study by Mathus-Vliegen in 303 patients in an attempt to answer the question "Is Endoscopy Really Necessary for Placing Intragastric Balloons?" is clinically relevant [142]. She demonstrated that a careful history can identify patients who may have contraindications for balloon therapy and that balloons can be placed safely under fluoroscopy after taking a careful history without screening endoscopy. As far as the most important exclusion criterion, i.e. hiatal hernia, is concerned, X-ray with contrast was actually more effective in identifying small anatomical abnormalities such as hiatal hernia. Moreover, screening endoscopy was not useful in predicting balloon intolerance or potential complications [142].

Obalon Intragastric Balloon (Obalon Therapeutics, Carlsbad, CA)

The Obalon intragastric balloon is a 250 mL, gas-filled balloon (Table 2.4, Fig. 2.2d). The balloon is compressed, folded and fitted in a large porcine gelatine capsule that has to be swallowed and that is attached to a slender tube that allows filling of the balloon after fluoroscopy has verified that the capsule has entered the stomach. The gelatine dissolves, freeing the balloon. The catheter is connected to a dispenser that contains a can filled with nitrogen-sulphur hexafluoride gas mixture to inflate the balloon controlled by a pressure gauge. The balloon contains a self-sealing valve that closes upon detachment and removal of the tube. If the balloon is tolerated, a second balloon can be swallowed at 4 weeks and a third balloon at 8 weeks. Upper endoscopy is still needed to puncture and remove the balloon(s). It should be noticed that unique contraindications for the gas-filled balloons are scuba diving and travel in unpressurised airplane cabins [38]. The Obalon website mentions that one should not live 1200 m (4000 feet) higher or 760 m (2500 feet) lower than the physician placing the balloons.

Seventeen subjects (BMI between 27 and 35 kg/m^2) ingested a first balloon, 16 a second balloon and 10 a third balloon; 98% of balloons were swallowed successfully [143]. Weight loss after 12 weeks was 5 kg, 36.2% EW and 2.5 BMI units. All balloons were removed successfully by endoscopy at 12 weeks.

In a US pivotal multicentre randomised blinded clinical trial (SMART trial: "Six Month Adjunctive Weight Reduction Therapy"), including 387 subjects who all underwent moderate-intensity lifestyle modification ($n = 185$ in the Obalon capsule arm, $n = 181$ in the sham capsule arm), two co-primary endpoints were defined: the difference in mean percent total body weight loss (% TBWL) between the treatment group and control group, and a responder rate, defined as ≥5% TBWL, achieved in ≥35% of participants [144, 145]. The TBWL was 6.81% and 3.59% in the treatment and control groups, respectively, at 6 months from first balloon insertion (three balloons inserted at 0, 3, 9 or 12 weeks) accounting for a difference of 3.23% TBWL ($P = 0.0338$) [33, 38, 144]. The responder rate was 64.3% and 32.0% in the treatment and control groups, respectively, so both co-primary endpoints were met. Significant improvements in systolic blood pressure, fasting glucose, LDL cholesterol and triglycerides occurred in the treatment group but not the control group. No unanticipated device events occurred. Adverse events, mostly due to accommodation of the stomach such as abdominal cramps and nausea, occurred in 89.9% of subjects and 99.7% of these complaints were rated as mild or moderate. One case of gastric ulcer was seen as ulcer in a patient concomitantly taking non-steroidal anti-inflammatory drugs against study protocol [144]. The Obalon system was approved by the FDA in September 2016 for BMI 30–40 kg/m^2 [145]. Note that the Obalon is indicated in Europe for use at a lower BMI than other IGBs (at 27 kg/m^2 as opposed to 30 kg/m^2) [38].

Elipse Swallowable Balloon (Allurion Technologies Inc., Natick, MA, USA)

The Elipse is a swallowable fluid-filled balloon (Table 2.4, Fig. 2.2e). This is not truly an *endoscopic* bariatric therapy device as it does not require endoscopy for placement or removal but endoscopic facilities should be available in case of unforeseen problems or an early request of removal. The balloon is covered in a biodegradable vegetal capsule and is fixed to a slender flexible tube. Once the balloon is swallowed, its placement is confirmed via X-ray or ultrasound and then inflated with 550 mL of fluid, and while the self-sealing valves close the catheter is removed through the mouth. This device is designed to decompress spontaneously after a planned period of 4 months. During gastric residence, a resorbable material inside the balloon degrades. The resorbable material must completely degrade before a release valve opens and allows the balloon to empty instantaneously and to pass out through the stool. Eight Elipse devices used in a proof-of-concept pilot study were swallowed without the need for endoscopy and all passed uneventfully [146]. Twice an endoscopy was needed: once to puncture the balloon with a needle and forceps because of intolerance and once to puncture a balloon that appeared to be partially collapsed on ultrasound after 11 days. Both were left in the stomach and passed spontaneously per rectum. A recent prospective, open-label, observational study in 2 European centres with 34 patients (mean BMI 34.8 kg/m^2) reported a 10% TBWL and a 3.9 kg/m^2 reduction in BMI units at 4 months in the 25 patients (BMI 34.4 kg/m^2) who completed the study [124]. Reductions in HbA1c, systolic and diastolic blood pressure were statistically significant. In these patients, the mean residence time of the balloons was 117 days. Of the 34 patients included, 6 received an experimental balloon, and of the remaining 28 patients 3 required endoscopy, 2 patients requested endoscopic deflation owing to intolerance and in 1 patient the capsule did not enter the stomach and remained at the lower oesophageal sphincter. All 34 balloons passed in the stool (88%) or through emesis (12%) [124]. No serious adverse events occurred and expected balloon-related gastrointestinal adverse events, mainly rated as mild, occurred in 86%, such as nausea (54%), vomiting (64%) and abdominal pain (25%). Other complaints consisted of constipation (18%), diarrhoea (14%) and gastro-oesophageal reflux (11%) despite twice-daily 20 mg omeprazole. Importantly, a combination of ondansetron and the NK1 antagonist aprepitant dramatically decreased the side effects associated with balloon therapy [124]. A pivotal randomised multicentre trial to support regulatory approval is currently being planned in the USA.

Orally Ingested Balloon with Unknown Status

Ullorex Oral Intragastric Balloon (Obalon Therapeutics Inc., Carlsbad, CA)

Already in 2007 preliminary results with an orally ingested balloon were published but since then no further studies could be retrieved. The idea is very similar to that of the Elipse balloon. The Ullorex is a large capsule that is injected with citric acid and swallowed within 4 min. A carbon dioxide generator in the balloon uses the injected citric acid to release CO2, which after a 4-min delay slowly inflates a 300 cm^3 round balloon. Two capsules can be swallowed to achieve a volume of 600 mL. The balloon has a plug that is degraded by stomach acid over 25–30 days. This causes the balloon to deflate spontaneously and pass harmless in the stools. A feasibility study was performed in 12 obese subjects, who swallowed up to three balloons at a time [147]. Participants who received the balloon lost 1.5 kg more weight than sham-treated subjects over 2 weeks. It is unclear what prevents the capsule from passing through the pylorus into the small bowel before full inflation, and there are concerns about unintended expansion within the oesophagus if the capsule should become lodged [27, 29, 147].

Mechanisms of Action of Intragastric Balloons

Almost every investigation on the mechanism of action of intragastric balloons has been performed with the Orbera balloon. Intragastric balloons are hypothesised to mediate satiety peripherally, by being a physical impediment of food intake, by reducing the gastric capacity and by delaying gastric emptying, and centrally by activating gastric stretch receptors that transmit signals via afferent vagal nerves, solitary tract and paraventricular nuclei, to the ventromedial and lateral hypothalamus [148]. Short-term satiety is primarily affected by gastric distension and gastric volume. Short-term food intake is affected by the weight and volume of the food rather than its energy content [149]. This volume-regulated satiety is thought to result primarily from gastric distension. Mechanical gastric balloon distension to a volume greater than 400 mL during meals significantly reduces oral intake [150, 151].

Changes in gut peptides and hormones such as cholecystokinin (CCK), pancreatic polypeptide (PP) and ghrelin, affecting appetite control and gastric emptying, work in concert herewith [152, 153]. In two randomised sham-controlled studies, there was no difference between sham control and active subjects with an IGB on fasting or postprandial ghrelin concentrations [58, 153]. Interestingly, despite substantial weight losses during 26 weeks of balloon treatment, ghrelin levels did not show the expected rise seen after prolonged fasting and weight loss [153]. Authors, however, do not agree on fasting ghrelin levels which have been reported to remain unchanged to decrease or fail to increase despite weight loss or ghrelin suppression by meals was not always investigated [58, 153–155]. Konopko-Zubrzycka et al. studied ghrelin, leptin and adiponectin after IGB and found a significant decrease in body weight of 17.1 kg (12.3% TBWL) in IGB patients, compared with only 3.5 kg (2.3% TBWL) in the control group treated with diet and physical exercise [155]. The IGB group showed a significant increase in ghrelin after 1 and 6 months that returned to baseline values 3 months after balloon removal. They also noticed a significant decrease in leptin, related to the weight loss. Unexplained is the fact that adiponectin levels did not change in the IGB group [155]. Other gut hormones such as CCK and PP have been barely investigated. In a sham-controlled design Mathus-Vliegen and de Groot examined fasting and postprandial CCK and PP levels in two groups: one sham group who started with a 13-week sham period and then received their first balloon for 13 weeks and an IGB group who started with a 13-week IGB and continued with a second 13-week IGB therapy [152]. In the sham group, basal CCK levels decreased, explained by the effect of dieting, but meal-stimulated responses remained unchanged after 13 weeks of sham treatment. In the IGB group, basal and meal-stimulated CCK levels decreased after 13 weeks of balloon treatment. By the end of the second 13-week period, when the sham group had their first balloon treatment, they duplicated the initial 13-week results of the IGB group, whereas the IGB group continued their balloon treatment and reduced meal-stimulated CCK release. These findings are compatible with a delayed gastric emptying, which was not measured in this study. The authors alluded to their clinical findings of delayed gastric emptying by stressing the significant retention of food in the stomach on top of the balloon seen endoscopically upon balloon removal [152]. Both groups showed reduced meal-stimulated pancreatic polypeptide (PP) secretions at the start, after 13 weeks of sham or balloon treatment and after a second period of IGB in everyone. Improvements in glucose tolerance and insulin sensitivity partly explained the PP results. Changes in diet composition and visual analogue scores of satiety were similar [152].

Although the literature on gastric emptying over the years has been very inconsistent, more consistent findings have emerged recently [154, 156, 157]. A small prospective study by Su et al. demonstrated by scintigraphy that gastric emptying half-times for solids and liquids were significantly longer after IGB placement, with a significant positive correlation between gastric emptying times and body weight loss [158]. A randomised controlled trial of the Orbera intragastric balloon in 27 subjects who all received lifestyle modification therapy (LMT) with 13 receiving a balloon and 14 having sham endoscopy studied gastric emptying at baseline, after 8 and 16 weeks while the balloon was still present and at 27 and 39 weeks when the balloon was out for 1 and 13 weeks [69]. A highly significant increase in retained gastric contents 2 h after a ^{99}Technetium-labelled meal ingestion was observed in the IGB group compared with the control group at 8 weeks (61.4% and 25.7% retained, respectively, $P = 0.0003$) and 16 weeks (62.1% and 18.7% retained, respectively, $P < 0.001$) [69]. After balloon removal gastric emptying returned to the pretreatment baseline levels. No difference was seen in retained gastric contents in the IGB group compared with the control group at baseline or 1 and 13 weeks post-IGB removal, supporting an independent role of IGB on gastric motility. Moreover, weight loss was correlated with the change in gastric retention. Subjects in the IGB group (6 out 13) with 50% or more increase in gastric retention at 8 weeks after IGB insertion had significantly higher % TBWL compared with subjects (7 out of 13) with <50% increase in gastric retention [69]. Moreover, the amount of gastric retention correlated with weight loss, not only at balloon removal but also in the period after balloon removal, suggesting that some of the physiologic changes, which resulted in delayed gastric emptying during intragastric balloon treatment, continue to exert some effect even after the device is removed. This might also explain the weight maintenance and very gradual weight regain in contrast to the immediate weight gain that is seen after cessation of obesity medications in the previously mentioned studies over up to 6 years [5]. In a larger multicentre study, published in abstract form [70] and for some parts in articles [69, 159], 118 subjects had paired scintigraphic gastric emptying studies before and after endoscopic bariatric therapy (EBT) including 15 undergoing a sham endoscopic procedure, 14 lifestyle modification only, 45 gastric injections of botulinum toxin A (BTA), 15 saline-filled intragastric balloon (IGB), 25 duodenal-jejunal bypass sleeve (DJBS) and 4 endoscopic sleeve gastroplasty (ESG) [70]. Sham procedures and lifestyle modification therapy were not associated with delay in gastric emptying (median % increase in gastric retention at 2 h of −1%) compared to a 9% increased retention after BTA injection, 24% after DJBS, 30.5% after ESG and 47% after IGB. Interestingly, rapid baseline gastric emptying and degree of slowing in gastric emptying after EBTs were associated with % TBWL at 6 months on univariate and multivariate analysis after adjusting for age, sex, BMI, diabetes and intervention [70]. Subjects in the EBT group in the highest gastric emptying quantile lost four times more weight than non-EBT-treated controls. Both baseline gastric emptying and change in gastric emptying after EBT significantly predicted achieving ≥15% TBWL at 6 months [70]. One may conclude from this study that in tailoring the EBT method to the characteristics of the patient, pretreatment measurement of gastric emptying might be of help to assign an IGB to patients with rapid gastric emptying at the start.

Balloons may stay for 6 months; only the Spatz adjustable balloon system is allowed for a 12-month period. Interestingly, studies suggest that the first month's weight loss is predictive for successful weight loss, defined as ≥10% weight loss after 6, 12 and 18 months [160]. At 3 months the majority of the weight loss achieved after 6 months is obtained, while satiety levels are maximally at 1–3 months and delayed gastric emptying tends to return back to accelerated pretrial values after 3 months [52, 58, 157]. Also the review by Gaur et al. demonstrated that 80% of the weight loss at 6 months was achieved already at 3 months [85]. The fact that most weight is lost in the first 3–4 months with a plateauing thereafter has been supposed to relate to an adaptation effect of the stomach to the balloon. After 30 years of balloon treatment it is still not clear if gastric adaptation occurs [151, 161, 162].

Remarks for Use of Balloons in Clinical Practice

As mentioned earlier, the FDA approved the Orbera, ReShape Duo and Obalon balloons for a 6-month period being imbedded in a 12-month comprehensive weight management programme [67, 141, 145]. The ASMBS mentioned in their position statement, endorsed by SAGES, that the efficacy of an intragastric balloon intervention has at least two components: (1) the behavioural (diet and lifestyle) effect and (2) the balloon effect [46]. The ASMBS and SAGES support the use of balloons regarding the evidence level 1 data on the clinical utility, efficacy and safety of intragastric balloon therapy for obesity. They also emphasised the temporary treatment of 6 months and the 12-month multidisciplinary approach around balloon therapy [46]. The context of the workplace and working programme determine the outcome and therefore a comparison of the US pivotal studies with the three-decade experience in European and some South American centres is appropriate. An average result can be obtained from meta-analyses.

Comparison of US Studies with Non-US Studies

The weight loss seen in the three US pivotal trials is lower than what is seen in clinical practice outside of the USA by as much as 50% [33]. For Orbera balloons, the active group in the US pivotal study achieved a 10.2% TBWL and 79.2% achieved a ≥5% TBWL or ≥25% EWL [68]. In the Imaz meta-analysis the TBWL was 12.3% and the % EWL was 32.1% [56]. The meta-analysis by Abu Dayyeh et al. with mostly European and South American studies reported these same figures at 12 months, so 6 months after balloon removal: a TBWL of 11.3% and an % EWL of 25.4. The three RCTs that were analysed showed a 26.9% greater EWL in the active group [41]. In the US pivotal ReShape Duo trial the active group showed a 6.8% TBWL and 48.8% achieved a ≥5% TBWL or ≥25% EWL [140]. One pilot study in 21 patients with the ReShape Duo balloon showed a 32% EWL [138]. A clinical case series of 60 patients with the ReShape Duo balloon demonstrated a 15.4% TBWL and a 47.1% EWL at IGB removal [139].

Another conspicuous finding is the very different rate of early removal of balloons. Early retrieval of balloons in the Orbera US study was 18.9% with 50% on own request [68]. In the ReShape Duo US trial there were 15.0% early retrievals [140]. Vomiting occurred in 86.9% and 86.7% of Orbera and ReShape Duo balloons, respectively, and nausea was reported by a respective 75.6% and 61.0% and abdominal pain in 57.5% and 54.5%, respectively [68, 140]. Data from the Imaz meta-analysis showed an early removal in 4.2%, 43% on own request [56]. In Abu Dayyeh's meta-analysis the early removal was 7.5%, nausea was present in 29% and abdominal pain was present in 33.7% [41]. Lopez-Nava et al. reported a 1.7% early removal [139]. So, also here there is a large difference between pivotal US studies and the year-long experience from elsewhere.

There are almost no data on the air-filled Obalon balloon, but comparison of other air-filled with fluid-filled balloons reported a much better tolerance of the air-filled balloon [129, 130, 163, 164]. Also, in the US pivotal Obalon study, the air-filled balloon was much better tolerated with vomiting in 17.3% and nausea in 56.0%, but still abdominal pain was present in 72.6% of cases [144]. Early removal was 9.6% for the Obalon device, yet higher than the Imaz and Abu Dayyeh meta-analysis data [41, 56, 144]. It is important to recognise that the investigators in these US trials had no or limited experience with managing patients with IGBs and certainly did not realise the impact of – especially fluid filled – IGBs in the first 3 days on well-being and may therefore have been less aggressive in the treatment of these symptomatic patients. This assumption is verified by the lower numbers in the meta-analyses of clinical trials performed by more experienced practitioners.

More information on the everyday practice is given by the study of Mathus-Vliegen et al. who noticed that much of the data collected on balloons has been in the context of clinical trials in academic medical centres or in large obesity centres, or as a bridge to bariatric surgery in obesity bariatric centres [165]. Moreover, virtually no reports have been published on patients who are treated exclusively outside the academic or hospital settings, and outside the setting of a clinical trial. They recognised the challenge of balloon placement in an everyday practice by gastroenterologists or surgeons with less experience than their academic colleagues or bariatric surgeons, and to take up the gage of realising a similar degree of efficacy and safety as has been published in the scientific literature. They had access to efficacy and safety data in a private practice setting, where compliance with dietary advice, physical exercise, behavioural modification and frequency of follow-up visits were left to the wishes of the patient [165]. A total of 815 consecutive patients were included (131 males, mean body weight 111.7 kg, mean BMI 38.1 kg/m^2). In 672 patients the mean weight loss at 6 months was 20.9 kg, and the BMI decreased by 7.2 BMI units. Of these, over 50% (372 patients) were only seen once at balloon placement and after 6 months for balloon removal. These patients, despite not receiving any dietary support or counselling, achieved a weight loss of 19.4 kg (6.6 BMI units). A total of 326 patients attended for weight consultation at 3 months and had lost 15.8 kg and 5.4 BMI units, again bearing out the statement of the largest weight loss in the first 3 months. Three months after balloon removal, 65 patients remained 6.6 BMI units (18.8 kg) lower than at baseline level. Successful weight loss after 6 months as defined by internists (≥10% total body weight loss) was achieved by 571 patients (85.0%). Successful weight loss as defined by surgeons (≥50% EWL) was achieved by 299 patients (44.5%). A total of 53 patients (6.5%) requested balloon removal during the first month. Nine balloons (1.1%) were removed for medical reasons [165]. There were four serious adverse events (0.5%): two cases of severe dehydration and two cases of balloon deflation who required surgery. The high rate of self-requesting balloon removal, 6.5% in the current study, compared with only 1.8% in the meta-analysis of Imaz suggests that patients may not have been well informed about the initial side effects of balloon therapy and the need for adequate medication to overcome symptoms [56, 165]. Every patient ($n = 815$) showed up for balloon removal, 807 on the agreed 6-month appointments and eight patients who returned after 9 months. Inspection of the stomach revealed abnormalities in 69 patients (8.5%), with clinical irrelevant abnormalities in 57, severe asymptomatic oesophagitis was present in 12 patients (1.5%) [165].

Meta-analysis

Two meta-analyses examined the outcomes of Orbera balloons and have been discussed earlier [41, 56]. Both included RCTs and open studies. A Cochrane review which included many studies with older balloon designs such as the Garren Edwards Gastric Bubble (GEGB) that were withdrawn from the market because of unsafety had a very negative tenor [53]. Three very recent meta-analyses only included RCTs and two of them included some of the older studies with the Garren Edwards Gastric Bubble that set the world of balloon treatments in stir and commotion [166–168]. One meta-analysis only reviewed studies with balloons filled with >400 mL, and thereby automatically excluded the older balloon versions [168]. This meta-analysis included 9 studies with 669 patients using either the Orbera, ReShape Duo or air-filled balloons. The meta-analysis favoured the IGB group with a 1.4 kg/m^2, 3.6 kg and 14% EWL greater weight loss compared with the sham/diet group. There were no differences between air-filled and fluid-filled balloons. Zheng et al. excluded all crossover trials and thereby excluded a great deal of available studies [166]. They included the older balloon versions and reported the results separately for those having less than 6 months and 6 months of balloon treatment. Those with less than 6-month therapy showed 1.5 kg and 1.2 kg/m^2 greater losses with balloons over controls, but when carefully looking at their data these results came all from the older balloons that are not available anymore. The 6-month results, so with larger size balloons and either air filled or fluid filled, reported a 8.9 kg, 3.1 kg/m^2 and 21.0% greater weight loss compared with controls [166]. Saber et al. also included the crossover trials and as these crossed over after 3 months they had to divide their data into overall, 3 months and >3 months' data. Older balloon studies were included as well [167]. Twenty studies involving 1195 patients were analysed. Also, their data were in favour of IGBs as they showed greater weight losses over controls of 1.59 and 1.34 kg/m^2 for overall and 3-month BMI loss, respectively; 14.3% and 11.2% for overall and >3-month percentage of excess weight loss, respectively; 4.6 and 4.8 kg for overall and 3-month weight loss, respectively; and 2.8%, 1.6% and 4.1% TBWL for overall, 3-month and >3-month, respectively. Interestingly, they demonstrated that fluid-filled balloons were significantly more effective than air-filled balloons [167]. Complaints of flatulence, abdominal pain, abdominal distension and general discomfort were significantly more prevalent after IGBs. They also found gastric ulcers in 12.5% versus 1.2% in controls ($P < 0.001$) but although they did not find a different risk of ulcers in air-filled and fluid-filled balloons, the unfavourable data on gastric ulcers and the better performance of fluid-filled balloons have to be viewed in the context of their decision to consider all balloons, also the old ones that proved to be ineffective and dangerous, the reason why they were taken from the market. Albeit Saber's meta-analysis is very recent from 2017, there is still room for a new meta-analysis of only the new and currently available balloons.

In view of the fact that balloon-induced weight loss occurs predominantly in the first 3–4 months, a new treatment modus may be developed by the availability of the new orally ingested and rectally excreted balloons. The limited durability of prior balloon treatments and FDA approval for 6 months only can now be extended if a single balloon is followed by the use of multiple balloons. Repeated therapy may become the most common paradigm for this device to obtain and maintain long-term effects and this will be facilitated by balloons that do not require endoscopy for placement or removal. Whether this has to be done with a period of adaptation of the stomach during a balloon-free period in between to rest the stomach and reset its normal motility before repeating therapy should be investigated further.

2.3.1.2 Miscellaneous Endoscopic Techniques

AspireAssist Gastric Aspiration (Aspire Bariatrics, King of Prussia, PA, USA)
Endoscopic aspiration therapy involves the placement of a percutaneous endoscopic gastrostomy (PEG) tube via the pull technique for PEG placement (Figs. 2.1 and 2.5). The A-tube of the AspireAssist system is a gastrostomy tube, which has a 15 cm fenestrated intragastric portion to allow aspiration of gastric contents. After maturation of the gastrostomy tract after approximately 10–14 days, the proximal end of the A-tube is cut within 1 cm of skin level and attached to a Skin-Port. For aspiration the connector of the AspireAssist siphon is connected to the Skin-Port, herewith opening the Skin-Port valve. The AspireAssist siphon consists of a water reservoir for gastric infusion and a drain for stomach contents to drain into the lavatory, which are opened and closed by flipping a lever. The aspiration process involves infusing water into the stomach from a reservoir of 600 mL and then reversing the flow by flipping the lever and flushing food particles out of the stomach through the A-tube into the lavatory. This process is repeated (typically 3–8 infusions) until food particles are no longer seen in the aspirate. The aspiration process usually takes 10–15 min to perform and is done about 20 min after each of three main meals daily. Usually, ≈30% of the ingested meal can be aspirated. To

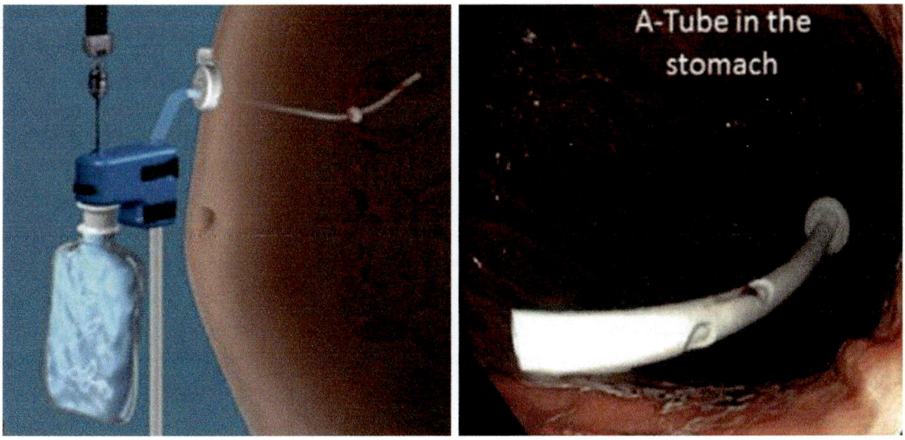

Fig. 2.5 AspireAssist system with A-tube in the stomach and the AspireAssist siphoning system plugged onto to the Skin-Port, herewith opening the Skin-Port valve. Reprinted from Clin Endosc 2017; 50: 42–66, Bazerbachi F, Vargas Valls EJ, Abu Dayyeh BK. Recent clinical results of endoscopic bariatric therapies as an obesity intervention (Open Access Article)

safeguard long-term unsupervised and overzealous use the connector has a counter-mechanism which allows 115 times the opening of the Skin-Port valve; thereafter it can no longer open the Skin-Port valve and the patient has to visit the physician to obtain a new connector. Exclusion criteria, additionally to those mentioned in Table 2.2, consisted of eating disorders, major depression and usual contraindications for a PEG procedure. In a pilot trial, Sullivan et al. randomised 18 obese subjects to 1 year of aspiration therapy plus lifestyle ($n = 11$) or lifestyle only ($n = 7$) [169]. Ten of the 11 and 4 of the 7 completed the first year. Weight losses after the first year were 18.6% TBWL and 49% EWL in the aspiration group (initial BMI 42.0 kg/m^2) and 5.9% TBWL and 14.9% EWL in the lifestyle group (initial BMI 39.3 kg/m^2) ($P < 0.05$). Seven of the ten completed another year and maintained their weight loss with 20.1% TBWL and a 54.6% EWL [169]. No adverse effect on eating behaviours or compensation for aspirated calories was seen. Initially abdominal pain at the aspiration tube site was frequently reported, which improved after the device was redesigned. Once a hypokalaemia and three peristomal infections occurred despite a 7-day course of antibiotics. Five tubes became blocked. Four patients had their tubes removed and one had a persistent gastrocutaneous fistula. In a subsequent study, 25 patients with a BMI of 39.8 kg/m^2 were enrolled after a 4-week run-in period of a very-low-calorie diet (VLCD) in a 6-month aspiration treatment period by Forssell and Norén [170]. In the per protocol analysis (22 patients), weight loss at 6 months after aspiration therapy was 16.5 kg including the VLCD period and 8.0 kg without VLCD-induced weight loss. Total excess weight loss was 40.8% with 14.8% TBWL, which is very much in line with Sullivan's data [169, 170]. There was a trend towards improved fasting glucose and haemoglobin A1c, and significant improvement in fasting glucose in the seven patients with type 2 diabetes mellitus [170]. Three of five patients taking medication for diabetes were able to discontinue it. Early adverse events included post-procedure abdominal pain, intra-abdominal fluid collection and skin breakdown around the stoma; a later skin infection required treatment with antibiotics. Moderate abdominal pain was reported by 52% of patients in the first week, and severe pain by 12% [170]. In each study, three patients discontinued therapy: because of relocation, pain and personal life issues in Sullivan's study, and because of inability or unwillingness to spend 45 min per day on aspiration therapy in the study by Forssell and Norén [169, 170]. To meet criticism of creating eating disorders, both studies offered lifestyle therapy or cognitive behavioural therapy. The claim of inducing adverse eating behaviours could not be substantiated by Sullivan et al. [169]. Patients also did not compensate for the energy lost by aspiration. In the US pilot trial, bomb calorimetry of gastric aspirate from aspiration therapy after a meal was compared with an identical unconsumed meal and it revealed that 25–30% of calories were removed with each aspiration session [169]. This only accounted for 80% of the weight loss achieved in the subjects undergoing aspiration therapy if they aspirated 25–30% of all consumed calories, which they apparently did not as they did not aspirate snacks and frequently aspirated only twice a day. This means that another explanation likely accounts for a part of the weight loss, and indeed, patients self-reported a decrease in food intake as they have to change their eating behaviour considerably. They must take more time to thoroughly chew food and drink sufficient water with meals to ensure that food will be successfully aspirated and will not clog the tube, which may lead to smaller portions of food consumed [169]. So, by itself the AspireAssist promotes key elements of behaviour modification therapy.

The US pivotal multicentre study ("Pivotal Aspiration Therapy with Adjusted Lifestyle", the PATHWAY trial) randomised subjects in a 2:1 ratio to AspireAssist with lifestyle counselling, or lifestyle counselling alone [171]. The main eligibility criteria were age 21–65 years and a body mass index of 35.0–55.0 kg/m^2. A total of 207 participants were randomised, 137 to AspireAssist (BMI 42.2 kg/m^2) and 70 to lifestyle counselling alone (BMI 40.9 kg/m^2). Of these, 111 in the AspireAssist group and 60 in the lifestyle counselling group were enrolled and 82 AspireAssist (74% of those enrolled) and 31 lifestyle counselling participants (52% of those enrolled) completed the entire 52-week study. A modified intention-to-treat (mITT) and a completer's analysis (CA) were performed. Successful endoscopic placement of the A-tube was achieved in 97% of attempts. The co-primary endpoints were mean percent excess weight loss which had to be at least 10% higher in the AspireAssist group and the proportion of participants who achieved at least a 25% excess weight loss, which had to be at least 50% higher in the AspireAssist group. Both primary endpoints were reached as the % EWL in the AspireAssist group (31.5% in mITT and 37.2% in CA) was 22% greater than the % EWL achieved in the lifestyle counselling-only group (9.8% in mITT and 13.0% in CA). Moreover, 58.6% of the AspireAssist group (68.3% in CA) lost at least 25% of their excess body weight, which was more than the 50% pre-specified criterion. This was the case for 22.0% of the mITT and 25.8% of the CA analysis in the lifestyle counselling-only group. At 52 weeks, based on an mITT analysis, mean percent body weight loss at 52 weeks was 12.1% (14.2% for completers only) in the AspireAssist group and 3.5% (4.9% for completers only) in the lifestyle counselling group [171]. Early responsiveness with the AspireAssist, defined as 5% or more body weight loss at week 14, was predictive of weight loss at week 52. Ninety percent of the study-related adverse events were associated with the gastrostomy tube and half of them occurred in the first week after placement. Five (3.6%) severe adverse events were reported: one case of mild peritonitis, twice severe abdominal pain, one prepyloric ulcer related to the A-tube and once an A-tube malfunctioning. Four instances of hypokalaemia were noticed. There were no differences in comorbidities between the groups, and eating patterns remained undisturbed and there was no evidence of a compensatory increase in food intake. Of the 29 subjects who had their A-tubes removed before the end of the 52-week study, one had a persistent fistula that was clipped successfully [171]. An additional small European trial of 11 subjects (average BMI 66.5 kg/m^2 and body weight 196.1 kg) demonstrated a 21.4% TBWL included on purpose super-superobese subjects to investigate aspiration therapy as a bridge-to-surgery. After 1 year a weight loss of 41.1 kg, 21.4% TBWL and 33.9% EWL were obtained in these 11 patients [172]. After 2 years in 6 subjects these figures were 45.0 kg, 23.3% TBWL and 38.8% EWL. Three minor skin infections were seen which were treated with antibiotics [172].

In June 2016, the device was approved by the FDA for long-term implantation in patients with a BMI between 35 and 55 kg/m^2 [173].

TransPyloric Shuttle (BAROnova, Goleta, CA, USA)
The TransPyloric Shuttle (TPS) consists of a large silicone spherical bulb attached to a smaller cylindrical bulb by a flexible tether (Figs. 2.1, 2.2f, and 2.6a–c). The smaller cylindrical sphere is small enough to enter the duodenal bulb with peristalsis, and pulls the larger spherical bulb into the pylorus where it occludes the pylorus intermittently to reduce gastric emptying. The TPS is preloaded in its delivery system in a coil configuration. The device delivery system is inserted through an overtube into the stomach. Under fluoroscopic view, the coil is deployed, and the TPS is constructed and locked into its treatment profile for gastric residence. Removal is by endoscopy using the same type of gastric overtube (Fig. 2.6b, c). Once the overtube is in position, an endoscope is used to locate the TPS and with a standard endoscopic rat tooth forceps the lock-release mechanism to deconstruct the device is actuated and after retrieval of the locking device the device can be unfolded by a polypectomy snare into the overtube and removed. Two groups of ten patients (BMI of 36 kg/m^2) were treated, ten patients for 3 and ten for 6 months [174]. Three-month patients had mean % EWL of 25.1%, mean % excess BMI loss of 33.1% and mean TBWL of 8.9%. Six-month patients had mean % EWL of 41.0%, mean % excess BMI loss of 50.0% and mean TBWL of 14.5%. Both the 3- and 6-month patients had statistically significant improvements in the overall quality-of-life score. Mild complaints in the first 30 days were pharyngeal/laryngeal irritation due to the overtube, a sore throat, nausea, vomiting and abdominal pain. Endoscopic observations of mucosal erosion and/or granulated tissue were noted in 15/20 patients. A gastric ulcer, defined as ≥5 mm in diameter, was noted in ten patients and ulcers were all located in the antrum. Eight of ten ulcers were asymptomatic endoscopic findings and resolved by medication such as proton pump inhibitors and sucralfate, but in two patients persistent ulcers with acute-onset epigastric pain and epigastric pain and vomiting led to early device removal [174]. Symptoms resolved immediately after device removal. A surface feature on the device appeared to be associated with the development of ulceration. This prompted changes in the design to the current generation of the TPS. A US pivotal study (ENDOBESITY II) is in progress.

Botulinum Toxin A (BTA) Injection (Botox; Allergan, Irvine, CA, USA)
Botulinum toxin A (BTA) is produced by *Clostridium botulinum*. It inhibits acetylcholine release at the neuromuscular junction and selectively inhibits the activity of cholinergic nerves, and smooth and striated muscles. When injected in the antrum it delays gastric emptying and induces satiety by means of a pharmacologically induced gastroparesis. When injected in the fundus, BTA was hypothesised to decrease gastric accommodation and ghrelin secretion and to induce an early sensation of satiety and fullness [175]. The first meta-analysis of six studies, three open studies and three RCTs, in 2008 evaluated the effect of intragastric injection of BTA by endoscopy on obesity [176]. These six studies yielded conflicting results and part

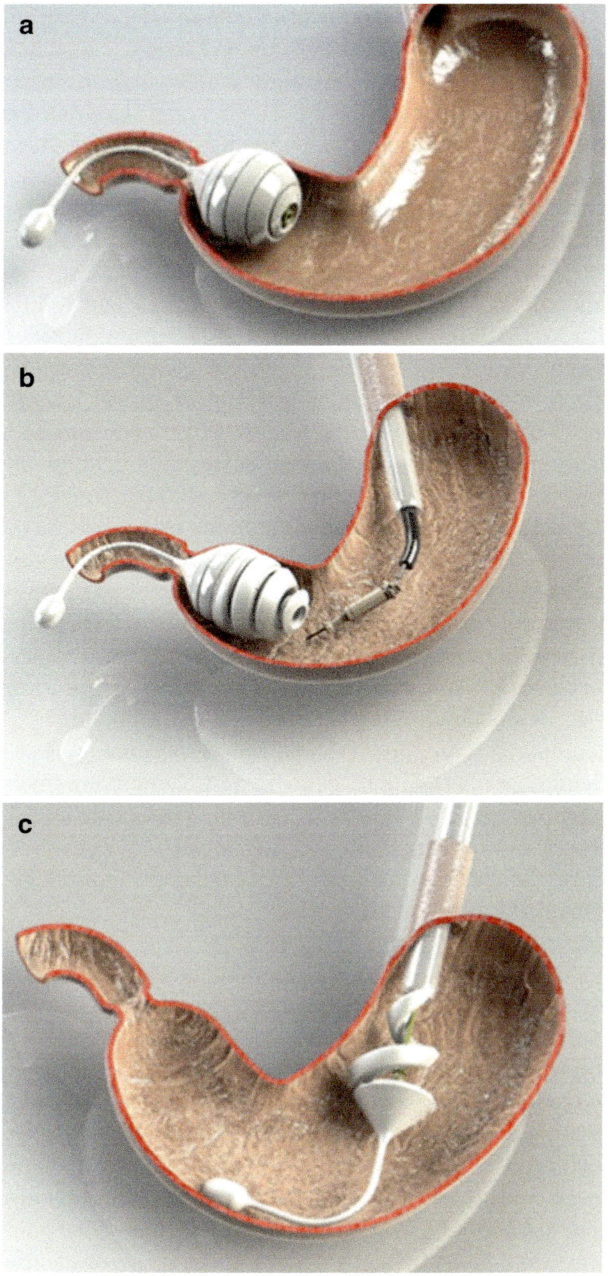

Fig. 2.6 Transpyloric shuttle: (**a**) Position of the large silicone spherical bulb in the stomach which is attached to a smaller cylindrical bulb in the duodenum; (**b**, **c**) deconstruction of the device by activating the lock-release mechanism and unfolding of the device after retrieval of the locking device [174]. Reprinted from Surg Obes Relat Dis 2014; 10: 929–935, Marinos G, Eliades C, Muthusamy R, Greenway F. Weight loss and improved quality of life with a nonsurgical endoscopic treatment for obesity: clinical results from a 3- and 6-month study with permission from Elsevier

of the inconsistency was due to differences in patient selection, injected BTA doses (100–300 IU), method of application (number and depth of injections) and area of application (antrum, antrum combined with fundus). Of these six studies, five reported negative and one positive results. The positive study used eight injections in both the antrum and fundus. Recently, in 2015, a new meta-analysis of eight studies (4 RCTs, 4 open, 115 patients, 79 treated vs. 36 placebo) encountered the same methodological problems but adapted the method of statistical analysis [177]. They found a significant effect on weight both between and within subjects. Sensitivity analysis learned that a wider area of injection (fundus and body vs. antrum only) and multiple injections (>10) but not the dose of BTA (> or <500 IU) were associated with weight loss [177]. Multiple injections showed significant efficacy, and the reason for this efficacy seems to be the enhanced intramuscular diffusion of toxin. Botulinum toxin A is known to spread by diffusion to an area as large as 3 cm from the injection site. The meta-analysis only reports effect sizes and does not report the percentage of weight lost, which is relevant for the treating physician [177]. Furthermore, the method is expensive (100 IU cost 300 euro) and the duration of the effect is limited to 3–6 months. Not included in the meta-analysis is a recent study reported in a letter where 118 patients were treated with follow-up in 75% [178]. Treatment consisted of 100 IU BTA per area of antrum, body and fundus and each 100 IU BTA was given in five spaced injections. Patients lost 14 kg after 4 months and regained 2 kg at 6 months. Mainly complaints of vomiting (12.5%) and diarrhoea (3.4%) occurred [178]. So, the application of BTX-A injections remains very controversial. To demonstrate the effects on gastric emptying 45 BTA injection patients were compared with patients with sham procedures (n = 15) and lifestyle modification therapy (n = 14) with no delay in gastric emptying (median % increase in gastric retention at 2 h of −1%) and BTA-treated patients showed a 9% increase in gastric retention, a rather small effect [70].

Techniques with Unknown Status

SatiSphere (Endosphere, Columbus, OH, USA)

The SatiSphere is an endoscopically implantable device designed to delay transit time of nutrients through the duodenum which may alter satiety hormone levels and glucose metabolism [179]. It consists of a 1 mm preformed memory nitinol wire with several polyethylene terephthalate mesh spheres mounted along its course. It is released in the duodenum and made to stay in place by pigtail endings in the antrum and down to the ligament of Treitz, mimicking the anatomy of the duodenal C-loop configuration. A trial of 31 patients with an average BMI of 41.3 kg/m^2 compared 21 SatiSphere patients with 10 controls, with a scheduled device removal after 3 months. Device migration was reported in 10 of 21 implanted patients and emergency surgery was necessary in two patients which led to the termination of the trial due to safety concerns. Weight loss after 3 months was 4.6 kg in the ITT analysis and 6.7 kg in the group completing the therapy (n = 12) versus 2.2 kg in controls. The EWL was 18.4% compared with 4.4% in the control group. The differences in weight loss with controls were only significantly higher for the completers. SatiSphere was associated with delayed glucose absorption, delayed insulin secretion and altered GLP-1 kinetics [179]. It is unknown whether the European study is still ongoing.

Full Sense Device (Baker, Foote, Kemmeter, Walburn LLC, Grand Rapids, MI, USA)
The Full Sense Device is a modified fully covered metal stent with a cylindrical oesophageal component and a gastric disc component connected by struts that is placed across the gastro-oesophageal junction and that is removed endoscopically. By residing in the cardia, it induces satiety and feelings of fullness. There are only some data on the Internet but no peer-reviewed data or abstracts have been published to date.

2.3.2 Invasive Endoscopic Bariatric and Metabolic Therapies

In contrast to the previously discussed endoscopic options to treat obesity, which are mostly at the disposal of and practicable by endoscopist but have the disadvantage of limited durability, the gastric volume reduction devices require high endoscopic skills and much time and some are still in its infancy of development. The methods are more invasive and not reversible and in the analogy of surgery also named endoscopic bariatric and metabolic therapy (EBMT) [180]. As these procedures use stitches and sutures or staples which cannot be removed, they should always have to consider the feasibility of bariatric surgery if needed in the near future. The endoscopic procedures may mimic bariatric surgical interventions such as the vertical banded gastroplasty, gastric band, gastric plication and sleeve gastrectomy (Table 2.5) [180]. As is the case with bariatric surgery, the principles underlying the mechanisms of action are being unravelled. Some of these EBMTs fell into disfavour, but in view of the insights obtained and lessons learned from these methods they will be reported as well. There are two main methods of making plications: by suturing and by stapling.

Table 2.5 Endoscopic bariatric and metabolic therapy and their surgical analogues [180]

Endoscopic bariatric and metabolic therapy	Surgical analogues
Stomach	
Endoluminal vertical gastroplasty (EVG)	Vertical banded gastroplasty (VBG)
Transoral gastric volume reduction (TGVR)	Laparoscopic gastric plication
Primary Obesity Surgery Endolumenal (POSE)	Laparoscopic gastric plication
Endoscopic sleeve gastroplasty (ESG)	Laparoscopic gastric plication
TransOral Gastroplasty (TOGa)	Vertical banded gastroplasty (VGB)
Transoral endoscopic restrictive implant system (TERIS)	Laparoscopic gastric banding (LAGB)
Articulating circular endoscopy (ACE) stapler	Laparoscopic gastric plication
Small intestine	
Duodenojejunal bypass sleeve (DJBS)	Roux-en-Y gastric bypass (RYGB)
ValenTx bypass sleeve	Roux-en-Y gastric bypass (RYGB)
Duodenal mucosal resurfacing (DMR)	Roux-en-Y gastric bypass (RYGB)
Incisionless magnetic anastomotic system (IMAS)	Modified duodenal switch/ileal transposition

2.3.2.1 Gastric Suturing

Several systems of endoluminal suturing have been investigated with both disappointing and promising results. The EndoCinch suturing system and its modified version, the RESTORe Suturing System device, do not provide durable sutures and plications because they do not acquire the required full-thickness and transmural suturing and have been abandoned. The Primary Obesity Surgery Endolumenal (POSE) and the endoscopic sleeve gastroplasty (ESG) on the other side are so promising that US pivotal trials to support regulatory approval are in progress or just finished. Both companies (USGI-POSE and Apollo-Overstitch) have their systems already approved by the FDA for tissue apposition in the management of post-bariatric complications [31] (see Chaps. 5 and 6).

Endoluminal Vertical Gastroplasty (EVG) (Bard EndoCinch Suturing System – Bard Inc., Murray Hill, NJ, USA; Product Currently Discontinued)

Fogel et al. used the EndoCinch Suturing system which is mounted on an endoscope and fires a straight-threaded needle through a tissue fold formed by suction. One continuous suture, following a specific woven pattern, runs through anterior and posterior parts of the gastric wall from the proximal fundus to the distal body. When tightened the suture approximates anterior and posterior walls of the stomach creating an endoluminal vertical gastroplasty (EVG) from fundus to distal corpus. The EVG reduces the capacity of the stomach and gives a functional restrictive component. The EVG differs from its surgical analogue, the vertical banded gastroplasty (VBG), in some aspects: the plication does not start at the angle of His, it is not parallel to the lesser curvature and there is no formation of a narrow outlet to delay gastric emptying [180] (Table 2.5). Fogel et al. treated 64 patients (BMI of 39.9 kg/m^2) without any significant adverse event apart from one case with vomiting [181]. After 12 months 59 of these 64 patients had an EWL of 58% and a significant 9.3 units reduction in BMI. Follow-up endoscopy was done when they reported loss of satiety. Fourteen endoscopies were done and revealed an intact EVG in five, a loosened but still intact EVG in six and a disrupted EVG in three. Two of the three had a repeat stitching procedure [181]. The device was then modified and named the RESTORe (Davol, Murray Hill, NJ, USA), and was capable of both full-thickness suturing and suture reloading in vivo.

Transoral Gastric Volume Reduction (TGVR) (RESTORe – Davol, Murray Hill, NJ, USA; Product Currently Discontinued)

Brethauer et al. used the RESTORe Suturing System device in their TRIM study – "Transoral gastric volume Reduction as Intervention for weight Management" [182, 183]. It is a single-intubation, multi-stitch, endoscopic suturing system. The suction capsule is placed at the end of the endoscope and the suturing system and suture fastening system are placed through the working channel of the endoscope. The system used interrupted sutures, apposing directly opposite tissues by suction of the mucosa into the device and deploying a suture through the gastric tissue. When the desired numbers of stitches have been made, the suture delivery device is removed. A suture fastening system is positioned over the free suture ends, pulling them together and fastening them. An average of six gastric plications is desired to approximate the anterior and posterior wall of the stomach to achieve restriction of the upper stomach and to decrease gastric compliance. Diabetic gastroparesis and diabetes for >10 years are additional exclusion criteria (Table 2.2). The TGVR was more similar to the laparoscopic gastric plication [180] (Table 2.5). In the 18 included patients the desired number of plications were placed in 16; in two poor visibility, too much tension and insufficient place to flex the endoscope resulted in less than six plications. Four patients withdrew. A mean % EWL of 27.7% and a weight loss of 11.0 kg and 4.0 units in BMI were observed. Half of the patients had a ≥30% EWL. Average waist circumference declined by 12.6 cm and systolic and diastolic blood pressure decreased significantly. The endoscopy at 1 month revealed completely intact plications in only two subjects, a partial release was seen in 15 and plications could not be well visualised in 1. Endoscopy at 12 months showed complete release of plications in five and partial release in eight patients [183]. There were no serious adverse events and one adverse event of moderate diarrhoea. Disappointingly, although the RESTORe Suturing System proved to be safe and well tolerated, the plications were not full-thickness stitches and not durable. Both this system and its predecessor have been discontinued.

Primary Obesity Surgery Endolumenal (POSE) (IOP, USGI Medical, San Clemente, CA, USA)

The Primary Obesity Surgery Endoluminal (POSE) procedure uses the incisionless operating platform (IOP) which gained FDA approval in 2006 for grasping, mobilisation and approximation of soft tissue in minimally invasive gastroenterological procedures [31]. The Primary Obesity Surgery Endolumenal (POSE) procedure is done perorally with the incisionless operating platform (IOP), a stable platform with four working ports, which is steerable in four directions with a 360-degree rotation and has a 73 cm insertion length (Fig. 2.7a). One channel allows a 4.9 mm endoscope for endoscopic visualisation. Three channels are for the three specialised instruments: the g-ProxEZ Endoscopic Grasper with 33 mm stainless steel jaws, for grasping, mobilising and approximating full-thickness (serosa-to-serosa) tissue folds and to cut the suture; the g-Lix Tissue Grasper, a helix, to grasp tissue and pull it into the jaws of the g-Prox; and the g-CathEZ Suture Anchor Delivery system, a catheter system that penetrates the target tissue with a needle at its distal tip, installs a pair of preloaded tissue anchors and cinches the anchored tissue fold (Fig. 2.7b, c). The sutures are snow-shoe shaped. The device can be reloaded in vivo.

To perform the POSE procedure, the IOP is retroflexed and used to create two parallel rows with 4–5 plications each. This reduces the fundic apex of the stomach to the level of the gastro-oesophageal junction. After the forward view is restored and the distal gastric body is visualised, a ridge of 3–4 plications is then created at the intersection of the gastric body and gastric antrum, opposite the incisura [184] (Fig. 2.1). Care should be taken to avoid deep g-Lix insertion in this area, in order to avoid injury of adjacent viscera. The plicated area restricts contact with ingested food. The anchored plications may more rapidly activate gastric stretch receptors in response to food and the plications in the fundus are thought to defunctionalise the fundus by limiting the ability to accommodate a meal. Additional distal plications are expected to slow antral mill contractions and to delay gastric emptying. Plicating both the fundus and distal antrum is supposed to induce early fullness and prolonged satiety. Its surgical analogue is the laparoscopic gastric plication, POSE being a partial plication with separated transmural stitches and anchors placed along the upper part and the antrum (Table 2.5). To date, there have been two open-label, prospective, single-arm trials and two randomised controlled trials assessing the

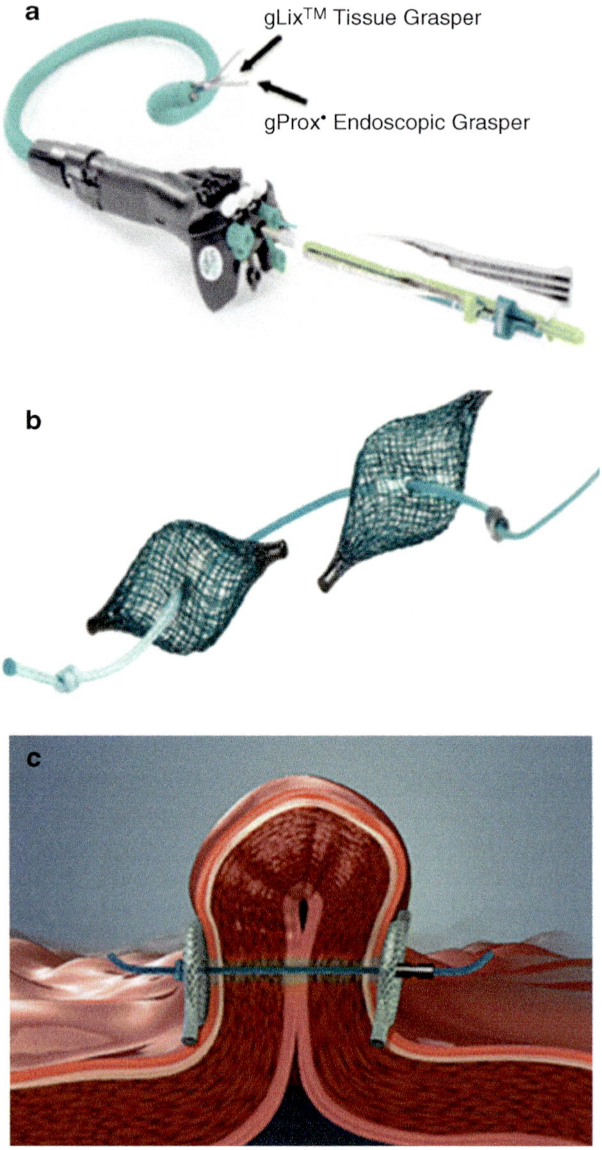

Fig. 2.7 The Primary Obesity Surgery Endolumenal (POSE) procedure: (**a**) The incisionless operating platform (IOP), a stable platform with four working ports: one channel for the endoscope and three channels for the three specialised instruments: the g-ProxEZ Endoscopic Grasper, the g-Lix Tissue Grasper and the g-CathEZ Suture Anchor Delivery system. (**b**) The sutures are snow-shoe shaped. (**c**) An anchored tissue plication [184]. Reprinted from Obes Surg 2013; 23: 1375–1383.186, Espinos JC, Turro R, Mata A, Cruz M, da Costa M, Villa V, et al. Early experience with the Incisionless Operating Platform (IOP) for the treatment of obesity: the Primary Obesity Surgery Endolumenal (POSE) procedure with permission from Springer

Fig. 2.7 (continued)

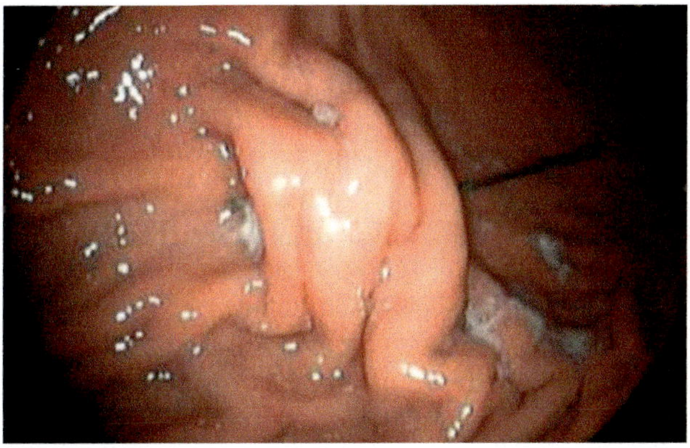

safety and efficacy of the POSE procedure [184–187]. POSE is under FDA review for approval.

Transmural plications were successfully performed in 45 subjects (BMI 36.7 kg/m^2), 8.2 in the fundus and 3 along the distal body wall by Espinos et al. [184]. After 6 months, 27 patients were available for follow-up and reported a 6-month excess weight loss of 49.4%, a weight loss of 16.3 kg or 15.5% and a BMI decrease by 5.8 kg/m^2. Over 80% of patients achieved ≥25% EWL at 6-month follow-up. There were no major adverse events and adverse events associated with the procedure included one case of low-grade fever and one case of chest pain. Lopez-Nava et al. reported the 1-year results from a study of 147 patients with class 1 and 2 obesity (BMI 38.0 kg/m^2) and showed in 116 patients a 44.9% EWL and a TBWL of 15.1% or 16.6 kg [185]. Fifty-nine patients (50.9%) had at least 15% of TBWL at 1 year post-intervention. Only minor complications were reported, including minor bleeding. One patient had a prolonged hospital stay because of a low haematocrit value. No long-term complications have been reported. Patients reported satisfaction with weight loss results, and they were found to have a 50% decrease in hunger and 60% decrease in gastric capacity. Predictive for success were age (younger patients) and BMI (higher initial BMI) [185]. Lopez-Nava also reported the top four serious adverse events reported after 1500 POSE procedures which are immediate post-operative bleeding requiring transfusion, perforation of the stomach, pneumothorax, and perihepatic/perisplenic abscess. The frequency of adverse events is 1.0% overall (15 of 1500), with 0.33% (5 of 1500) of patients requiring hospitalisation with surgery and 0.67% (10 of 1500) requiring rehospitalisation after the procedure or requiring a prolonged stay after the procedure without a surgical intervention [185].

The MILEPOST study, a "Multicentre Study of an Incisionless Operating Platform for Primary Obesity vs. Diet and Exercise", is a prospective, unblinded RCT of 30 months' duration and the 1-year result was reported very recently [186]. Subjects with class I–II obesity were randomised in a 3:1 ratio to POSE or diet/exercise guidance only. Forty-four subjects (BMI 36.5 kg/m^2) were randomised to POSE ($n = 34$) or control ($n = 10$) groups in three centres. All procedures were carried out successfully with serious adverse events; only two minor bleedings required prolonged hospitalisation. Weight losses were 13.0% TBWL and 45.0% EWL in the POSE versus 5.3% TBWL and 18.1% EWL in the controls ($P < 0.01$) at 12 months. At 6 months, 93.8% of POSE group subjects had achieved ≥5.0% TBWL compared with 40% of controls ($P < 0.001$). At 12 months, these percentages were 90.0% in POSE versus 55.6% in controls [186].

The ESSENTIAL trial ("A Randomised, Subject and Evaluator-blinded, Parallel-group, Multicentre Clinical Trial Using an Endoscopic Suturing Device (G-Cath EZ™ Suture Anchor Delivery catheter) for Primary Weight Loss") is a multicentre, randomised, sham-controlled double-blind trial to compare the POSE procedure with a sham procedure with an initial follow-up of 12 months, which has recently been completed [187]. Patients with a BMI between 30 and 34.9 kg/m^2 with one obesity-related comorbidity or 35 and 40 kg/m^2 with no requirement for an obesity-related comorbidity were eligible. Thirty-four patients (BMI 36.5 kg/m^2) were included in a lead-in group for the purpose of investigator training and they also followed the study protocol. In total, 332 subjects were randomised (active $n = 221$, BMI 36.0 kg/m^2; sham $n = 111$, BMI 36.2 kg/m^2) [187]. Aftercare was limited to six visits in active and sham groups, consistent with a low-intensity lifestyle therapy. Co-primary efficacy endpoints were the difference in mean percent of total body weight loss (% TBWL) and the difference in responder rate, response being defined by reaching ≥5% TBWL between the groups. A super superiority design was followed, meaning that the lower limit of the two-sided 95% confidence interval (CI) for the observed difference in % TBWL between groups had to be greater than 3% and that at least 50% of active treatment subjects should obtain a ≥5% TBWL. The 34 patients who participated in the lead-in open-label portion of the study achieved 7% TBWL at 12 months. TBWL was 4.95% in the active and 1.38% in the sham groups ($P < 0.0001$), with a mean weighted difference of 3.57% (95% CI 2.08 to 5.05; $P = 0.2256$). Mean weight loss in the active group was 3.6-fold that of the sham group but the 95% CI lower limit needed to be greater than 3% to have met the predefined super superiority efficacy endpoint which was not the case. The responder rate was 41.6% in active and 22.1% in sham groups, respectively ($P < 0.0001$); however, the super superiority margin of ≥50% of active subjects as set forth in the study design was not met [187]. The procedure success rate was 99.5%; in one patient an abnormal oesophageal anatomy precluded safe insertion of the IOP system. The rate of serious adverse events was 5.0%: 4% ($n = 8$) due to vomiting, nausea and pain, all requiring longer hospitalisation, and one extragastric bleeding requiring open surgical exploration, and one liver abscess requiring percutaneous drainage [187]. Improvement in comorbidities was only significant for diabetes with trends for serum lipids and hypertension. The authors concluded that the POSE procedure is safe and results in statistically significant and clinically meaningful weight loss over sham through 1 year, but they do not discuss the deficiency to demonstrate super superiority.

Mechanism of Action of the POSE Procedure

Espinos et al. tried to explain the working mechanism of the POSE procedure [188]. Caloric intake capacity with standardised nutrient drink test was significantly decreased from baseline (901 kcal) by 48% ($P < 0.001$) at 2 months (473 kcal) and by 36% ($P < 0.001$) at 6 months (574 kcal) in 18 patients with the POSE procedure [188]. Gastric emptying was delayed at 2 months, but returned to normal by 6 months. Changes in hormones including ghrelin and PYY occurred, with an increase in fasting ghrelin and a greater depression of 7% at 2 months and 15% at 6 months ($P = 0.003$) following a meal. Basal PYY also decreased but after a meal the release increased by 15% and 34% at 2 and 6 months, respectively, but it is unclear if these changes are due to the procedure or due to weight loss from the procedure, as 83% obtained a ≥25% EWL at 6 months. Sixty-six percent of the variance in the 15-month weight loss could be explained by pre-procedure BMI, gastric emptying and PYY postprandial change 2 months post-procedure. Thus, weight loss at 15 months was greater in lower weight patients, those who experienced a greater delayed gastric emptying at 2 months and those who experienced a higher PYY postprandial change at 2 months. Also, the MILEPOST study showed a decreased gastric capacity during the standardised nutrient drink test [186]. The standardised nutrient drink test showed that to reach maximum satiation, POSE subjects drank on average 1176 kcal prior to the procedure and 568 kcal 12 months after it, constituting a mean change of 608 kcal ($P < 0.001$) [186].

Comparison of US Studies with Non-US Studies

As has been previously discussed in the intragastric balloon section also here, in the US pivotal study weight losses were lower. The two open and the European multicentre randomised controlled trial showed all three excess weight losses between 45% and 49%, a body weight loss around 16.5 kg and a TBWL between 13.0% and 15.5%, so rather uniform findings [184–186]. Defining a certain weight loss as successful resulted in 80% achieving a ≥25% EWL, 15% achieving a ≥15% TBWL and 93.8% achieving a ≥5% TBWL [184–186]. TBWL was only 4.95% in the blinded part and 7.0% in the unblinded part of the POSE trial with only 41.6% achieving a ≥5% TBWL [187]. Physicians should be aware of these differences and they have to put these figures into the perspective of their field of clinical activity.

Endoscopic Sleeve Gastroplasty (ESG) (OverStitch Suturing System (Apollo Endosurgery Inc., Austin, Texas, USA)

The Apollo OverStitch can place full-thickness stitches in a variety of interrupted or running patterns. Sutures can be reloaded without removal of the endoscope (Fig. 2.8). The OverStitch includes a curved needle driver attached to the tip of the endoscope, a catheter-based suture anchor and an actuating handle attached to the handle of the endoscope. A double-channel endoscope is necessary. The OverStitch can be used to perform endoscopic sleeve gastroplasty, creating a sleeve along the lesser curvature. Two parallel rows of interrupted sutures from the antrum to the fundus are applied. To create a suture, a catheter is passed through one channel of the endoscope to function as a suture anchor and through the other channel a tissue helix screw is placed that is screwed full thickness through the wall and is then retracted, pulling the gastric tissue into the device for full-thickness tissue acquisition. The same is done on the opposite site, using the free suture end of the same

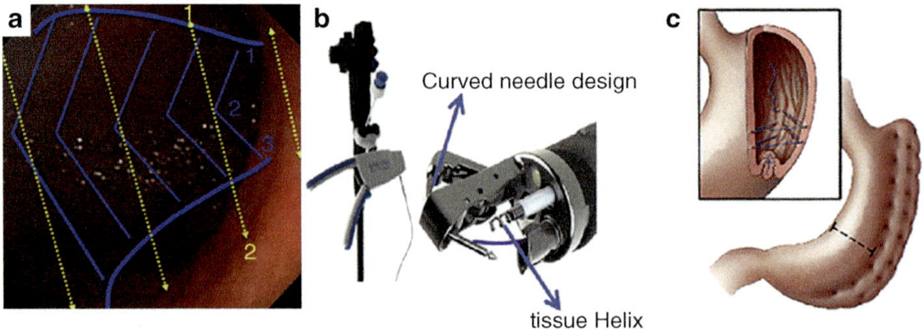

Fig. 2.8 The OverStitch suturing system with the endoscope and the suturing device in the middle, the triangular suturing mode to the left and the two rows of gastric plication to the right, mimicking a laparoscopic gastric plication surgery [189]. Reprinted from Gastrointest Endosc 2013; 78: 530–535, Abu Dayyeh BK, Rajan E, Gostout CJ. Endoscopic sleeve gastroplasty: a potential endoscopic alternative to surgical sleeve gastrectomy for treatment of obesity with permission from Elsevier

suture. The suture is tightened by using a cinching device, thereby creating a full-thickness plication. By this method, approximately 25 sutures are needed to accomplish a full reduction of the gastric capacity (Fig. 2.1). In 2013, Abu Dayyeh et al. described in a single-centre pilot trial a method in four patients (BMI 35.9 kg/m^2) to mimic the surgical sleeve [189]. They used closely spaced interrupted sutures through the gastric wall from the prepyloric antrum to the gastro-oesophageal junction in two parallel rows of anterior and posterior suture placement. Approximately ten interrupted full-thickness, opposing sutures are delivered to reduce the gastric body and create the central length of the sleeve. Finally, closure of the fundus is established with a two-layer set of as many as five sets of opposing sutures and the last suture plication in the sequence is placed at the level of the squamocolumnar junction. It was a lengthy procedure of 170–245 min [189]. About 1 year later, Kumar et al. demonstrated the feasibility and safety of a modified method in five patients [190]. Running sutures with 6–12 stitches each were placed in a triangular fashion at the anterior wall, greater curvature and posterior wall, beginning in the antrum upwards to avoid the need for retroflexion and, once the fundus was reached and closed, it was sutured to the lower oesophageal sphincter. These five patients changed their BMI from 37.4 kg/m^2 at the time of the procedure to 34.8 kg/m^2 after 5 months. The procedure was continued in a further 23 patients (BMI 34.2 kg/m^2) [190]. A median of 8 running sutures, each with 6–12 tissue stitches, was used per procedure. The procedure time was 120 min. There were no significant adverse events. Weight loss at 1 month was 8.0 kg, at 6 months 14.5 kg and at 12 months 13.1 kg. The BMI had decreased to 28.9 kg/m^2 after 6 and to 29.4 kg/m^2 after 12 months [190]. Some prefer to reinforce the suture line with interrupted stitches. The goal of the procedure is to reduce the gastric cavity to resemble a tubular lumen along the lesser curvature, with the greater curvature replaced by a line of cinched plications. It may thus be compared to a bariatric surgical plication [180] (Table 2.5).

Lopez-Nava et al. referred to this novel technique as endoscopic endoluminal greater curvature plication [191]. They also emphasised that the suturing technique is intended not only to reduce the stomach diameter, but also to shorten it substantially through an accordion effect.

Indeed, Sharaiha et al. who described their experience in the first ten patients measured the length of the stomach and found a decreased length of the stomach from 36.6 to 26.1 cm [192]. These ten patients (BMI 45.2 kg/m^2) lost 33 kg, 4.9 BMI units and an excess weight of 30% after 6 months. Eight patients had post-operative abdominal pain and two had chest pain [192]. Lopez-Nava et al. treated 20 patients (BMI 38.5 kg/m^2) [191]. There were no adverse events, except for an intra-procedural bleeding in two patients that was controlled with injection therapy. These 20 patients had a 19.3 kg weight loss, a 17.8% TBWL and a 53.9% EWL and their BMI decreased with 6.6 BMI units after 6 months. On oral contrast studies and on endoscopy performed on a voluntary basis in 10 of the 20 patients an intact gastroplasty with intact sutures was seen [191]. In a further extension of the study in 25 patients they tried to find predictors of weight loss and found the frequency of nutritional and psychological contacts to be associated with TBWL [193]. They also reported the feasibility of an endoscopic revision and repeat procedure in one patient who demonstrated loosened plications on an oral contrast study.

Abu Dayyeh et al. investigated the outcome of 25 patients undergoing ESG for up to 20 months [159]. The % EWL was 53% ($n = 25$) at 6 months, 56% ($n = 17$) at 9, 54% ($n = 13$) at 12 and 45% ($n = 10$) at 20 months after ESG. Five of eight available participants (62.5%) with 20 months of follow-up had an excellent durable response to ESG with % EWL of 72% but three of eight (37.5%) regained all the weight lost at 20 months. Repeat upper endoscopy was performed at 3 months in nine sequential patients to evaluate integrity of the ESG. Six of nine (67%) had a durable, intact ESG with formation of fibrotic bridges. Three of nine (33%) had a partially intact ESG; two of the three non-responders at 20 months were among them. Complaints of pain and/or nausea required hospitalisation for eight patients. Three serious immediate adverse events occurred; one participant developed a perigastric inflammatory serous fluid collection that resolved with percutaneous drainage and antibiotics, another developed a pulmonary embolism 72 h after the procedure and a third developed pneumoperitoneum and pneumothorax requiring chest tube placement.

ESG results were also reported in a registry study, which collected data on 126 patients from 9 sites across 4 countries [194]. Of these, 82 reached 6-month follow-up and 40 reached 1-year follow-up. There were no significant adverse events. BMI decreased from 36.2 kg/m^2 at the time of the procedure to 30.9 kg/m^2 at 6 months and 29.8 kg/m^2 at 1 year. Weight loss and % TBWL at 6 months were 18.1 kg and 17.8%, respectively. These figures were 19.3 kg and 19.0% at 1 year [194].

The largest study of ESG is a clinical case series including 242 consecutive patients at two US centres and one centre in Spain but some of these data might have been included in the mentioned registry study [195]. The procedure success was 100% and ESG was associated with 16.8% (n = 137), 18.2% (n = 53) and 19.8% (n = 30) TBWL at 6, 12 and 18 months, respectively. Five (2%) severe adverse events occurred, all within 30 days of the procedure: two perigastric inflammatory fluid collections (adjacent to the fundus) that resolved with percutaneous drainage and antibiotics, one self-limited haemorrhage from a splenic laceration, one pulmonary embolism 72 h after the procedure and one pneumoperitoneum and pneumothorax requiring chest tube placement. All five patients recovered fully with no need for surgery. Post-procedure symptoms such as nausea, vomiting or abdominal pain were frequent but mostly transient [195].

The OverStitch device has not been specifically approved by the FDA to perform ESG; however, it does have broad approval by the FDA for tissue apposition in the gastrointestinal tract [31]. No randomised controlled trials have been completed with ESG. The PROMISE trial, the "Primary Obesity Multicenter Incisionless Suturing Evaluation" trial to study efficacy of endoscopic sleeve gastroplasty using OverStitch, is currently ongoing.

Mechanism of Action of the Endoscopic Sleeve Gastroplasty

Abu Dayyeh et al. subjected 4 of their 25 patients undergoing ESG to a very detailed assessment of gastric motility and fasting and meal-released hormone levels prior to and 3 months after ESG [159]. A significant delay in gastric emptying of solids with an increase in time with 90 min for 50% emptying of solids was observed compared with pretreatment values without a significant change in the gastric emptying of liquids. During a standardised nutrient drink test ESG was found to decrease caloric intake needed to reach maximum satiety by 59%, signifying earlier satiation and reduced calorie intake and leading to a decrease of meal duration from 35.2 to 11.5 minutes. Despite significant weight loss, fasting and postprandial ghrelin levels decreased by 29.4% 3 months after ESG. ESG significantly improved insulin sensitivity and postprandial glucose values, measured by using the area under the curve, demonstrated a significant decrease (36%). There were no statistically significant changes in leptin, GLP-1 and PYY levels [159].

Techniques with Unknown Status

Two new techniques have been reported. The transoral mucosal excision sutured gastroplasty has been described in a first-in-man study in four patients and the second, the transoral anterior-to-posterior greater curvature plication (Endolumina), reports their preliminary data in 11 patients.

Transoral Mucosal Excision Sutured Gastroplasty (SafeStitch Medical Inc., Miami, USA)

Aiming for full-thickness durable plications the method is used both for obesity and for GORD. The procedure consists of mucosal excision, suturing of the excision beds for apposition and suture knotting at the level of the gastro-oesophageal junction. An excision device retracts gastric tissue of the greater curvature by applying a vacuum. A hypertonic saline and adrenaline solution is injected in the retracted tissue for vasoconstriction and the (sub)mucosa is excised. This is repeated twice to create a confluent adjacent excision bed. Two sets of full-thickness sutures are placed on the sides of the excision bed. The sutures are tightened and knotted using a stitch knotter. The plication of the treated area also partially closes the gastro-oesophageal junction. By injecting hypertonic saline in the proximal lesser curvature a restrictive fibrotic ring ensues. Three patients with GORD and four obese patients have been treated but the first two GORD patients had incomplete procedures due to instrument malfunction [196]. After the procedure the endoscopist rated the suture and excision not optimal in three and satisfactory in one. One of these patients suffered from a pneumoperitoneum without evidence of a perforation at laparoscopy and was treated conservatively. She developed repeated vomiting and at 6 and 12 months the gastroplasty integrity was disturbed with small gaps of 2 mm; she also had the least beneficial weight loss outcomes. No gaps were observed in the other three patients. Weight losses at 3 months varied between 2 and 19% EWL, at 6 months between 4 and 25%, at 12 months between −0.08 and 37% and at 24 months between 0 and 68% EWL. One patient suffered from intermittent dysphagia [196]. The current status of the technique is unknown.

The Transoral Anterior-to-Posterior Greater Curvature Plication (Endomina, EndoTool SA [STT], Gosselies, Belgium)
This system creates transoral anterior-to-posterior greater curvature plications to reduce gastric volume, using an over-the-scope triangulation platform capable of delivering a single interrupted suture anchored by two T-tags. Two guidewires are introduced down to the duodenum. Then, the Endomina platform system is gently introduced over the guidewires into the stomach. The endoscope follows the system and when arrived in the stomach the guidewires are retrieved, the system is opened like the jaws of a crocodile and between them the endoscope is inserted and fixed to the system. Next, a 5 French needle preloaded with a T-tag fixed at a suture (Transmural Anterio-Posterior Endoscopic Suture [TAPES, ETT, Gosselies, Belgium]) is introduced into the flexible arm of the platform. This arm is bent perpendicular to the axis of vision. The stomach wall is grasped with a forceps via the endoscope and pulled back into the platform. The needle is pushed through the wall, under visual control, and a first T-tag, attached to the suture and a pre-tied knot are released. The needle is retracted, the first plication is released and a second plication is made with a second T-tag at the opposite wall of the stomach. APC is applied around the two wire entry points to destroy the mucosa and ensure adhesion of tissue apposition. Then, the pre-tied knot is grasped with a hook and tightened until both plications are firmly apposed. The double plication involves now two serosa-to-serosa appositions and one mucosa-to-mucosa apposition at the level of the coagulation. Huberty et al. reported 6-month weight loss outcomes of 11% TBWL in ten patients with no major adverse events [197]. Although the results are encouraging and in par with those of other gastric remodelling techniques, final data on the safety of this device as well as long-term efficacy are still unavailable.

2.3.2.2 Gastric Stapling

Three systems of endoscopic stapling exist but, in contrast to the USGI-POSE and the Apollo OverStitch which were first applied in patients with post-bariatric complications and had their systems already approved by the FDA for tissue apposition for this indication, and thus easily rolled into the application of their method as primary treatment, these systems had to make a fresh start with a lot of development costs. To demonstrate this more in detail, BaroSense first explored a range of device prototypes and design implants, surgical technique and gastric attachment schemes in over 200 dogs. Then safety and durability of the plication method over time were demonstrated in a series of 18 animals, and finally the ability to transorally create and cannulate plications, place anchors, and deliver and attach the restrictive implant needed an additional series of 50 animals [198]. The high development costs and the costs of different human trials, with many adaptations and subsequent new animal work, and in the end, despite all the work, negative outcomes, are the reasons why these companies went into bankruptcy. Only one, the ACE stapler, was promising enough to be taken over by another company.

TransOral Gastroplasty (TOGa) (Satiety Inc., Palo Alto, CA, USA)
The TransOral Gastroplasty uses an endoscopic stapling device, the TOGa Sleeve Stapler, to create full-thickness, serosa-to-serosa, plications of the anterior and posterior walls in the proximal stomach. The TOGa system is composed of a flexible 18 mm shaft device that is introduced into the proximal stomach over a guidewire. The endoscope is passed through a special channel within the shaft. Once its position is confirmed endoscopically, a "sail septum" is deployed to stabilise the anterior and posterior walls of the body and greater curvature and to prevent their incorporation into the sleeve. Suction pods located within the stapling device are activated, bringing lesser curvature tissue within the jaws of the device. The stapler is then fired and three rows of 11 titanium staples each are delivered to create a transmural suture, with serosa-to-serosa apposition. This process is repeated to create a sleeve of the desired length extending over a length of 8–9 cm distally from the oesophagus beginning at the angle of His and parallel to the lesser curve. The sleeve outlet is then constricted from 20 mm to approximately 12 mm using the TOGa restrictor which clamps and staples gastric folds together after acquiring tissue via suction. The surgical analogue of this operation is the vertical banded gastroplasty [180] (Table 2.5). Devière et al. reported the first results in 21 patients (BMI 43.3 kg/m^2) with a weight loss of 12 kg, an EWL of 24.4% and BMI loss of 4.8 BMI units at 6 months [199]. There were no serious adverse events, although pain, nausea, vomiting and temporary dysphagia were reported. However, at the 6-month endoscopy, gaps between the two staple lines were evident and a fully intact sleeve was present in only 5 of 21 patients. A re-restriction was allowed but only one patient underwent a re-restriction. With improved techniques and perioperative administration of methylprednisolone and diclofenac, a second trial in 11 patients demonstrated a 24.0 kg weight loss, a 46.0% EWL and a decrease in BMI with 8.5 units at 6 months [200]. An intact sleeve persisted in 7 of the 11 patients at 6 months. Two patients underwent additional restrictions at 3 months because of insufficient weight loss and five restrictions could be placed. The TOGa multicentre study involved 67 patients who underwent the procedure successfully with two complications of a respiratory insufficiency and an asymptomatic pneumoperitoneum [201]. Fourteen patients did not complete the follow-up: 53 patients showed a weight loss of 19.5 kg,

a 7.6 kg/m^2 decrease in BMI, a 44.8% excess BMI loss and 38.7% EWL at 12 months. Patients with a BMI ≥40 kg/m^2 had 52.2% EWL and patients with BMI <40 kg/m^2 had 41.3% EWL. There were significant improvements in haemoglobin A1c (decline from 7.0% to 5.7%), HDL cholesterol and triglycerides. Partial dehiscence of the staple line was seen in 25 at the 12-month endoscopy, 7 proximally and 16 distally, and 2 patients had the combination, without a deleterious effect on weight loss. The conversion of TOGa into a laparoscopic RYGB or sleeve was easy without excess time and difficulty [200, 201]. Nanni et al. reported the results of 29 patients enrolled in the FDA-approved pilot study "Endoscopic Bariatric Stapling Pilot Study (TOGa®)" which would include 86 patients [202]. The average weight loss was 16.8 kg, 14.9% TBWL and a loss of 6.2 BMI units. The pilot study was never completed and the application is at present interrupted because of bankruptcy of the company.

Transoral Endoscopic Restrictive Implant System (TERIS) (BaroSense, Redwood City, CA, USA)

The transoral endoscopic restrictive implant system (TERIS) is aimed at endoscopically implanting a prosthesis at the level of the cardia, to decrease the size of the food reservoir of the upper part of the stomach creating a restrictive pouch, with a 10 mm orifice for food entering the distal stomach, being an endoscopic equivalent to gastric banding [180, 203] (Table 2.5). Five plications were made at the level of the cardia, 3–5 cm under the gastro-oesophageal junction. These plications were used to attach the gastric restrictor using silicone anchors inserted in the plications. Each plication was made using an articulated endoscopic circular stapler. This stapler can acquire a full-thickness gastric plication through suction, compressing the tissue and then creating two concentric rings of 3.5 mm staples, and excise the tissue within the ring to create a plication hole. Then a silicone anchor was brought down and the proximal end was pulled under direct visualisation through the plication hole and then released. Four other anchors were placed in a similar fashion. Five locking anchor graspers were advanced through a multilumen guide and attached to the anchors. The multilumen tube was then removed and the restrictor was advanced into the cardia. The anchors were then pulled through the restrictor's attachment holes one by one. After each anchor had been attached the graspers were removed, and finally the position of the restrictor was inspected. If needed, the silicone implant is removable. For a device-removal procedure, a 22 mm endogastric tube was advanced and a specially designed removal instrument system was advanced through the endogastric tube. With the assistance of an endoscope, graspers were used to pull the head of an anchor into the shaft of the removal instrument. An internal cutting snare was activated to cut the anchor. The grasper removed the anchor and this process was repeated for all anchors. After all anchors were cut and removed, the restrictor was grasped with a grasper and withdrawn through the endogastric tube.

In total, 12 of 13 implantation procedures were successful with three complications in the first seven patients, once a gastric perforation due to stapler malfunction – this patient was operated and the perforation oversewn – and twice an asymptomatic pneumoperitoneum, once treated conservatively and once by deflation by a hollow 16-gauge needle placed in the left flank [204]. In one patient due to limited manoeuvrability only four anchors could be placed. The study was put on hold and after technical improvements restarted and no procedural adverse events were seen in the next five patients. At 3 months an EWL of 22.2%, a decrease in body weight of 16.9 kg and a decrease in BMI from 42.1 to 37.9 kg/m^2 were observed [204]. As the system was designed as a 6-month bridge to surgery, the safety and efficacy results were investigated in the total number of 18 patients [198]. At 6 months, weight loss was 15.1% and EWL and excess BMI loss were 30.1% and 37.7%, respectively, demonstrating that TERIS was feasible and effective as a bridge to surgery. Mean waist circumference decreased by 18.7 cm. HDL cholesterol increased and HbA1C decreased significantly at 6 months. Two insulin-dependent diabetic patients did not need any insulin injections during the course of the study, and two other diabetics lowered the doses of oral medication. Four patients underwent an uncomplicated surgical procedure (three a gastric bypass and one a gastric band procedure) [198]. However, at the 6-month endoscopy 6 of the 16 successfully implanted patients had 1–3 detached anchors (37.5%). Their implants were removed. Of those who wanted to continue the treatment till up to 12 months, only two had a fully attached and intact device on the 12-month endoscopy. The colours of the anchors helped in the orientation and showed that mainly the lesser curvature anchors appeared to detach. The lesser curve seems to be a difficult area to attach to due to the thin muscle layer in this area of the stomach [198]. This terminated the TERIS technique. However, the stapling system functioned well, firing circular staples at a pressure of 6 bar and guaranteeing a full-thickness stapling with serosa-to-serosa application. A redesigned version of the stapler could make even larger plications, and studies with the articulating circular endoscopic (ACE) stapler as a means of endoscopic gastric volume reduction continued.

Articulating Circular Endoscopy (ACE) stapler (BaroSense, Redwood City, CA, USA, acquisition by Boston Scientific Corporation, Marlborough, MA, USA)
The articulating circular endoscopic (ACE) stapler is an endoscopic stapler with a head capable of 360-degree rotation and complete retroflexion. Vacuum suction is used to acquire tissue. Full-thickness plications are created by firing 10 mm plastic rings with eight titanium staples. After the placement of an overtube the ACE system and an ultrathin endoscope used for visualisation are introduced. The stomach tissue is imbibed inside the cover of the stapler by applying a vacuum at 6 bar, the tissue is then compressed by hydraulics inside the stapler and a 10 mm plastic ring with eight staples is fired creating full-thickness plications. The procedure starts high in the fundus in retroflexion with eight plications in the fundus to reduce the gastric volume. Two plications are created in the antrum to delay gastric emptying. The technique resembles the laparoscopic gastric plication surgery (Table 2.5).

Verlaan et al. included 17 patients (median BMI 40.2 kg/m^2) of whom 15 were available after 12-month follow-up [205]. They reported the safe placement of 160 plications in 17 patients which were still evident and appeared durable at endoscopy 12 months later. At that time endoscopy in 11 of the 17 patients revealed 6–9 plications and an important gastric volume reduction. The % EWL after 3, 6 and 12 months were 16.0%, 25.6% and 34.9%, respectively. Median BMI fell from 40.2 kg/m^2 to 34.5 kg/m^2 and median TBWL was 15.3% at 12 months. There were no serious adverse events and the most common adverse event was abdominal pain (seven patients). A sore throat, diarrhoea, nausea, constipation and vomiting were also reported but all were self-limited. Comorbidities including dyslipidaemia, hypertension, diabetes and obstructive sleep apnoea improved [205]. Van der Wielen et al. studied 10 of these 17 morbidly obese patients (BMI 39.8 kg/m^2) to gain insight into the long-term effects and underlying mechanisms of gastroplication [206]. Plasma adiponectin, HbA1c, and number of interleukins such as IL-1β, IL-6, IL-7, IL-8, tumour necrosis factor α (TNF-α), interferon-γ (IFN-γ), monocyte chemoattractant protein-1 (MCP-1), transforming growth factor-1 (TGF-1) and C-reactive protein (CRP) levels were determined at the start and after 12 months. At these times, also mucosal biopsies were collected from the fundus, antrum and duodenum and studied for gene expression using microarray analysis. After 12 months the BMI decreased to 33.4 kg/m^2 and the % EWL was 37.9%. Glycated haemoglobin (HbA1c) was significantly decreased ($P = 0.004$) by the treatment from 6.17% to 5.32%. Adiponectin showed a 1.64-fold increase and plasma IL-6 showed a tendency to decrease following ACE stapler treatment by a factor of 1.47. MCP-1 levels also showed a decrease (1.3-fold), but this effect did not reach statistical significance [206]. Fasted plasma ghrelin increased but on biopsies of the fundus there was a downregulation of MBOAT4, the gene encoding the ghrelin-activating enzyme GOAT4 and a trend for downregulation of ghrelin expression itself. Downregulation of inflammatory genes and gene sets was also observed on biopsies which coincided with improved HbA1c and adiponectin levels [206]. They could, however, not establish – by lack of a control group with a similar weight loss without the device – whether the reduction of inflammatory tone in the upper gastrointestinal tract might be a consequence of an improved metabolic health status and weight loss or alternatively caused by the procedure itself. Unfortunately, studies are at present on hold because the company went into bankruptcy and is taken over by Boston Scientific Corporation.

2.4 Intestinal Endoscopic Bariatric and Metabolic Therapies

2.4.1 Non-invasive Endoscopic Bariatric and Metabolic Therapies

2.4.1.1 The Duodenojejunal Bypass Sleeve (DJBS) or Duodenojejunal Bypass Liner (DJBL) or Endobarrier (GI Dynamics, Boston, MA, USA)

Until recently, the second-in-line in frequency and ease of application after balloon treatment was certainly the bypass of duodenum and proximal jejunum by the duodenojejunal bypass sleeve, also known as EndoBarrier gastrointestinal liner or simply the Endobarrier (Fig. 2.1). This is a totally different concept when compared to the gastric EMBTs, which, in addition to early satiety and delayed gastric emptying, aims at creating a duodenojejunal bypass. As the nutrients flow inside the sleeve and the pancreatobiliary secretions remain at the outside, it creates a barrier to nutrient absorption in the duodenum and proximal jejunum and delays the mixing of food with pancreaticobiliary secretions until more distally in the jejunum. Its surgical analogue is the Roux-en-Y gastric bypass (Table 2.5). The device is a 60 cm long, ultrathin, impermeable Teflon sleeve that is anchored in the duodenal bulb and extends into the proximal jejunum. By endoscopy a guidewire is introduced into the duodenum. After removal of the endoscope, the device which consists of a capsule at the distal end, holding the sleeve and the anchor, is advanced into the small bowel under fluoroscopy. First, the impermeable 60 cm Teflon sleeve is deployed by pushing the inner sheath of the catheter with an atraumatic ball at the end into the proximal jejunum. The ball and the sleeve are then released from the inner catheter and the ball passes under peristalsis. Once the sleeve is fully extended, a self-expanding 5.5 cm nitinol (nickel-titanium alloy) stent or crown with barbs is released into the duodenal bulb, 5 mm distally from the pylorus, to hold the device in place, under direct endoscopic visualisation. Ten barbs allow for stent or crown stabilisation and secure the crown to the muscularis propria. To remove the DJBS polypropylene drawstrings attached to the stent allow for collapse of the stent and retraction of the barbs from the duodenal bulb. The collapsed stent is then withdrawn into a protective plastic foreign-body retrieval hood mounted on the endoscope to avoid trauma to the stomach or oesophagus, and the entire device is withdrawn from the gastrointestinal tract along with removal of the endoscope. Escalona et al. modified the DJBS with a proximal flow-restricting orifice of 4 mm diameter in a small study of ten patients with an average BMI of 40.8 kg/m^2 which resulted in a percentage of EWL of 40% at 24 weeks [207]. Episodes of nausea, vomiting and abdominal pain required endoscopic dilation of the restrictor orifice in eight patients, with no clinically significant adverse events.

A systematic review by Patel et al. and a meta-analysis by Zechmeister-Koss et al. reviewed the ten available studies [208, 209]. There were six open studies [207, 210–214] and four randomised studies [215–218]. Of the four randomised studies, two are truly double blind and sham controlled [215, 217]. The 4 RCTs involved 95 DJBS patients, of whom two-thirds (61 patients) completed the study duration of 12–24 weeks, and 60 controls, 25 on a diet and 35 having sham placement, of whom 75% (43 patients) completed the trial [215–218]. Three of the four studies were designed to achieve preoperative weight loss and one to treat diabetic patients. The meta-analysis of these four RCTs concluded that in patients with obesity ≥grade I (BMI 30–34.9 kg/m^2) and type 2 diabetes there was a marginal greater reduction in weight loss (8 kg vs. 7 kg, NS) and in patients with obesity ≥grade II (BMI of 35–39.9 kg/m^2) (+ comorbidities) a significant and clinically relevant reduction in excess weight (12–22%) up to 12 weeks was seen, but effects on metabolic function expressed in terms of HbA1c and fasting blood glucose were unclear [209]. The 4 RCTs and the 6 non-RCTs were included in the safety analysis with in total 282 patients [209, 219]. Positioning of the device failed in 18 and succeeded only after several attempts in five. Mainly a too short duodenal bulb or a sharp angulation hindered successful positioning. There was a high number of early removals ($n = 60$; 24%) because of migration or rotation in 27, dislocation in 5, obstruction in 5, bleeding in 9 and intolerance in 10. Incompliance was the reason of early removal in four. The meta-analysis concluded that "While promising, the DJBS is not recommended for routine use but should be restricted to research settings only" [209]. Despite this scientific statement, the device was launched – outside the USA – as a metabolic intervention for those with a BMI >30 kg/m^2 and type 2 diabetes for the duration of 12 months. A recent meta-analysis in 2016 included 5 randomised controlled trials (235 subjects) and 10 observational studies (211 subjects) [220]. The risk of bias was evaluated as high in all studies. DJBS treatment compared with diet and/or lifestyle modifications alone resulted in a higher weight loss in obese subjects with significant mean differences in body weight loss of 5.1 kg and a 12.6% greater excess weight loss. The reductions in HbA1c and fasting plasma glucose were not significantly different and no changes in antidiabetic medication among the groups of obese patients were seen. In 20 patients the devices were not implanted. Adverse events were dominated by abdominal pain, nausea and vomiting. A total of 33 serious adverse events occurred. Additionally, 66 devices (19%) were explanted earlier than planned because of device migration, gastrointestinal bleeding, obstruction and abdominal pain or on investigator request. Furthermore, mucosal laceration during device removal was reported in three cases [220]. With respect to the many biases and distorting factors in the study design and data reporting, the authors requested future high-quality long-term RCTs to further assess efficacy and safety.

An important point to know is that the device did not interfere with subsequent gastric bypass or gastric banding in 12 patients and that intra-abdominal changes due to the device, as has been observed in animals, were not seen [217]. An interesting observation in the largest randomised study to date by Koehestani et al. requires further study: they found that significant differences in % EWL (19.8% in DJBS vs. 11.7% in controls) and HbA1c levels between the groups persisted for 6 months after the study completion [221]. A recent study by Vilarassa et al. confirmed these findings: 26 patients achieved a weight loss of 14.9% at the end of the 12-month DJBS period and retained 6.5% weight loss 12 months later [222]. At that time their HbA1c returned to pretreatment baselines, but of the 26.3% of patients who attained a HbA1c level of $\leq$7% during the DJBS period, 40% sustained this level over the next 12 months and the remainder experienced a lower increase of 0.7% [222].

The PIVI thresholds (Preservation and Incorporation of Valuable endoscopic Innovations (PIVI)) were also examined for the EndoBarrier/DJBS as this was the only device that had enough studies to evaluate (11 studies), besides the Orbera balloon with 82 studies [41]. For the DJBS meta-analyses, 11 studies met inclusion criteria. Of these, 9 reported adverse events and early removal rates, 3 reported % EWL at 12 months, 4 RCTs reported % EWL compared with a sham or control group at device removal, 9 reported changes in glycosylated haemoglobin (HbA1c) and three reported changes in HbA1c compared with a sham or control group in RCTs. Three studies enrolling 105 patients indicated that the DJBS may exceed the PIVI threshold of 25% EWL at 12 months by achieving a % EWL of 35.3% at

12 months. Four RCTs compared 12 to 24 weeks of treatment with the DJBS (90 subjects) with a sham or control arm (84 subjects). The mean % EWL difference compared with a control group was significant at 9.4%. However, the pooled % EWL of the DJBS over control did not meet the 15% PIVI threshold. So, the criteria for primary obesity treatment were not met [41]. Both of the above findings were associated with a high degree of heterogeneity. The DJBS demonstrated an impact on diabetic control after implantation, with decreases in HbA1c from 0.7% (NS) at 12 weeks to 1.7% ($P < 0.001$) at 24 weeks, and 1.5% ($P < 0.001$) after 52-week implantation. This improvement in HbA1c is statistically significant compared with a sham or control diabetic group, whereas it resulted in an additional 1% ($P = 0.001$) improvement in HbA1c compared with that seen in normal controls [41]. The published safety profile of the DJBS appears favourable based on experience with 271 implantations detailed in the literature (Fig. 2.9). Pain occurred in 58.7%, and nausea/vomiting in 39.4%. Early removal was needed in 18.4%. Serious adverse events included migration (4.9%), pain requiring early removal (4.2%), gastrointestinal bleeding (3.9%), sleeve obstruction (3.5%), liver abscess (0.13%), cholangitis (0.13%), acute cholecystitis (0.13%) and oesophageal perforation (0.13%) secondary to trauma from an uncovered barb at withdrawal [41].

Enrolment in the multicentre US pivotal trial, the ENDO trial, which compares the EndoBarrier DJBS with a sham endoscopic procedure in which no sleeve is

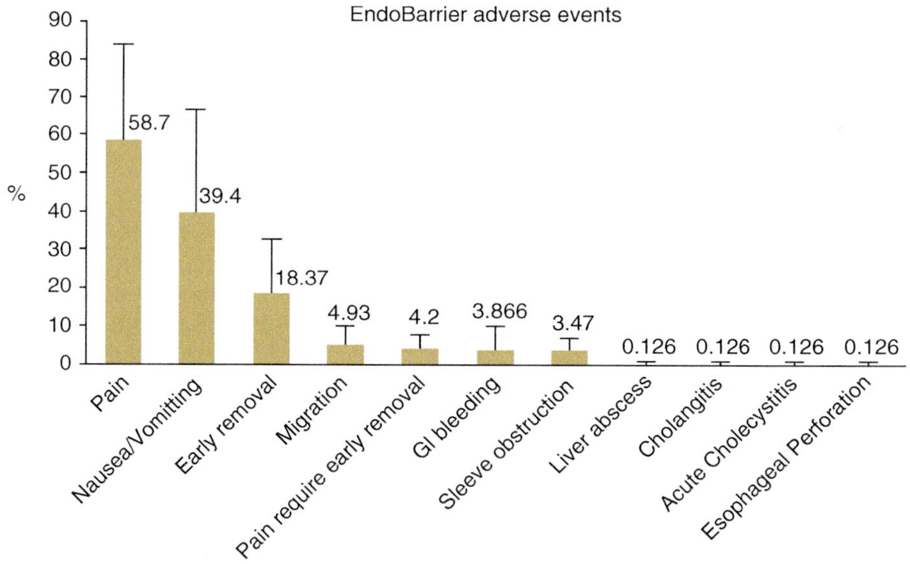

Fig. 2.9 Adverse events with the duodenojejunal bypass liner balloon as retrieved from 271 implantations detailed in the literature [41]. Reprinted from Gastrointest Endosc 2015; 82: 425–438, ASGE Bariatric Endoscopy Task Force and ASGE Technology Committee. Abu Dayyeh BK, Kumar N, Edmundowicz SA, Jonnalagadda S, Larsen M, Sullivan S, et al. ASGE Bariatric Endoscopy Task Force systematic review and meta-analysis assessing the ASGE PIVI thresholds for adopting endoscopic bariatric therapies with permission from Elsevier

inserted, was placed on hold in March 2015 by the US FDA, because of a higher-than-expected incidence of liver abscesses (i.e. 3.5%, so higher than the established safety threshold of 2%). These adverse events, adequately managed with intravenous antibiotics and percutaneous drainage, were most likely related to translocation of bacteria from the anchoring system but posed a prohibitive risk for continuing the trial. Brethauer et al. reported a worldwide incidence of liver abscesses of 0.9% (29/3000) [111]. At the time of suspension of the study, 325 of the needed 500 subjects (active group $n = 216$, sham control $n = 109$; starting values HbA1c 8.8%; BMI 38.3 kg/m^2) had been included [223]. With two-third enrolment, subjects who received the DJBS lost significantly more weight compared with the sham group at 12 months (7.7% TBWL vs. 2.1%; $P < 0.001$) and had more significant improvement in HbA1c level (−1.1% vs. -0.3%) [223]. Efficacy endpoints were met with 60% of the DJBS patients losing 5% or more TWL and 34.8% achieving a HbA1c level of 7% or less (compared with 20% and 9.8% in the sham arm, respectively) [223]. Ninety-four percent of active subjects had successful DJBS placement. Early device retrieval owing to adverse events was present in 11% of patients [223].

Second-generation DJBSs with atraumatic anchoring and retrieval systems are currently investigated in clinical human trials.

2.4.1.2 Valen-Tx Bypass Sleeve (ValenTx, Inc., Carpinteria, CA, USA)

The ValenTx is an implantable sleeve that runs from the oesophagus down to the jejunum and is 120 cm in length (Fig. 2.1). The device acts to mimic the effects of the traditional gastric bypass by restricting the amount of food intake, excluding food from the stomach, the ghrelin-secreting gastric fundus and small intestine, and leaving undigested food exposed to the jejunum (Table 2.5). The procedure begins with placement of a long overtube, extending through the pylorus, into the duodenal bulb. Through this overtube the gastroduodenojejunal bypass sleeve (GJBS) is delivered via a delivery catheter under fluoroscopic guidance into the proximal jejunum. Once the sleeve is adequately deployed downstream into the bowel, the delivery catheter is removed, and the overtube is exchanged for a shorter overtube. The polyester proximal cuff is then positioned endoscopically at the gastro-oesophageal junction. The attachment is performed with eight endoscopically delivered, nitinol suture anchors, deployed circumferentially, with the assistance of laparoscopic visualisation to ensure transmural anchor placement and to avoid any visceral injury. Future applications will aim to secure the device by endoscopy alone. When removal is needed the device can be explanted with endoscopic cutting of the sutures.

In 24 patients (BMI 42 kg/m^2) the device was successfully delivered in 22 and endoscopically retrieved in all 22 [224]. Two patients had no placement, one because of non-compliance, and the other had severe inflammation at the gastro-oesophageal junction. Of the 22 patients with successful implantation, 17 retained the device for 12 weeks; these patients had 39.7% EWL or a 16.8 kg weight loss. Early post-operative dysphagia was the main reason for removal in five. Seven patients with diabetes had normal glucose levels and did not require medication. All four with elevated HbA1c had significantly improved levels. In 2015, Sandler et al. reported the results of 1 year in 13 morbidly obese subjects (BMI 42 kg/m^2), meeting the

NIH criteria for bariatric surgery [224]. One patient had no placement and two did not tolerate the device. In ten patients, the ValenTx remained in place for 1 year, six patients had fully attached and functional sleeves at the 1-year follow-up evaluation, and four patients had partial cuff detachment seen at follow-up endoscopy. For these ten patients, the mean percentage excess weight loss at 1 year was 35.9% whereas it was 54% EWL among the six patients with intact sleeves [225]. 70% of all comorbidities resolved or significantly improved. Upon endoscopic removal, no cuff ingrowth was noted at the gastro-oesophageal junction, no adhesions were noted between the sleeve and mucosa in the stomach or small bowel and the mucosa appeared healthy and normal. No significant bleeding, erosion or oesophageal leakage was experienced at the time of removal. Of the six patients with a fully attached device, five were followed for an average of 14 months post-explant, so 26 months from the time of device implant. These five patients maintained an average percentage EWL of 30% at the 14-month post-explant follow-up [225]. In contrast to the DJBS, liver abscesses are not to be expected but due to its position at the gastro-oesophageal junction complaints of dysphagia and odynophagia may occur. The company is currently planning a US trial.

2.4.1.3 Mechanisms of Action of Endoscopic Bypass Procedures

The duodenojejunal and the gastroduodenojejunal bypass sleeves mimic the effects of a gastric bypass by creating a physical barrier that allows food to bypass the duodenum and proximal jejunum without mixing with bile and pancreatic enzymes until later in the gut, thus potentially altering the incretin pathways and the entero-insular system [148]. In gastric bypass surgery, the rapid improvement of diabetes before any weight reduction has occurred can be explained by two hypotheses: the foregut and the hindgut hypothesis [226–228]. De Jonge et al. have shown that after 24 weeks of implantation of the DJBS, patients had lost 12.7 kg ($P < 0.01$), while haemoglobin A1c had improved from 8.4% to 7.0% ($P < 0.01$) [229]. Both fasting glucose levels and the postprandial glucose response were decreased at 1 week after implantation and remained decreased at 24 weeks. The foregut hypothesis suggests that improved glycaemic control results from a reduced secretion of diabetogenic hormones or anti-incretin factors due to the absence of nutrients in the proximal small intestine. Intestinal glucagon synthesis and gastric inhibitory peptide or glucose-dependent insulinotropic polypeptide (GIP) have been suggested to decrease after exclusion of the proximal small intestine [226]. In accordance with the foregut hypothesis de Jong et al. discovered that prevention of digestion and uptake of nutrients by the DJBS were associated with a decreased secretion of glucagon, a diabetogenic factor, as well as a decreased secretion of GIP, which is secreted in the proximal small intestine and affects glucagon secretion [229]. The second hypothesis is the hindgut hypothesis which attributes the improved glycaemic control to the enhanced secretion of incretins such as glucagon-like peptide-1 (GLP-1) and enhanced secretion of peptide YY (PYY) in response to undigested nutrients in the distal small bowel [227, 228]. The observed increased GLP-1 secretion of de Jong et al. is in agreement with the hindgut hypothesis [229]. Furthermore, they investigated whether the early improvement of diabetes could be explained by a decreased inflammatory state which was not the case [230]. One other study found an increase in fasting peptide YY (PYY), a gut hormone involved in appetite suppression [222]. However, increased fasting ghrelin levels, a gut hormone which stimulates hunger, was identified in two studies and could be related to the fasting state or to the decrease in weight, which both increase the orexigenic ghrelin levels [222, 231]. These two studies were also at variance with the study of de Jonge et al. as they could not demonstrate an effect on GLP-1 [222, 229, 231]. Moreover, whereas de Jonge et al. found a decreased secretion of glucagon in their 6-month DJBS treatment, fasting plasma glucagon concentrations in Vilarassa's study decreased at month 1 and were found to be increased at the end of their 12-months DJBS study, but unfortunately no data are available at the 6-month point of time [222, 229]. Parallel herewith HbA1c decreased 1.3% in the first month, but at the end of the 12-month study, the reduction was only 0.6% [222]. The primary endpoint of success, a HbA1c $\leq$7%, was achieved in only 26.3% of patients [222]. These conflicting findings may be the result of small sample sizes, difference in duration of DJBS treatment, differences in characteristics of patients regarding their diabetes such as duration, oral medication or insulin requirement, and differences in hormone level measurements either as fasting values or repeated samples before and during a standardised meal.

Gastric emptying was also studied in 25 patients with DJBS treatment [232]. While there was a significant decrease in gastric emptying, 16 weeks after DJBS implantation, compared to the basal situation, this recovered almost completely to normal after DJBS removal [232]. However, the delayed gastric emptying provoked by the DJBS did not correlate with glycated haemoglobin concentrations or weight loss success but might explain the abdominal side effects. The delayed emptying was explained by duodenal irritation and duodenal distension by the anchor of the sleeve, resulting in gastric relaxation [222, 232]. Unfortunately, no blood samples for gut hormones were taken, as cholecystokinin (CCK), GLP-1 and PYY are particularly important in the control of gastric emptying and are known to delay the gastric emptying. A delayed gastric emptying was also found when 15 sham patients and 14 patients with lifestyle modification therapy were compared with 25 DJBS patients: while the former had a normal gastric emptying (median % increase in gastric retention at 2 h of −1%) the DBJS had a 24% increase in gastric retention [70]. Further studies are necessary to elucidate the mechanisms responsible for weight loss and improved blood glucose control with the DJBS.

2.4.2 Invasive Endoscopic Bariatric and Metabolic Therapies

These rather new techniques are invasive as in the case of duodenal mucosa resurfacing they destroy temporarily the normal anatomy of the duodenum by burning the mucosa, and in the case of an incisionless magnetic anastomosis system they divert the digestive flow partly from the normal way through a jejunoileal shortcut.

2.4.2.1 Duodenal Mucosa Resurfacing (Revita, Fractyl Laboratories, Cambridge, MA, USA)

Duodenal mucosal resurfacing (DMR) or the Revita procedure is an endolumenal procedure, consisting of determination of the duodenal size, saline expansion of the submucosal space and hydrothermal ablation of the superficial mucosa layers. The duodenal mucosa is abnormal in patients with diabetes and exhibits abnormal hypertrophy and endocrine hyperplasia. From bariatric Roux-en-Y gastric bypass surgery, the beneficial effects of exclusion of an abnormal duodenal surface in type 2 diabetes from nutrient contact were known, perhaps through the reduction of putative anti-incretin mechanisms [148, 180, 226] (Table 2.5). By mucosa ablation at denaturation temperatures the triggering of a rejuvenative healing response was hypothesised [233]. First, a catheter with a terminal balloon is passed into the duodenum that has three needles spaced at 120° around the balloon's circumference. The needles are used to inject saline into the submucosal space in order to circumferentially separate and lift the mucosa from underlying tissues in the duodenal wall from 1 cm distal to the ampulla of Vater to proximal to the ligament of Treitz (Fig. 2.10a). After removal of the initial catheter, a second balloon catheter was introduced to perform thermal ablations of ≈10 s each at temperatures of ≈90 °C on the lifted area (Fig. 2.10b). A total of 39 patients out of 44 included with type 2 diabetes (screening HbA1c 9.5% [80 mmol/mol]; BMI 31 kg/m^2) could be treated: 28 had a long duodenal segment ablated (LS; ~9.3 cm) and 11 had a short segment ablated (SS; ~3.4 cm) [233]. Overall, DMR was well tolerated with minimal gastrointestinal symptoms of transient abdominal pain in 20%. Three patients experienced duodenal stenosis treated successfully by balloon dilation. HbA1c was reduced by 1.2% at 6 months in the full cohort ($P < 0.001$). At 6 months 29 of the 39 had some HbA1c reduction. More potent effects were observed among the LS cohort, who experienced a 2.5% reduction in mean HbA1c at 3 months versus 1.2% in the SS group ($P < 0.05$) and a 1.4% reduction at 6 months versus 0.7% in the SS group ($P = 0.3$) [234]. Interestingly, these beneficial effects were obtained without a dietary energy restriction and without any significant weight body loss (4.6% TBWL at 3 months and 3% TBWL at 6 months). The mixed meal data suggest that an insulin-sensitising mechanism is responsible for the effects on fasting glucose and HbA1c [233].

However, a very critical comment touched the authors on the raw: the observed reduction of HbA1c can also be achieved by medication and the effect on HbA1c is waning as it was less at 6 months compared with 3 months [234]. Five of the 44 patents were not suited for the treatment (10%) and 10 of the 39 patients (26%) were primary failures. Furthermore, the effects of the very-low-calorie diet immediately after the procedure which was built up over 2 weeks and the weight loss which are both adequate to restore insulin sensitivity might have been partly responsible for the observed changes [228, 234].

There are two ways of thermal ablation, either through the use of radiofrequency or through a recirculating hot-water-filled balloon. Currently, a multicentre study is being conducted in Europe and after modification and optimisation of the DMR procedure, by avoiding overlap of burns and adequate attention to the lifting of the mucosa at all sites, no additional duodenal stenosis or other serious adverse events have developed [235]. A US pivotal trial is planned.

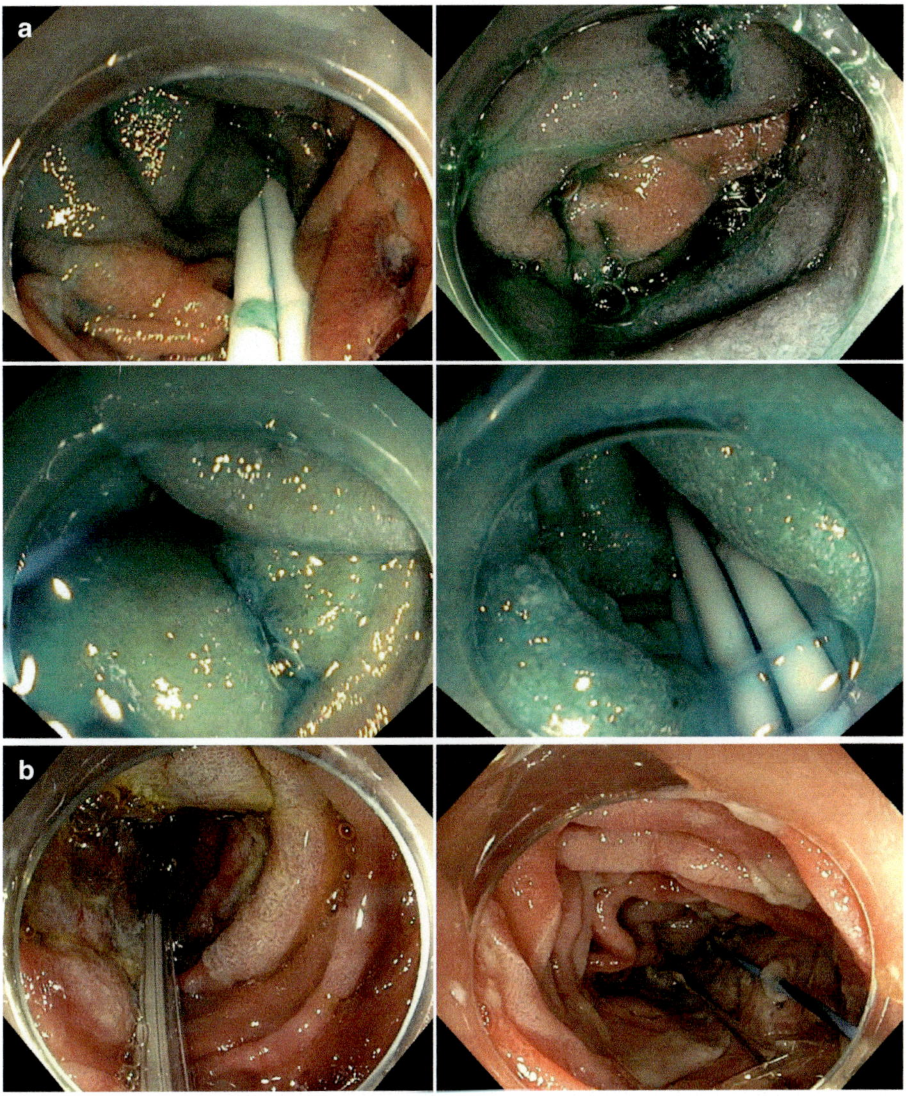

Fig. 2.10 Duodenal mucosa resurfacing: (**a**) the lifting of the mucosa with submucosal saline and methylene blue; (**b**) the white areas of mucosal ablation by heat. Pictures by courtesy of professor Dr. Jacques Bergman et al., Department of Gastroenterology and Hepatology, Academic Medical Centre, University of Amsterdam, the Netherlands

2.4.2.2 Incisionless Magnetic Anastomotic Systems (IMAS) (GI Windows, West Bridgewater, MA, USA)

An endoscopic incisionless magnetic anastomotic system (IMAS) has been developed using self-assembling magnets [236, 237]. The IMAS is preloaded into the instrumentation channel of the endoscope and by using simultaneous enteroscopy and colonoscopy two magnets are deployed in the gastrointestinal tract in the jejunum and ileum under endoscopic and fluoroscopic visualisation and they form octagonal rings (Fig. 2.11a, b). Laparoscopic assistance confirms the adequate mating of the magnets and measures the end position of the anastomosis. The magnets mate, apply compressive force to the tissue between them, and create pressure necrosis and a large-bore compression anastomosis over several days. The magnets then disassemble and pass down the gastrointestinal tract. The magnets were expelled fully intact without pain at a mean of 23 days, without obstruction. The result is a large-bore anastomosis and a dual-path enteral bypass with the flow of food down both limbs via the native anatomy and through the jejunoileal anastomosis (Fig. 2.11c). The surgical analogue is the modified duodenal switch or ileal transposition (Table 2.5). A trial in ten subjects (six males) with BMI of 41 kg/m^2 reported successful device placement and anastomosis formation in all cases [238, 239]. Anastomoses owere widely patent at the 2 and 6 month's control endoscopy. Transient nausea and diarrhoea were reported in most cases. Diarrhoea, that persisted in a few cases, could be managed by diet adjustments. Without any lifestyle intervention or calorie-restricted diet, mean weight loss at 6 months was 12.9 kg, 10.6% TBWL or 28.3% EWL. Four patients with type 2 diabetes experienced a 1.8% haemoglobin A1c reduction and a 3.6 mmol/L lower fasting glucose. Three patients with prediabetes normalised their HbA1c and glucose levels. All diabetic patients were able to reduce or discontinue their diabetic medication within 6 months [240].

The theory behind this technology is that nutrient delivery to the distal small bowel will induce an ileal break phenomenon by PYY release, which will delay the gastric emptying and decrease food intake. The diversion of nutrients and bile to the terminal ileum will also activate bile-signalling pathways and enhance incretin secretion with an increase in GLP-1 levels postprandially [180, 240]. It is functionally similar to the biliopancreatic diversion with duodenal switch (without the sleeve or partial gastrectomy) and mechanistically similar to ileal transposition [180, 240].

2.5 Perspective of Endoscopic Bariatric and Metabolic Therapies

Because of the obesity epidemic and the obesity-associated diseases a large number of individuals will need treatment. Endoscopic treatment has the advantage of being cheap, minimally invasive, moderately time consuming, reversible and feasible as an ambulant procedure, without a steep learning curve as is the case with bariatric surgery. It has the disadvantage of limited durability. Endoscopic bariatric therapy appears well suited to bridge the current management gap between medical treatment, which consists of intensive lifestyle treatment and pharmacotherapy at the one side and bariatric surgery on the other. EBTs offer an effective weight loss intervention with potentially lower risks, lower costs and higher patient acceptability than bariatric surgery. Many EBTs also offer the potential added advantages of reversibility and repeatability, depending on the individual therapy.

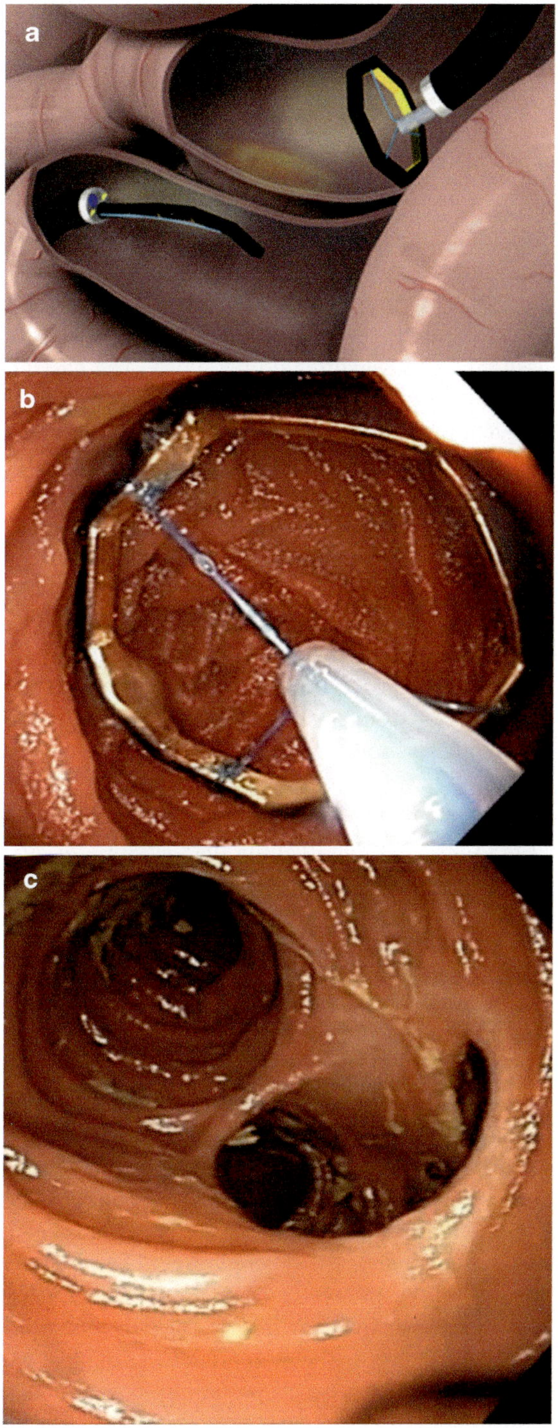

Fig. 2.11 The incisionless magnetic anastomotic system: (**a**, **b**) The deployment of two magnets by simultaneous enteroscopy and colonoscopy and the octagonal ring of the deployed magnet. (**c**) The large-bore anastomosis and a dual-path enteral bypass with the flow of food down both limbs via the native anatomy and through the jejunoileal anastomosis [240]. Reprinted from Gastrointest Endosc 2017 [published online ahead of print] doi: https://doi.org/10.1016/j.gie.2017.07.009.242, Machytka E, Bužga M, Zonca P, Lautz DB, Ryou M, Simonson DC, et al. Partial jejunal diversion using an incisionless magnetic anastomosis system: 1-year interim results in subjects with obesity and diabetes with permission from Elsevier

There are endoscopic gastric options such as balloons and aspiration therapy, which are all at the disposal of and practicable by endoscopists, but some have the disadvantage of limited durability. Yet, a 10% weight loss with improvement of obesity-associated comorbidities can be maintained after balloon removal by almost 50% for 1 year and by one-quarter of patients over 2.5 years. The FDA approved the Orbera balloon, the ReShape Duo balloon and the swallowable Obalon balloon for 6 months in subjects with a BMI between 30 and 40 kg/m^2. They also approved the AspireAssist aspiration therapy for patients with a BMI between 35 and 55 kg/m^2. Pivotal randomised multicentre trials to support regulatory approval in the USA are in progress or are planned for a number of devices.

Gastric suturing and gastric plication enable very skilled endoscopists to mimic gastric restrictive surgical operations. The gastric volume reduction devices mimic bariatric surgical interventions, but the mechanism of action of the existing endoscopic mimicry of bariatric surgery should be further investigated.

Endoscopic intestinal options are the duodenojejunal bypass sleeve, which is not available anymore because of the development of liver abscesses, but further modifications are awaited. Furthermore, data of duodenal resurfacing and jejunoileal bypass by magnet-induced wall apposition and pressure necrosis are very preliminary but look promising.

It may well be that future research will focus on the tandem and sequential use of a combination of endoscopic devices and obesity pharmacotherapies in addition to a comprehensive lifestyle intervention programme to augment and enhance the durability of weight loss with a lasting effect on obesity and its related comorbidities. However, cost-benefit analyses should always accompany these cost-enhancing combinations. Having all this information absorbed, the question "Are endoscopist definitely stepping into the arena of weight loss therapy?" which was answered with "I hope they will and I think they should" in 2015 [241] should now definitely be answered with a whole-hearted yes, when one sees what has been achieved over a period of only 2 years with four FDA approvals and two pending FDA approvals. The future is bright for "bariatric" endoscopists!

2.6 Laparoscopic Minimally Invasive Techniques

Neuromodulation represents a group of new surgical approaches to the treatment of obesity and associated metabolic disorders that involve the application of a small patterned electrical impulse to a target organ. The target organ may include true organs such as the stomach, duodenum, small intestine, adrenal glands, or brain, but also the vagal nerves. Changing the pattern and amount of energy delivered can also alter the desired effect. The impulse can augment or modify normal physiologic responses or block them. There is a growing body of research to suggest that the technology is safe. In addition, at least some of the neuromodulatory technologies have the potential to provide beneficial weight loss and positive effects on the associated metabolic conditions. To date, the published data with neuromodulation suggests that there may be potential for benefit with some of these technologies. Neuromodulation is supposed to offer safe and less complex options to the conventional surgical approaches to morbid obesity. Although being a known part of the current bariatric armamentarium and not anymore belonging to the research field, the cost of these devices, with issues of battery replacement (which have been improved), renders them unavailable for a routine use worldwide.

Neuromodulation has the potential to evolve towards endoscopic applications. Because of extreme downsizing of current cardiac stimulators (and leads) being a reality nowadays, an endoscopic application of gastric stimulation is no challenge to conceive, albeit quite expensive. So far, this is a highly speculative topic, owing to the already important costs of current devices. Our guess is that these devices will be reconsidered as soon as downsized stimulators have been proven cost effective in the cardiology field, and pending other technical issues (such as the fixation of the device inside the gastric lumen) have been solved.

Several systems are currently competing. Two of them (Abiliti™ and Tantalus™) deal with a satiety-inducing stimulation that is monitored through gastric distension measurement, thus allowing a theoretical fine-tuning of electrical stimulation. A third one (V-Bloc™) aims at direct vagal stimulation, which has been suspected for a long time of being instrumental in decreasing hunger and enhancing satiety (as well as vagotomy). Trials are being conducted with each of these devices, some of them focusing more specifically on comorbidities such as T2DM.

2.6.1 Gastric Pacing

2.6.1.1 Surgical Implantation of Electrodes

The technical details of the positioning of the electrodes differ according to different existing devices, some of them being implanted directly on the vagal nerves, others on their branches at a variable location on the anterior part of the stomach: antrum, pes anserinus - i.e. final vagal branches on the lesser curve - or even fundus. Multiples sources are possible for implementing neurostimulation (several electrodes or just one) as well as multiple parameters of stimulation (frequency, pulse width and amplitude). Most often, the fixation of the electrode is mandatory, to avoid dislodgement or intragastric penetration, ending up with a failure to stimulate. With one current system (Abiliti), a sensor is inserted in the fundus, which is supposed to allow fine-tuning of the stimulation. These electrodes are connected to a subcutaneous pacemaker that is comparable in size and potential side effects (e.g. haematoma) to the cardiac devices, routinely implanted in the left upper quadrant of the abdomen. The device is then verified on a routine basis, a dedicated software allowing modifications of the stimulation parameters.

2.6.1.2 Involvement of an Endoscopist

While waiting for devices that can theoretically be implanted endoscopically, gastroenterologists are quite instrumental in dealing with these patients for the time being. Assessment of the gastroesophageal junction, detection of *H. pylori*, etc. are part of the routine screening. Some devices require an intraoperative check during the implantation of the electrode/sensor. Finally, endoscopy is necessary if one suspects an electrode dislodgement or a transgastric erosion of the device.

2.6.1.3 Abiliti System (Intrapace Inc., San José, CA, USA)

This system is the direct continuation of a device initiated by Cigaina in 1999 in Italy [242], that produced variable outcomes [243]. It includes a simple stimulation electrode inserted approximately 4 cm from the gastro-oesophageal junction and 1.5 cm from the lesser curvature in the anterior wall (Fig. 2.12). This site corresponds with the point where the anterior vagal nerve (Latarjet nerve) divides into 3 branches. A transgastric food sensor is implanted in the body fundus region, about 3 cm from the greater curve with a distance between both electrodes of 3–4 cm. Peroperative endoscopy is performed to confirm the intragastric probe extension. The transgastric food sensor detects the entry of food into the stomach by distension and then triggers the gastric stimulator [244]. Horbach et al. assessed closed-loop gastric electrical stimulation (CLGES) versus laparoscopic adjustable gastric banding (LAGB) for the treatment of obesity, in a randomised 12-month multicentre

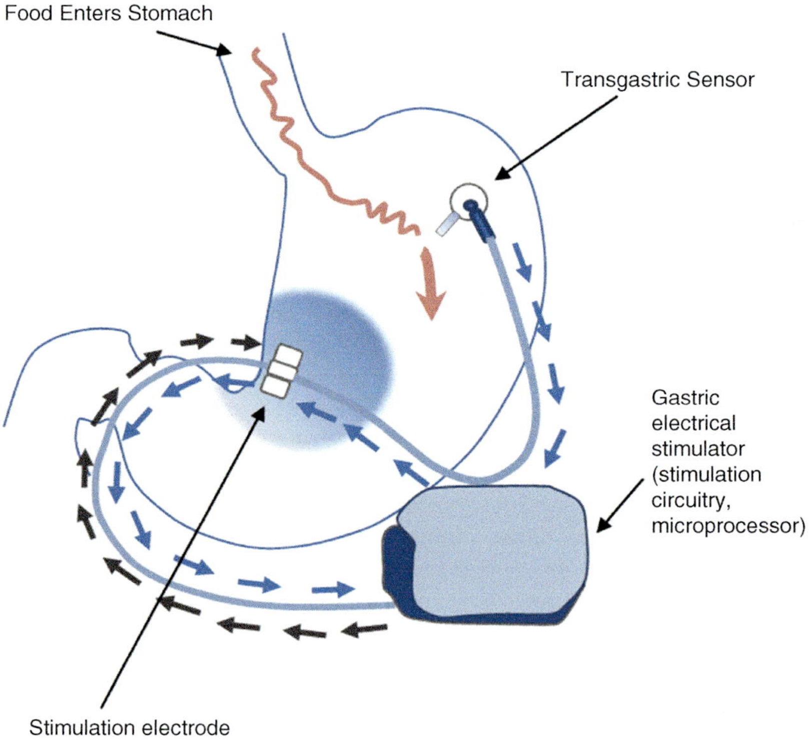

Fig. 2.12 Ability system with the transgastric sensor and gastric electrical stimulator [244]. Reprinted from Obes Surg 2015; 25: 1779–1787, Horbach T, Thalheimer A, Seyfried F, Eschenbacher F, Schuhmann P, Meyer G. Ability® closed loop gastric electrical stimulation system for treatment of obesity: clinical results with a 27-month follow-up (Open Access Article)

study [245]. This non-inferiority trial assigned the patients in a 2:1 ratio to laparoscopic CLGES versus LAGB and followed them for 1 year; 210 patients were enrolled, of whom 50 were withdrawn preoperatively. Among 160 remaining patients (age 39 years; BMI 43 kg/m^2), 106 received CLGES and 54 received LAGB. The first primary endpoint was the demonstration of non-inferiority of CLGES versus LAGB, ascertained by the proportion of patients who, at 1 year, fulfilled a ≥20% excess weight loss (EWL); no major device- or procedure-related adverse event (AE); and no major, adverse change in QOL, assuming a difference of <10% between the two procedures. The second primary endpoint was that ≥50% of patients had to reach ≥25% EWL in the CLGES group. At 1 year, the proportions of patients who reached all components of the primary study end-point were 66.7% and 73.0% for the LAGB and CLGES group, respectively, with a difference of −6.3% (upper limit of the 95% CI 7.2%, so non-inferiority proven). The second primary endpoint was also met, as 61.3% of patients in the CLGES group reached ≥25% EWL (lower 95% CI = 52.0%; $P < 0.01$). The quality of life improved significantly and similarly in both groups. Adverse events were significantly fewer and less severe in the CLGES (31%) than in the LAGB group (81%) ($P < 0.001$). More importantly, device-related adverse events were not different, 4.7% in the CLGES group and 13.0% in the LAGB group. Device replacement and lead fracture were seen in 4 subjects (4%), discomfort of the surgical pocket in eight (8%) and eight patients (8%) perceived the stimulation as painful.

2.6.1.4 Tantalus System (Metacure Inc., Australia)

The Tantalus system, now called DIAMOND, a meal-initiated gastrointestinal (GI) stimulator, aims at treating obese patients with T2DM (Fig. 2.13). Three year results were presented by Lebovitz et al. [246]. The aim was to investigate long-term benefit of non-excitatory gastric electrical stimulation (GES) by the DIAMOND device on glycaemic control and body weight in obese patients with T2DM inadequately controlled with oral agents, and to determine the magnitude of the modulating effects of fasting plasma triglyceride levels on the effects of GES. Sixty-one patients with T2DM (HbA1c between 7.0% and 10.5%) were implanted with the DIAMOND GES device and treated with meal-mediated antral electrical stimulation for up to 36 months. GES reduced mean HbA1c by 0.9% and body weight by 5.7% after 12 months. The effects were greater in patients with normal fasting plasma triglycerides (NTG, triglycerides ≤1.7 mmol/L) as compared to those with hypertriglyceridaemia (HTG, triglycerides >1.7 mmol/L). The mean decrease in HbA1c in patients with NTG averaged 1.1% and was durable over 3 years of follow-up. Improvement in HbA1c was a function of both baseline triglycerides ($P = 0.02$) and HbA1c ($P = 0.001$). However, the attrition rate was high as only 29 of the 61 device-implanted patients completed the 2 years and 8 the 3 years. There was a significantly different weight loss in NTG versus HTG patients. Whereas at 24 months a ≥10% weight loss was achieved by 7/13 patients in the NTG group; this was 0/16 in the HTG group. Also, weight losses at 12 months and 24 months were different: −4.7% and −9.4% in the 33 and 13 NGT patients, respectively, and −2.6% and −2.8% in the 24 and 16 HTG patients, respectively. One patient required device

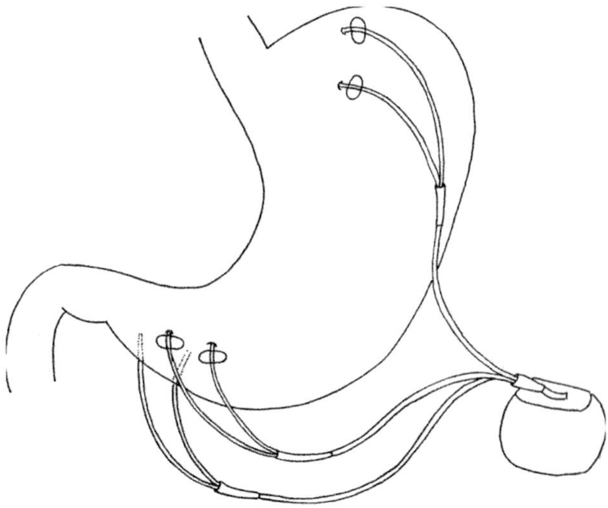

Fig. 2.13 Tantalus system with the sensing electrodes and the electrical stimulation electrodes

removal because of repeated infections around the implanted pulse generator. The authors postulated that GES creates a gut-brain interaction that modulates effects on the liver and pancreatic islets.

2.6.2 Vagal Blockade (Enteromedics Inc., St-Paul, MN, USA)

Truncal vagotomy has been suggested as an obesity treatment [247], and then advocated as an adjunct to a bariatric surgical technique such as vertical banded gastroplasty [248], but has become obsolete or had limited effects in the long term with sometimes persisting chronic side effects such as diarrhoea and vomiting. Yet, gastric pacing has taken this path, at least partially, with the vagal block stimulation from Enteromedics.

An active implantable device connected to 2 C-shaped electrodes positioned by laparoscopy on the anterior and posterior vagal trunks near the gastro-oesophageal junction is designed to induce intermittent sub-diaphragmatic vagal blocking for 12 hours or more per day in cycles of 5 minutes blockage and 5 minutes rest to allow the nerve to recover and to avoid tachyphylaxis [249]. This method has demonstrated clinically important weight loss and glycaemic control in obese T2DM subjects. Initial results were published by Shikora et al. [250]. VBloc-DM2 was a prospective, observational study of 28 subjects with T2DM and BMI 30–40 kg/m^2 to assess mid-term safety and weight loss and improvements in glycaemic parameters, and other cardiovascular risk factors with vagal blocking (VBloc) therapy. At 24 months, the mean percentage of excess weight loss was 22%, or 7.0% total body weight loss, both highly significant changes. Haemoglobin A1c decreased by 0.6 percentage points on average from 7.8% at baseline (significant). Fasting plasma glucose declined by 15 mg/dL (0.83 mmol/L) on average from 151 mg/dL (6.38 mmol/L) at baseline (non-significant). Among subjects who were hypertensive at baseline, systolic blood pressure declined by 10 mmHg, diastolic blood pressure declined by 6 mmHg and mean arterial pressure declined by 7 mmHg (all $P < 0.05$). Waist circumference was significantly reduced by 7 cm from a baseline of 120 cm. The most common adverse events were mild or moderate heartburn, implant site pain, and constipation. Improvements in obesity and glycaemic control were largely sustained after 2 years of treatment with VBloc therapy with a well-tolerated risk profile. These results have been confirmed very recently by a large study in 162 patients of whom 123 remained in the trial at 24 months [251]. Of the withdrawals, 9 withdrew because of adverse events such as pain at the neurostimulation site in 5, the need for a MRI in 2, and heartburn and abdominal pain each in one. In the first year of the study 8 patients required nine revisions. In follow-up after this year there were only 4 revisions, 2 due to pain at the neurostimulation site, one had twisted leads and one had the inability to recharge the device. Weight loss at 24 months was 8%, and 58% of patients had a ≥5% TBWL and 34% a ≥10% TBWL. In patients with abnormal values LDL-cholesterol levels decreased, HDL-cholesterol levels increased and a significant improvement was shown in HbA1c, systolic and diastolic blood pressure. The FDA approved the device in the USA, and an ASMBS position statement acknowledged the role of vagal neurostimulation in the treatment of obesity, in a BMI range of 35–45 kg/m^2 [249].

2.7 Perspectives of Laparoscopic Minimally Invasive Techniques

It is difficult to foresee the future of gastric stimulation, but one can guess that more research will tell if current techniques have an "electrical counterpart" that could be exploited further. An important contributing information comes from sleeve gastrectomy, which results in the resection of the gastric natural pacemaker, creating aberrant ectopic pacemaker impulses or even bioelectrical quiescence, which persists long after SG, inducing chronic dysmotility [252]. It is too early to correlate these findings to potential new applications of neurostimulation, but building accurate models is an interesting start.

The main focus here is to find therapies for the treatment of T2DM by affecting the autonomic system and in particular the afferent vagal activity, whose nerves project on the brainstem on the nucleus tractus solitarius and information gathered here is translated into vagal efferent outputs that control the splanchnic organs. Biasi depicted the important role of the nucleus tractus solitarius in the treatment of T2DM and the future prospects in surgical and pharmacological modulation of the vagal transmission [253]. Among different leads, there are some examples of current clinical and experimental research. Non-invasive neurostimulation, e.g. transcranial, has been tested as a mild treatment of craving; vagal branches can also be a target, i.e. if applied to the intra-auricular cutaneous area [254]. The role of vagal nerve has even been further investigated: signalling fullness to the brain may be de-activated after long-term consumption of a high-fat diet in rats [255]. Finally, other parts of the digestive tract are being targeted, and for instance the duodenum can be an interesting location: it has been shown that stimulation of this part of the digestive tract delayed gastric emptying and accelerated small-bowel transit while enhancing GLP-1 secretion in animal models [256].

Acknowledgments The author acknowledges J. Dargent for his help with the laparoscopic minimally invasive techniques.

References

1. World Health Organization. Obesity: preventing and managing the global epidemic. Report of a WHO Consultation on Obesity, Geneva, 3–5 June 1997. Report 1998 No.: WHO/NUT/NCD/98.1.
2. National Institutes of Health, National Heart, Lung and Blood Institute. Clinical guidelines on the identification, evaluation, and treatment of overweight and obesity in adults-the evidence report. Obes Res. 1998;6(Supplement 2):1S–209S.
3. National Institute for Health and Care Excellence. Obesity: guidance on the prevention, identification, assessment and management of overweight and obesity in adults and children. London, United Kingdom: National Institute for Health and Care Excellence; 2006. www.NICE.org.uk.
4. Jensen MD, Ryan DH, Apovian CM, Ard JD, Comuzzie AG, Donato KA, et al. 2013 AHA/ACC/TOS guideline for the management of overweight and obesity in adults: a report of the American College of Cardiology/American Heart Association Task Force on Practice Guidelines and The Obesity Society. J Am Coll Cardiol. 2014;63:2985–3023.
5. Apovian CM, Aronne LJ, Bessesen DH, McDonnell ME, Murad MH, Pagotto U, et al. Pharmacological management of obesity: an Endocrine Society clinical practice guideline. J Clin Endocrinol Metab. 2015;100:342–62.
6. Carvajal R, Wadden TA, Tsai AG, Peck K, Moran CH. Managing obesity in primary care practice: a narrative review. Ann N Y Acad Sci. 2013;1281:191–206.
7. Tuomilehto A, Lindström J, Eriksson JG, Valle TT, Hämäläinen H, Ilanne-Parikka P, et al. for the Finnish Diabetes Prevention Study group. Prevention of type 2 diabetes mellitus by changes in lifestyle among subjects with impaired glucose tolerance. N Engl J Med. 2001;344:1343–50.
8. Knowler WV, Barret-Connor E, Fowler SE, Hamman RF, Lachin JM, Walker ED, et al. Diabetes Prevention Program Research Group. Reduction in the Incidence of Type 2 Diabetes with Lifestyle Intervention or Metformin. N Engl J Med. 2002;346:393–403.
9. Wadden TA, Volger S, Tsai AG, Sarwer DB, Berkowitz RI, Doewald LH, et al. POWER-UP Research Group. Managing obesity in primary care practice: an overview with perspective from the POWER-UP study. Int J Obes. 2013;37(Suppl 1):S3–S11.
10. Langeveld M, DeVries JH. The long-term effect of energy restricted diets for treating obesity. Obesity. 2015;23:1529–38.
11. Sacks FM, Bray GA, Carey VJ, Smith SR, Ryan DH, Anton SD, et al. Comparison of weight-loss diets with different compositions of fat, protein, and carbohydrates. N Engl J Med. 2009;360:859–73.
12. Loveman E, Frampton GK, Shepherd J, Picot J, Cooper K, Bryant J, et al. The clinical effectiveness and cost-effectiveness of long-term weight management schemes for adults: a systematic review. Health Technol Assess. 2011;15:1–182.
13. Sumithran P, Prendergast LA, Delbridge E, Pursell K, Shulkes A, Krikelos A, et al. Long-term persistence of hormonal adaptations to weight loss. N Engl J Med. 2011;365:1597–604.
14. Yanovski SZ, Yanovski JA. Long-term drug treatment for obesity: a systematic and clinical review. JAMA. 2014;311:74–86.
15. Hampp C, Kang EM, Borders-Hemphill V. Use of prescription anti-obesity drugs in the United States. Pharmacotherapy. 2013;33:1299–307.

16. Padwal R, Kezouh A, Levine M, Etminan M. Long-term persistence with orlistat and sibutramine in a population-based cohort. Int J Obes. 2007;31:1567–70.
17. Xia Y, Kelton CM, Guo JJ, Bian B, Heaton PC. Treatment of obesity: pharmacotherapy trends in the United States from 1999 to 2010. Obesity. 2015;23:1721–8.
18. Buchwald H, Oien D. Metabolic/bariatric surgery worldwide 2011. Obes Surg. 2013;23:427–736.
19. Afonso BB, Rosenthal R, Li KM, Zapatier J, Szomstein S. Perceived barriers to bariatric surgery among morbidly obese patients. Surg Obes Relat Dis. 2010;6:16–21.
20. Padwal R, Chang H-J, Klarenbach S, Sharma A, Majumdar S. Characteristics of the population eligible for and receiving publicly funded bariatric surgery in Canada. Int J Equity Health. 2012;11:54.
21. Gregory DM, Temple Newhook J, Twells LK. Patients' perceptions of waiting for bariatric surgery: a qualitative study. Int J Equity Health. 2013;12:86.
22. Mathus-Vliegen EMH. Endoscopic treatment: the past, the present and the future. Best Pract Res Clin Gastroenterol. 2014;28:685–702.
23. Tsesmeli N, Coumaros D. The future of bariatrics: endoscopy, endoluminal surgery, and natural orifice transluminal endoscopic surgery. Endoscopy. 2010;42:155–62.
24. Abu Dayyeh BK, Thompson CC. Obesity and bariatrics for the endoscopist: new techniques. Therap Adv Gastroenterol. 2011;4:433–42.
25. Delegge MH. Endoscopic approaches for the treatment of obesity: fact or fiction? Nutr Clin Pract. 2011;26:534–8.
26. Espinet-Coll E, Nebreda-Duran J, Gomez-Valero JA, Munoz-Navas M, Pujol-Gebelli J, Vila-Lolo C, et al. Current endoscopic techniques in the treatment of obesity. Rev Esp Enferm Dig. 2012;104:72–87.
27. Singhal S, Le DL, Duddempudi S, Anand S. The role of endoscopy in bariatrics: past, present, and future. J Laparoendosc Adv Surg Tech A. 2012;22:802–11.
28. Kumar N. Endoscopic therapy for weight loss: gastroplasty, duodenal sleeves, intragastric balloons, and aspiration. World J Gastrointest Endosc. 2015;7:847–59.
29. Fanelli RD, Andrew BD. Is endoluminal bariatric therapy a new paradigm of treatment for obesity? Clin Gastroenterol Hepatol. 2016;14:507–15.
30. Davis M, Kroh M. Novel endoscopic and surgical techniques for treatment of morbid obesity. A glimpse into the future. Surg Clin N Am. 2016;96:857–73.
31. Kumar N. Weight loss endoscopy: development, applications, and current status. World J Gastroenterol. 2016;22:7069–79.
32. Neylan CJ, Dempsey DT, Tewksbury CM, Williams NN, Dumon KR. Endoscopic treatments of obesity: a comprehensive review. Surg Obes Relat Dis. 2016;12:1108–15.
33. Sullivan S, Edmundowicz EA, Thompson CC. Endoscopic bariatric and metabolic therapies: new and emerging technologies. Gastroenterology. 2017;152:1791–801.
34. Dargent J. Novel endoscopic management of obesity. Clin Endosc. 2016;49:30–6.
35. Abu Dayyeh BK, Edmundowicz S, Thompson CC. Clinical practice update: expert review on endoscopic bariatric therapies. Gastroenterology. 2017;152:716–29.
36. Gleysteen JJ. A history of intragastric balloons. Surg Obes Relat Dis. 2016;12:430–5.
37. Thompson CC. Endoscopic therapy of obesity: a new paradigm in bariatric care. Gastrointest Endosc. 2010;72:505–7.
38. Laing P, Pham T, Taylor LJ, Fang J. Filling the void: a review of intragastric balloons for obesity. Dig Dis Sci. 2017;62:1399–408.
39. Ginsberg GG, Chand B, Cote GA, Dallal RM, Edmundowicz SA, Nguyen NT, et al. ASGE/ASMBS Task Force on Endoscopic Bariatric Therapy: White paper: a pathway to endoscopic bariatric therapies. Surg Obes Relat Dis. 2011;7:672–82.
40. Abu Dayyeh BK, Edmundowicz SA, Jonnalagadda S, Kumar N, Larsen M, Sullivan S, et al. ASGE Bariatric Endoscopy Task Force and ASGE Technology Committee. Endoscopic bariatric therapies. Gastrointest Endosc. 2015;81:1073–86.
41. Abu Dayyeh BK, Kumar N, Edmundowicz SA, Jonnalagadda S, Larsen M, Sullivan S, et al. ASGE Bariatric Endoscopy Task Force and ASGE Technology Committee. ASGE Bariatric Endoscopy Task Force systematic review and meta-analysis assessing the

ASGE PIVI thresholds for adopting endoscopic bariatric therapies. Gastrointest Endosc. 2015;82:425–38.
42. Society of American Gastrointestinal and Endoscopic Surgeons. Position statement on endolumenal therapies for gastrointestinal diseases. 2009. http://www.sages.org/publications/guidelines/position-statement-on-endolumenal-therapies-for-gastrointestinal-diseases/. Accessed 16 Aug 2017.
43. Emerging Technologies and Clinical Issues Committees of the ASMBS. American Society of Metabolic and Bariatric Surgery Position Statement on emerging endosurgical interventions for the treatment of obesity. Surg Obes Relat Dis. 2009;5:197–298.
44. Kethu SR, Banerjee S, Barth BA, Desilets DJ, Kaul V, Perosa MC, et al. ASGE Technology Committee. Report on emerging technology: endoluminal bariatric techniques. Gastrointest Endosc. 2012;76:1–7.
45. Sullivan S, Kumar N, Edmundowicz SA, Abu Dayyeh BK, Jonnalagadda SS, Larsen M, et al. ASGE Bariatric Endoscopy Task Force. ASGE position statement on endoscopic bariatric therapies in clinical practice. Gastrointest Endosc. 2015;82:767–72.
46. Ali MR, Moustarah F, Kim JJ, on behalf of the American Society for Metabolic and Bariatric Surgery Clinical Issues Committee. American Society for Metabolic and Bariatric Surgery position statement on intragastric balloon therapy endorsed by the Society of American Gastrointestinal and Endoscopic Surgeons. Surg Obes Relat Dis. 2016;12:462–7.
47. Schapiro M, Benjamin S, Blackburn G, Frank B, Heber D, Kozarek R, et al. Obesity and the gastric balloon: a comprehensive workshop. Tarpon Springs, Florida, March 19–21, 1987. Gastrointest Endosc. 1987;33:323–7.
48. Frank BB, Stern WR, Fisher AH. Survey of gastric bubble usage in the United States. Rockville, MD: Fisher; 1987.
49. Delport A, Harvey BH, Petzer A, Petzer JP. The monoamine oxidase inhibition properties of selected structural analogues of methylene blue. Toxicol Appl Pharmacol. 2017;325:1–8.
50. Top WM, Gillman PK, de Langen CJ, Kooy A. Fatal methylene blue associated serotonin toxicity. Neth J Med. 2014;72:179–81.
51. Kapadia K, Cheung F, Lee W, Thalappillil R, Florence FB, Kim J. Methylene blue causing serotonin syndrome following cystocele repair. Urol Case Rep. 2016;9:15–7.
52. Mathus-Vliegen EM, Tytgat GN. Intragastric balloon for treatment-resistant obesity: safety, tolerance, and efficacy of 1-year balloon treatment followed by a 1-year balloon-free follow-up. Gastrointest Endosc. 2005;61:19–27.
53. Fernandes M, Atallah AN, Soares BG, Humberto S, Guimaraes S, Matos D, et al. Intragastric balloon for obesity. Cochrane Database Syst Rev. 2007;1:CD004931.
54. Mathus-Vliegen EM. Intragastric balloon treatment for obesity: what does it really offer? Dig Dis. 2008;26:40–4.
55. Dumonceau JM. Evidence-based review of the Bioenterics intragastric balloon for weight loss. Obes Surg. 2008;18:1611–7.
56. Imaz I, Martinez-Cervell C, Garcia-Alvarez EE, Sendra-Gutierrez JM, Gonzalez-Enriquez J. Safety and effectiveness of the intragastric balloon for obesity. A meta-analysis. Obes Surg. 2008;18:841–6.
57. Genco A, Cipriano M, Bacci V, Cuzzolaro M, Materia A, Raparelli L, et al. BioEnterics Intragastric Balloon (BIB): a short-term, double-blind, randomised, controlled, crossover study on weight reduction in morbidly obese patients. Int J Obes. 2006;30:129–33.
58. Martinez-Brocca MA, Belda O, Parejo J, Jimenez L, del Valle A, Pereira JL, et al. Intragastric balloon-induced satiety is not mediated by modification in fasting or postprandial plasma ghrelin levels in morbid obesity. Obes Surg. 2007;17:649–57.
59. Abou Hussein BM, Khammas AA, Al Ani AM, Swaleh AH, Al Awadhi SA, El Tayyeb YH, et al. Gastric perforation following intragastric balloon insertion: combined endoscopic and laparoscopic approach for management: case series and review of literature. Obes Surg. 2016;26:1127–32.
60. Cubattoli L, Barneschi C, Mastrocinque E, Bonucci P, Giomarelli PP. Cardiac arrest after intragastric balloon insertion in a super-obese patient. Obes Surg. 2009;19:253–6.

61. Rossi A, Bersani G, Ricci G, Petrini C, DeFabritiis G, Alvisi V. Intragastric balloon insertion increases the frequency of erosive esophagitis in obese patients. Obes Surg. 2007;17:1346–9.
62. Mathus-Vliegen EM, Tygat GN. Gastro-esophageal reflux in obese subjects: influence of overweight, weight loss and chronic gastric balloon distention. Scand J Gastroenterol. 2002;37:1246–52.
63. Mathus-Vliegen EM, van Weeren M, van Eerten PV. LOS function and obesity: the impact of untreated obesity, weight loss, and chronic gastric balloon distention. Digestion. 2003;68:161–8.
64. Hirsch DP, Mathus-Vliegen EM, Holloway RH, Fakhry N, D'Amato M, Boeckxstaens GE. Role of CCK(A) receptors in postprandial lower esophageal sphincter function in morbidly obese subjects. Dig Dis Sci. 2002;47:2531–7.
65. Hirsch DP, Mathus-Vliegen EM, Dagli U, Tytgat GN, Boeckxstaens GE. Effect of prolonged gastric distention on lower esophageal sphincter function and gastroesophageal reflux. Am J Gastroenterol. 2003;98:1696–704.
66. Bazerbachi F, Vargas Valls EJ, Abu Dayyeh BK. Recent clinical results of endoscopic bariatric therapies as an obesity intervention. Clin Endosc. 2017;50:42–50.
67. FDA. ORBERA™ Intragastric balloon system-P140008 [Internet]. Silver Spring: U.S. Food and Drug Administration; 2015. http://www.fda.gov/medicaldevices/productsandmedicalprocedures/deviceapprovalsandclearances/recently-approveddevices/ucm457416.htm.
68. Courcoulas A, Abu Dayyeh BK, Eaton L, Robinson J, Woodman G, Fusco M, et al. Intragastric balloon as an adjunct to lifestyle intervention: a randomized controlled trial. Int J Obes. 2017;41:427–33.
69. Gómez V, Woodman G, Abu Dayyeh BK. Delayed gastric emptying as a proposed mechanism of action during intragastric balloon therapy: results of a prospective study. Obesity. 2016;24:1849–53.
70. Abu Dayyeh BK, Woodman G, Acosta A, Lopes GS, Gostout C, De Moura E, et al. Baseline gastric emptying and its change in response to diverse endoscopic bariatric therapies predict weight change after intervention. Gastroenterology. 2016;150:S86.
71. Kumar N, Bazerbachi F, Rustagi T, McCarty TR, Thompson CC, Galvao Neto MP, et al. The influence of the Orbera intragastric balloon filling volumes on weight loss, tolerability, and adverse events: a systematic review and meta-analysis. Obes Surg. 2017;27(9):2272–8. https://doi.org/10.1007/s11695-017-2636-3.
72. Puglisi F, Antonucci N, Capuano P, Zavoianni L, Lobascio P, Martines G, et al. Intragastric balloon and binge eating. Obes Surg. 2007;17:504–9.
73. Melissas J, Malliaraki N, Papadakis JA, Taflampas P, Kampa M, Castanas E. Plasma antioxidant capacity in morbidly obese patients before and after weight loss. Obes Surg. 2006;16:314–20.
74. Ricci G, Bersani G, Rossi A, Pigo F, De Fabritiis G, Alvisi V. Bariatric therapy with intragastric balloon improves liver dysfunction and insulin resistance in obese patients. Obes Surg. 2008;18:1438–42.
75. Chan AO, Chow WS, Lam KF, Hsu A, Hung I, Chan P, et al. The effect of intragastric balloon placement on weight loss and type 2 diabetes control. Aliment Pharmacol Ther. 2008;28:162–4.
76. Forlano R, Ippolito AM, Iacobellis A, Merla A, Valvano MR, Niro G, et al. Effect of the BioEnterics intragastric balloon on weight, insulin resistance, and liver steatosis in obese patients. Gastrointest Endosc. 2010;71:927–33.
77. Mui WL, Ng EK, Tsung BY, Lam CH, Yung MY. Impact on obesity-related illnesses and quality of life following intragastric balloon. Obes Surg. 2010;20:1128–32.
78. Musella M, Milone M, Bellini M, Fernandez ME, Fernandez LM, Leongito M, et al. The potential role of intragastric balloon in the treatment of obese-related infertility: personal experience. Obes Surg. 2011;21:426–30.
79. Fuller NR, Pearson S, Lau NS, Wlodarczyk J, Halstead MB, Tee HP, et al. An intragastric balloon in the treatment of obese individuals with metabolic syndrome: a randomized controlled study. Obesity. 2013;21:1561–70.

80. Lopez-Nava G, Rubio MA, Prados S, Pastor G, Cruz MR, Companioni E, et al. BioEnterics® Intragastric Balloon (BIB®): single ambulatory center Spanish experience with 714 consecutive patients treated with one or two consecutive balloons. Obes Surg. 2011;21:5–9.
81. Genco A, Bruni T, Doldi SB, Forestieri P, Marino M, Busetto L, et al. BioEnterics intragastric balloon: the Italian experience with 2,515 patients. Obes Surg. 2005;15:1161–4.
82. Herve J, Wahlen CH, Schaeken A, Dallemagne B, Dewandre JM, Markiewicz S, et al. What becomes of patients one year after the intragastric balloon has been removed? Obes Surg. 2005;15:864–70.
83. Dastis NS, Francois E, Deviere J, Hittelet A, Ilah MA, Barea M, et al. Intragastric balloon for weight loss: results in 100 individuals followed for at least 2.5 years. Endoscopy. 2009;41:575–80.
84. Kotzampassi K, Grosomanidis V, Papakostas P, Penna S, Eleftheriadis E. 500 intragastric balloons: what happen 5 years thereafter? Obes Surg. 2012;22:896–903.
85. Gaur S, Levy S, Mathus-Vliegen L, Chuttani R. Balancing risk and reward: a critical review of the intragastric balloon for weight loss. Gastrointest Endosc. 2015;81:1130–6.
86. Roman S, Napoleon B, Mion F, Bory RM, Guyot P, D'Orazio H, et al. Intragastric balloon for "nonmorbid" obesity: a retrospective evaluation of tolerance and efficacy. Obes Surg. 2004;14:539–44.
87. Loffredo A, Cappuccio M, De Luca M, de Werra C, Galloro G, Naddo M, et al. Three years' experience with the new intragastric balloon, and a preoperative test for success with restrictive surgery. Obes Surg. 2001;11:330–3.
88. Crea N, Pata G, Della Casa D, Minelli L, Malfredi G, Di Betta E, et al. Improvement of metabolic syndrome following intragastric balloon: 1 year follow-up analysis. Obes Surg. 2009;19:1084–8.
89. Angrisani L, Lorenzo M, Borrelli V, Guiffré M, Fonderico C, Capece G. Is bariatric surgery necessary after intragastric balloon treatment? Obes Surg. 2006;16:1135–7.
90. Genco A, López-Nava G, Wahlen C, Maselli R, Cipriano M, Sanchez MM, et al. Multi-centre European experience with intragastric balloon in overweight populations: 13 years of experience. Obes Surg. 2013;23:515–21.
91. Genco A, Maselli R, Cipriano M, Lorenzo M, Basso N, Redler A. Long-term multiple intragastric balloon treatment – a new strategy to treat morbid obese patients refusing surgery: prospective 6-year follow-up study. Surg Obes Relat Dis. 2014;10:307–12.
92. Jebb SA, Goldberg GR, Coward WA, Murgatroyd PR, Prentice AM. Effects of weight cycling caused by intermittent dieting on metabolic rate and body composition in obese women. Int J Obes. 1991;15:367–74.
93. Reed GW, Hill JO. Weight cycling: a review of the animal literature. Obes Res. 1993;1:394–402.
94. Wing RR. Weight cycling: the public concern and the scientific data. Obes Res. 1993;1:390–1.
95. Jeffery RW. Does weight cycling present a health risk? Am J Clin Nutr. 1996;63(Suppl 3):452S–5S.
96. Kajioka T, Tsuzuku S, Shimokata H, Sato Y. Effects of intentional weight cycling on non-obese young women. Metabolism. 2002;51:149–54.
97. Riess KP, Baker MT, Lambert PJ, Mathiason MA, Kothari SN. Effect of preoperative weight loss on laparoscopic gastric bypass outcomes. Surg Obes Relat Dis. 2008;4:704–8.
98. Pasulka PS, Bistrian BR, Benotti PN, Blackburn GL. The risks of surgery in obese patients. Ann Intern Med. 1986;104:540–6.
99. Liu RC, Sabnis AA, Forsyth C, Chand B. The effects of acute preoperative weight loss on laparoscopic roux-en-Y gastric bypass. Obes Surg. 2005;15:1396–402.
100. Gottig S, Weiner RA, Daskalakis M. Preoperative weight reduction using the intragastric balloon. Obes Facts. 2009;2(Suppl 1):20–3.
101. Busetto L, Segato G, DeLuca M, Bortolozzi E, MacCari T, Magon A, et al. Preoperative weight loss by intragastric balloon in super-obese patients treated with laparoscopic gastric banding: a case-control study. Obes Surg. 2004;14:671–6.

102. Frutos MD, Morales MD, Lujan J, Hernandez Q, Valero G, Parrilla P. Intragastric balloon reduces liver volume in super-obese patients, facilitating subsequent laparoscopic gastric bypass. Obes Surg. 2007;17:150–4.
103. Zerrweck C, Maunoury V, Caiazzo R, Branche J, Dezfoulian G, Bulois P, et al. Preoperative weight loss with intragastric balloon decreases the risk of significant adverse outcomes of laparoscopic gastric bypass in super-super obese patients. Obes Surg. 2012;22:777–82.
104. Busetto L, Enzi G, Inelmen EM, Costa G, Negrin V, Sergi G, et al. Obstructive sleep apnea syndrome in morbid obesity: effects of intragastric balloon. Chest. 2005;128:618–23.
105. Spyropoulos C, Katsakoulis E, Mead N, Vagenas K, Kalfarentzos F. Intragastric balloon for high-risk super-obese patients: a prospective analysis of efficacy. Surg Obes Relat Dis. 2007;3:78–83.
106. Yorke E, Switzer NJ, Reso A, Shi X, de Gara C, Birch D, et al. Intragastric balloon for management of severe obesity: a systematic review. Obes Surg. 2016;26:2248–54.
107. Coffin B, Maunoury V, Pattou F, Hébuterne X, Schneider S, Coupaye M, et al. Impact of intragastric balloon before laparoscopic gastric bypass on patients with super obesity: a randomized multicenter study. Obes Surg. 2017;27:902–9.
108. Jones M, Healey AJ, Efthimiou E. Early use of self-expanding metallic stents to relieve sleeve gastrectomy stenosis after intragastric balloon removal. Surg Obes Relat Dis. 2011;7:e16–7.
109. de Goederen-van der Meij S, Pierik RG, Oudkerk PM, Gouma DJ, Mathus-Vliegen LM. Six months of balloon treatment does not predict the success of gastric banding. Obes Surg. 2007;17:88–94.
110. Khan O, Irukulla S, Sanmugalingam N, Vasilikostas G, Reddy M, Wan A. Simultaneous intra-gastric balloon removal and laparoscopic sleeve gastrectomy for the super-super obese patients – a prospective feasibility study. Obes Surg. 2013;23:585–7.
111. Brethauer SA, Chang J, Galvao Neto M, Greve JW. Gastrointestinal devices for the treatment of type 2 diabetes. Surg Obes Relat Dis. 2016;12:1256–61.
112. Genco A, Lorenzo M, Baglio G, Furbetta F, Rossi A, Lucchese M, et al. Does the intragastric balloon have a predictive role in subsequent LAP-BAND surgery? Italian multicenter study results at 5-year follow-up. Surg Obes Relat Dis. 2014;10:474–8.
113. Dumonceau JM, Francois E, Hittelet A, Mehdi AI, Barea M, Deviere J. Single vs repeated treatment with the intragastric balloon: a 5-year weight loss study. Obes Surg. 2010;20:692–7.
114. Genco A, Cipriano M, Bacci V, Maselli R, Paone E, Lorenzo M, et al. Intragastric balloon followed by diet vs intragastric balloon followed by another balloon: a prospective study on 100 patients. Obes Surg. 2010;20:1496–500.
115. Genco A, Maselli R, Frangella F, Cipriano M, Paone E, Meuti V, et al. Effect of consecutive intragastric balloon (BIB(R)) plus diet versus single BIB(R) plus diet on eating disorders not otherwise specified (EDNOS) in obese patients. Obes Surg. 2013;23:2075–9.
116. Deliopoulou K, Konsta A, Penna S, Papakostas P, Kotzampassi K. The impact of weight loss on depression status in obese individuals subjected to intragastric balloon treatment. Obes Surg. 2013;23:669–75.
117. Coskun H, Bostanci O. Assessment of the application of the intragastric balloon together with sibutramine: a prospective clinical study. Obes Surg. 2010;20:1117–20.
118. Farina MG, Baratta R, Nigro A, Vinciguerra F, Puglisi C, Schembri R, et al. Intragastric balloon in association with lifestyle and/or pharmacotherapy in the long-term management of obesity. Obes Surg. 2012;22:565–71.
119. Dargent J, Mion F, Costil V, Ecochard R, Pontette F, Mion V, et al. Multicenter randomized study of obesity treatment with minimally invasive injection of hyaluronic acid versus and combined with intragastric balloon. Obes Surg. 2015;25:1842–7.
120. Peker Y, Coskun H, Bozkurt S, Cin N, Atak T, Genc H. Comparison of results of laparoscopic gastric banding and consecutive intragastric balloon application at 18 months: a clinical prospective study. J Laparoendosc Adv Surg Tech A. 2011;21:471–5.

121. Milone L, Strong V, Gagner M. Laparoscopic sleeve gastrectomy is superior to endoscopic intragastric balloon as a first stage procedure for super-obese patients (BMI ≥ 50). Obes Surg. 2005;15:612–7.
122. Genco A, Cipriano M, Materia A, Bacci V, Maselli R, Musmeci L, et al. Laparoscopic sleeve gastrectomy versus intragastric balloon: a case-control study. Surg Endosc. 2009;23:1849–53.
123. Genco A, Dellepiane D, Baglio G, Cappelletti F, Frangella F, Maselli R, et al. Adjustable intragastric balloon vs non-adjustable intragastric balloon: case-control study on complications, tolerance, and efficacy. Obes Surg. 2013;23:953–8.
124. Machytka E, Klvana P, Kornbluth A, Peikin S, Mathus-Vliegen LE, Gostout C, et al. Adjustable intragastric balloons: a 12-month pilot trial in endoscopic weight loss management. Obes Surg. 2011;21:1499–507.
125. Brooks J, Srivastava ED, Mathus-Vliegen EM. One-year adjustable intragastric balloons: results in 73 consecutive patients in the U.K. Obes Surg. 2014;24:813–9.
126. Carvalho GL, Barros CB, Okazaki M, Novaes ML, Albuquerque PC, Almeida NC, et al. An improved intragastric balloon procedure using a new balloon: preliminary analysis of safety and efficiency. Obes Surg. 2009;19:237–42.
127. Carvalho GL, Barros CB, Moraes CE, Okazaki M, Ferreira MN, Silva JS, et al. The use of an improved intragastric balloon technique to reduce weight in pre-obese patients—preliminary results. Obes Surg. 2011;21:924–7.
128. Bužga M, Machytka E, Klvaňa P, Kupka T, Zavadilová V, Zonča P, et al. Effects of the intragastric balloon Medsil® on weight loss, fat tissue, lipid metabolism, and hormones involved in energy balance. Obes Surg. 2014;24:909–15.
129. De Castro ML, Morales MJ, Del Campo V, Pineda JR, Pena E, Sierra JM, et al. Efficacy, safety, and tolerance of two types of intragastric balloons placed in obese subjects: a double-blind comparative study. Obes Surg. 2010;20:1642–6.
130. Giardiello C, Borrelli A, Silvestri E, Antognozzi V, Iodice G, Lorenzo M. Air-filled vs water-filled intragastric balloon: a prospective randomized study. Obes Surg. 2012;22:1916–9.
131. Caglar E, Dobrucali A, Bal K. Gastric balloon to treat obesity: filled with air or fluid? Dig Endosc. 2013;25:502–7.
132. Lecumberri E, Krekshi W, Matia P, Hermida C, de la Torre NG, Cabrerizo L, et al. Effectiveness and safety of air-filled balloon Heliosphere BAG(R) in 82 consecutive obese patients. Obes Surg. 2011;21:1508–12.
133. Forestieri P, De Palma GD, Formato A, Giuliano ME, Monda A, Pilone V, et al. Heliosphere Bag in the treatment of severe obesity: preliminary experience. Obes Surg. 2006;16:635–7.
134. Mion F, Gincul R, Roman S, Beorchia S, Hedelius F, Claudel N, et al. Tolerance and efficacy of an air-filled balloon in non-morbidly obese patients: results of a prospective multicenter study. Obes Surg. 2007;17:764–9.
135. Trande P, Mussetto A, Mirante VG, De Martinis E, Olivetti G, Conigliaro RL, et al. Efficacy, tolerance and safety of new intragastric air-filled balloon (Heliosphere BAG) for obesity: the experience of 17 cases. Obes Surg. 2010;20:1227–30.
136. Lopasso FP, Sakai P, Gazi BM, Artifon EL, Kfouri C, Souza JP, et al. A pilot study to evaluate the safety, tolerance, and efficacy of a novel stationary antral balloon (SAB) for obesity. J Clin Gastroenterol. 2008;42:48–53.
137. Gaggiotti G, Tack J, Garrido AB Jr, Palau M, Cappelluti G, Di Malteo F. Adjustable totally implantable intragastric prosthesis (ATIIP)-Endogast for treatment of morbid obesity: one-year follow-up of a multicenter prospective clinical survey. Obes Surg. 2007;17:949–56.
138. Ponce J, Quebbemann BB, Patterson EJ. Prospective, randomized, multicenter study evaluating safety and efficacy of intragastric dual-balloon in obesity. Surg Obes Relat Dis. 2013;9:290–5.
139. Lopez-Nava G, Bautista-Castaño I, Jimenez-Baños A, Fernandez-Corbelle JP. Dual intragastric balloon: single ambulatory center Spanish experience with 60 patients in endoscopic weight loss management. Obes Surg. 2015;25:2263–7.
140. Ponce J, Woodman G, Swain J, Wilson E, English K, Ikramuddin S, et al. REDUCE Pivotal Trial Investigators. The REDUCE pivotal trial: a prospective, randomized controlled piv-

otal trial of a dual intragastric balloon for the treatment of obesity. Surg Obes Relat Dis. 2015;11:874–81.
141. FDA. ReShape integrated dual balloon system-P140012 [Internet]. Silver Spring: U.S. Food and Drug Administration; 2015. http://www.fda.gov/medicaldevices/productsandmedical-procedures/deviceapprovalsandclearances/recently-approveddevices/ucm456293.htm.
142. Mathus-Vliegen. EMH Is endoscopy really necessary for placing intragastric balloons? Obes Surg. 2017.; published online, ahead of print; https://doi.org/10.1007/s11695-017-2812-5.
143. Mion F, Ibrahim M, Marjoux S, Ponchon T, Dugardeyn S, Roman S, et al. Swallowable Obalon gastric balloons as an aid for weight loss: a pilot feasibility study. Obes Surg. 2013;23:730–3.
144. Sullivan S, Swain JM, Woodman G, Edmundowicz S, Hassanein TI, Shayani V, et al. The Obalon swallowable 6-month balloon system is more effective than moderate intensity lifestyle therapy alone: results from a 6- month randomized sham controlled trial. Gastroenterology. 2016;150:S1267.
145. FDA. Obalon balloon system-P160001 [Internet]. Silver Spring: U.S. Food and Drug Administration; 2016. http://www.fda.gov/medicaldevices/productsandmedicalprocedures/deviceapprovalsandclearances/recently-approveddevices/ucm520741.htm.
146. Machytka E, Chuttani R, Bojkova M, Kupka T, Buzga M, Stecco K, et al. Elipse, a procedureless gastric balloon for weight loss: a proof-of-concept pilot study. Obes Surg. 2016;26:512–6.
147. Martin CK, Bellanger DE, Rau KK, Coulon S, Greenway FL. Safety of the Ullorex oral intragastric balloon for the treatment of obesity. J Diabetes Sci Technol. 2007;1:574–81.
148. Camilleri M. Peripheral mechanisms in appetite regulation. Gastroenterology. 2015;148:1219–33.
149. Ello-Martin JA, Ledikwe JH, Rolls BJ. The influence of food portion size and energy density on energy intake: implications for weight management. Am J Clin Nutr. 2005;82(1 Suppl):236S–41S.
150. Geliebter A, Westreich S, Gage D. Gastric distention by balloon and test-meal intake in obese and lean subjects. Am J Clin Nutr. 1988;48:592–4.
151. Geliebter A, Melton PM, McCray RS, Gage D, Heymsfield SB, Abiri M, et al. Clinical trial of silicone-rubber gastric balloon to treat obesity. Int J Obes. 1991;15:259–66.
152. Mathus-Vliegen EMH, de Groot GH. Fasting and meal-induced CCK and PP secretion following intragastric balloon treatment for obesity. Obes Surg. 2013;23:622–33.
153. Mathus-Vliegen EM, Eichenberger RI. Fasting and meal-suppressed ghrelin levels before and after intragastric balloons and balloon-induced weight loss. Obes Surg. 2014;24:85–94.
154. Mion F, Napoleon B, Roman S, Malvoisin E, Trepo F, Pujol B, et al. Effects of intragastric balloon on gastric emptying and plasma ghrelin levels in non-morbid obese patients. Obes Surg. 2005;15:510–6.
155. Konopko-Zubrzycka M, Baniukiewicz A, Wroblewski E, Kowalska I, Zarzycki W, Gorska M, et al. The effect of intragastric balloon on plasma ghrelin, leptin, and adiponectin levels in patients with morbid obesity. J Clin Endocrinol Metab. 2009;94:1644–9.
156. Tosetti C, Corinaldesi R, Stanghellini V, Pasquali R, Corbelli C, Zoccoli G, et al. Gastric emptying of solids in morbid obesity. Int J Obesity Rel Metab Dis. 1996;20:200–5.
157. Bonazzi P, Petrelli MD, Lorenzini I, Peruzzi E, Nicolai A, Galeazzi R. Gastric emptying and intragastric balloon in obese patients. Eur Rev Med Pharmacol Sci. 2005;9(5 suppl 1):15–21.
158. Su HJ, Kao CH, Chen WC, Chang TT, Lin CY. Effect of intragastric balloon on gastric emptying time in humans for weight control. Clin Nucl Med. 2013;38:863–8.
159. Abu Dayyeh BK, Acosta A, Camilleri M, Mundi MS, Rajan E, Topazian MD, et al. Endoscopic sleeve gastroplasty alters gastric physiology and induces loss of body weight in obese individuals. Clin Gastroenterol Hepatol. 2017;15:37–43.
160. Dogan UB, Gumurdulu Y, Akin MS, Yalaki S. Five percent weight lost in the first month of intragastric balloon treatment may be a predictor for long-term weight maintenance. Obes Surg. 2013;23:892–6.
161. Geliebter A, Schachter S, Lohmann-Walter C, Feldman H, Hashim SA. Reduced stomach capacity in obese subjects after dieting. Am J Clin Nutr. 1996;63:170–3.

162. Pappas TN. Physiological satiety implications of gastrointestinal antiobesity surgery. Am J Clin Nutr. 1992;55:571S–2S.
163. Mathus-Vliegen EMH, Tytgat GNJ, Veldhuyzen-Offermans EAML. Intragastric balloon in the treatment of super-morbid obesity. Double-blind, sham-controlled, crossover evaluation of 500-milliliter balloon. Gastroenterology. 1990;99:362–9.
164. Mathus-Vliegen LM, Tytgat GN. Twenty-four-hour pH measurements in morbid obesity: effects of massive overweight, weight loss and gastric distension. Eur J Gastroenterol Hepatol. 1996;8:635–40.
165. Mathus-Vliegen EMH, Alders PRH, Chuttani R, Scherpenisse J. Outcomes of intragastric balloon placements in a private practice setting. Endoscopy. 2015;47:302–7.
166. Zheng Y, Wang M, He S, Ji G. Short-term effects of intragastric balloon in association with conservative therapy on weight loss: a meta-analysis. J Transl Med. 2015;13:246.
167. Saber AA, Shoar S, Almadani MW, Zundel N, Alkuwari MJ, Bashah MM, et al. Efficacy of first-time intragastric balloon in weight loss: a systematic review and meta-analysis of randomized controlled trials. Obes Surg. 2017;27:277–87.
168. Moura D, Oliveira J, DeMoura EG, Bernardo W, GalvãoNeto M, Campos J, et al. Effectiveness of intragastric balloon for obesity: a systematic review and meta-analysis based on randomized control trials. Surg Obes Relat Dis. 2016;12:420–9.
169. Sullivan S, Stein R, Jonnalagadda S, Mullady D, Edmundowicz S. Aspiration therapy leads to weight loss in obese subjects: a pilot study. Gastroenterology. 2013;145:1245–52.
170. Forssell H, Norén E. Results after 6-months use of the AspireAssist system, a novel endoscopic weight loss therapy. Endoscopy. 2015;47:68–71.
171. Thompson CC, Abu Dayyeh BK, Kushner R, Sullivan S, Schorr AB, Amaro A, et al. Percutaneous gastrostomy device for the treatment of class III and class III obesity: results of a randomized controlled trial. Am J Gastroenterol. 2017;112:447–57.
172. Machytka E, Turro R, Huberty V, Buzga M, Boykova M, Espinos JC, et al. Aspiration therapy in super obese patients - pilot trial. Gastroenterology. 2016;150:S822–3.
173. FDA Summary of Safety and Effectiveness Data (SSED) for the Aspire Assist weight loss system. http://www.accessdata.fda.gov/cdrh_docs/pdf15/p150024b.pdf.
174. Marinos G, Eliades C, Muthusamy R, Greenway F. Weight loss and improved quality of life with a nonsurgical endoscopic treatment for obesity: clinical results from a 3- and 6-month study. Surg Obes Relat Dis. 2014;10:929–35.
175. Foschi D, Lazzaroni M, Sangaletti O, Corsi F, Trabucchi E, Bianchi Porro G. Effects of intramural administration of Botulinum Toxin A on gastric emptying and eating capacity in obese patients. Dig Liver Dis. 2008;40:667–72.
176. Garcia-Compean D, Maldonado GH. Intragastric injection of botulinum toxin for the treatment of obesity. Where are we? World J Gastroenterol. 2008;14:1805–9.
177. Bang CS, Baik GH, Shin IS, Kim JB, Suk KT, Yoon JH, et al. Effect of intragastric injection of botulinum toxin A for the treatment of obesity: a meta-analysis and meta-regression. Gastrointest Endosc. 2015;81:1141–9.
178. Ahmad SS, Sherpa G, Ahmed AR, Ahmad S. Intragastric botolinum toxin-a injection as a treatment for obesity in comparison to gastric balloon. Obes Surg. 2016;26:2235–6.
179. Sauer N, Rosch T, Pezold J, Reining F, Anders M, Groth S, et al. A new endoscopically implantable device (SatiSphere) for treatment of obesity—efficacy, safety, and metabolic effects on glucose, insulin, and GLP-1 levels. Obes Surg. 2013;23:1727–33.
180. Jirapinyo P, Thompson CC. Endoscopic bariatric and metabolic therapy: surgical analogues and mechanisms of action. Clin Gastroenterol Hepatol. 2017;15:619–30.
181. Fogel R, De Fogel J, Bonilla Y, De La Fuente R. Clinical experience of transoral suturing for an endoluminal vertical gastroplasty: 1-year follow-up in 64 patients. Gastrointest Endosc. 2008;68:51–8.
182. Brethauer SA, Chand B, Schauer PR, Thompson CC. Transoral gastric volume reduction for weight management: technique and feasibility in 18 patients. Surg Obes Relat Dis. 2010;6:689–94.

183. Brethauer SA, Chand B, Schauer PR, Thompson CC. Transoral gastric volume reduction as intervention for weight management: 12-month follow-up of TRIM trial. Surg Obes Relat Dis. 2012;8:296–303.
184. Espinos JC, Turro R, Mata A, Cruz M, da Costa M, Villa V, et al. Early experience with the Incisionless Operating Platform (IOP) for the treatment of obesity: the Primary Obesity Surgery Endolumenal (POSE) procedure. Obes Surg. 2013;23:1375–83.
185. López-Nava G, Bautista-Castaño I, Jimenez A, de Grado T, Fernandez-Corbelle JP. The Primary Obesity Surgery Endolumenal (POSE) procedure: one-year patient weight loss and safety outcomes. Surg Obes Relat Dis. 2015;11:861–5.
186. Miller K, Turró R, Greve JW, Bakker CM, Buchwald JN, Espinós JC. MILEPOST multicenter randomized controlled trial: 12-month weight loss and satiety outcomes after *poses*[m] vs. medical therapy. Obes Surg. 2017;27:310–22.
187. Sullivan S, Swain JM, Woodman G, Antonetti M, De La Cruz-Munoz N, Jonnalagadda SS, et al. Randomized sham-controlled trial evaluating efficacy and safety of endoscopic gastric plication for primary obesity: the ESSENTIAL trial. Obesity. 2017;25:294–301.
188. Espinós JC, Turró R, Moragas G, Bronstone A, Buchwald JN, Mearin F, et al. Gastrointestinal physiological changes and their relationship to weight loss following the POSE procedure. Obes Surg. 2016;26:1081–9.
189. Abu Dayyeh BK, Rajan E, Gostout CJ. Endoscopic sleeve gastroplasty: a potential endoscopic alternative to surgical sleeve gastrectomy for treatment of obesity. Gastrointest Endosc. 2013;78:530–5.
190. Kumar N, Peña Sahdala HN, Shaikh S, Wilson EB, Galvao Neto M, Zundel N, et al. Endoscopic sleeve gastroplasty for primary therapy of obesity: initial human cases. Gastroenterology. 2014;146:S571–2.
191. Lopez-Nava G, Galvão MP, da Bautista-Castaño I, Jimenez A, De Grado T, Fernandez-Corbelle JP. Endoscopic sleeve gastroplasty for the treatment of obesity. Endoscopy. 2015;47:449–52.
192. Sharaiha RZ, Kedia P, Kumta N, DeFilippis EM, Gaidhane M, Shukla A, et al. Initial experience with endoscopic sleeve gastroplasty: technical success and reproducibility in the bariatric population. Endoscopy. 2015;47:164–6.
193. Lopez-Nava G, Galvao M, Bautista-Castaño I, Fernandez-Corbelle JP, Trell M. Endoscopic sleeve gastroplasty with 1-year follow-up: factors predictive of success. Endosc Intern Open. 2016;04:E222–7.
194. Kumar N, Lopez-Nava G, Peña Sahdala HN, Galvao Neto M, Sharaiha RZ, Wilson EB, et al. Endoscopic sleeve gastroplasty: multicenter weight loss results. Gastroenterology. 2015;148:S179.
195. Lopez-Nava G, Sharaiha RZ, Galvao Neto M, Kumta NA, Topazian M, Shukla A, et al. Endoscopic sleeve gastroplasty for obesity: a multicenter study of 242 patients with 18 months follow-up. Gastroenterology. 2016;150:S26.
196. Legner A, Altorjay A, Juhasz A, Stadlhuber R, Reich V, Hunt B, et al. Transoral mucosal excision sutured gastroplasty: a pilot study for GERD and obesity with two-year follow-up. Surg Innov. 2014;21:456–63.
197. Huberty V, Ibrahim M, Hiernaux M, Chau A, Dugardeyn S, Devière J. Safety and feasibility of an endoluminal-suturing device for endoscopic gastric reduction (with video). Gastrointest Endosc. 2017;85:833–7.
198. Verlaan T, de Jong K, de la Mar-Ploem ED, Veldhuyzen EA, Mathus-Vliegen EM, Fockens P. Trans-oral Endoscopic Restrictive Implant System: endoscopic treatment of obesity? Surg Obes Relat Dis. 2016;12:1711–8.
199. Deviere J, Ojeda VG, Cuevas HL, Closset J, Le Moine O, Eisendrath P, et al. Safety, feasibility and weight loss after transoral gastroplasty: first human multicenter study. Surg Endosc. 2008;22:589–98.
200. Moreno C, Closset J, Dugardeyn S, Barea M, Mehdi A, Collignon L, et al. Transoral gastroplasty is safe, feasible, and induces significant weight loss in morbidly obese patients: results of the second human pilot study. Endoscopy. 2008;40:406–13.

201. Familiari P, Costamagna G, Blero D, Le Moine O, Perri V, Boskoski I, et al. Transoral gastroplasty for morbid obesity: a multicenter trial with a 1-year outcome. Gastrointest Endosc. 2011;74:1248–58.
202. Nanni G, Familiari P, Mor A, Iaconelli A, Perri V, Rubino F, et al. Effectiveness of the Transoral Endoscopic Vertical Gastroplasty (TOGa®): a good balance between weight loss and complications, if compared with gastric bypass and biliopancreatic diversion. Obes Surg. 2012;22:1897–902.
203. Biertho L, Hould FS, Lebel S, Biron S. Transoral endoscopic restrictive implant system: a new endoscopic technique for the treatment of obesity. Surg Obes Relat Dis. 2010;6:203–5.
204. de Jong K, Mathus-Vliegen EM, Veldhuyzen EA, Eshuis JH, Fockens P. Short-term safety and efficacy of the Trans-oral Endoscopic Restrictive Implant System for the treatment of obesity. Gastrointest Endosc. 2010;72:497–504.
205. Verlaan T, Paulus GF, Mathus-Vliegen EMH, Veldhuyzen EAML, Conchillo JM, Bouvy ND, et al. Endoscopic gastric volume reduction with a novel articulating plication device is safe and effective in the treatment of obesity. Gastrointest Endosc. 2015;81:312–20.
206. van der Wielen N, Paulus G, van Avesaat M, Masclee A, Meijerink J, Bouvy N. Effect of endoscopic gastroplication on the genome-wide transcriptome in the upper gastrointestinal tract. Obes Surg. 2017;27:740–8.
207. Escalona A, Yanez R, Pimentel F, Galvao M, Ramos AC, Turiel D, et al. Initial human experience with restrictive duodenal-jejunal bypass liner for treatment of morbid obesity. Surg Obes Relat Dis. 2010;6:126–31.
208. Patel SR, Hakim D, Mason J, Hakim N. The duodenal-jejunal bypass sleeve (EndoBarrier Gastrointestinal Liner) for weight loss and treatment of type 2 diabetes. Surg Obes Relat Dis. 2013;9:482–4.
209. Zechmeister-Koss I, Huic M, Fischer S. The duodenal-jejunal bypass liner for the treatment of type 2 diabetes mellitus and/or obesity: a systematic review. Obes Surg. 2014;24:310–23.
210. Rodriguez-Grunert L, Galvao Neto MP, Alamo M, Ramos AC, Baez PB, Tarnoff M. First human experience with endoscopically delivered and retrieved duodenal-jejunal bypass sleeve. Surg Obes Relat Dis. 2008;4:55–9.
211. de Moura EG, Orso IR, Martins BC, Lopes GS, de Oliveira SL, Galvao-Neto MP, et al. Improvement of insulin resistance and reduction of cardiovascular risk among obese patients with type 2 diabetes with the duodenojejunal bypass liner. Obes Surg. 2011;21:941–7.
212. de Moura EG, Martins BC, Lopes GS, Orso IR, de Oliveira SL, Galvao Neto MP, et al. Metabolic improvements in obese type 2 diabetes subjects implanted for 1 year with an endoscopically deployed duodenal-jejunal bypass liner. Diabetes Technol Ther. 2012;14:183–9.
213. Escalona A, Pimentel F, Sharp A, Becerra P, Slako M, Turiel D, et al. Weight loss and metabolic improvement in morbidly obese subjects implanted for 1 year with an endoscopic duodenal-jejunal bypass liner. Ann Surg. 2012;255:1080–5.
214. Cohen RV, Neto MG, Correa JL, Sakai P, Martins B, Schiavon CA, et al. A pilot study of the duodenal-jejunal bypass liner in low body mass index type 2 diabetes. J Clin Endocrinol Metab. 2013;98:E279–82.
215. Rodriguez L, Reyes E, Fagalde P, Oltra MS, Saba J, Aylwin CG, et al. Pilot clinical study of an endoscopic, removable duodenal-jejunal bypass liner for the treatment of type 2 diabetes. Diabetes Technol Ther. 2009;11:725–32.
216. Tarnoff M, Rodriguez L, Escalona A, Ramos A, Neto M, Alamo M, et al. Open label, prospective, randomized controlled trial of an endoscopic duodenal-jejunal bypass sleeve versus low calorie diet for pre-operative weight loss in bariatric surgery. Surg Endosc. 2009;23:650–6.
217. Gersin KS, Rothstein RI, Rosenthal RJ, Stefanidis D, Deal SE, Kuwada TS, et al. Open-label, sham-controlled trial of an endoscopic duodenojejunal bypass liner for preoperative weight loss in bariatric surgery candidates. Gastrointest Endosc. 2010;71:976–82.
218. Schouten R, Rijs CS, Bouvy ND, Hameeteman W, Koek GH, Janssen IM, et al. A multicenter, randomized efficacy study of the EndoBarrier Gastrointestinal Liner for presurgical weight loss prior to bariatric surgery. Ann Surg. 2010;251:236–43.

219. Mathus-Vliegen EM. Endobarrier: a unique but still premature concept. Ned Tijdschr Geneeskd. 2012;156:A4590.
220. Rohde U, Hedbäck N, Gluud LL, Visboll T, Knop FK. Effect of the EndoBarrier Gastrointestinal Liner on obesity and type 2 diabetes: a systematic review and meta-analysis. Diabetes Obes Metab. 2016;18:300–5.
221. Koehestanie P, de Jonge C, Berends FJ, Janssen IM, Bouvy ND, Greve JW. The effect of the endoscopic duodenal-jejunal bypass liner on obesity and type 2 diabetes mellitus, a multicentre randomized controlled trial. Ann Surg. 2014;260:984–92.
222. Vilarrasa N, Ruiz de Gordejuela AG, Casajoana A, Duran X, Toro S, Espinet E, et al. Endobarrier® in grade I obese patients with long-standing type 2 diabetes: role of gastrointestinal hormones in glucose metabolism. Obes Surg. 2017;27:569–77.
223. Kaplan LM, Buse JB, Mullin C. EndoBarrier therapy is associated with glycemic improvement, weight loss and safety issues in patients with obesity and type 2 diabetes on oral antihyperglycemic agents. Diabetes. 2016;65(sup A):326-LB.
224. Sandler BJ, Rumbaut R, Swain CP, Torres G, Morales L, Gonzales L, et al. Human experience with an endoluminal, endoscopic, gastrojejunal bypass sleeve. Surg Endosc. 2011;25:3028–33.
225. Sandler BJ, Rumbaut R, Swain CP, Torres G, Morales L, Gonzales L, et al. One-year human experience with a novel endoluminal, endoscopic gastric bypass sleeve for morbid obesity. Surg Endosc. 2015;29:3298–303.
226. Rubino F, Forgione A, Cummings DE, Vix M, Gnuli D, Mingrone G, et al. The mechanism of diabetes control after gastrointestinal bypass surgery reveals a role of the proximal small intestine in the pathophysiology of type 2 diabetes. Ann Surg. 2006;244:741–9.
227. Le Roux CW, Aylwin SJB, Batterham RL, Borg CM, Coyle F, Prasad V, et al. Gut hormone profiles following bariatric surgery favor an anorectic state, facilitate weight loss, and improve metabolic parameters. Ann Surg. 2006;243:108–14.
228. Grams J, Garvey WT. Weight loss and the prevention and treatment of type 2 diabetes using lifestyle therapy, pharmacotherapy, and bariatric surgery: mechanisms of action. Curr Obes Rep. 2015;4:287–302.
229. de Jonge C, Rensen SS, Verdam FJ, Vincent RP, Bloom SR, Buurman WA, et al. Endoscopic duodenal-jejunal bypass liner rapidly improves type 2 diabetes. Obes Surg. 2013;23:1354–60.
230. de Jonge C, Rensen SS, D'Agnolo HM, Bouvy ND, Buurman WA, Greve JW. Six months of treatment with the endoscopic duodenal-jejunal bypass liner does not lead to decreased systemic inflammation in obese patients with type 2 diabetes. Obes Surg. 2014;24:337–41.
231. Koehestanie P, Dogan K, Berends F, Janssen I, Wahab P, Groenen M, et al. Duodenal-jejunal bypass liner implantation provokes rapid weight loss and improved glycemic control, accompanied by elevated fasting ghrelin levels. Endosc Int Open. 2014;2:E21–7.
232. de Moura EG, Lopes GS, Martins BC, Orso IR, Coutinho AM, de Oliveira SL, et al. Effects of duodenal-jejunal bypass liner (Endobarrier®) on gastric emptying in obese and type 2 diabetic patients. Obes Surg. 2015;25:1618–25.
233. Rajagopalan H, Cherrington AD, Thompson CC, Kaplan LM, Rubino F, Mingrone G, et al. Endoscopic duodenal mucosal resurfacing for the treatment of type 2 diabetes: 6-month interim analysis from the first-in-human proof-of-concept study. Diabetes Care. 2016;39:2254–61.
234. Garvey WT. Ablation of the duodenal mucosa as a strategy for glycemic control in type 2 diabetes: role of nutrient signaling or simple weight Loss. Diabetes Care. 2016;39:2108–10.
235. Baar AV, Deviere J, Costamagna G, Galvao Neto M, Rodriguez L, Haidry R, et al. Early experience of duodenal mucosal resurfacing treatment for type 2 diabetes when expanding from single to multiple sites. Gastroenterology. 2016;150:S232.
236. Ryou M, Cantillon-Murphy P, Azagury D, Shaikh SN, Ha G, Greenwalt I, et al. Smart Self-Assembling MagnetS for ENdoscopy (SAMSEN) for transoral endoscopic creation of immediate gastrojejunostomy (with video). Gastrointest Endosc. 2011;73:353–9.
237. Ryou M, Aihara H, Thompson CC. Minimally invasive enteroenteral dual-path bypass using self-assembling magnets. Surg Endosc. 2016;30:4533–8.

238. Machytka E, Bužga M, Ryou MK, Lautz DB, Thompson CC. Endoscopic dual-path enteral anastomosis using self-assembling magnets: first-in-human clinical feasibility. Gastroenterology. 2016;150:S232.
239. Machytka E, Bužga M, Lautz DB, Ryou M, Simonson D, Thompson CC. A dual-path enteral bypass procedure created by a novel incisionless anastomosis system (IAS): 6-month clinical results. Gastroenterology. 2016;150:S26.
240. Machytka E, Bužga M, Zonca P, Lautz DB, Ryou M, Simonson DC, et al. Partial jejunal diversion using an incisionless magnetic anastomosis system: 1-year interim results in subjects with obesity and diabetes. Gastrointest Endosc. 2017;86(5):904–12. https://doi.org/10.1016/j.gie.2017.07.009.
241. Mathus-Vliegen EMH. Are endoscopists definitely stepping into the arena of weight-loss therapy? Endoscopy. 2015;47:8–10.
242. Cigaina V. Gastric pacing as therapy for morbid obesity: preliminary results. Obes Surg. 2002;12(Suppl 1):12S–16.
243. Dargent J. Gastric pacing as a therapy for morbid obesity: preliminary results from the French study. Obes Surg. 2002;12(Suppl 1):21S–25.
244. Horbach T, Thalheimer A, Seyfried F, Eschenbacher F, Schuhmann P, Meyer G. ability® closed loop gastric electrical stimulation system for treatment of obesity: clinical results with a 27-month follow-up. Obes Surg. 2015;25:1779–87.
245. Horbach T, Meyer G, Morales-Conde S, Alarcón I, Favretti F, Anselmino M, et al. Closed-loop gastric electrical stimulation versus laparoscopic adjustable gastric band for the treatment of obesity: a randomized 12-month multicenter study. Int J Obes. 2016;40:1891–8.
246. Lebovitz HE, Ludvik B, Yaniv I, Schwartz T, Zelewski M, Gutterman DD. Treatment of patients with obese type 2 diabetes with Tantalus-DIAMOND® gastric electrical stimulation: normal triglycerides predict durable effects for at least 3 years. Horm Metab Res. 2015;47:456–62.
247. Smith DK, Sarfeh J, Howard L. Truncal vagotomy in hypothalamic obesity. Lancet. 1983;1:1330–1.
248. Kral JG, Gortz L, Hermansson G, Wallin GS. Gastroplasty for obesity: long-term weight loss improved by vagotomy. World J Surg. 1993;17:75–9.
249. Papasavas P, El Chaar M, Kothari SN. American Society for Metabolic and Bariatric Surgery (ASMBS) position Statement on vagal blocking therapy for obesity. Surg Obes Relat Dis. 2016;12:460–1.
250. Shikora SA, Toouli J, Herrera MF, Kulseng B, Brancatisano R, Kow L, et al. Intermittent Vagal Nerve Block for improvements in obesity, cardiovascular risk factors, and glycemic control in patients with type 2 diabetes mellitus: 2-year results of the VBLOC DM2 Study. Obes Surg. 2016;26:1021–8.
251. Apovian CM, Shah CM, Wolfe BM, Ikramuddin S, Miller CJ, Tweden KS, et al. Two-year outcomes of vagal nerve blocking (vBloc) for the treatment of obesity in the ReCharge trial. Obes Surg. 2017;27:169–76.
252. Berry R, Cheng LK, Du P, Paskaranandavadivei N, Angeli TR, Mayne T, et al. Patterns of abnormal gastric pacemaking after sleeve gastrectomy defined by laparoscopic high-resolution electrical mapping. Obes Surg. 2017;27:1929–37.
253. Biasi C. The role of the vagal nucleus tractus solitaries in the therapeutic effects of obesity surgery and other interventional therapies on type 2 diabetes. Obes Surg. 2016;26:3045–57.
254. Kassir R, Barthelemy JC, Roche F, Perrot JL, Tiffet O. Letter to the editor. Effect of vagal nerve blockade on moderate obesity with an obesity-related comorbid condition: the recharge study. Obes Surg. 2016;26:2221–2.
255. Kentish SJ, O'Donnell TA, Frisby CL, Li H, Wittert GA, Page AJ. Altered gastric vagal mechanosensitivity persists on return to normal chow and is accompanied by increased food intake. Int J Obes. 2014;38:636–42.
256. Li S, Chen JDZ. Pulse width-dependent effects of intestinal electrical stimulation for obesity: role of gastro-intestinal motility and hormones. Obes Surg. 2017;27:70–7.

Bariatric Surgery

3

Contents

Abbreviations

AGB	Adjustable Gastric banding
BMI	Body mass index
BPD	Biliopancreatic diversion
BPD-DS	BPD-duodenal switch
CD	Crohn's disease
CC	Concomitant cholecystectomy
CPAP	Continuous positive airway pressure
DSS	Diabetes Surgery Summit
ERAS	Enhanced recovery after surgery
ERCP	Endoscopic retrograde cholangiopancreatography
EWL	Excess weight loss

E. M. H. Mathus-Vliegen, J. Dargent, *Bariatric Therapy*,
https://doi.org/10.1007/978-3-319-90074-2_3

FU	Follow-up
GI	Gastrointestinal
GIP	Gastric inhibitory peptide
GLP-1	Glucagon-like peptide-1
GORD	Gastro-oesophageal reflux disease
HbA1c	Glycated haemoglobin A1c
HH	Hiatal hernia
HRIM	High-resolution impedance manometry
IIGP	Increased intragastric pressure
IBD	Inflammatory bowel disease
IFSO	International Federation for the Surgery of Obesity
IWL	Insufficient weight loss
JIB	Jejunoileal bypass
LAGB	Laparoscopic adjustable gastric banding
LGCP	Laparoscopic greater curve plication
LRYGB	Laparoscopic Roux-en-Y gastric bypass
LSG	Laparoscopic sleeve gastrectomy
MIIpH	24-h Multichannel intraluminal impedance pH-metry
NAFLD	Non-alcoholic fatty liver disease
NASH	Non-alcoholic steatohepatitis
NOTES	Natural orifice translumenal endoscopic surgery
OAGB	One-anastomosis gastric bypass
PIVI	Preservation and Incorporation of Valuable endoscopic Innovations
PYY	Polypeptide YY
QOL	Quality of life
RCT	Randomised control trials
SADI-S	Single-anastomosis duodenoileal bypass with sleeve gastrectomy
SAGI	Single anastomosis gastroileal bypass
SGIT	Sleeve gastrectomy combined with ileal transposition
SILS	Single-incision laparoscopic surgery
SOS	Swedish Obese Subjects
TB	Transit bipartition
TBWL	Total body weight loss
T2DM	Type 2 diabetes
UC	Ulcerative colitis
UDCA	Ursodeoxycholic acid
VAS	Visual analogue scale
VBG	Vertical banded gastroplasty
WR	Weight regain

3.1 Introduction

Bariatric surgery comes a long way, since the first description of the jejunoileal bypass (JIB) in 1954 [1], which had deleterious outcomes in the long term, to the current operations with scientific proof of their efficacy and with long-term safety and efficacy data, thus gaining progressively credibility and popularity. Yet one should not take it for granted: while the shortcomings of early operations brought them on the verge of extinction, the combination of an "obesity epidemic" and great scientific improvements made them finally acceptable and supported by a host of solid arguments. The very success of bariatric procedures has yet become a kind of challenge, not only owing to constant controversies over evolutions or choice of a procedure, or issues like cost-effectiveness and complications, but also because the ever-growing population of eligible patients poses a threat to the allocation of resources worldwide. Do we have the capacity and can we afford to operate on all these eligible patients, and are we even in position of convincing them, in the same time as convincing public health leaders? Then the question may be asked "Is it time to turn ourselves towards less invasive operations" which will be tried to answer in this book that deals in great part with the possibilities of upper GI endoscopy.

In this part, we shall review the essential of what should be known about current interventions and their results. Whatever their destiny (some will thrive, some may disappear), they represent the most relevant benchmark to any other procedure, particularly if performed through endoscopic ways. In other words, we cannot exonerate ourselves from the review of historical techniques and results, when considering any new technology, whether acting on its own or as an adjuvant [2].

In this review, we keep in mind the general guidelines in effect in most countries, for the indication of bariatric surgery, already defined by the NIH in 1991 [3], that state that a patient is eligible for surgery if the body mass index (BMI) is above 40 or 35 kg/m^2 in the presence of associated comorbidities. They are effective in most countries, although debated with cut-off BMI values being lower in Eastern Asia for instance and lower BMI values allowed for patients with severe diabetes [4].

3.2 Bariatric Surgery

3.2.1 A Brief History

The first steps of obesity surgery appear retrospectively as full of surprises and unexpected trajectories! In April 1954, surgeons from Minneapolis had a focus on short-bowel syndrome after any kind of digestive surgery, and did experiments on dogs to evaluate the nutritional effects of small-bowel reduction. In the meantime, massively obese patients attracted their attention. Observing weight loss and lipid malabsorption as "by-products" from a specifically designed shortcut of the small intestine, they went to human trial, and called this operation the jejunoileal bypass (JIB) [1] (Fig. 3.1). There was a rapid success in the USA, which turned out detrimental owing to dramatic side effects, till complete banishment at the end of the 1970s, and a an ever-lasting negative reputation of the whole field of bariatric surgery. Nevertheless, during the same time, the fundamentals of a modern science of surgical weight loss were implemented [5].

After this dramatic and somewhat disturbing episode, the history of bariatric surgery unfolded in a reasonable way, with discussions and progresses that gained momentum, this being paralleled by the extension of the worldwide obesity epidemic. Gastrojejunal bypass, inaugurated by Edward Mason in 1967 [6], was the first operation that brought consensus, followed by purely restrictive operations: vertical banded gastroplasty (VBG) [7], and then laparoscopic

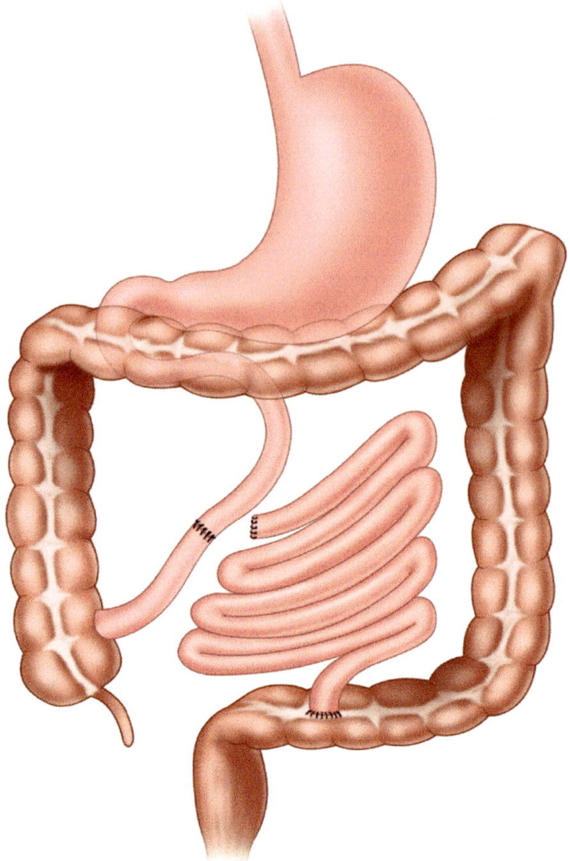

Fig. 3.1 Jejunoileal bypass

adjustable gastric banding (LAGB) [8]. After 1994, the entire spectrum of these operations became feasible through the laparoscopic approach, which attracted a significant proportion of morbidly obese patients. In the same time, credibility was obtained through evidence-based medicine in favour of surgery, starting with the Swedish Obese Subjects (SOS) Study initiated in 1994 [9], and the more fundamental approach unravelling the underlying metabolic effects of these procedures.

It is important to consider the history of the surgical techniques, since even discarded ones may survive for a long time as a niche (VBG being an example of this). We may also consider that history teaches us valuable lessons, and that a field of clinical research that has been opened cannot be entirely shut down. Moreover, obsolescence and technical upgrades are often intertwined, allowing old principles to find a second youth, as we have learned from many examples that are worth a quote in the context of this book: there was an endo-stapling device that could have been successful, but has been abandoned (TOGA device), while mimicking a VBG "from the inside"; there is now an endoscopic magnetic device that mimics jejuno-ileal bypass, etc. (see Chap. 2).

Finally, we shall also examine technical suggestions that might appear irrelevant or excessive, or even soon to be abandoned. Again, as to the field of bariatric techniques being evolving on a fast pace, there is no harm in putting under scrutiny successful and less successful operations in the same time!

3.2.2 Discussion of Bariatric Techniques with the Most Current Operations More in Detail

Most of the time and in a worldwide fashion, the surgical approach of obesity surgery focuses on the three major procedures that existed in 2017: the laparoscopic Roux-en-Y laparoscopic gastric bypass (LRYGB), the laparoscopic sleeve gastrectomy (LSG) and the laparoscopic adjustable gastric banding (LAGB). As emphasised in many recent surveys, there have been important shifts over the past few years, LSG becoming dominant and LAGB plummeting [10]: Fig. 3.2.

For example in the USA, LSG has been increasingly chosen as a primary bariatric procedure in recent years, superseding LAGB and RYGB [11]: The American College of Surgeons National Surgical Quality Improvement Program database has included 93,328 patients from 2010 to 2014: RYGB, LAGB and LSG comprised 58.4%, 28.8% and 9.3% of the procedures in 2010, which changed to 37.6%, 3.1% and 58.2% in 2014, respectively. Interestingly, the proportion of diabetic patients undergoing RYGB increased (30.4–33.2%, $P < 0.001$) but decreased among those having LSG (26.6–22.8%, $P = 0.001$).

These shifts have become more important than the issue of patient selection, which plays a minimal role for the present time, although one may prefer more malabsorptive operations (starting with RYGB) in super-obese patients (BMI > 50 kg/m^2) or patients with metabolic syndrome and/or type 2 diabetes mellitus (T2DM).

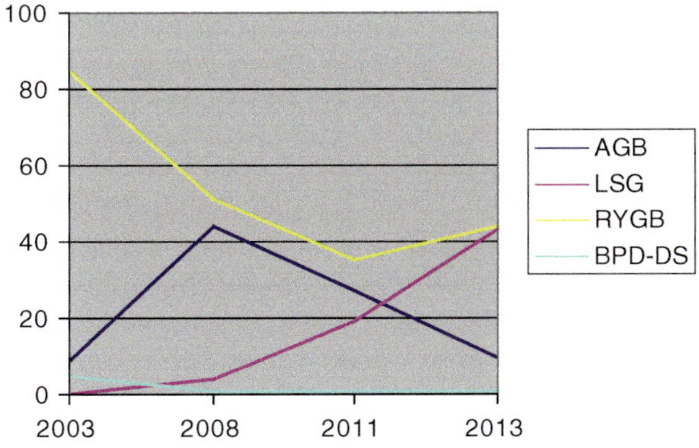

Fig. 3.2 Evolution of bariatric procedures, worldwide trends [10]

3.2.2.1 Three Leading Procedures and a Perpetual Outsider

Laparoscopic Roux-En-Y Gastric Bypass (RYGB) (Fig. 3.3)

This operation remains the golden standard of bariatric surgery, whatever new operations have come up ever since its inception and initial description by Mason and Ito (1966) [6], then modified with a Roux-en-Y shape (Griffen). Owing to pioneers, such as Wittgrove et al., the laparoscopic approach was possible as early as 1994 [12], and has become a routine in the hands of any young bariatric surgeon. It consists in creating a small upper gastric pouch of 50–80 cc, a gastrojejunal anastomosis, and then a side-to-side jejunojejunal anastomosis. The Y-shape of the procedure entails two bowel functional limbs: an alimentary limb of 1.5 m (with variations, especially in so-called long-limb gastric bypass), connected to a biliopancreatic limb of 0.5–0.75 m.

Early complications of LRYGB include post-operative bleeding (0–3%), leak with abscess or peritonitis (0–5%) and pulmonary embolism. Dumping syndrome is more an undesired effect than a complication, and lasts usually less than 2 years post-operatively. Late complications are marginal ulcer, stenosis of the gastrointestinal anastomosis, jejunoileal obstruction or volvulus. Most of these complications require an endoscopic expertise and/or treatment (see Chaps. 5 and 6), although surgical re-intervention is necessary in many occasions. Possible vitamin and nutrient deficiencies are addressed in Chap. 7 (post-operative guidance).

A significant variation of RYGB, introduced by Fobi in 1998 [13], consists of placing a nonadjustable ring around the gastric pouch above the gastrojejunal anastomosis. It claims to enhance short- and mid-term weight loss, and to prevent weight regain in the long run. Optionally, such a ring can be placed as a rescue in case of weight regain after a standard bypass. According to a recently published study with a long follow-up, banding the bypass could overcome insufficient weight loss and weight regain due to dilation of either the pouch, the pouch outlet or the proximal alimentary limb [14]: 432 patients (n = 254, non-banded RYGB; n = 178, banded RYGB) were followed up for 5 years. No significant differences between groups in the first year following surgery were observed in terms of weight loss; follow-up rates were 89.4% and 88.8%, respectively. Percentages of excess weight loss (% EWL) at 5 years were 65.2% in non-banded patients and 74.0% in banded patients. Weight regain was significantly higher in the non-banded group ($P < 0.0001$). The complication rate due to the band was rather low in this publication: slippage (1), stenosis (5: 2.8%), broken band (6: 3.4%) and intragastric migration (0 reported, but this is a sensitive issue since in some cases they may have to be removed endoscopically).

We may question these assertions since banded bypass has never become a routine procedure for most surgeons, although available and well known for almost two decades. The fact that it is also advised for redo surgery, namely in case of weight regain (or sometimes in case of intractable dumping syndrome), is also very interesting: in that case, it competes nowadays with endoscopic additional restriction, such as advocated with OverStitch or USGI POSE (see Chap. 6).

Fig. 3.3 Roux-en-Y gastric bypass

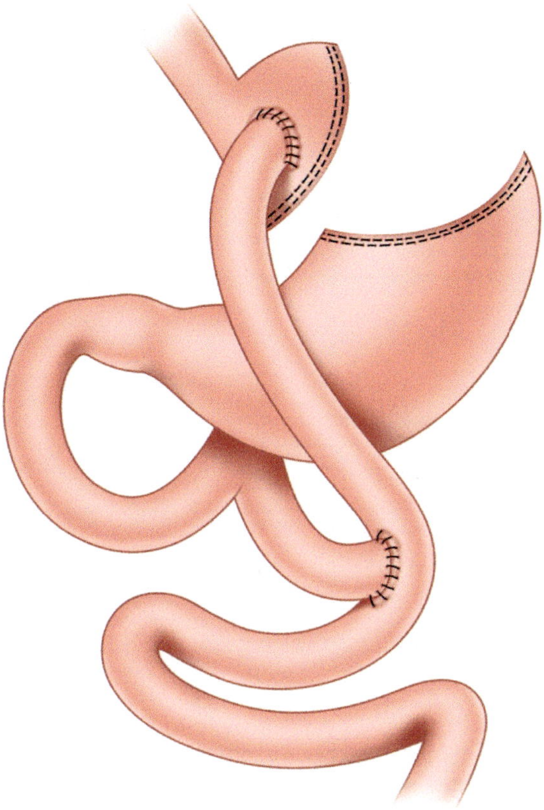

Laparoscopic Sleeve Gastrectomy (LSG) (Fig. 3.4)

Initially conceived as a first step before BPD (more precisely BPD with duodenal switch, described by Hess and Marceau in 1988) [15] or RYGB [16, 17], which was deemed dangerous in very obese patients at that time, LSG has become an operation on its own, with long-term acceptable weight loss. It consists of dividing the greater curve 3–10 from the pylorus up till the angle of His, and then creating a pouch with a sleeve shape, calibrated on a 32–38 French intragastric bougie or tube (inserted intra-operatively) and through a linear stapling. Some have advocated replacing this tube by an intra-operative endoscope, which might have the advantage of evaluating the suture line for bleeding and leak immediately after the procedure (see Chap. 5). A portion of the antrum is left in place, some surgeons suggesting keeping this portion very minimal, i.e. the resection coming few centimetres away from the pylorus.

Very commonly, the staple line is reinforced by buttressing material to minimise the risks of bleeding or leak, especially in the upper part of the sleeve. The gastric remnant has a usual 100–150 cc volume, while approximately two-thirds of the stomach are removed. The growing success of LSG is impressive worldwide, only

Fig. 3.4 Sleeve gastrectomy

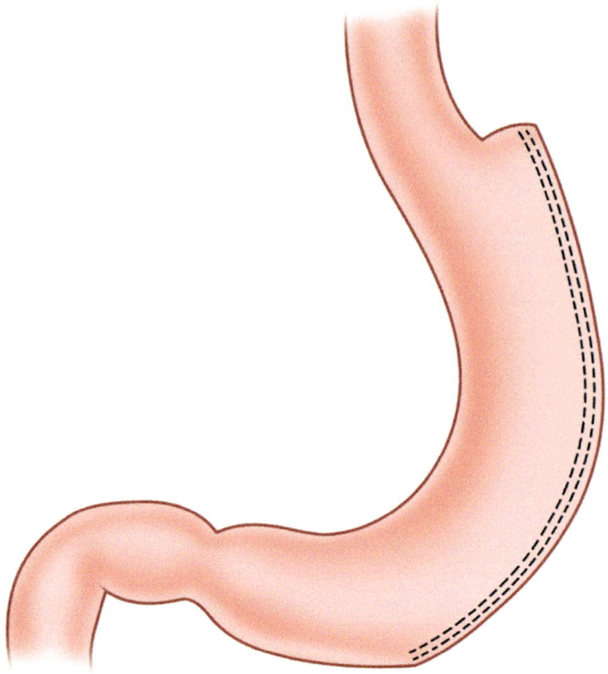

altered by the current rate of post-operative complications (1–5%), which although decreasing may be difficult to handle especially when dealing with sepsis and leaks, or more rarely stenosis. Some issues are discussed abundantly: What to do when sleeve fails? Does the size of the sleeve mechanically and automatically increase [18, 19]? Is LSG causing gastro-oesophageal reflux (GORD), with its late complications of Barrett's oesophagus, eventually oesophageal cancer? (See below, GORD issue.) Although RYGB seems to be the natural response/rescue to these issues, the debates are still going on. So far, 5-year and beyond weight loss numbers are still satisfactory in most series, and the rate of early and late complications is acceptable.

The success of LSG is perceived as being potentially limited by dilation of the remaining gastric tube during the follow-up. In a prospective study, gastric volumetry using 3D gastric computed tomography with gas expansion was performed in 54 successive LSG patients at 3 and 12 months post-operatively [18]. An increase of at least 25% of the total gastric volume was considered as sleeve dilation, and was observed in 61% of the subjects 1 year after surgery, the gastric tube being mainly involved in this process, especially in subjects with smaller total gastric volume at baseline (189 vs. 236 mL, $P = 0.02$). Dilation was not necessarily linked to an increase of daily caloric intake and insufficient weight loss during the first 18 months after LSG. Another prospective study of 112 LSG patients has used a radiological evaluation [19]. All patients showed a significant reduction in BMI (from 50.5 to 33.5 kg/m^2). Sleeve volume at 1 month was 68.39 cm^3 and 122.58 cm^3

at 12 months, again with no association between this increase and weight loss at 1-year follow-up. These findings may question the strategy of "re-sleeve gastrectomy" in case of weight regain with a significant enlargement of the gastric tube. Under these circumstances, it seems also.fair to acknowledge different mechanisms of action than pure restriction, which contribute to weight maintenance in the long term after LSG. Ghrelin suppression could be one of them.

Laparoscopic Adjustable Gastric Banding (LAGB) (Fig. 3.5)
Kuzmak invented in 1986 an adjustable band [20], which was then popularised by Belachew in its laparoscopic version [6]. This operation became the first laparoscopic bariatric procedure that was reproducible and performed on a routine basis. On a worldwide scale, it has been stressed that the number of LAGB declined substantially over the past decade: from 24.4% of the total in 2003 to 10% in 2013, with a temporary peak of 42.3% in 2008 [10].

LAGB became the most commonly performed bariatric surgical procedure in Europe during the years 1995–2005, and then in the USA, later than in Europe due to the late approval of the technique by the FDA. Although deemed effective in the long term [21], it is now performed less frequently. The reader should realise that the last version of a modified band is still one of the first options in countries such as Australia, where the band with its adjustments is well imbedded in the healthcare system with reimbursement of long-term follow-up and band adjustments, explaining their good results, compared with others being less dedicated and accessible for follow-up. The disadvantages of LAGB include flaws in some materials, the need for multiple reoperations and a lack of effectiveness over time. Oesophageal dilation can be a serious problem, but this can be resolved by downward adjustment of the band. The most commonly reported problems are related to long-term food intolerance or difficulties with band adjustments, resulting in band removal and

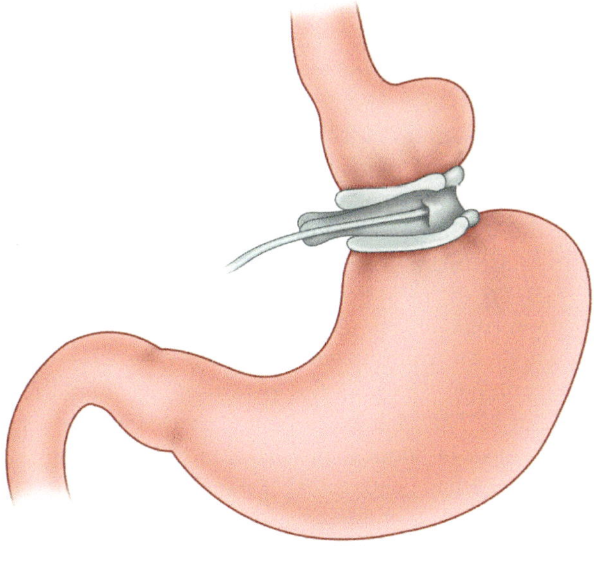

Fig. 3.5 Laparoscopic adjustable gastric banding

conversion to a different procedure, from 10% up to 60% of the cases. Repeated adjustments are initially useful, but the need for such adjustments is regarded as a disadvantage in the long term: the primary asset of this procedure, adjustability and turning into a liability. Over time, the band loses its ability to re-implement weight loss, along with food intolerance. Undeniable adverse effects explain why LAGB is no longer popular: short-term inefficacy for a variable number of patients, difficulties with adjustments and follow-up, and food intolerance complaints are the most cited. As shown in a French survey, including all adult patients operated on with LAGB between 2007 and 2013 (52,868 patients), 10,815 bands were removed [22]. The removal rates at 5, 6 and 7 years were 28%, 34% and 40%, respectively. Two-thirds of the patients needed revisional surgery after removal. This publication also emphasises the important discrepancy between low-volume centres and high-volume centres, the latter doing better in terms of "band survival".

Minor suggestions have been implemented and are still advocated, like banding a sleeve/bypass as an adjunction to the original operation or as a treatment of weight regain, and suggesting using LAGB for adolescents, all strategies that are unlikely to do more than buy some more years. More importantly, gastric banding could remain useful in combination with future techniques, particularly endoscopic techniques, and/or as a redo procedure after these techniques have been implemented. LAGB has increased our understanding of the mechanisms underlying effective restriction of food intake. It has represented a major step in the field of obesity treatment, and using it for a long period has been valid and sound. In general, we should maintain a set of options for obese patients that includes simpler operations than RYGB and even LSG; best candidates are endoscopic procedures such as gastric internal plication (see Chap. 2). In that sense, there is a strong legacy to the band, mostly playing the role of a "simple restrictive intervention" in comparison to more demanding procedures. When considering a larger spectrum of obesity treatments, for instance including class I obesity cases, there is a need for minimally aggressive techniques that would operate with a comparable status as LAGB did in the recent past.

BilioPancreatic Diversion and BPD-Duodenal Switch

(BPD and BPD-DS, Figs. 3.6 and 3.7)

Although a current outsider because of its complexity, barely representing 1–2% of the procedures worldwide, the fact that this operation exists since 1979 [23] makes it a prominent tool in weight-loss surgery. It was originally conceived by Scopinaro to avoid the most important side effects of the JIB (e.g. blind loop). The input of current modifications has brought a renewed interest to the concept of malabsorption. Being the most powerful and long-standing bariatric intervention is a privilege that unfortunately entails a super-close surveillance, and possible long-term adverse effects due to mineral and vitamin deficiencies. The BPD-DS results in superior excess weight loss with the lowest rate of weight regain [24] while achieving the best rate of T2DM resolution of all current bariatric surgeries. Owing to the considerable raise in surgical numbers, more long-term failures are observed after any given procedure, making BPD paradoxically more attractive in 2017. Under these circumstances, it comes as no surprise that technical variations are flourishing as well, with a trend in one-anastomosis operations, supposed to be simpler.

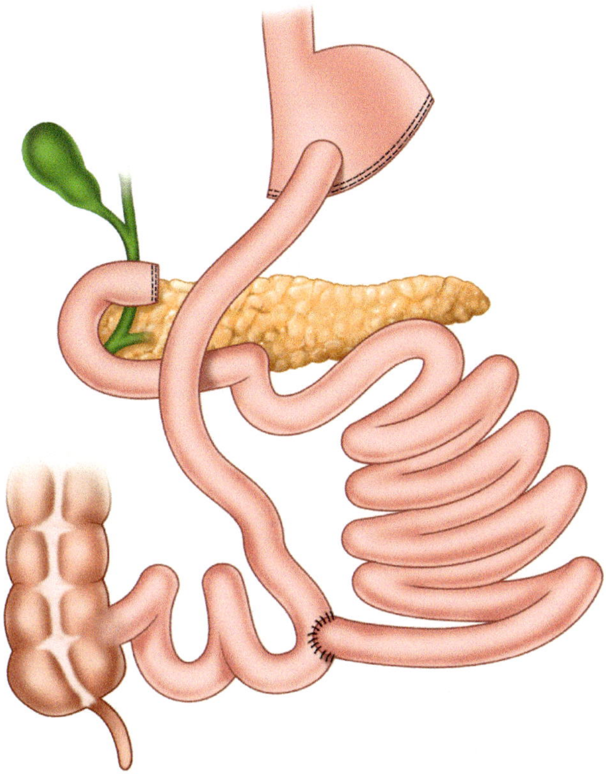

Fig. 3.6 Biliopancreatic bypass

The key feature of BPD compared to other bariatric surgeries is a partial gastrectomy with a gastroileal anastomosis, where in a short common channel of ileum of 1 m (70 cm in the primary version of BPD) the food "shares" the biliopancreatic enzymes after a biliopancreatic limb of usually more than 2.5 m [25]. In the duodenal switch not a partial gastrectomy but a sleeve gastrectomy is performed keeping the pylorus intact with a postpyloric duodenoileal anastomosis (hence the name "duodenal switch") [15].

Despite a high degree of malabsorption, BPD-DS is a viable option due to its flexibility. The standard common channel (75–100 cm) may be adjusted to 125–150 cm to avoid excessive bowel movements and excessive weight loss. One can adjust the size of the sleeve as well, and alter the impact of restriction that is added to the diversion. There is limited information on the multiple long-term effects of the biliopancreatic diversion with duodenal switch (BPD-DS). In a US series, patients who had a BPD-DS from 1999 to 2010 were evaluated for weight change [25]: 284 patients received a BPD-DS. Two hundred and seventy-five patients were available in year 1, 275 patients in year 3, 273 patients in year 5, 259 patients in year 7 and 228 patients in year 9, this good follow-up being a necessity given the risks associated with (micronutrient) deficiencies. BMI was 30.1 kg m^2 at 1 year and 32.0 kg m^2 at 9 years. Body fat was reduced to 26% after 2 years. Complications requiring surgery were significant. Nutritional problems developed in 29.8% of

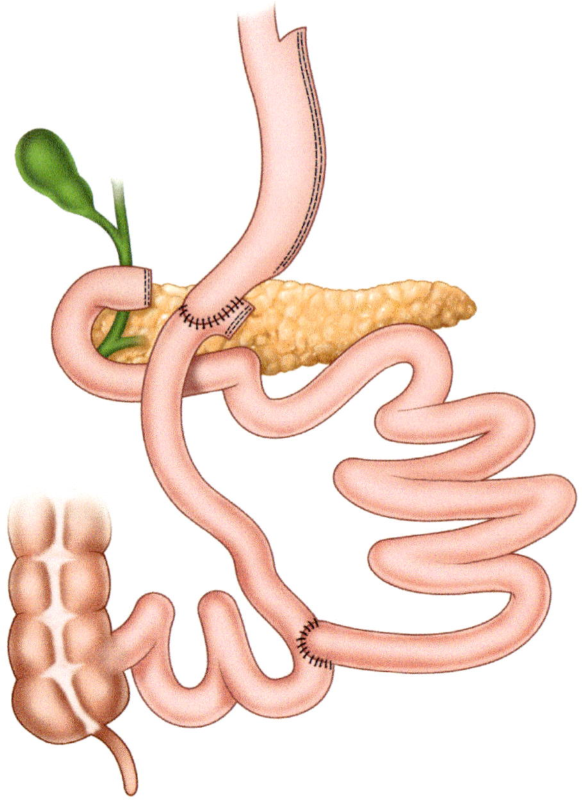

Fig. 3.7 Biliopancreatic bypass with duodenal switch

patients over the course of observation. After surgery, the resolution of comorbidities continued for the period of follow-up of 9 years. While rates of surgical complications resembled other bariatric procedures, long-term nutrient deficiencies represented a major concern.

3.2.2.2 Forgotten Heroes

Jejunoileal Bypass

JIB could have been one of the forgotten heroes, but is hardly remembered as such! On the other hand, BPD could be placed here in the opinion of many who deem the malabsorptive principle as such as obsolete. Yet it appears that one cannot escape the necessity of keeping long-standing operations for weight loss and resolution of comorbidities within the armamentarium, which obviously other surgeries do not provide. Moreover, this principle has been revitalised in many current malabsorptive operations, including the endoscopic dual-magnet JIB (see Chap. 2). However, many of the disasters related to the JIB were not related to the malabsorption as such but more to the excluded long limb with bacterial stasis and endotoxaemia. In the endoscopic JIB, the food can choose which way to go, either following the original anatomy or shortcutting the way down through the jejunoileal bypass (see Chap. 2).

Vertical Banded Gastroplasty (VBG), Fig. 3.8
VBG is the typical fallen hero. Historically, it has been the alternative option when a gastric bypass was deemed too aggressive in terms of surgical complications and/or necessity of a strict follow-up. This choice was even designed by the same surgeon at the origin of modern bariatric surgery, Edward Mason, and was extremely successful in the years 1980–2000. The most typical variation (VBG) uses a gastric pouch of 50–80 cc, and an outlet through a Marlex band, or a silastic ring of 4–6 cm diameter [7]. The staplers that are used for creating the pouch can either divide the stomach or not (which entailed a risk of staple disruption, with further weight regain). Technical variations were numerous and have lost their interest. Although still argued in favour, this operation became irrelevant when LAGB appeared, albeit feasible through laparoscopy, and practically ceased to exist when LSG came up.

3.2.2.3 Technical Variations and/or Experiments
Surgical novelties represent either novel procedures or the input of new technologies/devices in existing procedures. It has been pointed out that such innovations frequently did not benefit from the adequate scrutiny bariatric patients were entitled to; likewise, the dissemination of operations with dubious results, or at least insufficient assessment of their side effects, has been criticised [2, 26]. Some of the operations cited hereafter do not necessarily fulfil the ideal criteria of the bariatric standards. Some would answer that even the most established procedures face evolution and pitfalls; yet it seems fair to state that the techniques we shall describe should be considered investigational for their major part while eliciting highly interesting debates.

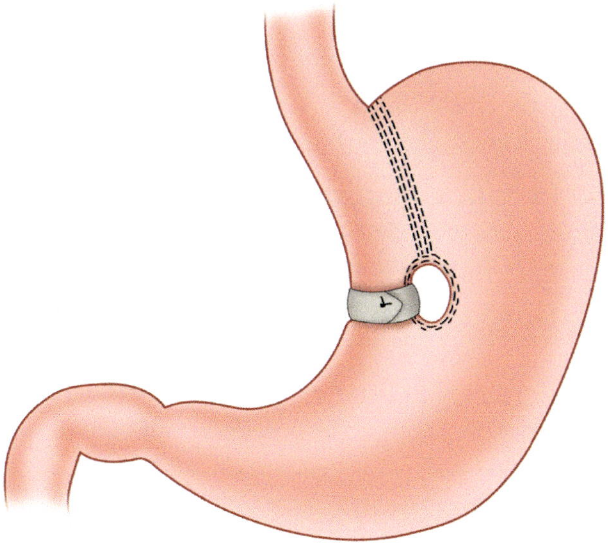

Fig. 3.8 Vertical banded gastroplasty

Single-Anastomosis Operations

Omega-Loop Gastric Bypass or One-Anastomosis Gastric Bypass (OAGB), Fig. 3.9
Sometimes abusively called "mini-bypass", the most significant variation of Roux-en-Y gastric bypass is paradoxically a return to the origin of bypass, as described by Mason, with a single gastrojejunal anastomosis. The admitted length of the biliary limb ranges from 150 to 250 cm, which could be held accountable for some of the side effects due to the shortness of the remaining alimentary limb, that are attributed to this operation: protein deficiency and malnutrition, and biliary reflux (leading rarely to a switch to regular RYGB). In experimented teams though, it does not seem than the rate of these complications exceeds 1–2%. Theoretically, biliary reflux could lead to an increased rate of oesophageal cancer in the long term, and the results of the background literature could seem contradictory in this regard [27].

From the current literature, we know that OAGB can be as efficient as RYGB, if not more efficient given the pronounced malabsorptive component [28]. In a Spanish series of 1200 patients (2002–2008), analysed after a 6–12-year FU, the highest mean EWL was 88% (at 2 years), and then 77% and 70%, 6 and 12 years post-operatively [29]. Mean BMI decreased from 46 to 26.6 6 kg/m^2 at 2 years and was 28.5 kg/m^2 and 29.9 kg/m^2 after 6 (55% of FU) and 12 years (21% of FU), respectively. Remission (18–100%) or improvement (4–100%) of comorbidities was achieved in most patients.

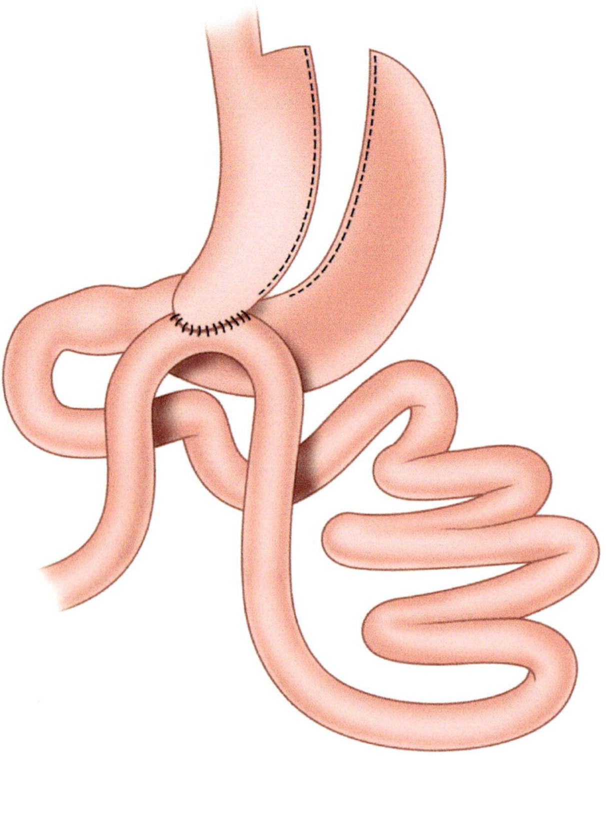

Fig. 3.9 Omega-loop gastric bypass

The technically easier OAGB is associated with similar metabolic improvements and weight loss as the RYGB. However, OAGB is controversial mostly because of a long biliopancreatic limb, and could result in greater malabsorption than RYGB. In a French study, macronutrient absorption and intestinal adaptation after OAGB or RYGB were compared in rats [30]. The OAGB and RYGB surgeries both resulted in a reduction of body weight and an improvement of glucose tolerance relative to sham rats. OAGB led to greater protein malabsorption and energy loss than RYGB.

Similarly, a case series of patients with nutrition complications after bariatric surgery has suggested that in case of complication after OAGB, the probability of the need of artificial nutrition was more likely than in LSG or RYGB [31].

There is a recent tendency to suggest the elimination of one anastomosis in malabsorptive procedures, which might reduce the operation time and possibly might decrease the rate of surgical complications (e.g. late obstruction, owing to the non-opening of the mesentery). In the same time, other surgeons have chosen to measure mainly the common limb, i.e. selecting the place of the gastrointestinal anastomosis, possibly responsible for the malabsorptive effect, starting from the ileocaecal valve. We will discuss two of the suggested current variations, the SADI-S and the SAGI.

Single-Anastomosis Duodeno-Ileal Bypass with Sleeve Gastrectomy (SADI-S), Fig. 3.10

The single-anastomosis duodeno-ileal bypass with sleeve gastrectomy (SADI-S) is based on the biliopancreatic diversion in which a sleeve gastrectomy is followed by an end-to-side duodeno-ileal diversion, and has been described by Sanchez-Pernaute et al. [32].

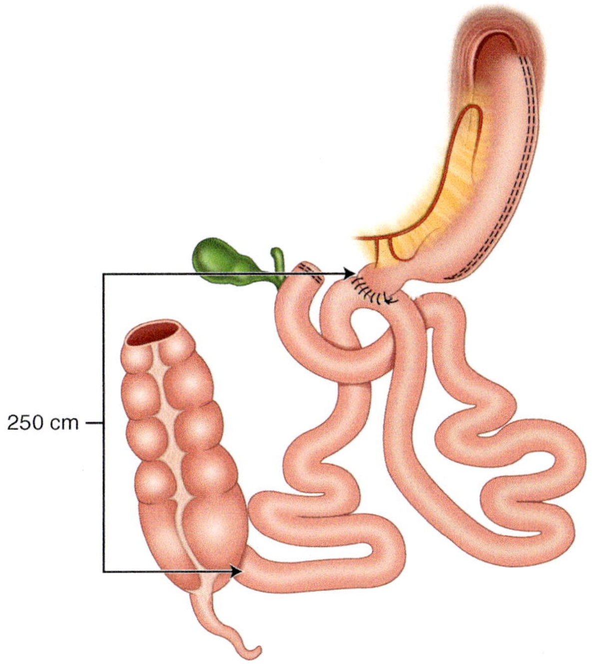

Fig. 3.10 Sleeve gastrectomy with duodenal switch (SADI)

The preservation of the pylorus makes possible the reconstruction in one loop, which reduces operating time and needs no mesentery opening. The initial experience comprised 50 patients. There were two gastric staple-line leaks and one subphrenic abscess. Excess weight loss reached 94.7% at 1 year, and it was maintained over the second and third years. At 1 year, mild anaemia has been detected in 10% of the cases. Albumin concentration was below normal in 8% of the patients in the first post-operative year, but all patients recovered to normal levels by the third post-operative year. All diabetic patients had normalised HbA1c levels at 6 months with no need of anti-diabetic therapy.

Single-Anastomosis GastroIleal Bypass (SAGI)

In OAGB, the measurement of the afferent limb starting at the angle of Treitz may result in insufficient absorptive surface of the intestine of the remaining efferent limb. As a variation of the SADI and to address this concern, some surgeons have recently modified the technique of OAGB by constructing the gastrointestinal anastomosis at a fixed distance from the ileocaecal valve (i.e. 300 cm), and called it the single-anastomosis gastroileal bypass (SAGI). Seven consecutive patients were operated on, with no intraoperative complications, a mean EWL of 55.1% at 3 months and 82.1% at 6 months [33].

Sleeve Gastrectomy with Intestinal Transposition, Fig. 3.11

This operation combines a sleeve gastrectomy with the latest possibility in metabolic surgery, transposing the initial and the most distal segments of the small intestine. It adds a significant malabsorption to the sleeve, with additional expected metabolic effects [34], which we shall also review (hereafter, section "mechanism of action").

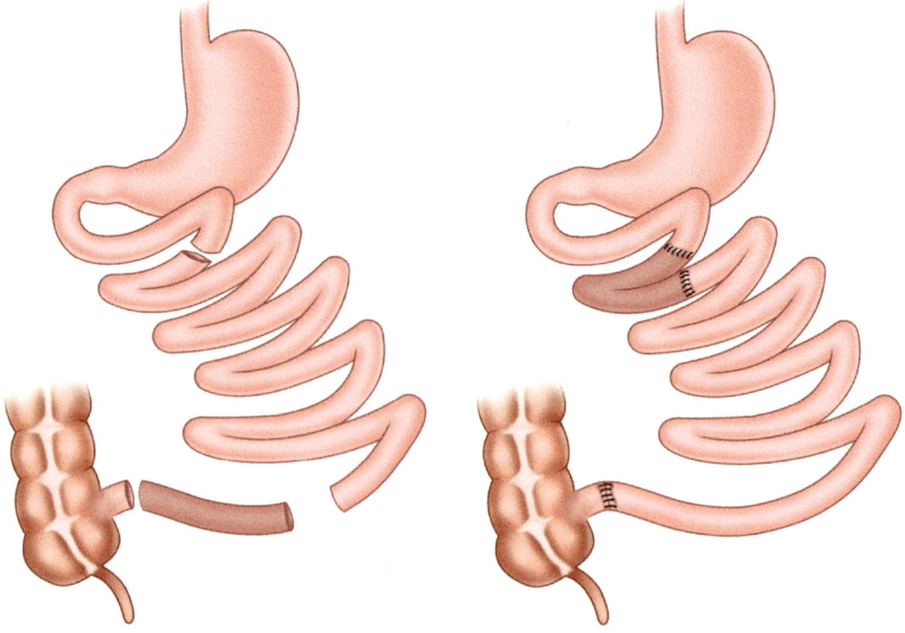

Fig. 3.11 Sleeve gastrectomy with ileal transposition

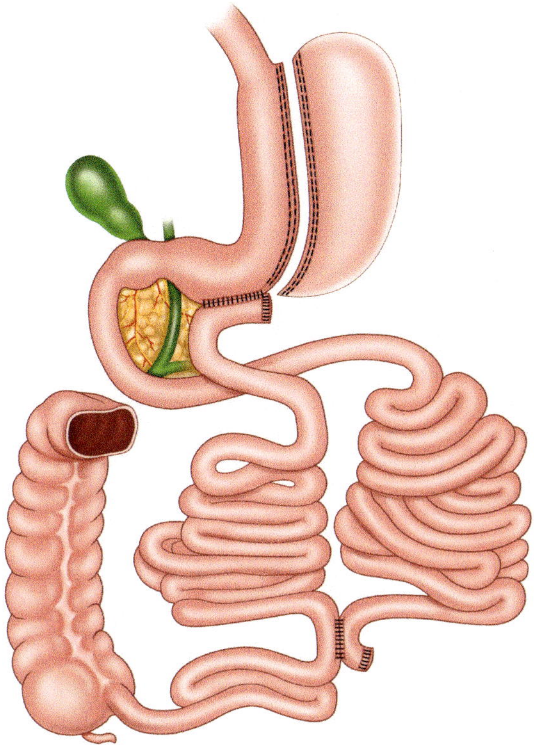

Fig. 3.12 Sleeve gastrectomy with transit bipartition

Sleeve Gastrectomy with Transit Bipartition, Fig. 3.12
A variation of malabsorption has been suggested in Brazil that keeps two outflow pathways starting from the stomach. The 5-year results of this technique have been presented, called transit bipartition (TB), associated with LSG [35]. It has been designed to counterbalance the hypothesis that high-glycaemic-index foods may lead to a hormonally hyperactive proximal gut, and in the same time a hypoactive distal gut, with subsequent metabolic syndrome. TB creates an additional gastroileal anastomosis in the antrum after the LSG; nutrient transit is maintained in the duodenum, avoiding blind loops and minimising malabsorption; a lateral entero-anastomosis connects both segments at 80 cm, proximal to the caecum like in BPD. A total of 1020 obese patients were operated on, with 91% and 74% excess BMI loss at 1 and 5 years. There were two deaths (0.2%), and 6% complications.

Laparoscopic Greater Curve Plication (LGCP)
This procedure is supposed to replicate the sleeve gastrectomy, while instead of dividing any part of the stomach, a running suture is carried out from the angle of His to the antrum; it is a debatable procedure but in endoscopy it has some relevant application analogues (see Chap. 2). A gastric plication has also been suggested as

an adjuvant to LAGB, but, LAGB being an obsolete operation for many surgeons, the combination of the LAGB with an unproven operation does not seem to make sense. LGCP has been described in Iran [36], with questionable data, and initially meant to counterbalance the costs of stapling! As stated in 2011 in an ASMBS statement [37], evidence is unclear regarding efficacy, safety and durability, revisional surgery following LGCP being common. In a retrospective study of 100 patients between 2009 and 2010, 42 had an EWL <50% and 38 had severe symptoms (vomiting) after a mean time of 13.5 months; 30 had revisional surgery with a BMI of 38.6 kg/m^2 before conversion into LSG in 17 and LRYGB in 13. At 18 months, those converted to a RYGBP had a higher % EWL (75.7%) than those converted to a LSG (61.4%, $P = 0.008$) [38].

In a recent meta-analysis, the comparison of LSG with LGCP was unfavourable for the LGCP [39]: 8 studies (3 RCTs, 4 retrospective studies and 1 prospective study) with 536 patients were included. Despite the limitations, results suggested that LSG was superior to LGCP in terms of % EWL at 3 ($P < 0.02$), 6 ($P < 0.01$), 12 ($P < 0.01$) and 36 months ($P < 0.01$). No significant difference was found in operation time, adverse events and resolution of obesity-related comorbidities.

It is currently not possible to foresee the future of LCGP, but we may already consider it a useful benchmark to endoscopic plication even it fails as a surgical technique (see Chap. 2).

3.2.2.4 Other Experimental Surgeries

Although we may state that all bariatric surgery in its incipience in general is experimental, and clearly did not need to follow the strict rules that govern the introduction of pharmacotherapy in the market, the now established surgical operations such as RYGB, SG, BPD-DS and to some extent also LAGB have earned their credibility over time, but some operations fall clearly under the category of experiments today, which may also be true for some of the above-mentioned operations.

Gastric Neuromodulation

Digestive neuro-stimulation can be applied directly to the vagus nerve, or to any other part of the digestive tract. Its mechanisms are different from malabsorption and restriction, and it is described in Chap. 2.

Gastric Clip

This new technique aims at reproducing the sleeve gastrectomy principle, with a vertically placed clip [40]. No resection takes place, and it is reversible. From 2012 to 2016, prospective collected data from 117 patients were included in a trial. The clip consists of a silicone-covered titanium backbone, with an inferior hinged opening that separates a medial lumen from an excluded lateral gastric pouch. The inferior opening allows the gastric juices to empty from the fundus and the body of the stomach into the distal antrum. Weight loss and comorbidities were evaluated over a 39-month period. EWL was 66.7%, with minimal adverse events. Average length of surgery was 69 min, and average length of hospital stay 1.3 days. Fifteen of the originally implanted clips were electively removed based on the original protocol, and the other two were removed for displacement of the device. We may consider

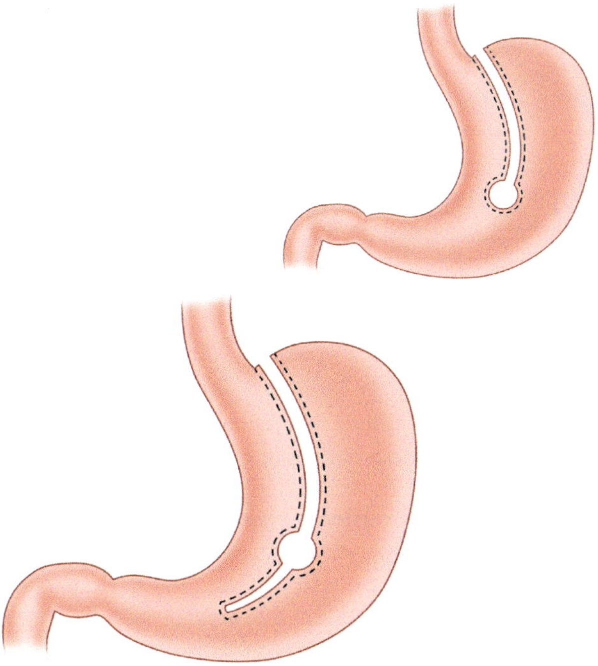

Fig. 3.13 Magenstrasse and Mill operation

that the clip is also inspired by the so-called Mill and Magenstrasse procedure [41], Fig. 3.13, consisting of a kind of sleeve gastrectomy without gastric removal—a technique that disappeared when LSG came out. We may have concerns about the possibilities of exploring a semi-blind segment during an upper GI endoscopy.

3.2.3 Adjuncts to Surgery

3.2.3.1 Enhanced Recovery After Bariatric Surgery (ERAS)

This protocol is well established in many surgical disciplines and leads to a decrease in the length of hospital stay and morbidity. It has a preoperative part, an intraoperative part and a post-operative part. It is important to mention in this bariatric surgery section the elimination of prolonged preoperative fasting to circumvent the insulin resistance provoked by the trauma of surgery, and during the operation not to overload the patient with fluids, and to remove the nasogastric tube before discharge to the ward. Post-operative measures are reviewed in detail in the part "post-operative guidance" (Chap. 7).

3.2.3.2 Robotics

Robotic assisted surgery represents an evolving platform that should be considered as an addition to our armamentarium instead of a wholly competitive technology. Numerous publications insist on advantages in terms of intraoperative enhanced skills, particularly concerning the suturing part of a bariatric procedure including one or several anastomoses, such as present in the gastric bypass [42]. In terms of post-operative recovery, or morbidity, no real benefit has been shown yet, not mentioning the costs.

In other procedures than bypass, the benefits seem more limited. In a systematic review and meta-analysis of robotic LSG, 19 studies have incorporated 29,787 patients [43]. Robotic LSG showed significantly higher mean operative time and increased length of hospital stay. Post-operative incidence of leakage, wound infection and bleeding, along with weight reduction, were comparable with non-robotic SG.

3.2.3.3 Three-Dimensional Imaging

3D and/or enhanced imaging (4K or ultra-high definition) augments the vision [44], hence diminishing the skills required for delicate operations. Dedicated glass is needed, while the 3D learning curve may also benefit from a special environment within training facilities (augmented reality). These tools are expensive for the time being, but progress is very rapid.

3.2.3.4 Single-Incision Laparoscopic Surgery (SILS)

Minimising post-operative pain and discomfort is a powerful incentive in digestive surgery, from which obese patients may benefit even more. The appeal of single incision has been important a few years ago, but seems today out of trend in most hands. As seen with many surgical variations, and despite efforts to promote such techniques, patients are not particularly in demand. Most surgeons complain about the tedious manoeuvers with minimal access to the intraoperative areas combined with ill-adapted instruments, albeit some claim otherwise. Moreover, the improved cosmetic effect is balanced against the increased likelihood of incisional hernia, while there is no decisive advantage in terms of post-operative pain or recovery. Yet most bariatric procedures have been proven feasible and reproducible through this access, including more demanding operations such as RYGB [45].

3.2.3.5 Natural Orifice Translumenal Endoscopic Surgery (NOTES) Procedures, Fig. 3.14

Like SILS, this field of research seems objectively less interesting than a few years ago, when many resources were pulled out and programmes implemented. NOTES, however, had a significant contribution in the development of new instruments and contributed a lot to the principle of thinking out of the box and beyond the narrow surgical or endoscopic scope. It appears that NOTES stays at the frontier between surgery and endoscopy, yet it might also appear that the line could be crossed one way or the other. For the time being, we believe that some of the NOTES concepts are better employed through purely endoscopic ways, while others still preferably require laparoscopic skills. The debate remains about bypass procedures, as exemplified in Fig. 3.14. Research is being carried out with gastrojejunal anastomosis through stents [46] or magnets [47]. Other approaches like transvaginal procedures (e.g. for LSG [48, 49]) are being discussed. Promising upgrades include single-use master slave NOTES robot and/or a flexible robotic platform, with a telemanipulation of the endoscope [50].

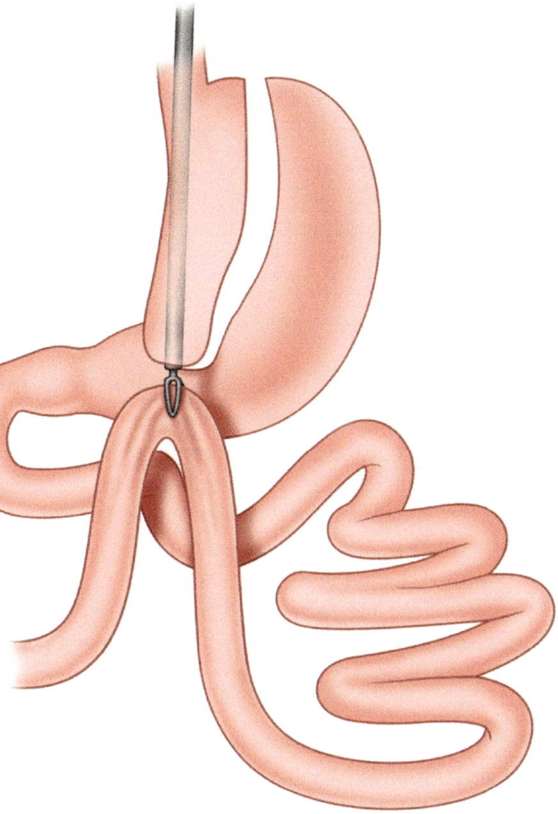

Fig. 3.14 Example of NOTES surgery: transgastric gastrojejunal anastomosis

3.2.4 Reoperations in Bariatric Surgery

Each bariatric technique faces a variable but inevitable rate of long-term failures. While some cases are not necessarily leading to further surgery and can be managed through diet counselling and various supports, a significant proportion are eligible for a bariatric re-intervention. Several options are available for each case, and guidelines are not clear most of the time. Countless publications can be quoted without dissipating a kind of "fog of war" when seeking to translate them into decisions. Nevertheless, there is a general agreement on carefully re-evaluating such patients, best candidates being sometimes the ones not asking for redo, and vice versa. Not all reoperations are requested because of weight regain solely, some resulting from technical flaws (e.g. band slippage or eroding the gastric lumen, gastrogastric fistula after RYGB, severe reflux after LSG) with or without weight regain.

Dealing with weight regain, it is common sense that LAGB can be transformed into a LSG or a RYGB, with a common interval of time of 3 months between removal of the band and redo. Conservative options after LAGB, such as band replacement, or re-suturing after reduction of a pouch, have become an exception. Likewise, LSG is often transformed into RYGB or one-anastomosis gastric banding

(OAGB), while "re-sleeving" is an alternative option. Dealing with the reoperation of the RYGB, an operation considered at "the end of the line", the question of what to do next remains tricky. Among current options, none has gained consensus: banding (usually with a nonadjustable band) of the gastric pouch, resizing (or "sleeve") of the pouch or lengthening of the alimentary limb. Endoscopic options are mainly the plication of the pouch and/or preferably the gastrojejunal anastomosis (see Chap. 6). BPD-DS and other malabsorptive operations are also "end-of-the-line operations" that may have a role but often are ruled out because of insufficient experience in many teams.

Deciding a reoperation requires an algorithm, at least informal, and follows a step-by-step process:

1. Establishing a state of the art regarding indications and contraindications. This is an uneasy task because variations exist, progresses are made and divergent opinions often collide one with another. Analysis of the literature is a tricky procedure, and most of the time ends up with no strong consensus amid surgeons. The mixture of several indications (e.g. RYGB after LSG or after LAGB, redo operations in primary "home" patients or patients having been primarily treated in another centres) and the difficulty to express weight loss results (excess weight loss, or loss by weight regain) have led to endless discussions with prejudices pertaining to the background of a given surgical team. The bottom line is that no formal guidelines have been established, and the inconstancy of procedures, with new possibilities coming up, makes it unlikely to have general guidelines soon.
2. Diagnostic means: Endoscopy and high-quality imaging (e.g. 3D CT scan) are most of the time mandatory. Evaluating the size of a pouch or a sleeve is necessary when choosing between a re-sleeve and a bypass for instance, or between a surgical pouch reduction and an endoscopic pouch/anastomosis plication.
3. Listing the possibilities: Restoration to a normal anatomy, usually a very long and tedious procedure, sometimes impossible (sleeve gastrectomy), but fortunately not requested often; restoration of the restrictive component; introducing a malabsorptive component to a restrictive operation or the other way around (i.e. adding restriction to a malabsorptive operation). Complex interactions make it almost impossible to come to a consensus and to establish a guideline, and one must realise that no proposal has reached a formal consensus so far, even over such a "simple choice" between further restriction and adding a mild or strong malabsorptive component. Purely endoscopic means are often criticised because they fail to provide a long-term weight maintenance, yet more aggressive surgical options also have limited effect in the long term and entail their own morbidities.
4. Last item: What to do with patients having had an obsolete operation (forgotten heroes … and acknowledging that some current operations may become obsolete sooner than anticipated, e.g. LAGB)? Again, choices are most of the time made on a case-to-case basis, depending on the surgical experience.
5. For the time being, the best advice to be given in any situation results from the strong habits in a dedicated centre, with a solid and coherent multidisciplinary team choosing among several redo options, according to the patient's preferences and informed consent, and the team's experience.

6. Evidence-based medicine may be found in some cases; we shall give three significant examples:
   (a) Conversion of failed LAGB is currently the main topic for redo. A review and meta-analysis of LRYGB versus LSG as revisional procedure after LAGB have included 8 studies with 635 patients [51]. Both procedures were associated with comparable complications (leaks, abscess and bleeding being the complications occurring in both operations), conversions, mean hospital stay and weight loss at 6 and 12 months. In the LRYGB group, the %EW and BMI reduction after 24 months were higher.
   (b) Conversion of failed LSG is a growing issue, keeping in mind that LSG was initially conceived as a first step to RYGB or BPD-DS. The conclusion of a recent small study on conversion of LSG to RYGB is that there is a positive effect on GORD but not on further weight loss [52]. In this small series, outcomes in patients converted to RYGB for insufficient weight loss or weight regain (IWL/WR) were evaluated separately from the outcomes of conversion because of GORD. 22 LSG were converted to RYGB between 2012 and 2015, with a mean follow-up of 16 months. Indication for conversion was GORD in 10/22 patients and IWL/WR in 11/22 patients. Patients undergoing conversion for GORD were significantly less obese (BMI 30.5 kg/m^2) than those converted for IWL/WR (BMI 43.3 kg/m^2) at the time of conversion. The conversion was very effective for GORD with 100% patients reporting improvement in symptoms, and 80% able to stop their antacid medications, whatever the weight loss. In contrast, the IWL/WR group achieved a further BMI drop of 2.5 points 2 years after surgery (final BMI 40.8 kg/m^2) in comparison with 2.0 points BMI drop achieved by the GORD group (final BMI 28.5 kg/m^2). This study also emphasises that redo interventions solely based on requests of IWL and WR must be surrounded by careful preoperative evaluation and by explaining to patients that realistic goals may include underachievements, whatever the preliminary and secondary techniques! Moreover, when the LSG has taken place after a failed LAGB, further conversion adds risks, with the sequelae of multiple procedures, because of adhesions, tissue impairment, etc.
   (c) We stated previously that RYGB, and not BPD, was the usual "end-of-the-line operation", which results from the observation of worldwide trends [10], thus entailing difficult choices of reoperation. Let us eventually examine what happens with the alternative and real "end-of-the-line operation", namely BPD and BPD-DS. A literature review has shown that the necessity of revision was not uncommon, but limited [53]. The range varies from 0.5 to 18.5%, more frequently with BPD than with BPD-DS. Approximately 50% of the revisions are caused by protein malnutrition, 30% by diarrhoea or flatus and few due to bone demineralisation. Three-quarters of the revisions take place within 18 months after initial surgery. Revisions here mean that the operation was "too drastic", and so the usual revisional procedure consists of increasing the common channel by 100–150 cm; a complete reversal is rarely necessary. Likewise, revision for insufficient weight loss is rare (0.5–2.78%), with usually a re-gastrectomy.

3.2.5 Indications and Contraindications for Bariatric Surgery

Although widely discussed and frequently revised or amended regarding age and weight, the NIH guidelines still apply when evaluating a bariatric candidate [3]:

- Body mass index above 40 kg/m^2 or a BMI >35 kg/m^2 with coexisting medical problems, or more obsolete: 45 kg above 100% desirable weight
- Failure of non-surgical methods of weight reduction
- Absence of endocrine disorder that can cause massive obesity (e.g. neuroendocrine disorders like craniopharyngioma, genetic obesity)
- Psychological stability, and readiness and commitment to the surgical process, defined as basic understanding of how surgery can produce weight loss; realisation that surgery cannot guarantee an excellent result if not surrounded by a multidisciplinary approach including diet support and exercise; absence of ongoing drug/alcohol abuse.

3.2.5.1 Contraindications

Contraindications regarding age and weight are relative. With respect to the prevention of comorbidities such as T2DM and metabolic syndrome in adolescents and the increased life expectancy in the elderly, there is room for addressing these age classes.

The existence of a chronic disease can be regarded as a contraindication in some cases and on the other hand can reinforce the arguments in favour of a bariatric procedure, when substantial weight loss may alleviate the burden of a given impairment. Common sense dictates that an ongoing disease with no relation to obesity, and continuing to progress regardless of patient's weight, should be considered a contraindication. On the other hand, diseases under control, e.g. multiple sclerosis or previous malignancy in profound remission, are no contraindication, provided that a multidisciplinary screening has established that indeed the disease is medically controlled.

The psychological contraindications are listed in Table 3.1, with the level of evidence and grade of recommendation. With extreme caution, some of these conditions can be considered indications on a case-to-case basis when cured.

Table 3.1 Psychological contraindications to bariatric surgery, with level of evidence and grade of recommendation

Condition	Level of evidence	Grade of recommendation
Mood and anxiety disorders[a]	2	A
Severe and untreated bipolar disorder, schizophrenia and psychosis[b]	2	C
Active/recent substance abuse or dependence (e.g. alcohol)	3	C
Binge-eating disorder	3	B
Bulimia nervosa	2	B
Night-eating syndrome[a]	3	C

[a]Mood and anxiety disorders are considered negative predictors for the outcome of bariatric surgery, but not a contraindication if the patient benefits from the proper treatment

[b]Optimal control of these conditions, including medication absorption, may lead to surgery in highly selected cases

3.2.5.2 Special Indications

The BMI criteria for bariatric surgery and contraindication have been discussed but certain groups with special indications should be mentioned as well.

3.2.5.3 Class I Obesity and Comorbidities

Numerous observational studies and RCTs have shown that obesity surgery is effective in patients with BMI 30–35 kg/m^2 (class I obesity). Therefore, a statement from IFSO has claimed in 2011 that obesity surgery should not be denied for patients within this BMI range suffering from comorbidities and willing to undergo such procedures [54]. In the context of this book, we are aware that this new frontier may elicit discussions. While claiming further territory, surgery faces competition from bariatric endoscopic techniques, which claim different and less strict definitions for success in less obese subjects compared with surgeons in more heavy patients. For instance, the American Society for Gastrointestinal Endoscopy [55] has issued a document on Preservation and Incorporation of Valuable endoscopic Innovations (PIVI), which states the following goals: success is defined by an excess weight loss (EWL) of more than 25% or a total body weight loss (TBWL) >5%. The usual surgical threshold is 50% EWL, and it is usually required to be sustained for 5 years. This might create some conflict, since the initial requirements in terms of bariatric efficacy should be the same whatever the technical approach: for the time being, endoscopic techniques apply and are approved by the FDA for use in patients with a BMI 30–40 kg/m^2, but we may consider their application in more obese patients in the near future. Should then the definition of the gastroenterologist or the surgeon be valid? On the one hand, surgery entails more risks and endoscopy rightly claims that the benefit/risk ratio could be superior if the procedures are kept minimally invasive; on the other hand, long-term results are essential when evaluating any kind of bariatric technique. Confusion might also arise, as candidates for endoscopy are often requiring a surgical therapy but are not willing to undergo it, while occasionally less severely obese patients are seeking surgery (see also Chap. 2).

3.2.5.4 Elderly Patients

There are no clear boundaries in older patients, despite a relative consensus on picking them up as bariatric candidates on a case-to-case basis after the age of 60. Physiological age represents undeniably the best criteria when figuring post-operative quality of life and life-expectancy predictions, hence requiring the full expertise of the multidisciplinary team. Yet somehow, patients with the worst general conditions might also benefit the most from aggressive procedures and numerous publications have stressed a non-prohibitive rate of complications in older patients, provided that cardiologic, pulmonary and anaesthesiology evaluations have been conducted thoroughly.

Casillas et al. compared the effectiveness of sleeve gastrectomy with that of Roux-en-Y gastric bypass for weight loss and safety outcomes in older adults [56]. Nine different bariatric surgery centres with 23 surgeons dealing with over 30,000 bariatric patients were addressed and patients ≥65 years of age who had a LSG or RYGB between 2010 and 2015 were investigated. There were 177 LRYGB and 252 LSG patients ($n = 429$). Patients were female (70%), a mean of 67 years old with a

BMI of 42.6 kg/m^2. After 4 years data were available in 322 subjects (75%). LRYGB patients lost significantly more weight than LSG ($P < 0.001$), mortality was similar and LRYGB had higher overall complication rates (30.5%) than LSG (15.4%).

A matched case-control study of post-operative outcomes in older obese patients has been recently published in France [57]. Despite less weight loss, a higher post-operative complication rate and less improvement of QOL scores, bariatric surgery had in their hands an acceptable benefit/risk balance in selected older patients and should not be rejected on the sole argument of age. Patients ≥60 years of age (n = 55) who were operated on between 2009 and 2014 were matched to patients <40 years and patients 40–59 years (n = 55 each). The elderly underwent 40 times a LSG, 14 an OAGB and 1 a RYGB. As expected, patients ≥60 years presented more obesity-related comorbidities at baseline. Except for bleeding ($P = 0.01$), no difference in major complication rate was observed ($P = 0.43$). At 24 months, % EWL was lower in older patients compared to others (76.3%, 89.7% and 82.2%, respectively, $P = 0.009$). Iron and vitamin B12 deficiencies were less prevalent in patients ≥60 years, which may be attributed to a better adherence to supplementation. After a mean follow-up of 27 months, QOL score was lower in patients ≥60 years ($P = 0.01$).

3.2.5.5 Adolescents

Operating on non-adult obese patients has always been a matter of dispute, since preoperative and post-operative management are delicate matters, requiring the experience of dedicated paediatricians and more generally of a specialised team for both preoperative assessment and follow-up. The fact that any kind of procedure poses a natural challenge in terms of eventual failures or long-term complications has elicited various debates on the choice of a technique in adolescents, keeping in mind the possibilities of redo. This debate is far from finished, and finally there is no consensus over a primary choice among current established procedures. Other authors still consider that other incentives to weight loss should be proposed to adolescents, including intragastric balloon, before they reach maturity and full ability to formal consent.

Based on a national registry, Benedix et al. have looked into the results of LSG [58]: LSG represented the most common bariatric procedure in Germany with a proportion of 48.1% in adolescents and 48.7% in adults in 2014, and was performed in 362 adolescents and 15,428 adults. Complication rates and mortality (0% vs. 0.2%) did not differ significantly. Adolescents achieved a BMI reduction of 16.8 and 18.0 units at 12 and 24 months, respectively, compared with 15.4 and 16.6 BMI units in the adult group. There was a significantly higher BMI reduction in late adolescents (19–21 years) compared with patients ≤18 years at 24 months (19.8 vs. 13.6 BMI units, respectively).

3.2.5.6 Transplantation

The necessity of any kind of transplantation in obese patients is a complicated issue, and for instance in case of renal failure BMI over 32 kg/m^2 is a common contraindication for kidney transplantation. In general, obesity surgery acts as a useful bridge to a successful transplantation, e.g. heart transplantation in patients with end-stage heart failure.

Bariatric surgery is an effective option with an acceptable rate of complications and post-operative mortality for both patients with obesity awaiting organ transplantation and patients who have received an organ transplantation, as reviewed by Lazzati et al. regarding liver transplantation [59]. Previously, many morbidly obese patients were denied liver transplantation because of the higher operative risk. However, nowadays, 5 and 10 years of graft survival is the rule. Patients whose lives can be prolonged with transplantation are dying of obesity-related comorbidities, but weight reduction in patients awaiting transplantation would improve their long-term survival. The dilemma is clearly demonstrated in the liver-transplantation patients: bariatric surgery is contraindicated in patients with decompensated cirrhosis, while post-transplant bariatric intervention is associated with increased technical difficulty. In a very small series by Nesher et al. three patients underwent simultaneous liver transplantation and sleeve gastrectomy; one patient had a mild post-operative renal failure and a biliary leak. After a median 13 months of follow-up, all patients were having normal allograft function and significant weight loss [60].

3.2.5.7 Inflammatory Bowel Syndromes

Many if not all bariatric procedures entail a radical modification of the digestive tract, which might be problematic in inflammatory bowel disease (IBD). IBD represents difficulties in choosing, implementing and following obese patients affected by this condition. Bariatric surgery is usually considered as being contraindicated in morbidly obese IBD patients because most techniques will affect the bowel to some degree (see also Chap. 1). Series have been reported, where LSG or LAGB was deemed safe and effective, for instance by Keidar et al. [61], who performed a LAGB in one and a LSG in nine morbidly obese patients suffering from Crohn's disease in eight and ulcerative colitis in two with a mean age of 40 years, and a mean BMI of 42 kg/m^2.

A systematic review has included 7 studies with 43 morbidly obese IBD patients (31 F, 11 M) with an age of 30–64 years and a BMI varying between 35.7 and 71 kg/m^2 [62]. Twenty-five patients had Crohn's disease (CD) (58.2%) and 18 ulcerative colitis (UC) (41.8%). The small bowel was the most common involved gastrointestinal segment in 27.3% of patients. CD patients more commonly underwent sleeve gastrectomy (72%), while UC patients similarly underwent sleeve gastrectomy and Roux-en-Y gastric bypass (44.4%). After a follow-up of 8–77 months, EWL was 71.4% and BMI loss was 14.3 BMI units. There were 9 early (21.4%) and 10 late (23.8%) post-operative complications related to the bariatric procedure. IBD remitted in 20 patients (47.6%), improved in 2 patients (4.8%), but exacerbated in 7 patients (16.7%).

3.3 Effect of Bariatric Surgery Through Weight Loss and Metabolic Changes on Obesity-Associated Comorbidities

If weight loss seems the primary target of any bariatric procedures, the alleviation of obesity-related diseases is the core objective of these operations. A strong level of evidence exists for the improvement of a series of comorbidities, which have been listed by the International Federation for the Surgery of Obesity (IFSO) by De Luca et al. in a position statement in 2016 [63], to which we cordially invite our

Table 3.2 Improvements of obesity-related morbidities after bariatric surgery, with level of evidence and grade of recommendation

Comorbidity	Level of evidence	Grade of recommendation
Management of T2DM with obesity (improvement/resolution)	1	A
Improvement of components of the metabolic syndrome	2	A
Reduction of cardiovascular risks and cardiovascular events	1	A
Improvement/resolution of obstructive sleep apnoea syndrome	1	A
Improvement of respiratory function/asthma	3	C
Reduction of pain/disability from joint disease/osteoarthritis	1	A
Controlling GORD	2	B
Improvement of non-alcoholic fatty liver disease and steatohepatitis	2	B
Treatment of infertility	2	B
Reduction of malignancies occurrence and mortality	3	B/C
Improvement of physical functioning (exercise and training participation)	2	A
Quality of life improvement	1	A

reader and that we will not cite into details. This paper has also stated that the expression "metabolic and bariatric surgery" should be replaced by "surgery for obesity and weight-related diseases", which implies that surgery is able to dramatically improve obesity and weight-related conditions.

Weight loss results are highly variable among published series, also depending on the rate of follow-up. Ten-year results seem the most important and significant parameter, with usually a premium for RYGB, and then LSG and LAGB, roughly 60% EWL, versus 50% and 40% EWL, respectively. Quality of life (QOL) results and details of the follow-up will be addressed in Chap. 7 (post-operative guidance).

The most important effects on comorbidities, as described in the IFSO statement [63], are summarised in Table 3.2, with related level of evidence and grade of recommendation.

3.3.1 Mechanisms of Action

In the recent past, it seemed that bariatric surgery was determined and divided by two strong principles, possibly intertwined, but whose respective parts were not actually open for discussion: food restriction versus food malabsorption. On the one end, the limitation of food ingestion creates satiety over the long term and limits the capacity for calorie intake; on the other, in malabsorption, ingested food, whatever its amount, is less absorbed in specific parts of the digestive tract, artificially creating a deficit in absorbed macronutrients such as lipids. This theoretical separation has never been a dogma, albeit initial JIB had no restrictive component at all. Subsequent and current malabsorptive operations have a strong if not dominant restrictive part; some restrictive operations and some unclassified operations claim a "metabolic effect" (acting favourably upon elements of the metabolic syndrome) that is also an added and more recently studied component to the two others.

In between the two stays gastric bypass, with complex mechanisms that have not yet been fully elucidated. However, it represents a good example of the interaction of most of the meaningful mechanisms that contribute to weight loss and improvement of comorbidities after any kind of bariatric technique. The restrictive component of bypass is now presented as of utmost importance, and the typical 100 cc pouch that was primarily advised is nowadays replaced by a 20–50 cc pouch. Modifications of eating behaviour come next, due to the exclusion of trans-pyloric and duodenal food passage. Finally, and in connection to this exclusion (as shown experimentally), the endocrine metabolic component plays the major part. They are mediated by two important hormones identified as incretins: gastric inhibitory peptide (GIP, also named gastric insulinotropic peptide), and glucagon-like peptide-1 (GLP-1), in conjunction with other hormones like ghrelin and polypeptide YY (PYY). These mechanisms account for the major part of the metabolic effects, particularly the improvement of insulin sensitivity, and eventually diabetes remission or even diabetes resolution in some cases.

There are two global mechanisms that compete and account for the most important effect of a bypass operation: the foregut and the hindgut hypothesis; the first one relates to the under-stimulation of the duodenum and proximal jejunum (food being diverted from it), and the second relates to overstimulation of the hindgut (distal small bowel and colon), with early and rapid exposure to partially digested food. The foregut hypothesis has been suggested by Rubino et al. [64], while the hindgut hypothesis was formulated by Mason in 1999 [65].

Sophisticated neurohormonal pathways have been discovered and interact with several other mechanisms that are being assessed through fundamental studies, e.g. pertaining to the microbiota, with exploration of the "host metabolic-microbial crosstalk" after bariatric procedures. Magouliotis et al. reviewed the literature on obese patients treated with bariatric procedures with respect to their effect on the metabolic and gut microbiota profiles. Twenty-two articles could be included in the systematic review (562 patients) and 15 in the meta-analysis [66]. This review pointed to significant amelioration of post-operative levels of glucose, insulin, triglycerides, total cholesterol, LDL cholesterol, HDL cholesterol, HOMA-IR as a measure of insulin sensitivity, food intake and T2DM remission. Post-operative gut microbiota was significantly affected and became close to that of lean, and less obese objects. Other important changes relate to the bile acids and their impact on metabolism [67], partially in conjunction with the microbiota.

Metabolic effects are not the sole privilege of gastric bypass operations. Cavin et al. have shown that both RYGB and LSG modified alimentary glucose absorption and intestinal disposal of blood glucose in animals and humans: while RYGB increases intestinal glucose disposal through a hyperplasia of the Roux limb, with an increased number of incretin-producing cells, LSG delays glucose absorption [68].

3.3.2 Beneficial Effects on Diseases

3.3.2.1 Type 2 Diabetes (T2DM)

Weight loss induced by obesity surgery improves glycaemic control and glycosylated haemoglobin, and diminishes the need for diabetes medications. It is superior to optimal medical and lifestyle treatment alone. This has been supported by several randomised control trials (RCT) that have proven that surgery achieved better glycaemic control than optimal medical and lifestyle treatment alone.

In the RCT reported by Schauer et al., 5-year outcome data showed that, among patients with T2DM and a BMI of 27–43 kg/m^2, bariatric surgery (RYGB or LSG) plus intensive medical therapy was more effective than intensive medical therapy alone in decreasing or, in some cases, resolving T2DM [69]. The primary outcome was a glycated haemoglobin A1c (HbA1c) of 6.0% or less with or without the use of diabetes medications. At baseline, the mean HbA1C level was 9.2%, and the mean BMI was 37 kg/m^2. At 5 years, the criterion of the primary end point was met by 2 of 38 patients (5%) who received medical therapy alone, as compared with 14 of 49 patients (29%) who had RYGB (adjusted $P = 0.03$, $P = 0.08$ in the intention-to-treat analysis), and 11 of 47 patients (23%) who had LSG (adjusted $P = 0.07$, $P = 0.17$ in the intention-to-treat analysis). Patients who underwent surgical procedures had a significantly greater mean percentage reduction from baseline in HbA1c level than did patients who received medical therapy alone (2.1% vs. 0.3%, $P = 0.003$). At 5 years, changes from baseline observed in the RYGB and LSG groups were superior to the changes seen in the medical therapy group with respect to body weight (−23%, −19% and −5% in the RYGB, LSG and medical therapy groups, respectively), triglyceride level (−40%, −29% and −8%, respectively), HDL cholesterol level (+32%, +30% and +7%, respectively), use of insulin (−35%, −34% and −13%, respectively) and quality-of-life measures (general health score increases of 17, 16 and 0.3) ($P < 0.05$ for all comparisons). No major late surgical complications were reported except for one reoperation.

The study by Mingrone et al. compared bariatric-metabolic surgery versus conventional medical treatment in obese patients with T2DM, with 5-year follow-up in an open-label, single-centre RCT [70]. Patients aged 30–60 years with a body mass index of 35 kg/m^2 or more and a history of T2DM lasting at least 5 years were randomly assigned to receive either medical treatment or RYGB or BPD. The primary end point was the rate of T2DM remission at 2 years, defined as a HbA1c 6.5% or less, and fasting glucose concentration 5.6 mmol/L or less, without active pharmacological treatment for 1 year. Between April and October 2009, 60 patients had either medical treatment ($n = 20$), RYGB ($n = 20$) or BPD-DS ($n = 20$). Nineteen (50%) of the 38 surgical patients achieved T2DM remission at 5 years, compared with none of the 15 medically treated patients ($P = 0{\cdot}0007$). Eight (42%) patients who underwent gastric bypass and 13 (68%) patients who underwent BPD-DS had an HbA1c concentration of 6.5% or less with or without medication, compared with 4 (27%) of medically treated patients ($P = 0{\cdot}0457$). Surgical patients lost more weight than medically treated patients, but weight changes did not predict diabetes remission or diabetes relapse after surgery. Both surgical procedures were associated with significantly lower plasma lipids, cardiovascular risk and medication use. Five major complications of diabetes (including one fatal myocardial infarction) arose in four (27%) patients in the medical group compared with only one complication in the RYGB group and no complications in the BPD-DS group. No late complications or deaths occurred in both surgery groups. These studies resulted in a level of evidence of 1 and a grade of recommendation A (Table 3.2). It has also been proven that surgery was cost effective and in some instances cost saving. Although less common, also type 1 diabetes mellitus is eligible for bariatric surgery that often reduces daily insulin requirements along with weight loss, as well as associated comorbidities.

Eventually, a joint statement by several diabetes organisations has been presented and published by Rubino et al., introducing metabolic surgery in the treatment algorithm for T2DM, and called healthcare regulators to introduce appropriate reimbursement policies [71]. The 2nd Diabetes Surgery Summit (DSS-II), an international consensus conference, was convened in collaboration with leading diabetes organisations to develop global guidelines to inform clinicians and policymakers about benefits and limitations of metabolic surgery for T2DM. Numerous randomised clinical trials, albeit mostly short/midterm, have demonstrated that metabolic surgery achieved excellent glycaemic control and reduced cardiovascular risk factors. Based on such evidence, metabolic surgery should be recommended to treat T2DM in patients with class III obesity (BMI $\geq$40 kg/m^2) and in those with class II obesity (BMI 35.0–39.9 kg/m^2) when blood glucose levels are inadequately controlled by lifestyle and optimal medical therapy. Surgery should also be considered for patients with T2DM and BMI 30.0–34.9 kg/m^2 if glucose blood levels are inadequately controlled despite optimal treatment with either oral or injectable medications. These BMI thresholds should be reduced by 2.5 kg/m^2 for Asian patients.

3.3.2.2 Metabolic Syndrome

This includes insulin resistance, hypertension, impaired glucose tolerance or T2DM, dyslipidaemia (high plasma triglycerides, low HDL cholesterol levels) and central weight distribution. RCTs have shown improvements, except regarding hypertension [72, 73].

3.3.2.3 Cardiovascular Diseases

Improvement has been reported in terms of atherosclerosis, myocardial infarction, stroke and death. In other words, surgery provides a very significant reduction of major cardiovascular events, and of the mortality related to these events [73]. This included microvascular and macrovascular events in patients with T2DM. Likewise, markers of atherosclerosis are improved. Pre-existing heart ischaemia with or without heart failure might be improved, but with no evidence on the long-term prognosis. However, when analysing RCTs only, results were more uncertain in terms of cardiovascular events, as shown in a recent meta-analysis [74].

3.3.2.4 Pulmonary Diseases

Obstructive sleep apnoea syndrome [75] and asthma [76] are relieved. When undiagnosed, a polysomnographic examination is strongly suggested to evaluate the necessity of a respiratory therapy device (CPAP) perioperatively. More generally speaking, restrictive pulmonary deficiencies associated with obesity are relieved [77].

3.3.2.5 Osteoarthritis

Disability resulting from joint diseases is improved, particularly hip and knee arthritis, a finding that is very relevant in older patients [78]. Moreover, a bariatric procedure facilitates further prosthetic joint replacement surgeries [79].

3.3.2.6 Hepatobiliary Disease

Non-alcoholic fatty liver disease (NAFLD) may be improved [80]. NAFLD ranges from simple fatty liver to hepatic steatosis with inflammation (non-alcoholic steatohepatitis, NASH), advanced fibrosis and cirrhosis. Steatohepatitis appears to improve [81, 82], but it is deemed premature to recommend bariatric surgery as an established option to specifically treat NASH [83].

3.3.2.7 Mental Health

Surgery is not contraindicated for patients with mood and anxiety disorders, binge-eating disorder and night-eating syndrome if well treated in the same time [84, 85]. On the contrary, other conditions are contraindications: severe bipolar disorders, unstable psychosis (e.g. schizophrenia), untreated bulimia nervosa and ongoing substance or alcohol abuse [86], as has been discussed in Table 3.1.

3.3.2.8 Endocrinopathy and Fertility

Endocrinopathy that is responsible for secondary obesity or that requires therapeutic interventions is usually a contraindication to obesity surgery. Infertility, with or without polycystic ovary syndrome, is ameliorated by weight loss, including weight loss by surgical means [87, 88].

3.3.2.9 Cancer

Weight loss, mediated by surgery or not, reduces the obesity-associated increased risks of gastrointestinal, genito-urinary, reproductive and haematopoietic malignancies [89, 90] (see also Chap. 1). Endometrial cancer risk and postmenopausal breast cancer risk are diminished [91].

3.3.2.10 Intracranial Hypertension

Weight loss is recommended for pseudotumour cerebri, and surgery may play a role [92].

3.3.2.11 Renal Function and Urinary Incontinence

These conditions are improved by weight loss. Chronic renal failure requiring dialysis is not a contraindication for obesity surgery [93].

3.3.3 Adverse Effects on Diseases

3.3.3.1 Gastro-Oesophageal Reflux Disease (GORD) and Bariatric Surgery

Although debated, bariatric surgery, particularly RYGB, may improve and sometimes cure GORD. It is debated whether preoperative GORD should be a contraindication for a specific procedure or not, e.g. LSG or LAGB. The choice of an operation in the presence of GORD, the necessity or not to modify a given bariatric procedure when there is GORD and the role of each operation in aggravating or alleviating GORD remain hot topics in the bariatric field! As mentioned in Chap. 4, the guideline states that preoperative endoscopy should be performed only when patients have GI complaints. But complaints of gastro-oesophageal reflux do not always imply oesophageal lesions and no complaints do not exclude abnormalities, especially not in Barrett patients where the Barrett's epithelium is resistant against acid and acid exposure so does not result in complaints. At least the surgeon should ask for GORD and Barrett's oesophagus in the family. Another problem is that motility disturbances are frequently found when looked after with manometry. A third problem is the fact that if severe dysplasia or cancerous changes occur after sleeve gastrectomy, an oesophagus resection with colon interposition remains the only choice or otherwise endoscopic methods such as radiofrequency ablation by Barrx Halo balloon system (Covidien, USA) or photodynamic therapy or more invasive techniques such as endoscopic mucosal resection (EMR) or endoscopic submucosal dissection (ESD) should be applied, although there are currently no data on application of these endoscopic methods in patients after bariatric surgery.

What should be the specific follow-up (when, which intervals of time, for which patients)? What exams? Should a hiatal hernia be repaired in the same time as a bariatric procedure and how (crus repair only, with or without plication)? What are the mechanisms and the relative proportion of aggravated GORD and *de novo* GORD? What is the role of bile reflux? Is Barrett's oesophagus more prone to cancer development under these circumstances? Many questions are with only poorly satisfying answers.

Does Bariatric Surgery Improve or Worsen GORD?

As a powerful weight-loss tool, bariatric surgery aims at the relief of GORD symptoms, which are also connected to the overweight status. De Groot et al. have presented a review of the literature on the effects of bariatric surgery, diet and lifestyle interventions, and weight loss on GORD [94]. Lifestyle interventions improved GORD in four of seven studies. RYGB improved GORD in all studies; VBG did not affect GORD, and LAGB results were conflicting. It seems that the amount of excess weight loss plays an important role in the improvement.

When and How to Repair Hiatal Hernia in the Context of Bariatric Surgery?

It occurs to many surgeons that weight loss achieved through bariatric procedures may be insufficient to cure GORD when present at the time of the surgery. The question of repair of a hiatal hernia (HH) during a bariatric procedure has been asked ever since bariatric procedures exist, yet the question remains largely unanswered, while it is commonly done concomitantly with laparoscopic RYGB, LSG and LAGB to decrease GORD. A United States Nationwide Inpatient Sample 2004–2009 was reviewed to compare mortality risk, prolonged length of stay and perioperative adverse events using propensity score-matched analysis [95]. There were 42,272 patients undergoing RYGB alone and an additional 1945 undergoing RYGB and HH repair. For LAGB, there were 10,558 records and 1959 had LAGB combined with HH repair. Thirty-eight per cent of the patient in the RYGB-only group had GORD compared to 55% in the RYGB and HH repair group. After LAGB only, GORD was present in 31% of cases, compared to 44% in the LAGB and HH repair group. Although not commented by the authors, it seems that both the preoperative presence of GORD and the peroperative finding of a hiatal hernia were decisive in adding a hiatal hernia repair to the RYGB and LAGB surgery.

The repair of HH combined with LSG could theoretically prevent the development of GORD. There is no consensus on how to best manage HH at the time of LSG or how to repair a HH once identified. However, 83% of participants in the International Sleeve Gastrectomy Expert Panel favoured an aggressive approach to identify and repair HH at the time of LSG [96]. Nonetheless, participants did not comment on how to aggressively identify HH or repair a HH once identified.

What Are the Differences Among Current Bariatric Operations Regarding GORD?

RYGB and OAGB

Being the current gold standard of bariatric surgery RYGB confers many advantages to obese patients including delivering the best anti-reflux effect. This is typically the case when a regular RYGB is performed, in which most of the acid-secreting cells are out of the food circulation and in which biliary and pancreatic secretions become excluded from the alimentary tract owing to a secondary jejuno-jejunal anastomosis 150 cm away from the gastrojejunal anastomosis, on the alimentary limb. OAGB has a single gastrojejunal anastomosis, and a 150–250 cm biliopancreatic limb, therefore putting the gastric pouch and the lower oesophagus at risk of inflammation due to bile reflux on top of acid reflux. Yet the necessity of an "en-Y" anastomosis as a second stage is a necessity in 1–2% of the cases only. The question of a predisposition of OAGB to exacerbating or provoking GORD increased by bile reflux and depending on the preliminary status of the oesophagogastric junction remains, like it does for LSG.

LSG

While LSG is becoming an increasingly popular stand-alone bariatric operation, one of its limitations according to some authors is the development of *de novo* GORD in patients with no reflux symptoms prior to the procedure, in addition to the worsening of GORD symptoms if existing previously. On the other hand, others have noted an improvement in GORD symptoms due to weight loss or other factors, following LSG.

Accurate evaluation of GORD post-operatively may require reliable exams, such as 24-h multichannel intraluminal impedance pH-metry (MIIpH). In a study assessing GORD post-LSG, 12 asymptomatic obese patients were studied prospectively by using (MIIpH) pre- and 12 months post-LSG [97]. At 1 year post-LSG, 83.3% of patients suffered from GORD as indicated by an abnormal DeMeester score. The mean DeMeester score 1 year post-LSG was 47, almost 2.5 times higher than the preoperative score ($P = 0.072$). The percentage of total time with pH lower than four was statistically significant higher post-operatively (13.3% vs. 3.9%, $P = 0.048$). Given these results, the authors recommended a close post-operative monitoring for GORD with the use of pH testing and upper gastrointestinal endoscopy to identify possible mucosal injury.

To document increased intragastric pressure (IIGP) and reflux after LSG, other authors have evaluated the impact of LSG on oesophagogastric motility with high-resolution impedance manometry (HRIM) [98]. A retrospective analysis of 53 cases showed that IIGP occurred very frequently in patients after LSG (77%) and was not associated with any upper GI symptoms, a specific oesophageal manometric profile, or impedance pH-metry. Impedance pH-metry reflux episodes were also frequently observed (52%), and significantly associated with GORD symptoms and ineffective oesophageal motility. The sleeve volume and diameters were also significantly smaller in patients with reflux episodes detected by impedance pH-metry ($P < 0.01$).

Longer term results have brought the issue of permanent damage to the oesophagogastric junction forward, and possibly the development of cancer of the lower oesophagus, preceded by the stage of Barrett's oesophagus. In that case, the usual therapeutic options are radio-frequency ablation of the lesions, photodynamic therapy or EMR or ESD, and ultimately considering a redo with RYGB. This has been emphasised recently by Genco et al. [99]: From 2007 to 2010, 162 patients underwent primary LSG, and the follow-up rate has been 69.1%. At a mean 58 months of follow-up, the incidence of GORD symptoms (68.1% vs. 33.6%), complaints based on a visual analogue scale (VAS) mean score (3 vs. 1.8) and PPI intake (57.2% vs. 19.1%) significantly increased compared with preoperative values. At endoscopy, an upward migration of the Z line and a biliary-like oesophageal reflux was found in 73.6% and 74.5% of the cases, respectively. A significant increase in the incidence and in the severity of erosive oesophagitis was seen, whereas non-dysplastic Barrett's oesophagus was newly diagnosed in 19 patients (17.2%). No significant correlations were found between GORD symptoms and endoscopic findings.

LAGB

Does banding necessarily result in irreversible damage to the oesophagogastric junction and oesophageal motility? The placement of a gastric band near the oesophagogastric junction may be associated with partial or total slippage, pouch dilation, oesophagitis, Barrett's oesophagus, GORD, food intolerance, oesophageal dilation and band erosion. So, these complications should be ruled out before studying the influence of LAGB on GORD as they may all cause GORD in themselves. Burton et al. used high-resolution video manometry to compare patients with an optimally adjusted band fill volume, 20% less than the optimal fill volume and 20% more than the optimal fill volume, and patients in the waiting list as control [100]. Patients who had undergone LAGB had a mean intraluminal pressure of 26.9 mm Hg below the LOS. LOS pressure was reduced compared with the control group

(10 mmHg vs. 18 mmHg, $P < 0.01$) but the LOS relaxed normally. Oesophageal motility was better in patients with an optimal gastric volume compared with patients with a higher volume (normal swallowing rate 77% vs. 51%, $P = 0.08$). A pause in adjustments is required in cases of significant dilation, but may also be useful in other patients, resulting in attenuation of GORD symptoms. Some issues remain unresolved, such as the causes of persistent food intolerance in patients without abnormal X-ray or endoscopic findings, although high-resolution manometry has not systematically been applied in these patients and oesophageal abnormalities either already present before or provoked by the operation may explain these complaints.

Can We Draw Lessons from GORD Endoscopic Treatment if We Move to Minimally Invasive Bariatric Techniques?

Endoscopic therapy for GORD has been a leading research procedure for more than 20 years, but there is a competition between PPI treatment and laparoscopic surgery. Various techniques have been described that reinforce the oesophagogastric junction.

It is likely that minimally invasive bariatric procedures (via natural orifices) will be performed more frequently in the future, although surgeons may consider that most of the current endoscopic methods are not yet cost efficient, and that long-term outcomes are uncertain. Among the different procedures that have been developed for endoscopic treatment of GORD, some can be applied to the treatment of obesity, provided that they target the appropriate anatomical area. However, data on obese patients treated after bariatric surgery are not yet available.

As a conclusion to this part, it may seem futile to discuss thoroughly the pros and cons of hiatal hernia repair while doing a bariatric procedure. Yet, finding a consensus over the optimal surgical strategy is of utmost importance if we aim at moving forward to better solutions. A more complete understanding of the oesophagogastric junction physiology after bariatric surgery will be highly useful when implementing new types of operations, e.g. through endoscopic channels. Creating gastric restriction without durably impairing oesophagogastric junction anatomy and function will be a key challenge when designing relevant procedures.

3.3.3.2 Cholelithiasis and Bariatric Surgery

Weight loss following bariatric surgery facilitates the development of gallstones. Several issues have been addressed: Should a routine cholecystectomy - even in the absence of cholelithiasis - be performed in bariatric procedures including a malabsorptive component, i.e. with a digestive shortcut that will limit the access to the common bile duct later? Is cholecystectomy mandatory in case of cholelithiasis (gallstones) without symptoms, should it be performed in a later stage, or not at all, in the absence of symptoms? Is ursodeoxycholic acid recommended to prevent cholelithiasis after any bariatric procedure?

The indication and safety of concomitant cholecystectomy (CC) during bariatric surgical procedures are topics of controversy. Although it is not widely recommended to perform CC in the absence of biliary symptoms, some argue otherwise.

There exists a retrospective analysis of the American College of Surgeons National Surgical Quality Improvement Program database 2010–2013 [101]. Between 2010 and 2013, 21,137 patients underwent LSG; of those 422 (2.0%) underwent CC (LSG + CC), and the majority (20,715 = 98%) underwent LSG alone. The average surgical time was significantly higher, by 33 min, in the LSG + CC cohort. No differences were noted in terms of overall 30-day mortality and length of hospital stay. CC increased the odds of any adverse event (5.7% versus 4.0%), but the difference did not reach statistical significance (odds ratio 1.49). Two complications were noted to be significantly higher with LSG + CC, namely bleeding and pneumonia.

The idea of prophylactic cholecystectomy during gastric bypass has been challenged, because the risk of further cholelithiasis may be lower than reported earlier and because cholecystectomy during laparoscopic gastric bypass may be more difficult and risky. Yet, Nougou and Suter reviewed 772 patients with primary LRYGB between 2000 and 2007 and concluded that CC can be performed safely in most patients during laparoscopic gastric bypass and does not prolong hospital stay [102]. Fifty-eight (7.5%) patients had had previous cholecystectomy, and in the remaining patients ultrasound showed gallstones or sludge in 81 (11.3%). Cholecystectomy was performed at the time of gastric bypass in 665 patients (91.7%). Cholecystectomy was not associated with a procedure-related complication, prolonged the duration of surgery by a mean of 19 min and had no effect on the duration of hospital stay. When a cholecystectomy was deemed too risky or was nor performed for any other reason, a 6-month course of ursodeoxycholic acid was prescribed.

More extensively, the Swedish Register for Cholecystectomy and Endoscopic Retrograde Cholangiopancreatography (n = 79,386) and the Scandinavian Obesity Surgery Registry (n = 36,098) were cross-matched for the years 2007 through 2013 and compared with the National Patient Register [103]. The standardised incidence ratio for cholecystectomy before RYGB was 3.42 (range, 2.75–4.26, $P < 0.001$); the ratio peaked at 11.4 (range, 10.2–12.6, $P < 0.001$) 6–12 months after RYGB, which was 3.54 times the baseline incidence level (range, 2.78–4.49, $P < 0.001$). After 36 months, the incidence ratio had returned to baseline. The post-RYGB group demonstrated a highly significant increased risk of 30-day post-operative complications after cholecystectomy (odds ratio 2.13), including reoperation (odds ratio 3.84) compared with the background National Patient Register population. The post-RYGB group also demonstrated a higher risk of conversion, acute cholecystectomy and complicated gallstone disease and a slightly prolonged operative time, adjusted for age, sex, American Society of Anaesthesiologists class and previous open RYGB. Compared with the background population, the incidence of cholecystectomy was substantially elevated already before RYGB and increased further 6–36 months after RYGB. Previous RYGB doubled the risk of post-operative complications after cholecystectomy and almost quadrupled the risk of reoperation, even when intraoperative cholangiography was normal.

This study thus suggested an adverse effect of not performing CC simultaneously with RYGB.

One more technical issue is the fact that a Roux-en-Y gastric bypass excludes the biliary tree from traditional evaluation and treatment with endoscopic retrograde cholangiopancreatography (ERCP). Various techniques to access the biliary tree have been described in Chap. 6, e.g. the introduction of an endoscope through the gastrojejunal anastomosis with inherent complexity, as it comprises a double balloon, and with varying results. For example, a study assessed the feasibility and outcome of an alternative, laparoscopic assisted transgastric ERCP in patients with gastric bypass, reviewing cases from 2010 to 2016 [104]. Thirty-one laparoscopic assisted transgastric ERCP procedures were performed in 29 patients for choledocholithiasis, with 100% success in cannulation of the common bile duct. Median hospital stay was 2 days (range 1–22). Perforation of the wall of the gastric remnant occurred in two patients. The overall post-operative complication rate was 36%. Surgical complications were bleeding, haematoma and intra-abdominal abscesses.

One should also evaluate the role of ursodeoxycholic acid (UDCA) in the prevention of cholelithiasis, e.g. after laparoscopic LSG. In a randomised study on 406 patients (age 32.1 years, BMI 50.1 kg/m^2), UDCA therapy was given for 6 months after LSG (247 patients, group II) or not (159 patients, group I). The two groups showed comparable demographics and a similar % EWL at 6 and 12 months [105]. Eight patients (5%) developed gallstones in Group I, whereas no patients in Group II did ($P = 0.0005$). Preoperative dyslipidaemia and rapid loss of excess weight within the first 3 months after LSG were risk factors that significantly predicted cholelithiasis post-operatively. Routine prescription of UCDA for 6 months post-operatively whatever the procedure was a sound strategy in 2017.

3.4 Economical Evaluation

Bariatric surgery is to date the most effective treatment for morbid obesity and it has been proven to reduce obesity-related comorbidities and total mortality. As any medical treatment with complex interactions, bariatric surgery is costly and doubts about its affordability have been raised. On the other hand, bariatric surgery may reduce the direct and indirect costs of obesity and related comorbidities. The appreciation of the final balance between financial investments and savings is critical from a health economic perspective. Cost-efficacy analyses included in a recent Italian review demonstrated that the additional years of life gained through bariatric surgery may be obtained at a reasonable and affordable cost. In groups of patients with very high obesity-related health costs, like patients with type 2 diabetes mellitus (T2DM), the use of bariatric surgery requires an initial economic investment, but may save money in a relatively short period of time [106].

Despite wide acknowledgement of cost-effectiveness, the provision of surgical services varies significantly between countries. While many adults who fulfil the eligibility criteria for bariatric surgery may not want or require it, the current level of need for bariatric surgery is often not being met, as shown in a recent Irish study [107]. Two separate evidence-based criteria categories for eligibility for bariatric surgery were established: (1) Those with a BMI $\geq$40 or $\geq$ 35 kg/m^2 were considered, and one or more of the following: T2DM, hypertension, previous myocardial infarction or sleep apnoea. (2) Patients with T2DM and BMI $\geq$35 kg/m^2 were considered, with one or more of the following: previous myocardial infarction, elevated urine albumin-creatinine ratio, retinopathy, neuropathy or peripheral vascular disease. Among adults aged ≥50 years, 7.97%, representing 92,573, met evidence-based criterion 1 and 0.97%, representing 11,231, met evidence-based criterion 2. With fewer than 1/100,000 population publicly funded surgeries taking place annually, current service provision meets much less than 0.1% of the need. It is uneasy to extrapolate from one country to another, since health systems and reimbursement processes differ widely around the world, even among countries with comparable gross incomes per habitant. Yet we acknowledge that bariatric surgery is most of the time insufficiently funded.

Conclusion

Although having gained merits and being supported by highly significant evidence-based medicine, bariatric surgery is in a state of constant evolution by definition, which makes it a thrilling field of clinical research. The fact that it could be challenged by purely endoscopic methods poses a problem in the view of some, while other considerations represent a much bigger threat to its very survival in the modern era. Almost every bariatric publication starts by saying that the worldwide epidemic justifies a solid development of surgical methods, whereas logic commands the opposite. The more obesity is growing, with a general shift to the right, signifying that obesity shifts to higher BMI values, the less resources can be effectively dedicated to such an expensive (even if cost-effective) way of handling it. Yet only time will tell if public health on its own may reverse the trends … till then, bariatric procedures will thrive!

References

1. Kremen AJ, Linner LH, Nelson CH. An experimental evaluation of the nutritional importance of proximal and distal small intestine. Ann Surg. 1954;140:439–44.
2. Dargent J, Vilallonga R, Katz L, Portenier D, Wilson E, Escalona A, et al. IFSO position statement on new technologies for treatment of obesity. Obes Surg. 2017. https://doi.org/10.1007/s11695-017-2780-9. [Epub ahead of print].
3. NIH conference. Gastrointestinal surgery for severe obesity. Consensus development conference panel. Ann Intern Med. 1991;115:956–61.
4. Lakdawala M, Bhasker A. Asian Consensus Meeting on Metabolic Surgery (ACMOMS) Report: Asian consensus meeting on metabolic surgery. Recommendations for the use of bariatric and gastrointestinal metabolic surgery for treatment of obesity and type II diabetes mellitus in the Asian population. August 9th and 10th, 2008, Trivandrum, India. Obes Surg. 2010;20:929–36.
5. Buchwald H, Buchwald JN. Evolution of operative procedures for the management of morbid obesity 1950–2000. Obes Surg. 2014;24(8):1126–35.
6. Mason EE, Ito C. Gastric bypass in obesity. Surg Clin North Am. 1967;47:1345–52.
7. Mason EE. Vertical banded gastroplasty for obesity. Arch Surg. 1982;117:701–6.
8. Belachew M, Legrand M, Jaquet N. Laparoscopic placement of adjustable silicone gastric banding in the treatment of morbid obesity: an animal model experimental study. Obes Surg. 1993;3:140.

9. Sjöström L, Lindroos AK, Peltonen M, Torgerson J, Bouchard C, Carlsson B, et al. Swedish obese subjects study scientific group. Lifestyle, diabetes, and cardiovascular risk factors 10 years after bariatric surgery. N Engl J Med. 2004;351(26):2683–93.
10. Angrisani L, Santonicola A, Iovino P, Vitiello A, Zundel N, Buchwald H, et al. Bariatric surgery and endoluminal procedures: IFSO worldwide survey 2014. Obes Surg. 2017;27(9):2279–89.
11. Khorgami Z, Shoar S, Andalib A, Aminian A, Brethauer SA, Schauer PR. Trends in utilization of bariatric surgery, 2010–2014: sleeve gastrectomy dominates. Surg Obes Relat Dis. 2017;13(5):774–8.
12. Wittgrove AC, Clark GW, Tremblay LJ. Laparoscopic gastric bypass, roux-en-Y: preliminary report of five cases. Obes Surg. 1994;4(4):353–7.
13. Fobi M, Lee H, Holness R, Cabinda D. Gastric bypass operation for obesity. World J Surg. 1998;22:925–35.
14. Lemmens L. Banded gastric bypass: better long-term results? A cohort study with minimum 5-year follow-up. Obes Surg. 2017;27(4):864–72.
15. Hess DS, Hess DW. Biliopancreatic diversion with a duodenal switch. Obes Surg. 1998;8(3):267–82.
16. Regan JP, Inabnet WB, Gagner M, Pomp A. Early experience with two stage laparoscopic roux-en-Y gastric bypass as an alternative in the super-super obese patient. Obes Surg. 2003;13(6):861–4.
17. Ren C, Patterson E, Gagner M. Early results of laparoscopic biliopancreatic diversion with duodenal switch: a case series of 40 consecutive patients. Obes Surg. 2000;10(6):514–23.
18. Disse E, Pasquer A, Pelascini E, Valette PJ, Betry C, Laville M, et al. Dilation of sleeve gastrectomy: myth or reality? Obes Surg. 2017;27(1):30–7.
19. Ferrer-Márquez M, García-Díaz JJ, Moreno-Serrano A, Garcia-Diez JM, Ferrer-Ayza M, Alarcon-Rodriguez R, et al. Changes in gastric volume and their implications for weight loss after laparoscopic sleeve gastrectomy. Obes Surg. 2017;27(2):303–9.
20. Kuzmak LI. A review of seven years'experience with silicone gastric banding. Obes Surg. 1991;1:403–8.
21. O'Brien PE, Brennan L, Laurie C, Brown W. Intensive medical weight loss or laparoscopic adjustable gastric banding in the treatment of mild to moderate obesity: long-term follow-up of a prospective randomised trial. Obes Surg. 2013;23(9):1345–53.
22. Lazzati A, De Antonio M, Paolino L, Martini F, Azoulay D, Iannelli A, et al. Natural history of adjustable gastric banding: lifespan and revisional rate: a nationwide study on administrative data on 53,000 patients. Ann Surg. 2017;265(3):439–45.
23. Scopinaro N, Gianetta E, Civalleri D, Bonalumi U, Bachi V. Biliopancreatic bypass for obesity. II. Initial experience in man. Br J Surg. 1979;66:619–20.
24. Marceau P, Biron S, Bourque RA, Potvin M, Hould FS, Simard S. Biliopancreatic diversion with a new type of gastrectomy. Obes Surg. 1993;3(1):29–35.
25. Strain GW, Torghabeh MH, Gagner M, Ebel F, Dakin GF, Abelson GS, et al. The impact of biliopancreatic diversion with duodenal switch (BPD-DS) over 9 years. Obes Surg. 2017;27(3):787–94.
26. Dixon JB, Logue J, Komesaroff J. Promises and ethical pitfalls of surgical innovation: the case of bariatric surgery. Obes Surg. 2013;23(10):1698–702.
27. Mahawar KK, Jennings N, Brown J, Gupta A, Balupari S, Small P. "Mini" gastric bypass: systematic review of a controversial procedure. Obes Surg. 2013;23(11):1890–8.
28. Bruzzi M, Chevallier JM, Czernichow S. One-anastomosis bypass: why biliary reflux remains controversial? Obes Surg. 2017;27(2):545–7.
29. Carbajo MA, Luque-de-León E, Jiménez JM, Ortiz-de-Solorzano J, Perez-Miranda M, Castro Alija MJ. Laparoscopic one-anastomosis gastric bypass: technique, results, and long-term follow-up in 1200 patients. Obes Surg. 2017;27(5):1153–67.
30. Cavin JB, Voitellier E, Cluzeaud F, Kapel M, Marmuse JP, Chevallier JM, et al. Malabsorption and intestinal adaptation after one anastomosis gastric bypass compared with Roux-en-Y gastric bypass in rats. Am J Physiol Gastrointest Liver Physiol. 2016;311(3):G492–500.

31. Bétry C, Disse E, Chambrier C, Barnoud D, Gelas C, Baubet S, et al. Need for intensive nutrition care after bariatric surgery: is mini gastric bypass at fault? JPEN J Parenter Enteral Nutr. 2016;41(2):258–62.
32. Sánchez-Pernaute A, Rubio MA, Cabrerizo L, Ramos-Levi A, Perez-Aguirre A, Torres A. Single-anastomosis duodenoileal bypass with sleeve gastrectomy (SADI-S) for obese diabetic patients. Surg Obes Relat Dis. 2015;11(5):1092–8.
33. De Luca M, Himpens J, Angrisani L, Di Lorenzo N, Mahawar K, Lunardi C, et al. A new concept in bariatric surgery. Single anastomosis gastro-ileal (SAGI): technical details and preliminary results. Obes Surg. 2017;27(1):143–7.
34. Celik A, Ugale S, Ofluoglu H, Vural E, Cagiltay E, Cat H, et al. Metabolic outcomes of laparoscopic diverted sleeve gastrectomy with ileal transposition (DSIT) in obese type 2 diabetic patients. Obes Surg. 2015;25(11):2018–22.
35. Santoro S, Castro LC, Velhote MC. Sleeve gastrectomy with transit bipartition. Ann Surg. 2015;256(1):104–10.
36. Niazi M, Maleki AR, Talebpour M. Short-term outcomes of laparoscopic gastric plication in morbidly obese patients: importance of postoperative follow-up. Obes Surg. 2013;23(1):87–92.
37. Brethauer S. ASMBS policy statement on gastric plication. Surg Obes Rel Dis. 2011;7(3):262.
38. Zerrweck C, Rodríguez JG, Aramburo E, Viscara R, Rodriguez JL, Solorzano A, et al. Revisional surgery following laparoscopic gastric plication. Obes Surg. 2017;27(1):38–43.
39. Ye Q, Chen Y, Zhan X, Wang Y, Zhu J. Comparison of laparoscopic sleeve gastrectomy and laparoscopic greater curvature plication regarding efficacy and safety: a meta-analysis. Obes Surg. 2017;27(5):1358–64.
40. Jacobs M, Zundel N, Plasencia G, Rodriguez-Pumarol P, Gomez E, Leithead J 3rd. A vertically placed clip for weight loss: a 39-month pilot study. Obes Surg. 2017;27(5):1174–81.
41. Johnston D, Dachtler J, Sue-Ling HM, King RF, Martin IG. The Magenstrasse and mill operation for morbid obesity. Obes Surg. 2003;13(1):10–6.
42. Economopoulos KP, Theocharidis V, McKenzie TJ, Sergentanis TN, Psaltopoulou T. Robotic vs. laparoscopic roux-en-Y gastric bypass: a systematic review and meta-analysis. Obes Surg. 2015;25(11):2180–9.
43. Magouliotis DE, Tasiopoulou VS, Sioka E, Zacharoulis D. Robotic versus laparoscopic sleeve gastrectomy for morbid obesity: a systematic review and meta-analysis. Obes Surg. 2017;27(1):245–53.
44. Curro G, La Malfa G, Caiazzone A, Rampulla V, Navarra G. Three-dimensional (3D) versus two-dimensional (2D) laparoscopic bariatric surgery: a single-surgeon prospective randomized study. Obes Surg. 2015;25(11):2120–4.
45. Stefanopoulos A, Economopoulos K, Kalles V. Single incision laparoscopic sleeve gastrectomy: a review. Obes Surg. 2015;25(8):1502–10.
46. Barthet M, Binmoeller KF, Vanbiervliet G, Gonzales JM, Baron TH, Berdah S. Natural orifice transluminal endoscopic surgery gastroenterostomy with a biflanged lumen-apposing stent: first clinical experience (with videos). Gastrointest Endosc. 2015;81(1):215–8.
47. Diana M, Mutter D, Lindner V, Vix M, Chung H, Demartines N, et al. A modular magnetic anastomotic device for minimally invasive digestive anastomosis: proof of concept and preliminary data in the pig model. Surg Endosc. 2014;28(5):1613–23.
48. Ramos AC, Zundel N, Neto MG, Maalouf M. Human hybrid NOTES transvaginal sleeve gastrectomy: initial experience. Surg Obes Relat Dis. 2008;4(5):660–3.
49. Erridge S, Sodergren MH, Darzi A, Purkayastha S. Natural orifice translumenal endoscopic surgery: review of its applications in bariatric procedures. Obes Surg. 2016;26:422–8.
50. Diana M, Chung H, Liu KH, Dallemagne B, Demartines M, Mutter D, et al. Endoluminal surgical triangulation: overcoming challenges of colonic endoscopic submucosal dissections using a novel flexible endoscopic surgical platform: feasibility study in a porcine model. Surg Endosc. 2013;27(11):4130–5.
51. Magouliotis DE, Tasiopoulou VS, Svokos AA, Svokos KA, Sioka E, Zacharoulis D. Roux-en-Y gastric bypass versus sleeve gastrectomy as revisional procedure after adjustable gastric band: a systematic review and meta-analysis. Obes Surg. 2017;27(5):1365–73.

52. Parmar CD, Mahawar KK, Boyle M, Schroeder N, Balupuri N, Small PK. Conversion of sleeve gastrectomy to roux-en-Y gastric bypass is effective for gastro-oesophageal reflux disease but not for further weight loss. Obes Surg. 2017;27(7):1651–8.
53. Topart PA, Becouarn G. Revision and reversal after biliopancreatic diversion for excessive side effects or ineffective weight loss: a review of the current literature on indications and procedures. Surg Obes Relat Dis. 2015;11(4):965–72.
54. Busetto L, Dixon J, De Luca M, Shikora S, Pories W, Angrisani L. Bariatric surgery in class I obesity. A position statement from the International federation for the Surgery of obesity and metabolic disorders (IFSO). Obes Surg. 2014;24(4):487–519.
55. ASGE Bariatric Endoscopy Task Force, Sullivan S, Kumar N, Edmundowicz SA, Abu Dayyeh BK, Jonnalagadda SS, et al. ASGE Bariatric Endoscopy Task Force systematic review and meta-analysis assessing the ASGE PIVI thresholds for adopting endoscopic bariatric therapies. Gastrointest Endosc. 2015;82(3):425–38.
56. Casillas RA, Kim B, Fischer H, Zelada-Getty JL, Um SS, Coleman KJ. Comparative effectiveness of sleeve gastrectomy versus roux-en-Y gastric bypass for weight loss and safety outcomes in older adults. Surg Obes Relat Dis. 2017;13(9):1476–83.
57. Bergeat D, Lechaux D, Ghaina A, Thibault R, Bouygues V. Postoperative outcomes of laparoscopic bariatric surgery in older obese patients: a matched case control study. Obes Surg. 2017;27(6):1414–22.
58. Benedix F, Krause T, Adolf D, Wolf S, Lippert H, Mangert T, et al. Perioperative course, weight loss and resolution of comorbidities after primary sleeve gastrectomy for morbid obesity: are there differences between adolescents and adults? Obes Surg. 2017;27(9): 2388–97.
59. Lazzati A, Iannelli A, Schneck AS, Nelson AC, Katsahian S, Gugenheim J, et al. Bariatric surgery and liver transplantation: a systematic review a new frontier for bariatric surgery. Obes Surg. 2015;25(1):134–42.
60. Nesher E, Mor E, Shlomai A, Naftali-Cohen M, Yemini R, Youssim A, et al. Simultaneous liver transplantation and sleeve gastrectomy: prohibitive combination or a necessity? Obes Surg. 2017;27(5):1387–90.
61. Keidar A, Hazan D, Sadot E, Kashtan H, Wasserberg N. The role of bariatric surgery in morbidly obese patients with inflammatory bowel disease. Surg Obes Relat Dis. 2015;11(1):132–6.
62. Shoar S, Shahabuddin Hoseini S, Naderan M, Mahmoodzadeh H, Ying Man F, Shoar N, et al. Bariatric surgery in morbidly obese patients with inflammatory bowel disease: a systematic review. Surg Obes Relat Dis. 2017;13(4):652–9.
63. De Luca M, Angrisani L, Himpens J, Busetto N, Scopinaro N, Weiner R, et al. Indications for surgery and weight-related disease: position statements from the International Federation for the Surgery of obesity and metabolic disorders (IFSO). Obes Surg. 2016;26(8):1659–96.
64. Rubino F, Forgione A, Cummings DE, Vix M, Gnuli D, Mingrone G, et al. The mechanism of diabetes control after gastrointestinal bypass surgery reveals a role of the proximal small intestine in the physiopathology of type 2 diabetes. Ann Surg. 2006;244:741–9.
65. Mason EE. Ileal transposition and enteroglucagon/GLP-1 in obesity and diabetic surgery. Obes Surg. 1999;9(3):223–8.
66. Magouliotis DE, Tasiopoulou VS, Sioka E, Chatedaki C, Zacharoulis D. Impact of bariatric surgery on metabolic and gut microbiota profile: a systematic review and meta-analysis. Obes Surg. 2017;27(5):1345–57.
67. Fouladi F, Mitchell JE, Wunderlich JA, Steffen KJ. The contributing role of bile acids to metabolic acids to metabolic improvements after obesity and metabolic surgery. Obes Surg. 2016;26(10):2492–052.
68. Cavin JB, Couvelard A, Lebtahi R, Ducroc R, Arapis K, Voitelier E, et al. Differences in alimentary glucose absorption and intestinal disposal of blood glucose after roux-en-Y gastric bypass vs sleeve gastrectomy. Gastroenterology. 2016;150:454–64.
69. Schauer PR, Bhatt DL, Kirwan JP, Wolski K, Aminian A, Brethauer SA, et al. Bariatric surgery versus intensive medical therapy for diabetes—5-year outcomes. N Engl J Med. 2017;376(7):641–51.

70. Mingrone G, Panunzi S, De Gaetano A, Guidone C, Iaconelli A, Nanni G, et al. Bariatric-metabolic surgery versus conventional medical treatment in obese patients with type 2 diabetes: 5 year follow-up of an open-label, single-centre, randomised controlled trial. Lancet. 2015;386(9997):964–73.
71. Rubino F, Nathan DM, Eckel RH, Schauer PR, Alberti KG, Zimmet PZ, et al. Metabolic surgery in the treatment algorithm for type 2 diabetes: a joint statement by international diabetes organizations. Obes Surg. 2017;27(1):2–21.
72. O'Brien PE, Dixon JB, Laurie C, Skinner S, Proietto J, Mc Neil J, et al. Treatment of mild to moderate obesity with laparoscopic adjustable gastric banding or an intensive medical program: a randomized trial. Ann Intern Med. 2006;144(9):625–33.
73. Sjöström L, Peltonen M, Jacobson P, Sjöström CD, Karason K, Wedel H, et al. Bariatric surgery and long-term cardiovascular events. JAMA. 2012;307(1):56–65.
74. Zhou X, Liu J, Li L, Gloy VL, Nordmann A, Tiboni M, et al. Effects of bariatric surgery on mortality, cardiovascular events, and cancer outcomes in obese patients: systematic review and meta-analysis. Obes Surg. 2016;26(11):2586–601.
75. Dixon JB, Schachter LM, O'Brien PE, Jones K, Grima M, Lambert G, et al. Surgical vs conventional therapy for weight loss treatment of obstructive sleep apnea: a randomized control trial. JAMA. 2012;308(11):1142–9.
76. Dixon JB, Chapmann L, O'Brien PE. Marked improvement in asthma after lap-band surgery for morbid obesity. Obes Surg. 1999;3(1):15–21.
77. Pannain S, Mokhlesi B. Bariatric surgery and its impact on sleep architecture, sleep-disordered breathing, and metabolism. Best Pract Res Clin Endocrinol Metab. 2010;24(5):745–61.
78. Christensen R, Bartels EM, Astrup A, Bliddal H. Effect of weight reduction in obese patients diagnosed with knee osteoarthritis: a systematic review and meta-analysis. Ann Rheum Dis. 2007;66(4):433–9.
79. Parvizi J, Trousdale RT, Sarr MG. Total joint arthroplasty in patients surgically treated for morbid obesity. J Arthroplast. 2000;15(8):1003–8.
80. Chavez-Tapia NC, Tellez-Avia FI, Barrientos-Gutierrez T, Mendez-Sanchez N, Lizardi-Cervera J, Uribe M. Bariatric surgery for non-alcoholic fatty liver disease in obese patients. Cochrane Database Syst Rev. 2010;1:CD007340.
81. Rabl C, Campos GM. The impact of bariatric surgery on nonalcoholic steatohepatitis. Semin Liver Dis. 2012;32(1):80–91.
82. Lassailly G, Caiazzo R, Buob D, Pigeyre M, Verkindt H, Labrenche J, et al. Bariatric surgery reduces features of nonalcoholic steatohepatitis in morbidly obese patients. Gastroenterology. 2015;149:379–88.
83. Chalasani N, Younossi Z, Lavine JE, Diehl AM, Brunt EM, Cusi K, et al. The diagnosis and management of non-alcoholic fatty liver disease: practice guide-line by the American Gastroenterological Association, American Association for the Study of Liver Diseases, and American College of Gastroenterology. Gastroenterology. 2012;142(7):1592–609.
84. de Zwaan M, Enderle J, Wagner S, Mühlhans B, Ditzen B, Gefeller O, et al. Anxiety and depression in bariatric surgery patients: a prospective, follow-up study using structured clinical interviews. J Affect Disord. 2011;133(1–2):61–8.
85. Mitchell JE, Selzer F, Kalarchian MA, Devlin MJ, Strain GW, Elder KA, et al. Psychopathology before surgery in the longitudinal assessment of bariatric surgery-3 (LABS-3) psychological study. Surg Obes Relat Dis. 2012;8(5):533–41.
86. Kalarchian MA, Marcus MD, Levine MD, Courcoulas AP, Pilkonis PA, Ringham RM, et al. Psychiatric disorders among bariatric surgery candidates: relationship to obesity and functional health status. Am J Psychiatry. 2007;164(2):328–34.
87. Motta AB. The role of obesity in the development of polycystic ovary syndrome. Curr Pharma Des. 2012;18(17):2482–91.
88. Crosignani PG, Colombo M, Vegetti W, Somigliana E, Gessati A, Ragni G. Overweight and obese anovulatory patients with polycystic ovaries: parallel improvements in anthropometric indices, ovarian physiology and fertility rate induced by diet. Hum Reprod. 2003;18(9):1928–32.

89. Casagrande DS, Rosa DD, Umpierre D, Sarmiento RA, Rodrigues CJ, Schaan BD. Incidence of cancer following bariatric surgery: systematic review and meta-analysis. Obes Surg. 2014;24(9):1499–509.
90. Afshar S, Kelly SB, Seymour K, Lara J, Woodcock S, Mathers JC. The effects of bariatric surgery on colorectal cancer risk: systematic review and meta-analysis. Obes Surg. 2014;24(10):1793–9.
91. McCawley GM, Ferriss JS, Gefel D, Northup CJ, Modesitt SC. Cancer in obese women: potential protective impact of bariatric surgery. J Am Coll Surg. 2009;208(6):1093–8.
92. Kupersmith MJ, Garnell L, Turbin R, Peck V, Spiegel P, Wall M. Effects of weight loss on the course of idiopathic intracranial hypertension in women. Neurology. 1998;105(12):2313–7.
93. Subak LL, King WC, Belle SH, Chen JY, Courcoulas AP, Ebel FE, et al. Urinary incontinence before and after bariatric surgery. JAMA Intern Med. 2015;175(8):1378–87.
94. De Groot NL, Burgerhart JS, Van De Meeberg PC, de Vries DR, Smout AJ, Siersema PD. Systematic review: the effects of conservative and surgical treatment for obesity on gastro-oesophageal reflux disease. Aliment Pharmacol Ther. 2009;30(11–12):1091–102.
95. Al-Haddad BJ, Dorman RB, Rasmus NF, Kim YY, Ikramuddin S, Leslie DB. Hiatal hernia repair in laparoscopic adjustable gastric banding and laparoscopic roux-en-Y gastric bypass: a national database analysis. Obes Surg. 2014;24(3):377–84.
96. Rosenthal RJ, International Sleeve Gastrectomy Expert P, Diaz AA, Arvidsson D, Baker RS, Basso N, et al. International Sleeve Gastrectomy Expert Panel Consensus Statement: best practice guidelines based on experience of >12,000 cases. Surg Obes Relat Dis. 2012;8(1):8–19.
97. Georgia D, Stamatina T, Maria N, Konstantinos A, Konstantinos F, Emmanouil A, et al. 24-h multichannel intraluminal impedance PH-metry 1 year after laparocopic sleeve gastrectomy: an objective assessment of gastroesophageal reflux disease. Obes Surg. 2017;27(3):749–53.
98. Mion F, Tolone S, Garros A, Savarino E, Pelascini E, Robert M, et al. High-resolution impedance manometry after sleeve gastrectomy: increased intragastric pressure and reflux are frequent events. Obes Surg. 2016;26(10):2449–56.
99. Genco A, Soricelli E, Casella G, Maselli R, Castagneto-Gissey L, Di Lorenzo N, et al. Gastroesophageal reflux disease and Barrett's esophagus after laparoscopic sleeve gastrectomy: a possible, underestimated long-term complication. Obes Surg. 2017;13(4):568–74.
100. Burton PR, Brown WA, Laurie C, Korin A, Yap K, Richards M, et al. Pathophysiology of laparoscopic adjustable gastric bands: analysis and classification using high-resolution video manometry and a stress barium protocol. Obes Surg. 2010;20(1):19–29.
101. Dakour-Aridi HN, El-Rayess HM, Abou-Abbass H, Abu-Gheida I, Habib RH, Safadi BY. Safety of concomitant cholecystectomy at the time of laparoscopic sleeve gastrectomy: analysis of the American College of Surgeons National Surgical Quality Improvement Program database. Surg Obes Relat Dis. 2017;13(6):934–41.
102. Nougou A, Suter M. Almost routine prophylactic cholecystectomy during laparoscopic gastric bypass is safe. Obes Surg. 2008;18(5):535–9.
103. Wanjura V, Sandblom G, Österberg J, Enochsson L, Ottosson J, Szabo E. Cholecystectomy after gastric bypass-incidence and complications. Surg Obes Relat Dis. 2016;13(6):979–87.
104. Frederiksen NA, Tveskov L, Helgstrand F, Naver L, Floyd A. Treatment of common bile duct stones in gastric bypass patients with laparoscopic transgastric endoscopic retrograde cholangiopancreatography. Obes Surg. 2017;27(6):1409–13.
105. Abdallah E, Emile SH, Elfeki H, Fikry M, Abdelshafy M, Elshobaky A, et al. Role of ursodeoxycholic acid in the prevention of gallstone formation after laparoscopic sleeve gastrectomy. Obes Surg. 2017;47(7):844–50.
106. Terranova L, Busetto L, Vestri A, Zappa MA. Bariatric surgery: cost-effectiveness and budget impact. Obes Surg. 2012;22(4):646–563.
107. O'Neill KN, Finucane FM, le Roux CW, Fitzgerald AP. Unmet need for bariatric surgery. Surg Obes Relat Dis. 2016;13(6):1052–6.

Endoscopists and Surgeons Playing in the Same Team: The Multidisciplinary Approach in Screening and Preoperative Workup

4

Contents

Abbreviations

AACE	American Association of Clinical Endocrinologists
ASA	American Society of Anaesthesiologists
ASGE	American Society for Gastrointestinal Endoscopy
ASMBS	American Society for Metabolic and Bariatric Surgery
BMI	Body mass index
C. difficile	*Clostridium difficile*
CAGS	Canadian Association of General Surgeons
CDAI	Crohn's Disease Activity Index
CT	Computed tomography

E. M. H. Mathus-Vliegen, J. Dargent, *Bariatric Therapy*,
https://doi.org/10.1007/978-3-319-90074-2_4

EAES	European Association of Endoscopic Surgery
EASO	European Association for the study of Obesity
FES	Fundamentals of endoscopic surgery
FLS	Fundamentals of laparoscopic surgery
GI	Gastrointestinal
GIST	Gastrointestinal stromal tumour
GORD	Gastro-oesophageal reflux disease
H. pylori	*Helicobacter pylori*
Hp	*Helicobacter pylori*
IBD	Inflammatory bowel disease
IFSO-EC	International Federation for the Surgery of Obesity-European Chapter
IGB	Intragastric balloons
IL	Interleukin
LAGB	Laparoscopic adjustable gastric banding
LOS	Length of stay
LOS	Lower oesophageal sphincter
LOSP	Lower oesophageal sphincter pressure
MALT	Mucosa-associated lymphoid tissue
MRI	Magnetic resonance imaging
NIH	National Institutes of Health
NSAID	Non-steroidal anti-inflammatory drug
OGD	Oesophagogastroduodenoscopy
OR	Odds ratio
PPI	Proton pump inhibitor
RCT	Randomised controlled trial
RYGB	Roux-en-Y gastric bypass
SAGES	Society of American Gastrointestinal and Endoscopic Surgeons
SG	Sleeve gastrectomy
SOReg	Scandinavian Obesity Register
TLOSR	Transient LOS relaxation
TNF-α	Tumour necrosis factor-alpha
TOS	The Obesity Society
VBG	Vertical banded gastroplasty
VLCD	Very-low-calorie diets
VLED	Very-low-energy diets

4.1 Introduction

In the multidisciplinary approach of a patient seeking surgical help for severe obesity, a team consisting of a bariatric surgeon, internist, anaesthesiologist, psychologist and a dietician is often involved. Other specialities are called up when needed such as a pulmonologist and cardiologist, and in this row the interventional radiologist, gastroenterologist and endoscopist figure as a second-hand assist. However, as endoscopists are often involved in complications associated with bariatric surgery and in attempts to rescue bariatric surgery, one should ask oneself if they should be part of the multidisciplinary team already from the onset. Several guidelines define the minimum requirements of preoperative workup. However, there is no consensus in the literature about the workup concerning the gastrointestinal tract and the routine performance of upper gastrointestinal (GI) endoscopy before bariatric surgery is highly controversial.

4.2 Preoperative Workup and the Role of Endoscopy

4.2.1 Guidelines

In 2005, the European Association of Endoscopic Surgery (EAES) recommended that the preoperative evaluation of obesity surgery patients should also include upper gastrointestinal endoscopy or radiographic evaluation with a barium meal, in addition to standard laboratory testing, chest radiography, electrocardiography, spirometry and abdominal ultrasonography [1]. Upper gastrointestinal endoscopy or upper gastrointestinal (GI) series was advisable for all bariatric patients (recommendation grade C), but was strongly recommended for gastric bypass patients (grade B). Ultrasound of the abdomen is usually done to detect cholelithiasis or choledocholithiasis. However, already in 1997 Ghassemian et al. demonstrated that 393 (59.8%) of the upper GI series were normal in 657 patients, who underwent gastric bypass surgery and who had a preoperative GI radiography [2]. The following abnormalities were discovered in the remaining 264 (40.2%): hiatal hernia (164), GE reflux (39), Schatzki's ring (18), small-bowel diverticula (4), renal stones (4), malrotation (3), gallstones (2), pyloric ulcer (1) and dysphagia lusoria (1). None of these findings resulted in cancellation or a delay in surgery. So, routine upper GI series appeared not justified in the preoperative evaluation of the morbidly obese. They were able to save $741 in charges and to spare their patients an ordeal that took 1–2 h.

In 2013, the American Association of Clinical Endocrinologists (AACE), The Obesity Society (TOS) and the American Society for Metabolic and Bariatric Surgery (ASMBS) updated their 2008 Clinical Practice Guideline [3, 4]. The preoperative evaluation should include a comprehensive medical history, psychosocial history, physical examination and appropriate blood testing and all patients should undergo a preoperative evaluation for the cause of obesity and for obesity-related comorbidities. Concerning the gastrointestinal tract they advised to screen for *Helicobacter pylori* in high-prevalence areas (grade C, based on inconsistent findings of reduced post-operative complications), to evaluate the gallbladder in the presence of symptomatic biliary disease and elevated liver function test (up to 2–3 times the upper limit of normal) (grade D) and to evaluate clinically significant gastrointestinal symptoms before bariatric surgery with imaging studies, upper GI series or endoscopy (grade D). Furthermore, patients should be followed by their primary physician and have age- and risk-appropriate cancer screening before surgery because of the fact that obesity is a risk factor for certain malignancies (endometrium, kidney, gallbladder, breast, colon, pancreas and oesophagus) and may adversely affect clinical outcomes.

The European guidelines of 2013 is an update of the 2008 Interdisciplinary European Guidelines on Surgery of Severe Obesity by the International Federation for the Surgery of Obesity-European Chapter (IFSO-EC) and the European Association for the Study of Obesity (EASO) [5, 6]. The guidelines state that patients in addition to the routine preoperative assessment may undergo further assessment for gastro-oesophageal disorders (*Helicobacter pylori*, etc.) without a clear indication about the necessity to perform an upper GI endoscopy.

In the guidelines thus far, the type of surgery was not taken into account. Most surgeons do not consider hiatal hernia and reflux oesophagitis to be clinically relevant. Both are thought to be a natural consequence of obesity and both will disappear after weight reduction [7]. However, some surgeons think that reflux is an important aspect of obesity which has consequences for the selection of the surgical procedure. Other lesions considered to be clinically relevant are Barrett's oesophagus, a large hiatal hernia $\geq$3.5 cm, erosions, erosive gastritis/duodenitis, ulcers and benign or malignant tumours [7, 8].

Furthermore, if specific pathological upper GI findings are known preoperatively, the chosen procedure might be changed, allowing the surgeon to plan the type of operation effectively, by notifying the operating room team of a change in the procedure and probably extending the length of time needed. This is the case for instance in known hiatal hernia or para-oesophageal hernia, where gastric banding should be avoided [9, 10]. Sleeve gastrectomy potentially carries an increased risk of developing de novo GORD symptoms and/or worsening reflux symptoms and oesophageal mucosa injury. The International Sleeve Gastrectomy Expert Panel Consensus Meeting in 2012 defined severe oesophagitis or Barrett's oesophagus as a contraindication to perform sleeve gastrectomy and Roux-en-Y gastric bypass (RYGB) should be considered instead [11]. At the 5th international consensus conference in 2016 the majority of experts tended to agree that Barrett's oesophagus precluded sleeve gastrectomy [12]. This means that most surgeons should propose a preoperative gastroscopy on all their patients. However, this was only done in 1.3%. Moreover 50% of experts in 2012 agreed that all patients should have 24-h pH measurement and manometry before laparoscopic sleeve gastrectomy (SG) if they complained of reflux; this agreement declined to 32.8% in 2016 [11, 12]. Peptic ulcers may be problematic in sleeve gastrectomy if the resection line runs through an ulcer and in RYGB if the ulcer is located in the gastric remnant and ulcer bleeding occurs in the post-operative period [9].

In 2015, the American Society for Gastrointestinal Endoscopy (ASGE) in conjunction with the Society of Gastrointestinal and Endoscopic Surgeons and the American Society for Metabolic and Bariatric Surgery (ASMBS) suggested that the decision to perform preoperative endoscopy should be individualised in patients scheduled to undergo bariatric surgery after a thorough discussion with the surgeon, taking into consideration the type of the procedure (low-quality evidence) [13]. Patients with symptoms of GORD or who use chronically H_2

blockers or PPIs should have an upper GI endoscopic evaluation. In contrast to the older guideline of 2008, the present guideline does no longer recommend routine *Helicobacter pylori* (Hp) screening and treatment due to conflicting data on its significance [13, 14].

Generally speaking, the guidelines are not clear nor consistent and leave room for doubt.

4.2.2 Arguments of Proponents and Opponents

Proponents of preoperative endoscopy argue that oesophago-gastro-duodenoscopy (OGD) may have several advantages:

1. Diagnostic purpose, i.e. identifying relevant lesions that may be different in relevance for different bariatric options, i.e. erosive oesophagitis, Barrett's oesophagus and a large hiatal hernia in sleeve gastrectomy, abnormalities in the inaccessible part of the stomach in the gastric bypass, etc.: Surgeons advocate hiatal hernia reduction and crural closure and thus it is useful for surgeons to know the measured size and length of the hiatal hernia reported in centimetre by the endoscopist. Indeed, this information about the length of the hiatal hernia and the gap between the diaphragmatic crura can be retrieved by laparoscopy, but in the super-obese patient it may be difficult to identify a hiatal hernia due to the large distal oesophageal fat pads. These hernias might be more easily visible by endoscopy or a barium swallow X-ray [15]. A major objection against the guidelines that advise an endoscopy in the presence of symptoms is the very obvious lack of correlation between symptoms and findings, as mentioned by many studies [8–10, 16–19]. Also, the correlation between endoscopic features and histology is poor. Guidelines also do not discuss influences of age and, more importantly, of ethnicity and race. Both Ng et al. and Lee et al. mentioned a high yield of oesophago-gastro-duodenoscopy in Asian populations which also have a higher upper GI cancer risk and incidence [20, 21].
2. Therapeutic purpose preoperatively: If findings are clinically relevant they may allow an optimisation of medical therapy preoperatively or they may change the choice and timing of the surgical procedure.
3. Preventive purpose: Lesions might be found that potentially may predict or cause complications in the immediate post-operative period or result in symptoms in the months or years following surgery. The relevance of Hp eradication in the prevention of marginal ulcer formation and perforation, as will be discussed later, is not yet clear.

Opponents suggest that routine OGDs do not alter the planned surgery sufficiently to warrant a potentially dangerous procedure. Indeed, the benefits of OGD should outweigh the potential risks of the procedure in this patient group. Large series on OGD report adverse event rates of 1 in 200 to 1 in 10,000 and mortality ranges from none to 1 in 2000 [22]. Adverse event rates related to diagnostic procedures are rare and include cardiopulmonary adverse events, infection, perforation and bleeding. The cardiopulmonary event rate is 1 in 170 and mortality rate 1 in 10,000 and is mainly related to sedation and analgesia. Patient-related risk factors are pre-existing cardiopulmonary disease, advanced age, American Society of Anaesthesiologist (ASA) class III or higher and a higher Goldman score. Procedure-related risk factors for hypoxia are difficult intubation of the oesophagus, a prolonged procedure and prone position. OGD may carry a higher risk in the morbidly obese due to a higher prevalence of diabetes and sleep apnoea, and electrocardiographic abnormalities. They may have a lower baseline oxygen saturation and thereby a higher probability of desaturation with sedation. Küper et al. found a 2.9% (two severe hypoxia) rate of critical events in morbidly obese subjects, and argued that upper endoscopy can be performed safely with careful monitoring and anaesthesiologist's support, realising that this event rate signified an approximately tenfold increase compared with the rates in large endoscopic series of normal-weight subjects [9]. Very recently, a retrospective study by McVay et al. examined the use of non-anaesthesia-administered propofol during upper GI endoscopy in control subjects (average BMI 21.9 kg/m^2, range 14–25; n = 265) and morbidly obese preoperative bariatric surgical patients (average BMI 45.8 kg/m^2, range 34–80; n = 130) [23]. The severely obese group had a significantly higher prevalence of sleep apnoea (62% vs. 8%), experienced more oxygen desaturations (22% vs. 7%) and received more chin-lift manoeuvers (20% vs. 6%) but advanced airway interventions were rarely required in either group and were not more frequent in the bariatric group. They concluded that with propofol sedation, given by appropriately trained personnel, outpatient upper endoscopy was safe in severely obese patients.

Alternatives to conventional OGD exist such as transnasal small-calibre upper endoscopy which does not require sedation, barium X-ray for the diagnosis of hiatal hernia and *Helicobacter pylori* testing by serology, stool antigen testing or ^{13}C urea breath test.

Moreover, preoperative endoscopy is associated with increased costs, capacity issues and pressure on available health resources because insurance companies will not reimburse the costs of these investigations. Yet, a randomised clinical study comparing a group that did undergo OGD or did not have OGD prior to surgery is lacking and also cost-effectiveness has been addressed in only a few retrospective studies. Sharaf et al. reported a high yield of endoscopic findings being cost effective: a low cost of almost 700$ per clinically important lesion detected [18]. Azagury et al. in Switzerland calculated the costs of three proposed strategies in asymptomatic obese patients before Roux-en-Y gastric bypass: (1) No investigation: This carried a cost of 39 euro per patient with four Helicobacter-positive ulcers being untreated, three potentially significant lesions being undetected and seven lesions being undetected and untreated. (2) Hp stool antigen testing and eradication: This cost 64 euro with no lesions untreated and two potentially significant lesions undetected. (3) Endoscopy with Hp testing and eradication which cost 389 euro with no lesions undetected or untreated but three workups prompted by irrelevant findings [19].

4.2.3 Skills and Training

Another aspect is the skills of the endoscopist and the standardisation of reporting. Most of the studies have been performed by surgeons. Surgeons performing the endoscopy report more small hernias than gastroenterologists do [8, 15]. Mohammed et al. performed a retrospective analysis of complaints of GORD/heartburn/use of PPIs or H_2 blockers, which they sought to be related to the presence of a hiatal hernia, and related the absence or presence of symptoms with subsequent findings of a hiatal hernia at OGD and the hiatal hernia repair during surgery [15]. In 1570 patients 857 patients received a diagnosis of GORD/heartburn (55%) and 713 (45%) did not. Of these symptomatic 857 patients, 240 (28%) demonstrated a hiatal hernia on OGD and 116 were repaired intra-operatively. Of those being negative for hiatal hernia on OGD, 37 (6%) needed intra-operatively a hiatal hernia repair. In 713 patients without symptoms, a hiatal hernia was found on OGD in 194 (27%) and 88 of these had an intraoperative repair. Of those 519 who did not show a hiatal hernia during OGD, 19 required an intraoperative hiatal hernia repair. So, hiatal hernia repair was performed in 153 (18%) of patients with GORD/heartburn and in 107 (15%) of patients without symptoms. Five large hiatal hernias found on OGD were not present on intraoperative inspection. In 56 patients (5%) without a preoperative finding of hiatal hernia on OGD, a hiatal hernia was diagnosed and repaired. The sensitivity of finding a repairable hiatal hernia by clinical symptoms was 55% and the specificity 46%. Similarly the sensitivity of finding a repairable hiatal hernia by OGD findings was 78% and the specificity 82%. The absence of a hiatal hernia on EGD had a high negative predictive value of 95% compared with clinical indicators. So, indeed small hiatal hernias were over-diagnosed by OGD as most did not require repair. However, moderate and large hiatal hernias were accurately detected. However, the decision to repair small hiatal hernias is also operator dependent, as small hernias in patients without symptoms and negative OGD were repaired in 4% of cases and small hernias in patients with negative OGD findings were repaired in 5% of cases.

There has also been some discussion about the endoscopic training [24–26]. Gastroenterologists have a formal 2–3-year subspecialty training, which is needed to recognise endoscopic manifestations of diseases and to acquire enough experience to perform advanced endoscopic techniques. Furthermore, a growing awareness of the need to assess the quality of endoscopy and the specifications thereof have resulted in sets of quality measures and of the volume of endoscopic case numbers. Surgical trainees typically receive 3 months of dedicated endoscopy training while in general at least 6 months of training is needed to provide the necessary level of training and to fully understand and put into practice other aspects of endoscopy such as contraindications, guidelines, risks, complications and management of adverse sequelae [26]. Asfaha et al. discovered that none of the surgical trainees met the minimum recommendations for endoscopic case numbers [25]. The Society of American Gastrointestinal and Endoscopic Surgeons (SAGES) has commented that surgeons are uniquely qualified to perform endoscopic procedures during and after a surgical operation [24]. SAGES recommends that training of surgeons should take into account their need to perform endoscopy in this unique situation. They appointed a task force similar to the SAGES FLS (Fundamentals of Laparoscopic Surgery) to create and validate a programme that measure basic knowledge and skills to perform a safe flexible endoscopy [27]. This programme, the Fundamentals of Endoscopic Surgery (FES) programme, consists of online materials and didactic and skill-based tests and is designed to measure the skills and knowledge required to perform safe flexible endoscopy. A virtual reality simulator is used in the training. As part of the FES project the minimum number of procedures required was set at 50 for upper endoscopies and 75 for colonoscopies and a decision to use a combined total of 100 procedures to define the passing score was made. The Canadian Association of General Surgeons (CAGS) also stated that training of surgical residents in endoscopy is essential for adequate patient care in Canada [26].

4.2.4 Meta-Analyses

Two meta-analyses tried to put the (routine) use of preoperative OGD into perspective [28, 29]. Clinical studies were not available and all but one were retrospective cohort studies in different populations of symptomatic or purposely chosen asymptomatic subjects or on less well-defined populations. Also, sizes of hiatal hernia were perceived differently, being relevant if of any size, >2 cm, >3.5 cm or >4 cm. Some studies divided their findings into four groups: group 0 normal study, group 1 abnormal findings that neither changed the surgical approach nor postponed surgery (mild oesophagitis, gastritis and/or duodenitis, oesophageal webs), group 2 abnormal finding that changed the surgical approach or postponed surgery (mass lesions, ulcers, severe oesophagitis, gastritis or duodenitis, Barrett's oesophagus, bezoar, hiatal hernia of any size, peptic stricture, Zenker's diverticulum, oesophageal diverticula, AV malformation) and finally group 3 absolute contraindication to surgery (upper GI cancer, varices) [18, 20]. The two meta-analyses come to the same conclusion that routine upper GI endoscopy is not warranted.

A first meta-analysis by Parikh et al. included 28 articles (18 publications, 10 abstracts) over the period 1997–2013 [28]. Patients were divided into two groups: group 1–OGD with negative findings or finding that did not alter management (included here hiatal hernia and presence of Hp), and group 2–OGD findings that delayed, altered or cancelled surgery. Since some surgeons may treat all cases of oesophagitis, regardless of severity, all oesophagitis patients were categorised in group 2 in a second calculation. Twenty-five studies performed OGD routinely. Overall 92.4% (n = 6112) of patients had a normal OGD or findings that did not change clinical management, and 7.6% (n = 504) had findings that delayed or altered surgery. Patient-level data were available in 4511 patients (Table 4.1). Because of the significant heterogeneity in the studies, a general estimating equation model was used to calculate a confidence interval. OGD findings delayed or cancelled surgery in 7.8% (95% confidence interval (95% CI) 4.6/12.4) and when all oesophagitis cases were regrouped into group 2 this proportion was 20.6% (14.5/28.2). Based on these meta-analysis findings, a routine endoscopy is not

Table 4.1 Endoscopic findings in two meta-analyses analysing the role of routine preoperative endoscopy

Parikh patient-level data [28]			Bennett all studies [29]		
$N = 4511$			$N = 12{,}261$		
OGD findings	Number of patients	Proportion % with OGD findings	Number of studies	Number of patients	Proportion % with OGD findings
Gastritis	1562	34.6	31	7598	37.6
Hiatal hernia	889	19.7	39	9723	21.1
H. pylori	888	19.7	23	5650	20.2
Oesophagitis, all grades	786	17	37	9129	37.0
Duodenitis	226	5	20	5074	5.2
Gastric ulcer	97	2	25	6356	3.6
Duodenal ulcer	14	0.3	16	3547	1.8
Barrett's oesophagus	45	0.1	19	5802	2.1
Cancer	4	0.08			
Oesophageal cancer			5	1278	0.2
Gastric cancer			12	3586	0.4
Gastric intestinal metaplasia			5	1126	2.2

warranted and a selective approach may be considered based on patient symptoms, risk factors and type of procedure planned.

The second meta-analysis of Bennett et al. covered 48 studies in the period 1996–2014 (30 articles and 18 abstracts); the total number of patients was 12,261 [29]. Change in surgical management was considered to be a delay (also for the institution of a medical treatment), cancellation, addition or alteration of a surgical procedure. A change in medical management was defined as the addition of medical treatment or additional diagnostic tests based on OGD findings. Twenty-three studies reported the proportion of cases where OGD resulted in a change of surgical management (n = 6845), yielding a proportion of 7.8% (6.1/9.5) with significant heterogeneity (Table 4.1). Of a total of 492 changes in surgical management, 221 (44.9%) were hiatal hernia repairs, 201 (40.8%) were delays in surgery due to gastritis or peptic ulcer disease, 37 (7.5%) were major changes in planned procedure such as switching from RYGB to SG or addition of a gastrectomy to RYGB, 4 (0.8%) were cancellations due to varices or oesophageal cancer, 3 (0.6%) were additional endoscopic dissection procedures and 3 (0.6%) were delays for reasons other than peptic ulcer disease. In one study a gastrostomy was added for peptic ulcer disease or polyps in 16 cases [30]. Sensitivity analysis was performed by excluding those findings that were of debatable importance in the preoperative setting (hiatal hernia) or related to benign disease (gastritis, peptic ulcer disease). After excluding these findings the proportion of OGDs resulting in a change of surgical management was 0.4% (0.2/0.6) with much less heterogeneity.

A 27.5% (20.2/34.8) change in medical management was reported in 20 papers (n = 5140) with significant heterogeneity. Of the 1239 changes in medical management, 946 (76.4%) were for Hp eradication, 291 (23.5%) were for initiation of PPIs or H_2 blockers for gastritis or reflux, 1 was for biopsy and 1 for gastric emptying studies. Sensitivity analysis was performed by excluding management due to Hp. Then the proportion of OGDs resulting in a change in medical management was 2.5% (1.7/3.2) with still significant heterogeneity remaining. Studies that specifically mentioned the three pathologies of Barrett's, oesophageal and gastric cancer were included but studies not specifically mentioning these three lesions were not included in the denominator. Malignant or premalignant lesions were reported to be Barrett's oesophagus in 2.1% in 19 studies (n = 5802), oesophageal cancer was mentioned in only 5 studies (n = 1278) to be present in 0.2% and gastric cancer was reported in 12 studies (n = 3586) and was found in 0.4%. Gastric intestinal metaplasia was mentioned in 2.2% and would probably change the choice from RYGB to SG to enable further surveillance. In Western countries the risk of gastric cancer remains low, even in the setting of intestinal metaplasia, with a standardised incidence ratio of only 2.23 in a low-risk population. This meta-analysis concluded that it appears reasonable to forego routine preoperative OGD as the incidence of significant findings is low.

Both meta-analyses were not taken into consideration in the guidelines and also did not stop the ongoing debate as studies continued to be reported, summarised in Table 4.2 [10, 20, 21, 31]. These studies showed the high yield of asymptomatic endoscopic findings and two recent Asian studies reported the repercussion of such findings on timing and type of surgery.

There was also a survey sent to the British Obesity and Metabolic Surgery Society members [32]. A response was obtained from 49 centres, covering 5000 patients/year. Forty-four (90%) included preoperative OGD routinely (30%) or selectively (60%). According to the results, 25 units (51%) changed the operative plans because of peptic ulcer (46%), hiatal hernia (43%), Barrett's oesophagus (32%) or gastrointestinal stromal tumour (GIST) (25%). Two centres (7%) found incidental cancer. When specifically asked, OGD was believed to be essential in pernicious anaemia (57%), familial history of GI cancer (61%) and reflux symptoms (54%). Four units (9%) found OGD extremely important in every patient and five units considered EGD completely unnecessary (10%). Eleven units would not be able to accommodate routine OGD in all patients [32].

4.2.5 Preoperative Endoscopy and Fear of Missing Cancers and Lesions

4.2.5.1 Preoperative Endoscopy and Fear of Missing Cancers

Another argument to perform preoperative endoscopy is the difficult accessibility of the gastric remnant after RYGB. Obesity as such is associated with a higher cancer risk and bariatric surgery may delay a timely diagnosis because symptoms such as dysphagia, food intolerance, vomiting and epigastric pain may be attributed to the effects of bariatric surgery. The patient may be happy with a–probably disproportionate–weight loss, thus delaying the access to medical assessment and diagnosis. Scozzari et al. performed a systematic review of all reported gastro-oesophageal

Table 4.2 Endoscopic findings preoperatively in studies not included in the two meta-analyses

Author Yr, Country	N/operation/age	UGIT normal	HH	Oesophagitis	Gastritis	Ulcer S/D–polyp	Other	Comment/statistics
Carabotti (2016), Italy [10]	142/?/41 years	75 (52.9%)	33 (23.2%) >3 cm	8 (5.6%)	9 (6.3%) erosive and duodenal	5 (3.5%)–0	Hp 34 (24%)	Patients with lesions had symptoms in only 40.3%; 87.5% of erosive oesophagitis and 60.6% of HH might have been missed being asymptomatic
Fernandes (2016), Portugal [31]	613/SG, LASGB, RYGB/46.5 years	268 (43.7%)	105 (30.4%) (57 > 3 cm)	47 (13.6%), 3 Barrett	230 (66.7%) 111 erosive	9 (2.6%)/3 (0.9%)–29 (8.4%)	Hp 114/236 (48.3%), duodenitis 65 (18.8%), erosive in 33	Hp was the strongest independent predictor of abnormal endoscopy RR 10.3 (4.6/23.2)
Ng (2016), Singapore [20]	208 asymptomatic/ SG, LASGB, RYGB/40 years	70 (33.6%)	33 (15.9%)	4 (1.9%) erosive	10 (4.8%) erosive	10 (4.8%)–12 (5.8%)	Leiomyoma, adenocarcinoma, GIST	High diagnostic yield with influence on procedure in 69 (33.2%) and contraindications for operation in 2
Lee (2017), China [21]	368/?/39.1 years	131 (48.9%)	48 (17.9%), 28 < 2 cm	20 (7.5%) erosive	87 (32.5%)	5 (3.6%)/1 (0.7%)–0	Hp 58/243 (23.7%), polyps oesophagus 3, gastric 10, duodenal 1	Clinical significant lesions in 27.2% in 73 patients, resulting in a delay in surgery in 20 (27%) and in a change in operation procedure (18 HH repair, 2 RYGB instead of SG) in 20 (27%)

S/D stomach/duodenum; *UGIT* upper gastrointestinal tract; *HH* hiatal hernia cancers [33]. Twenty-eight articles describing 33 patients were retrieved in the period 1991, when the first cancer was reported, to 2012. Neoplasms were discovered at a mean of 8.5 (range, 2 months–29 years) after bariatric surgery. There were 11 oesophageal and 22 gastric cancers; 29 cases (90.6%) were adenocarcinomas. Fifteen patients had undergone a restrictive operation (vertical banded gastroplasty (VBG) in 9, laparoscopic gastric banding (LAGB) in 5, sleeve gastrectomy (SG) in 1) with an oesophageal cancer in 5 and a gastric cancer in 10. Eighteen patients had had a Roux-en-Y gastric bypass (RYGB). Four loop gastric bypasses had tumours located in the gastric pouch; in the 14 standard RYGBs the cancer was located in the oesophagus in 6 and in the stomach in 8: 3 in the gastric pouch and 5 in the bypassed segment. In only five subjects a preoperative endoscopy was performed with once a normal appearance, one subject had gastric ulcerations, one had intestinal metaplasia, and two had a Barrett's oesophagus and they developed an adenocarcinoma 21 and 5 years later. In eight patients a tumour was diagnosed within 3 years after bariatric surgery, after a VBG in one, a gastric band in three, sleeve gastrectomy in one and RYGB in three. Of these eight patients, three patients did not have endoscopy, in another three no data were reported and in two the appearance at endoscopy was normal. Because of a paucity of data and because the denominator of Scozarri's study is not known, it is impossible to quantify the incidence of oesophagogastric cancer [33]. The incidence of gastric cancer in the excluded stomach does not seem to be greater than in the normal population but studies came from areas with a low oesophagogastric cancer incidence and results might be different in Asian populations.

4.2.5.2 Histology of Resected Specimen to Look for Missed Lesions

Another way to investigate the yield of endoscopy and the relationship with endoscopic findings and post-operative complications is to examine the gastric sleeve specimen. Also here, the question has arisen whether this should be done routinely. Available studies are condensed in Table 4.3 together with their country of origin [34–40]. In the most recent study by Safaan et al. Hp was eradicated before the operation by triple therapy and this might have influenced the histopathological findings [34]. The absence of pathological findings varied substantially, with no normal findings in the study of Almazeedi et al. from Kuwait and absence of pathology in 69% in the study by Ohanessian et al. from the USA [35, 38]. More important is to look for follicular gastritis and lymphoid aggregates associated with Hp and presumed to be precursors of mucosa-associated lymphoid tissue (MALT) lymphoma which was present in 4.1–31.2% of patients (Table 4.3). Intestinal metaplasia as a precursor of adenocarcinoma was present in 0.2–2.6% of patients and if Helicobacter gastritis was included the rate of diagnosis indicating increased cancer risk varied between 4.5% and 42.3%. Benign tumours with potential for malignancy, i.e. GIST tumours, were found in 0.2–1% of patients. None of the studies showed a malignancy. In Safaan's study, age was associated with GIST tumours and intestinal metaplasia; female gender with chronic active gastritis; and the presence of *Helicobacter pylori* with follicular gastritis, lymphoid aggregates, GIST, intestinal metaplasia and chronic active gastritis [34]. Older age, female gender and presence of Helicobacter were in this study associated with abnormal histopathology [34].

Table 4.3 Prevalence of histopathology (% of patients) of laparoscopic sleeve specimens, modified after Safaan et al. [34]

Author, year, N, country	Normal	Chronic (inactive) gastritis	Chronic active gastritis	Follicular gastritis and/ or lymphoid aggregates	Intestinal metaplasia	GIST	*H. pylori*	Preoperative OGD
Almazeedi, (2013), *n* = 656 Kuwait [35]	0	74.4	7.5	14.5	0.2	0.2	7.3	All patients
Clapp, (2015), *n* = 145 USA [36]	50.3	44.1	[b]	4.1	[b]	[b]	18	Selected patients
Raess, (2015), *n* = 248 USA [37]	35.2	24[a]	[b]	31.2	2	[b]	5.2	Selected patients
Ohanessian (2015), *n* = 310 USA [38]	69	13	1.6	[b]	1.3	1	3.2	Selected patients
Lauti (2016), *n* = 976 N-Zealand [39]	46.3	38.9	[b]	[b]	2.6	0.4	8.6	Selected patients
Gaffar (2016), *n* = 546 United Arabic Emirates [40]	54	45	8.4	[b]	0.7	[b]	10	All patients
Safaar (2017), *n* = 155 Qatar [34]	52	33	6.8	4.9 (2.7 and 2.2%, resp.)	1.4	0.7	40.9[c]	All patients

GIST gastrointestinal stromal tumour; *H. pylori Helicobacter pylori*; resp. respectively
[a]All chronic gastritis added together
[b]Not reported
[c]All patients received eradication therapy before the sleeve gastrectomy

The routine performance of histopathology is still questionable. On the one hand, 8.4% of 248 cases in the USA had unforeseen findings in the sleeve specimen and consisted of *H. pylori* gastritis, autoimmune gastritis, necrotising vasculitis and intestinal metaplasia that required additional clinical follow-up [37]. In Kuwait no normal specimen was reported in 656 young (33.6 years old) patients with 74.4% having chronic gastritis and 24 (3.7%) having pathologies that required an altered post-operative management and in New Zealand over 50% had histopathological abnormalities and therefore some required routine microscopic examination, also enabling the discovery of *H. pylori* [35, 39]. Conversely, others found only a minority of pathologic findings and claimed that routine microscopic examination was unnecessary [36, 38, 40]. Following that line of reasoning they would likely also have turned away a routine upper GI endoscopy. Gaffar et al. suggested that a selective microscopic examination guided by relevant clinical history and macroscopic examination is a better option but that a careful gross description is still necessary for potential future medicolegal implications [40].

Data on the excluded stomach after RYGB are scarce as the excluded stomach remnant is without the reach of a normal endoscopy. Vaz Safatle-Ribeiro et al. performed a double-balloon endoscopy at a mean of 78 months after the RYGB procedure and reached the stomach in 35 out of 40 patients aged 43 years [41]. Upon endoscopy 8/35 (22.8%) had a normal bypassed stomach, in 23 (65.7%) pangastritis was seen and 4 (11.4%) had antrum gastritis. In 2 (5.7%) intestinal metaplasia was seen. Upon biopsy, pangastritis was present in 33/35 (94.3%). Five cases presented with atrophy and four of these had intestinal metaplasia. *Helicobacter pylori* was detected in the excluded stomach in 7/35 (20%) of cases and in the gastric stump in 12/35 (34.3%). They advised to treat Hp because of the findings at endoscopy and histology, based on the fact that duodenogastric reflux of bile and pancreatic secretions is not any longer buffered by food and that both Hp and bile reflux have synergistic effects on the development of intestinal metaplasia and thus may increase the gastric cancer risk [41].

4.2.6 Predictors of Significant Endoscopic Findings in the Preoperative Period

As most guidelines trust surgeons to decide on the need of an endoscopy in the preoperative workup, characteristics predicting findings during endoscopy might be helpful in the decision.

Age, gender, ethnicity, BMI, GI symptoms, H_2 blocker or PPI use, cigarette or alcohol use, haemoglobin and glucose values did not predict the presence or absence of significant lesions preoperatively [7, 8, 19]. The only study that showed a correlation between GI symptoms and endoscopic findings was that of Korenkov et al. in Germany who found that GI symptoms had a sensitivity of 80% and specificity of 98% in predicting an GI abnormality [7]. Carabotti et al. in an Italian population found lower values of a sensitivity of 40.3% and specificity of 54.7% [10]. In Fernandes' study, the presence of Hp was a significant predictor of abnormal endoscopy (OR 10.3 (3.97/26.94)); age only slightly predicted abnormalities (OR 1.03 (1.00/1.06)) [31]. Lee et al. found in univariate analysis in a population in Singapore age, use of NSAIDs and presence of reflux symptoms to be significant risk factors for clinically relevant lesions [21]. After multivariate analysis NSAIDs and reflux symptoms remained.

4.3 Preoperative Workup and the Role of Manometry and pH Measurements

Analogous to the discussion about the role of preoperative endoscopy there has been a debate about preoperative manometry and 24-h pH measurements, mainly in the time when predominantly gastric banding was used but now also related to the use of sleeve gastrectomy.

Gastric banding and vertical banded gastroplasty are both restrictive procedures for the treatment of morbid obesity. These procedures have been reported to cause GORD while others described beneficial or no effects on gastro-oesophageal reflux [16, 42–46]. On the 3rd summit the reasons why sleeve gastrectomy may increase or reduce gastro-oesophageal reflux were discussed at length [47]. Promoting factors for gastro-oesophageal reflux are the gastric small volume of 100 mL, a disrupted phreno-oesophageal ligament and a resection or division of the sling fibres, thereby reducing the lower oesophageal sphincter pressure (LOSP), and also a narrow sleeve at the angularis might create an obstruction [48]. In contrast, there are also reasons why the sleeve may reduce gastro-oesophageal reflux: removal of the fundus with less transient LOS relaxations (TLOSRs), decreased acid production and accelerated gastric emptying. Also, a dilated upper sleeve and intrathoracic sleeve migration may result in persistent regurgitation. Himpens et al. reported a biphasic pattern of reflux, with an increase in the first 6 months supposed to be related to poor patient compliance, and then a decrease in GORD till 3 years, and between 3 and 6 years GORD symptoms increased to 21% [49]. As these symptoms were usually after meals and never at night, this may indicate stasis and not reflux. However, preoperative and post-operative functional data by manometry and 24-h pH measurements are lacking. At 6 years Himpens et al. found a regrowth of the fundus. Moreover, the 6-year increase in reflux paralleled the increase in BMI [49]. On the 3rd summit in 2011 50% of surgeons agreed that all patients should have 24-h pH measurements and manometry before a sleeve gastrectomy if they complained of reflux [47]. However, in the 5th summit only 32.8% agreed on the question whether patients should have a formal pH measurement and manometry study before having a laparoscopic sleeve gastrectomy [12].

Many small studies including less than 50 patients have reported on the abnormalities in 24-h pH recording and manometry and on the changes after LAGB and RYGB. Jaffin et al. and Greenstein et al. participated in the US multicentre

FDA-moderated study on gastric banding which required a routine upper GI barium study to exclude patients with a significant hernia [50, 51]. Also the function of the oesophagus to clear swallowed contrast water was documented. Concerns about operation-induced oesophageal (dys)function led them to evaluate oesophageal motility with well-defined definitions of abnormalities [50, 51]. A total of 111 patients were evaluated and in 68/111 (61%) abnormal manometric findings were observed. Forty of the 68 (58.8%) with motility abnormalities were asymptomatic. Twenty-eight patients (25%) had a hypotensive LOS (<10 mmHg), and 11 had a low LOSP as secondary diagnosis, so 39 (35.1%) had a hypotensive LOS. Sixteen patients (14%) had nutcracker oesophagus (amplitude >180 mmHg), 15 (14%) had non-specific oesophageal motility disorders (abnormal peristalsis occurring >30% and not assignable to any other category), 8 (7%) had diffuse oesophageal spasm (>30% simultaneous contractions with intermittent normal peristalsis) and 1 (1%) had achalasia (incomplete relaxation of the LOS and 100% aperistalsis). Symptoms of GORD occurred significantly more in patients with a lower LOSP (66% vs. 20%).There was a lack of correlation between the BMI and LOSP. So, a majority of patients had abnormal manometric patterns without oesophageal symptoms, which is uncommon in patients suffering from a nutcracker oesophagus or diffuse oesophageal spasms. Usually, these disorders are associated with either chest pain or dysphagia. The perception of sensations arising from the GI tract may be diminished in obese subjects and impaired visceral sensation, likely to be ascribed to a dysfunction of the autonomic nervous system, might explain the asymptomatic presence of manometric and endoscopic lesions [10]. In this context, only relying on symptoms for further workup as recommended by the guidelines may overlook the presence of clinically relevant abnormalities.

Suter et al. performed endoscopy, manometry and 24-h pH recording in a very large group of 345 subjects accepted for bariatric surgery [52]. They used the same definitions of manometric abnormalities as Jaffin et al. [50]. One hundred and nineteen patients (35.8%) reported at least monthly reflux symptoms such as heartburn or regurgitation. Endoscopy showed a hiatus hernia (defined as ≥1 cm) in 181 patients (52.6%) and reflux oesophagitis in 108 (31.4%). 24-h pH monitoring revealed an elevated DeMeester score in 163 patients (51.7%) and 213 patients (61.8%) had an increased number of reflux episodes. It is relevant to know that almost half of the patients, not reporting reflux symptoms, had abnormal findings at 24-h pH monitoring. Manometry was normal in 247 patients, but abnormal in 85/332 patients (25.6%), with an LOSP <10 mmHg in 59 (17.7%), incomplete LOS relaxations in 10 (3%), hypertensive LOS in 4 (1.2%), nutcracker oesophagus in 16 (4.8%) and a nonspecific motility disorder in 14 (4.2%). So, more than one-third of their patients had at least monthly symptoms suggestive of gastro-oesophageal reflux, more than half had a hiatus hernia and almost one-third had GORD, as proven by the presence of peptic oesophagitis. More than one-half of patients had abnormal pH measurements and one in four had an abnormal manometry. So, indeed the question arises what these findings mean in the context of bariatric surgery and to what extent they may improve by weight loss.

4.4 Role of the Gastroenterologist in Preoperative Workup

The gastroenterologist and endoscopist are on the one side struck by the many symptoms and comorbidities as discussed in the first chapter; on the other they are also fully aware that absence of symptoms does not guarantee the absence of lesions. They should consider how the above-mentioned endoscopic lesions and manometric abnormalities might interfere with decision-making and choice of the bariatric procedure. Therefore, they should have knowledge on the role of *Helicobacter pylori* in post-operative complications as this might require eradication before the procedure but also a check on effective eradication, on the impact of abnormal manometric findings on post-operative outcomes and on specific conditions such as inflammatory bowel disease. The gastroenterologist may also be consulted in case of cholelithiasis and abnormal liver tests and besides the usual workup and diagnosis he/she should also warn against a too fast weight loss to prevent liver function deterioration and in case of gallstones prescribe ursodeoxycholic acid and dissuade from total fat abstinence, as discussed in Chap. 1. Finally, the gastroenterologist may be asked to assist in preoperative weight loss, and so knowledge of the sense and nonsense of preoperative weight loss should be available.

4.4.1 Role of *Helicobacter pylori*

Although the gold standard for *H. pylori* detection has been the endoscopic biopsy, with CLO (campylobacter-like organisms) testing, histology and cultures, endoscopy is not needed anymore as other tests are available. Serology is less sensitive (85%) and specific (79%) than histology (>95% for both) and does not necessarily indicate active infection. The serum antibody remains positive irrespective of active or resolved infection and antibodies may persist for a substantial duration even after eradication and thus overestimate the true prevalence of Hp. Similar to histology, urea breath testing ($100) and faecal antigen testing ($125) detect active infection and both have sensitivity and specificity of >95% [53]. Apart from the inclusion of *Helicobacter pylori* in group 1 of human carcinogens in 1994 by the International Agency for Research on Cancer, two meta-analyses have concluded that *Helicobacter pylori* is related to gastric cancer which may be relevant in the excluded stomach after RYGB [54–56]. Many studies have confirmed the high prevalence of Hp varying between 20% and 97%, in Middle East countries such as Iran, Egypt, Libya, Saudi Arabia and Turkey, which is related to socioeconomic status, crowding and sanitation but not to BMI. The opinion is that patients undergoing weight loss surgery have a greater prevalence of Hp compared to the general population in Western countries [57]. However, the combined prevalence of Hp as calculated from 13 studies is 30.3% (range, 11–42%) comparable to the prevalence in industrialised countries [57].

The role of *H. pylori* in post-operative complications, if present, might be a reason to postpone surgery. The presence of a waiting list for bariatric surgery gives the opportunity, not only to diagnose and treat *H. pylori*, but also to confirm its eradication. Most of the studies investigating the role of Hp in complications dealt with RYGB and sleeve gastrectomy.

4.4.1.1 Roux-En-Y Gastric Bypass

Marginal ulcers: Patients tested and treated for *H. pylori* had a lower incidence of marginal ulcers (5/206, 2.4%) than patients not undergoing such testing (24/354, 6.8%) after RYGB [30]. Also Rasmussen et al. found Hp at more than twice the rate in patients developing marginal ulcers (32% vs. 12%) in a retrospective study of 260 patients [58]. Chronic gastritis and intestinal metaplasia induced by Hp infection are known to regress slowly, sometimes over 18 months [59]. Loewen et al. performed RYGB and 34 patients (13%) developed ulceration [60]. Gastritis and duodenitis but not Hp were related to ulcer formation which may implicate the need of a better and more effective preoperative medical therapy. In Fernandes' study, 43 out of 342 (12.6%) operated patients suffered from post-operative complications and 2 (0.6%) died [31]. Only endoscopic ulceration predicted post-operative complications (OR 11.1 (1.8/68.47)); all ulcers were infected with *Helicobacter pylori*. Post-operative fistula was associated with gastric (OR 13.3 (2.07/85.24)) and duodenal ulcers (OR 19.94 (1.19/333.46)), post-operative sepsis was associated with gastric ulceration (OR 10.28 (1.03/102.63)) and age was of influence in the advent of gastrointestinal bleeding (OR 1.10 (1.01/1.20)). However, confidence intervals are wide. Yangs' study included 82 patients out of 636 patients who developed gastrointestinal symptoms after bariatric surgery and who received gastroscopic examinations [61]. IgG antibodies against Hp were measured preoperatively. Hp positivity was similar among patients with (32/82, 39%) and without complaints (220/554, 39.7%). Twenty-two (26.8%) of 82 symptomatic patients had a gastric ulcer (stomal or marginal ulcer) and no differences as to age, gender, BMI and Hp status were found. Patients with laparoscopic RYGB had significant more ulcers than laparoscopic VBG patients (45.5% vs. 20.0%). So, Yang et al. concluded that gastric ulcers in symptomatic patients were related to the surgical procedures rather than to exposure to *H. pylori* [61]. A study of 422 patients also did not confirm the increased risk of marginal ulcers or pouch gastritis in those tested versus not tested [57]. Similarly, Marano et al. showed a rate of 52% of anastomotic ulcers in symptomatic patients after gastric bypass, representing 6% of all patients [62]. None of the ulcers found was associated with the presence of Hp and all ulcers healed after PPI treatment. Lee et al. showed that of the 12 marginal ulcers, found after RYGB, only 1 was Helicobacter positive and 2 patients admitted to use NSAIDs [63].

Perforations: Another retrospective study in 183 patients demonstrated a higher perforation rate in the unscreened/untreated group versus the Helicobacter-screened and -treated group (5% vs. 0%) and although not significant there was a trend towards reduction of post-operative foregut symptoms, perforated ulcers, GI bleeding, marginal ulcer, stricture and need for endoscopic evaluation in the untested and untreated group [64]. The prevalence of *Helicobacter pylori* in this study, however, was low (12%).

4.4.1.2 Gastric Sleeve

Five studies did not report an increased risk of surgical complications in sleeve gastrectomy when *H. pylori* was present [35, 39, 65–67]. In the retrospective study by Almazeedi et al. only symptomatic patients were evaluated by upper GI endoscopy and CLO testing for Helicobacter which, if positive, was followed by triple therapy [65]. Of the 286 (42.0%) symptomatic patients who had an upper GI endoscopy for diagnosis of their symptoms, quite a substantial number of 140 (49%) had *H. pylori* on the CLO test. 396 asymptomatic patients had no preoperative endoscopy; of these 30 (7.7%) were positive for *H. pylori*, demonstrated later by analysis of the removed sleeve specimen. On the specimen 629/682 were Hp negative (92.2%) and 53 (7.8%) were Hp positive. So, most of the Hp-positive patients (93.6%) who took triple therapy were rendered negative by the time of the surgery. Thirty-two patients (4.7%) had post-operative complications, such as 5 leaks (0.8%), 5 bleeds (0.8%), 5 collections (0.8%) and furthermore 8 cases of neuropathy (1.2%), 2 respiratory failure (0.3%) and 2 hair loss (0.3%). There was no association between Hp and these post-SG complications. In Lauti's study staple-line leaks occurred in 2.0%, a haemorrhage in 1.2% and both in 0.2% with no relation with Hp infection [39]. Atrophic gastritis and intestinal metaplasia were present in 28 (2.9%) of patients and if Hp gastritis is included the rate of diagnosis indicating an increased cancer risk is 12.4%. In sleeve gastrectomy the argument for a preoperative gastroscopy is less strong than for gastric bypass. Moreover, *H. pylori* can be diagnosed from the operative specimen which is cost-effective.

So, according to the 2007 Maastricht III Consensus Report *Helicobacter pylori* eradication is indicated in patients with peptic ulcer disease and low-grade MALT lymphoma, patients with atrophic gastritis, first-degree relatives of patients with gastric cancer, patients with unexplained iron-deficiency anaemia and patients with idiopathic thrombocytopenic purpura [68]. Arguments for routine *Helicobacter pylori* testing include the possible greater rate of anastomotic ulcer and GI bleeding in non-treated Hp-positive patients, the difficulty in assessing the gastric remnant after RYGB for peptic ulcer disease and gastric malignancy, and a potentially lower rate of post-operative dyspeptic symptoms [57]. Arguments against routine testing include the lack of consensus on screening the general population, no differences in anastomotic ulcer between those tested and not tested, the increased risk of *C. difficile* colitis by the treatment and the obligation to treat patients once tested positive [57]. It should be emphasised that effective eradication of *Helicobacter pylori* should always be documented, which is easy by stool antigen testing. In many surgical studies reported here, effective eradication was not checked.

4.4.2 Impact of Abnormal Manometry and 24-h pH Measurements on Post-bariatric Outcomes

4.4.2.1 Gastric Restrictive Operations

One of the criticisms of the laparoscopic adjustable gastric banding but also of the sleeve gastrectomy has been the potential to cause oesophageal dysmotility and dilation because of an increased outflow resistance and outlet obstruction caused by gastric banding. The four studies that performed manometry in obese subjects had some conspicuous findings: motility disorders already before the operation, a nutcracker oesophagus and contractions with an amplitude >180 mmHg, reminiscent

Table 4.4 Summary of manometric data in preoperative bariatric patients [50, 52, 69, 70]. Numbers of manometric data exceed the abnormal numbers as patients may have more than one manometric abnormality

Author	Abnormal N/total	Defective/ hypotensive LOS	Hypertensive-non-relaxing LOS	Diffuse spasms	Nutcracker oesophagus	Amplitude contractions >180 mmHg	Motility disorders unspecified
Hong '04 [69]	33/61	10	11	2	6	20	15
Jaffin '99 [50]	68/111	39	1	8	16	16	15
Suter '04 [52]	85/332	59	14	–	16	–	14
Valezi '12 [70]	37/81	7	11	–	–	16 (increased amplitude)	3

of a nutcracker-like distal oesophagus, often asymptomatic [50, 52, 69, 70] (Table 4.4). A possible mechanism for the latter observation was discussed: the high intra-abdominal-thoracic pressure gradient might cause a functional outlet obstruction of the oesophagus, creating a high-pressure zone within the oesophagus [69]. For the passage of oral contents into the stomach the distal oesophagus would have to produce high-amplitude contractions. Any additional restriction by a restrictive gastric procedure might aggravate this situation.

Greenstein et al. tried to correlate their manometric and endoscopic findings with reoperation and slippage after gastric banding. Two factors were identified to predispose to band slippage: a large hiatal hernia and oesophageal manometry abnormalities [51]. A combination of both hiatus hernia and oesophageal dysmotility potentiated the likelihood of requiring reoperation [51].

Korenkow et al. analysed oesophageal motility disorders and GORD before and after gastric banding and gastric bypass [71]. In contrary to the previously mentioned studies they did not find a high incidence of primary motility disturbances. In the LAGB group nine patients had a preoperative incompetent LOS sphincter; after surgery six of them had a normal function of the LOS. In the RYGB group four had an incompetent LOS function preoperatively; after surgery three of them had a normal function of the LOS. Out of a total of 50 patients analysed, 8 (16%) had reflux symptoms and a pathological DeMeester score and, although the LOS function was improved mainly after LAGB, neither the LAGB nor RYGB influenced GORD. Of note, in the LAGB group eight patients had achalasia-like symptoms after adjustment of the band post-operatively and symptoms were relieved by emptying the band and readjusting the volume. Also Bueter et al. could not demonstrate an adverse outcome after gastric banding because of the presence of a hiatal hernia, oesophagitis, abnormal pH-metry or presence of motility disorders [72].

Klaus and Weiss advise a preoperative oesophageal manometry in any restrictive procedures such as the LAGB and the SG because functional disorders of the oesophageal body and a lower oesophageal sphincter can be identified before surgery [73]. In patients with a weak oesophageal body LAGB should not be considered a therapeutic option because oesophageal dilation, oesophageal stasis and oesophagitis could occur. In patients with a weak LOS pressure, the angle of His is taken away after sleeve gastrectomy without increasing the pressure of the muscular high-pressure zone with a wrap as is done in a fundoplication procedure. They are at risk of developing GORD symptoms or have ongoing or worsening symptoms after the operation. The fact that with time GORD symptoms may improve may be related to the acceleration of gastric emptying as shown by Melissas et al. [74]. Klaus and Weiss considered the RYGB to be an excellent procedure for both morbid obesity and GORD, because both acid and bile are excluded from the upper GI tract and thereby no longer reach the distal oesophagus. The fact that nonetheless about 28% of patients after RYGB experience persisting or recurrent GORD symptoms may be explained by the aggregation of parietal cells in the cardia.

4.4.2.2 Roux-en-Y Gastric Bypass

Eighty-one patients undergoing RYGB had a manometry before and 1 year after the operation [70]. Before the operation 37 (45.6%) of patients had abnormal manometry findings: hypertensive LOS in 11 (29.8%), hypotensive LOS in 7 (18.9%), an increase in the wave amplitude of contractions in 16 (43.2%) and abnormal peristalsis in 3 (8.1%) [70]. One year after the RYGB operation manometry was repeated and was found to be abnormal in 51 (62.9%) with hypertensive and hypotensive LES in 6 (11.7%) and 8 (15.7%), respectively. In 27 (53%) the amplitude of contractions changed and in 10 (19.6%) abnormal peristalsis was seen. Although mean values of LOS decreased, amplitude of waves increased, duration of waves increased and normal peristalsis decreased significantly after RYGB in preoperatively asymptomatic patients, Valezi et al. did not recommend to perform routine manometry [70].

4.4.3 Gastrointestinal Conditions that May Interfere in the Decision-Making

Besides the gastrointestinal comorbidities that are associated with obesity, there are also certain conditions where obesity may offer an increased risk or may impact the outcome. Obesity is a chronic low-grade inflammatory state and a risk factor for inflammatory diseases such as cardiovascular disease, non-alcoholic steatohepatitis and pancreatitis (see Chap. 1). In retrospective studies an association between BMI and diverticular disease has been found. There are two large prospective studies in men: a prospective cardiovascular prevention trial in Sweden where the admission rate for symptomatic diverticular disease could be assessed over a period of 28 years, and the Health Professionals Study with self-reported diverticular disease in a follow-up of 18 years [75, 76]. In the Swedish study, admission rates were in 42.7% for diverticulitis, 14.3% for perforation and 14.3% for bleeding [75]. Men with a BMI 20–22.5 kg/m^2 had the lowest risk and risks increased by a factor of 3 in overweight and 4.4 with obesity. In the larger Health

Professionals Study, the risks of both diverticulitis and diverticula bleeding could be assessed [76]. When compared with those with a BMI <21 kg/m^2 subjects with a BMI $\geq$30 kg/m^2 had a 1.8 times higher risk of diverticulitis and a 3.2 times higher risk of a diverticular bleed. Subjects in the highest quintile of waist circumference and waist/hip ratio had a 1.6 times higher risk of diverticulitis and a 1.9 higher risk for diverticular bleed. Also, weight gain was an important predictor of risks: men who gained more than 45 lb. since age 21 years had an RR of 1.66 for diverticulitis and 2.44 for diverticular bleeding when compared with men who gained less than 5 lb. [76]. A Japanese study not only measured the BMI but also the visceral and subcutaneous fat areas by CT scanning [77]. This study showed that obesity, particularly visceral obesity, was a risk factor for left-sided diverticulitis in Japan.

The presence of diverticular disease will not interfere with the decision-making, but the presence of inflammatory bowel disease (IBD) and more specifically Crohn's disease certainly will interfere, for instance with the choice of the type of surgery, i.e. gastric or intestinal bariatric surgery, where outcomes should be weighed one against the other. Also, the prevalence of obesity among IBD patients, the impact of overweight and obesity on the disease course, the role of creeping fat and the outcomes after surgery should be taken into deliberation.

4.4.3.1 Prevalence of Overweight and Obesity Among IBD Patients

Previously held beliefs regarding patients with IBD commonly being underweight are no longer correct. Patients experiencing a flare of their disease have a significantly lower body weight than during remission because of a reduced caloric intake due to lack of appetite and abdominal pain, increased energy and protein requirements because of fever, inflammation and exudative enteropathy with protein loss, and catabolic side effects of treatment. On the other hand, the incidence of obesity is increasing worldwide and many recent studies have documented a growing prevalence of obesity in IBD patients. Whereas Blain et al. from France reported a prevalence of obesity of 3% in 2002, Steeda et al. reported 7 years later a prevalence of overweight in 38% and of obesity in 18% in a Scottish IBD population, without a difference between Crohn's disease (CD) and ulcerative colitis (UC) patients and being similar of slightly less than the prevalence in the normal population [78, 79]. Moran et al. reviewed 40 randomised controlled trials involving a total of 10,282 patients with Crohn's disease conducted between 1991 and 2008 and observed a significant increase in weight and body mass index over the time period [80].

Three recent studies from 2015 had BMI data on 202 UC patients and 581 and 1494 IBD patients [81–83]. UC patients were underweight in 5%, 55% had a normal weight, 26.7% were overweight and 13.4% were obese [81]. Of 581 identified IBD patients, 2.6% were underweight, only 29.9% had a normal weight, 34.8% were overweight and 32.7% obese [82]. The rate of obesity was 30.3% among CD patients and 35.2% among UC patients. Among 1494 patients with IBD, 71.9% were above their ideal BMI and 31.5% were obese [83]. Underweight patients with IBD were rare (1.8% of the cohort). In this study, obesity was more common in ulcerative colitis compared with patients with Crohn's disease. All studies agreed that IBD was diagnosed at an older age in obese subjects. So, most of the data suggest that the rates of obesity in IBD are equivalent to the general population and that underweight is the exception rather than the rule.

4.4.3.2 The Impact of Obesity on the Course of the Inflammatory Bowel Disease and on Treatment

The rise in the prevalence of IBD in Western countries has not been as dramatic as the rise in the prevalence of obesity. This suggests that obesity is not contributing to the pathogenesis of IBD and that the increase in the frequency of obesity in IBD patients merely reflects the rising frequency of obesity in the general population [84]. In support of this contention, obesity was not found to be associated with the development of IBD in a large cohort of 300,724 participants who were recruited into the European Prospective Investigation into Cancer and Nutrition study (IBD in EPIC study) [84]. In contrast, a recent large US prospective cohort study found obesity to be associated with an increased risk of CD but not UC [85].

Mendall et al. performed an adequately powered analysis to find a 2.25 higher risk of IBD by the presence of obesity which required 500 IBD subjects [86]. A total of 524 consecutive IBD patients and a control group of 480 community controls aged 50–70 were included. Obesity at diagnosis was twice as common in subjects with Crohn's disease versus ulcerative colitis and 3.2 times as common versus community controls. There was evidence of a "dose response" with increasing degrees of obesity associated with increased risk. Low BMI at diagnosis was also associated with the risk of Crohn's disease versus ulcerative colitis. So, there was a suggestion of a U-shaped relationship between body mass index at diagnosis and risk of CD versus UC with both high and low BMI being associated with risks [86].

As will be discussed later, obesity, being itself a chronic low-grade inflammatory state with chronic activation of the innate immune system within the adipose tissue, with actively secreting visceral fat and creeping fat around affected bowel segments, might increase the risk for IBD and IBD flares. It may also worsen outcome whereas, in contrast, it may also be a marker of less severe disease. Unfortunately, most of the studies only considered the WHO BMI classes without taking into account the distribution of fat stores.

Course of the Disease

Three studies in the era before the use of biologicals, in the period of 2002–2008, and a review of Moran et al. of 40 randomised controlled trials (RCTs) involving a total of 10,282 patients with CD conducted between 1991 and 2008 reported a negative outcome in patients with overweight and obesity [78, 80, 87, 88]. Blain et al. showed more and earlier onset of anorectal and perineal complications, a more marked year-by-year disease activity and the need of more hospitalisations for disease activity in obese patients, but without significant worsening of the long-term course [78]. Hass et al. compared patients with overweight (BMI $\geq$25 kg/m^2) to a non-overweight group (BMI <25 kg/m^2) and found no differences as to the number of surgeries, escalation of therapy and disease distribution between the two groups [87]. The median time to first surgery was not significantly different: 24 months for those with a BMI ≥25 kg/m^2 versus 72 months for those with a BMI <25 kg/m^2. However, on subgroup analysis, a significant difference for time to first surgery was found when patients with a BMI of less than 18.5 kg/m^2 were compared with those with a BMI ≥25 kg/m^2 or higher: 252 months versus 24 months [87]. The authors concluded that overweight and obese patients experienced a more severe disease course and/or less effective treatment. Kiran et al. retrospectively reviewed their results in ileoanal pouch anastomosis after colectomy [88]. There were 1671 patients in group A (median BMI 23.8 kg/m^2) and 345 patients (median BMI 32.7 kg/m^2) in group B. Group B patients had a significantly higher risk of the development of wound infection and anastomotic dehiscence, whereas group A patients had a higher rate of development of obstruction over time. The incidence of complications such as pouchitis, sepsis, haemorrhage and anastomotic stricture was similar in both groups. In the 40 RCTs study subjects demonstrated a significant increase in clinical disease activity as measured by the Crohn's disease activity index (CDAI) and disease duration over the same time period [80]. When analysing all subject data CDAI and weight did not correlate significantly. Restricting the analysis to subjects with a moderate-to-severe disease activity (CDAI >250) at baseline revealed a significant correlation between these two parameters.

Studies conducted at a time when biologic therapy for IBD was available show virtually the opposite [81–83]. In 202 UC patients in a matched-pair analysis of normal weight versus overweight/obesity the proportion of patients with pancolitis was inversely related to weight and BMI; a significantly higher proportion of years with chronic active disease and proportion of years with disease complications were found among normal-weight subjects versus overweight subjects and more overweight than normal-weight patients had no chronic active disease in any year [81]. In matched-pair analysis of underweight versus normal-weight patients, the disease activity and hospital admission rate were higher for underweight subjects. So, a high BMI had rather a favourable effect on the prognosis, whereas low BMI pointed to a more severe course of the disease [81]. Flores et al. came to the same conclusion in their cohort of 544 IBD patients and found that obesity was a marker of a less severe disease course in IBD [82]. Overall, obese patients were significantly less likely to receive anti-TNF treatment, undergo surgery or experience a hospitalisation for their IBD than their thinner counterparts. When looking at the 297 CD and 284 UC patients separately, obese or overweight CD patients and overweight and obese UC patients were less likely to have had either anti-TNF use, surgery or hospitalisation during the last decade [82]. Overweight and obesity appeared to be protective risk factors against experiencing one of the adverse outcomes, after being adjusted for the other predictors in the model [82]. In the largest study by Seminerio et al. in 1494 IBD patients, there was no association between increasing BMI and annual prednisone use, emergency department visits, hospitalisation and surgery [83]. In this study, patients with IBD who were overweight (BMI 25–30 kg/m^2) enjoyed the best clinical status with the best mean quality-of-life scores, the lowest rates of CRP elevation and the lowest rates of hospitalisation compared with the normal-weight and obese patients with IBD [83].

Need of (Adjustment of) Treatment

Anti-TNF agents are effective in inducing and maintaining remission in Crohn's disease. Infliximab by intravenous infusion is weight adjusted, and adalimumab is a subcutaneous injection, not weight adjusted and with a dose frequency based on clinical response. Bhalme et al. investigated whether obesity is a risk factor for early loss of response to anti-TNF treatment and whether weight-adjusted anti-TNF treatment is preferable [89]. An increased weight as measured by BMI appeared to be predictive of anti-TNF treatment failure, specifically in the case of adalimumab rather than infliximab. Dose escalation because of loss of response to adalimumab after a median time of 7.0 months was needed in 20% of patients [89]. A similar proportion developed loss of response to infliximab but after a median time of 13.0 months. An increase of 1 unit in BMI corresponded to an increase in hazard of loss of response of 8.2%. So, obesity is an independent predictor of loss of response to adalimumab which is not apparent for infliximab-treated patients, which may reflect the fact that infliximab is weight adjusted [89]. This study could, however, not answer the question whether the findings were related to the pharmacokinetic properties of such drugs in obese individuals, such as the volume of distribution and drug clearance, or were related to the excess of circulating pro-inflammatory adipokines in the obese.

Others have also suggested that obesity was associated with an earlier time to loss of response to infliximab or with decreased response over time to adalimumab requiring more dose escalations in patients with IBD [90, 91]. However, one study found that obese and overweight IBD patients had significantly less use of anti-TNF therapy than normal or underweight patients and another found that obese patients with IBD were receiving dosages of medications, which were overall below guidelines for actual body weight but were similar to calculated dosages targeting ideal body weight [82, 83]. The responsiveness to azathioprine was investigated in a multicentre study in 818 CD patients and 358 UC patients [92]. A negative correlation was observed between BMI and therapeutic efficacy in UC patients but not CD patients. However, after discontinuation of azathioprine, the incidence of flares was significantly lower in overweight and obese CD patients than in normal or underweight patients, whereas no weight-related differences were seen in UC patients.

Creeping Fat

Creeping fat or fat wrapping is a characteristic feature of Crohn's disease, where ectopic adipose tissue extending from the mesenteric attachment is wrapped around the diseased intestine. Its appearance is often used by surgeons as a measure of the extent of active disease, and it correlates with the degree of bowel inflammation and with the severity of colitis [93–95]. There are two hypotheses: 1. the accumulation of visceral fat is a response to impaired intestinal permeability with increased bacterial translocation and release of pro-inflammatory cytokines or 2. mediators released from the visceral fat increase the permeability of the mucosal barrier, thereby facilitating bacterial translocation and promoting inflammatory processes [94]. Taken together, creeping fat can be regarded as a consequence of, or as a cause of, intestinal inflammation in CD. In the latter situation, this mesenteric adipose tissue and creeping fat are not innocent bystanders but actively contribute to the intestinal and systemic inflammatory responses in patients with IBD [93, 94]. CD is associated with a Th1 T-cell-mediated response, characterised by enhanced production of IL-1, IL-2, IL-6, IL-12, IL-18, TNF-a and interferon gamma. In UC, the local immune response is less polarised, but there is enhanced production of Th2 cytokines IL-4, IL-5 and IL-10. In visceral fat, macrophage infiltration is two- to fourfold higher than in subcutaneous fat tissue [94, 96]. The infiltrating macrophage population harbours a broad spectrum of subtypes with two major subtypes of pro-inflammatory M1 macrophages and immune-regulatory M2 macrophages [96]. Obesity has been associated with an increase in M1 macrophages, characterised by enhanced production of IL-6 and TNF-α. Unfortunately, mostly BMI as a measure of general adiposity is used when studying the outcome of IBD. In a study by Buning et al. the ratio of visceral to total fat in Crohn's disease was studied and a higher ratio has been associated with increased disease activity, a stricturing/fistulising course of disease, higher serum levels of IL-6 and more short-term than long-term remission rates [97].

4.4.3.3 Post-bariatric Outcomes

Safety and Efficacy of Bariatric Surgery

A systematic review yielded seven studies reporting post-bariatric surgery outcomes in 43 inflammatory bowel disease (IBD) patients: 25 patients with Crohn's disease and 18 with ulcerative colitis with a BMI ranging between 35.7 and 71 kg/m^2 [98]. Sleeve gastrectomy was performed in 77% of Crohn's disease patients and RYGB and sleeve each in 44.4% of ulcerative colitis patients. Nine early (24.4%) and ten late (23.8%) complications occurred. Surgery was effective with a weight loss of 14.3 BMI units in a follow-up of 8 to 77 months. More importantly, IBD remitted in 20 patients (47.6%), improved in 2 patients (4.8%), showed no change in 12 (28.6%) but exacerbated in 7 (16.7%).

New Onset of Crohn's Disease after Bariatric Surgery

Both Bernstein and Pickett-Blakely and Korelitz et al. reviewed the literature and both found the same 7 reported cases of new-onset Crohn's disease after RYGB, to which they added 2 and 5 cases, respectively, to a summary of 14 cases [95, 99]. A conspicuous finding is that all cases, except one after jejunoileal bypass, were reported after RYGB with a delay of 4 weeks to 10 years. Most of the patients were female and aged between 28 and 69 years. The most common presenting symptoms were diarrhoea and abdominal pain, which are among the most common symptoms after gastric bypass, along with unexplained weight loss, particularly in a patient who had the procedure many years before or had a previously stable weight. The onset of CD might be a coincidence in time but might also be related to the pathophysiologic changes specific to the bypass. Altogether 3 of the 14 subjects had onset of symptoms soon after the bariatric surgery while 11 of the 14 developed the syndrome more than a year later, making an activation of a preclinical phase of the disease by the surgical intervention less likely. Korelitz et al. suggested that, as long as it is not clear whether de novo onset of Crohn's disease is due to rapid metabolism of fat during rapid weight loss with massive release of TNF-α from fatty tissue, or due to changes in the anatomy, with the loss of defence mechanisms of the stomach, changes in the microbiota or a direct presentation of food, toxins and chemicals to the small intestine, alternative bariatric procedures leaving the anatomy in its native state should probably be chosen to minimise the overall risk of developing IBD [95]. From the review by Shoar et al. it seemed that Crohn's disease patients were indeed more frequently considered for non-intestinal bariatric procedures such as sleeve gastrectomy [98].

4.4.4 Sense and Nonsense of Preoperative Weight Loss

Severely obese patients are at higher risk of developing perioperative and postoperative complications related to their surplus in weight with mechanical consequences and their obesity-related metabolic alterations. Moreover, from a technical standpoint of view, a laparoscopic surgical approach may be problematic or impossible in patients who have a very high body mass index, central obesity or a large liver (Table 4.5) [100]. Preoperative weight loss may facilitate the laparoscopic approach, by decreasing liver size and by reducing the visceral adipose tissue mass, enabling better visibility and easier access to the upper stomach and oesophagus. In addition to the potential to improve technical factors with reduced operation time and decreased complication risk, the response to energy restriction and even a modest decrease of 5% of body weight will improve insulin resistance and serum glucose concentrations and will decrease cardiovascular and thromboembolic complications, and inflammation [101, 102]. Requiring preoperative weight loss

Table 4.5 Potential advantages and disadvantages of medical weight management programmes (modified after Tewksbury et al.) [100]

Potential advantages	Potential disadvantages
• Opportunity to lose weight through less-invasive means • Greater post-operative or total weight losses • Improved technical aspects of surgery such as visibility • Decreased post-operative complications • Shorter operating time • Shorter length of stay • Opportunity to practice post-operative dietary and behaviour changes • Opportunity to improve aberrant metabolic parameters • Opportunity to increase cardiopulmonary fitness by exercise	• Inconsistent definition, treatment and measurement of medical weight management programmes • Unnecessary dieting by patients considered to be dietary veterans • Lack of insurance coverage for visits • Discouraging of patients • Possibly unnecessary delay of necessary treatment • Negative impact by pre-surgical catabolism

might also identify the most motivated patient, who will comply better with the dietary restrictions and lifestyle changes after surgery.

Moreover, most of the preoperative medical weight management programmes are not standardised and should take advantage of the opportunity to teach the dietary and behavioural changes required for bariatric surgery and to document the lack of understanding of these requirements or a lack of willingness to change behaviour which are considered contraindications for surgery [4]. However, potential negative effects include patient discomfort and increased costs and possibly an increased morbidity associated with undergoing surgery in a catabolic state (Table 4.5) [100]. Bariatric patients are "dieting veterans" as shown in 177 pre-bariatric patients who completed a questionnaire and were aided by health professionals in an aided recall [103]. They completed 4.7 ± 2.9 successful weight loss attempts, defined as those that resulted in a 10 lbs. (4.5 kg) or more weight loss but also numerous other efforts that were unsuccessful, totalling to an overall 14.6 ± 9.1 times they tried to lose weight. They reported a mean total lifetime weight loss of 61.1 ± 41.3 kg and despite their efforts their weight increased from 89.4 at age 21.2 years to 144.5 at the time of their pre-bariatric evaluation at age 43.0 years. So, both surgeons and gastroenterologist should have knowledge of the recommendations by guidelines, the evidence from meta-analyses and large cohorts and the several options that are available.

4.4.4.1 Guidelines

The task of the 1991 National Institutes of Health (NIH) panel and the 1998 NIH Expert Panel was to define candidates for surgery [101, 104]. They required the evaluation by an experienced clinician of having a low probability of successful weight loss with non-surgical weight loss methods and less radical means of weight loss should have been attempted prior to surgical intervention. The 2004 Consensus Conference of the ASMBS stated that bariatric surgery candidates should have attempted to lose weight by non-operative means, but should not be required to have completed formal non-operative obesity therapy as a precondition for the operation [105]. The position statement on preoperative supervised weight loss requirements by the ASMBS in 2011 was more rigorous by saying that prolonged preoperative diet efforts that delay, impede or interfere with bariatric surgery are unacceptable without supporting evidence [106]. The Bariatric Surgery Clinical Practice Guidelines issued by the AACE/TOS/ASMBS downgraded their 2008 grade B and the best evidence level of 2 conclusion, that preoperative weight loss should be considered in cases where it may improve technical aspects of the surgery, to grade B and the best evidence level of 1 in 2013 because of inconsistent results [3, 4]. The Canadian Clinical Guidelines for the management of obesity recommend a preoperative weight loss of 10% within 6 months prior to surgery [107].

Preoperative weight loss can be mandated by insurance companies or by the surgical team. Insurance companies require the documentation of failed efforts with conservative weight loss interventions before considering bariatric surgery, but more commonly dictate that patients attend nutritionist, behavioural therapy or physician-supervised sessions of a specific duration of 3–6 months or lose a 5–10% preoperative body weight in order to receive insurance approval and coverage for surgery [106]. The efficacy and justification of the insurance-mandated requirement to lose weight before bariatric surgery have been challenged and many feel that it is inappropriate for decisions regarding access to surgery to be left to insurance companies. Physician-mandated weight loss will be applied to decrease the surgical risk, reduce the size of the liver and visceral fat load, maximise the post-operative weight loss and also to evaluate a patient's ability to adhere to dietary changes and to comply with treatment. Weight losses needed are modest: already a 5% weight loss or greater results in significant changes in glucose metabolism, blood pressure and lipids [101, 102]. Although only one-third of bariatric services, a total of 28 centres, in the UK responded to a survey, a short-term preoperative energy-restrictive diet appeared to be widely adopted to enable surgery by reducing liver size, but the dietary approach was not standardised, with a total of 49 diets in current use [108].

4.4.4.2 Meta-Analyses and Reviews

A total of six meta-analyses and reviews have, all in a different way, tried to answer the question whether preoperative weight loss improved perioperative outcomes such as length and ease of the procedure and post-operative outcomes such as weight loss and complications. They, however, all point towards many differences in methodology such as reporting of operation time and weight loss period.

Tarnoff et al. included only a proportion of the available literature, primarily the four major studies that reported improvements in post-operative outcomes related to preoperative weight loss [109]. They suggested that preoperative weight loss because of decreased complications and shorter procedure times should be a necessary component of the preoperative process. A systematic review and meta-analysis by Livhits et al. included only those studies using post-operative weight loss as a primary outcome and thereby excluded data from a number of studies assessing other significant primary outcomes such as operative time and complication rate [110]. They included 15 studies with a 10–20 lb. preoperative weight loss: 1 randomised controlled trial, 4 prospective cohort studies and 10 retrospective studies. Of the 15 articles ($n = 3404$ patients) identified, 5 found a positive effect of preoperative weight loss on post-operative weight loss, 2 found a positive short-term effect that was not sustained in the long term, 5 did not find an effect difference and 1 found a negative effect. A meta-analysis of the 11 high-quality studies revealed a significant 5% excess weight loss increase in the 1-year post-operative weight for patients who had lost weight preoperatively. A meta-analysis of high-quality studies with significant heterogeneity revealed a 23.3-min decreased operative time for patients who had lost weight preoperatively. Two high-quality studies investigated the length of stay and found no differences; data were not pooled. The authors concluded that a 10% preoperative weight loss may enhance 1-year total weight loss and improve operative times.

Cassie et al. included a total of 27 studies [111]. A total of 17 trials ($N = 4611$) deemed preoperative weight loss to be beneficial and 10 studies ($N = 2075$)

deemed preoperative weight loss to be of no benefit. The operative time of the laparoscopic gastric bypass was 12.5 min shorter for the preoperative weight loss patients in eight trials. Preoperative weight loss was positively correlated with post-operative weight loss in 9 studies ($n = 2177$), and 15 ($n = 3252$) reported no benefit. Nine studies reporting perioperative complications (852 patients) revealed no difference in the complication rates, and two studies (1234 patients) suggested a significant decrease in those with preoperative weight loss. When the studies were pooled those with preoperative weight loss had significantly less, 18.8%, complications versus 21.4% in non-weight-losing patients. Five studies reported on hospital stay which was borderline significantly shorter after weight loss, 3.34 versus 3.98 days. Despite these significant differences, Cassie et al. concluded that variations in the methodology across studies precluded them from making strong statements on the relationship between preoperative weight loss and surgical complications and that there was insufficient data to support preoperative weight loss to improve post-operative weight loss [111]. Ochner et al. focused on the context and effectiveness of preoperative diets and post-operative weight loss outcomes in 29 studies [112]. Three conclusions were drawn: (1) current preoperative requirements held by the majority of third-party payer organisations in the USA are ineffective at fostering weight loss as shown by 3 studies; (2) making the receipt of surgery contingent upon weight loss may be effective in fostering preoperative weight loss: studies where surgery was reportedly withheld if patients did not lose weight reported higher mean preoperative weight loss (15% and 7% total body weight) relative to other comparable programmes; and (3) preoperative weight loss may lead to some improvements in post-operative outcomes: findings from studies of the relation between pre- and post-operative changes in body weight range from a positive relationship (5 studies) to a negative relationship (2 studies) and many in between (no relationship in 12, mixed results in 3). Gerber et al. identified 23 original publications including 2 RCTs, 7 prospective studies, 14 retrospective studies and the mentioned review article by Livhits et al. and Ochner et al. between January 1, 1995, to April 30, 2014 [110, 112, 113]. They concluded that it is not entirely clear whether preoperative weight loss predisposes persons undergoing bariatric surgery to do better. Inconsistent data were reported for operating time and intraoperative complications such as blood loss and recovery. However, beneficial effects following adherence to weight loss prior to bariatric surgery were seen for outcomes such as post-operative complications and weight development over time.

Livhits et al. tried to further identify preoperative psychosocial factors associated with weight loss following bariatric surgery [114]. One hundred and fifteen articles were included in the review. They used a cut-off of at least seven studies and when a domain had ≥ 7 studies it was defined as having sufficient evidence. Factors positively associated with weight loss after surgery included mandatory preoperative weight loss (7 of 14 studies with a positive association). Factors that may be negatively associated with weight loss include preoperative BMI (37 out of 62 studies with negative association), super-obesity (24 out of 33 studies) and personality disorders (7 out of 14 studies).

Summarising these six reviews there is little strong evidence to support or refute the recommendation for preoperative weight loss management [100]. The uncertainty is due to lack of consensus on how to implement and how to standardise preoperative weight loss programmes and also due to methodological concerns with previous studies on this subject. The goal of preoperative weight management should be better defined and may be that the focus should be more on nutrition, psychoeducation, physical activity and behaviour modification rather than on the current measure of preoperative weight loss.

4.4.4.3 Evidence from Large Cohorts

Two studies from the Scandinavian Obesity Register (SOReg), a large population-based cohort including over 22,000 patients with gastric bypass (96.5% laparoscopic), addressed both preoperative weight loss and post-operative complications [115, 116]. No standardised protocol for weight loss was used. The first study by Anderin et al. evaluated the relationship between preoperative weight loss and post-operative complications [115]. Patients were divided into percentiles based on preoperative weight loss, and median preoperative total weight change was 0.5%, −4.7% and −9.5% in the 25th, 50th and 75th percentiles, respectively. At a follow-up of 6 weeks after surgery, complications were noted in 9.1% of all patients. When comparing patients in the 75th to the 25th percentiles of preoperative weight loss in multivariate analysis, the risk of any complication was reduced by 13% (odds ratio (OR) 0.87, 95% CI 0.82–0.94). For specific complications, the corresponding risks were reduced for anastomotic leakage by 24% (OR 0.76, 0.64/0.91), deep infection/abscess by 37% (OR 0.63, 0.43/0.93) and minor wound complications by 54% (OR 0.46, 0.33/0.64). For patients in the 75th percentile range of BMI (>45.8 kg/m^2), the risk reduction associated with preoperative weight loss ranged from an odds ratio of 0.28 (minor wound complication) to 0.55 (post-operative bleeding), so much more pronounced than in patients with lower BMIs.

In the same cohort, 9570 patients with complete data on preoperative weight loss and 2 years post-operative weight loss were analysed [116]. Total preoperative weight loss in the 25th, 50th and75th percentiles was 0%, 4.5% and 8.6%, respectively. When patients in the 50th percentile for preoperative weight loss were compared with those in the 25th percentile, total post-operative weight loss was 5.0% and 5.3% higher at 1 and 2 years, respectively. There was a 42% increased probability (OR 1.42, 1.28/1.57) of losing more weight after 1 year and a 35% increased probability (OR 1.35, 1.23/1.51) of doing so after 2 years in the 50th percentile preoperative weight loss group. Similarly, patients in the 75th percentile for preoperative weight loss lost 11.8% and 10.1% more weight at 1 and 2 years, respectively. Corresponding values of increased probability to lose weight were 139% in the 75th percentile (OR 2.39, 2.10/2.72) after 1 and 88% (OR 1.88, 1.66/2.12) after 2 years. These effects were even more pronounced for patients in the 75th percentile of preoperative BMI (>45.7 kg/m^2). Thus, at 1 and 2 years post-operatively, patients in the 75th percentile of preoperative weight loss and BMI displayed 15.2% and 13.6% increased weight reduction, respectively, compared with patients within the 25th percentile.

So, these data strongly suggest that weight loss prior to bariatric surgery is associated with marked reduction in the risk of post-operative complications and increased chances of ongoing and higher post-operative weight loss [115, 116]. There was a positive dose-response relationship between pre- and post-operative weight loss and preoperative weight loss and complications, the most pronounced in the highest BMI region, signifying that especially patients in the higher range of BMI are likely to benefit most from preoperative weight loss measures.

4.4.4.4 Medical Weight Management Options

In a landmark study from 2006, Colles et al. demonstrated using serial magnetic resonance imaging (MRI) in obese individuals that very-low-calorie diet (VLCD) for 12 weeks was associated with a reduction in liver volume by 20% and 80% of this loss was achieved already during the first 2 weeks of treatment [117]. This relatively short period should enable patients to comply with such a protocol.

Commercial Very-Low-Energy Meal Replacements

Very-low-calorie diets (VLCD) or very-low-energy diets (VLED) consist of nutritionally complete commercially available meal replacement products with a total daily energy content of 1.8–3.8 MJ (450–800 kcal). Commonly, these diets are followed for a defined period (most commonly 8–16 weeks). A systematic review by Ross et al. included 15 studies (591 VLCD and 351 controls), and 13 studies ($n = 750$) involved bariatric patients [118]. The primary aims of the included studies were a 5–10% total body weight loss and a 10% liver shrinkage. Ten out of 14 studies achieved 5–10% total weight loss. Ten out of the 14 studies that reported on weight loss achieved greater than a 5% total weight loss compared to baseline weight. Seven of these studies achieved greater than 10% total weight loss. Two studies reported that the majority of liver volume reduction occurred in the first 2 weeks of intervention. All six studies that measured liver volume achieved reductions of greater than 10% (range 12–43%) and one study reported a reduction in liver size of 5%. However, a study by Andersen reported development of portal fibrosis with rapid weight loss [119]. In their study they provided a 400 kcal formula diet to 41 morbidly obese subjects and found that 24% developed slight portal inflammation and portal fibrosis. However, none of the patients who lost less than 1.6 kg/week developed fibrosis and they defined this to be a safe weight loss. Non-adherence and/or intolerance was calculated at 8%. End points for perioperative risks and outcomes were too varied to support definitive risk benefit and no significant difference in length of stay (LOS) was observed. Improvements in metabolic risk factors such as blood glucose in four studies, insulin in one and lipid levels in two studies were reported.

Exercise

To prescribe another diet to bariatric patients who are already "dieting veterans" may ask for revolt. The American Heart Association recommends that, before undergoing bariatric surgery, patients should perform mild exercises for 20 min/day 3–4 times per week to improve cardiorespiratory fitness, reduce surgical complications, facilitate healing and enhance post-operative recovery [120]. This stimulated Rejane Marcon et al. to investigate a 4-month low-intensity exercise programme with two weekly sessions of 25 min each in 66 morbidly obese individuals awaiting bariatric surgery [121]. Patients were randomised to exercise-only, exercise + behavioural treatment or a control group. The weight change was −7.4 kg, −4.2 kg and +2.9 kg and the BMI change was −2.7, −1.4 and +1.1 kg/m^2 for the groups exercise, exercise + behaviour treatment and control, respectively. Changes were significant when compared to the control group but there were no differences between the two intervention arms. Functional capacity and cardiometabolic parameters such as 6-min walk test, heart and respiration rate before and after exercise, dyspnoea, oxygen saturation and peak oxygen consumption significantly improved in both intervention arms and worsened in the control group. The adherence to the exercise programme in both groups was high and above 78%. A 5% weight loss was observed in 31% of the patients in the exercise group, in 35% of the patients in the exercise + behaviour therapy group and in none of the control group. After the intervention, HDL cholesterol, total cholesterol and glucose levels improved significantly in the exercise group. HDL cholesterol and triglycerides improved in the exercise + behaviour therapy group. Conversely, the control group showed a significant reduction in HDL cholesterol and increase in triglycerides and glucose levels. So, exercise alone or combined with behavioural treatment may achieve favourable weight losses and improved metabolic parameters before undergoing bariatric surgery.

Preoperative Intragastric Balloon

Many reports on the use of balloons in the preoperative period exist, mainly stemming from Italy and Southern American countries (see Chap. 2). Most of these studies used balloons to promote preoperative weight loss or more specifically used balloons in high-risk supermorbid patients. No control groups were available or a historical control group from the same clinic was considered. Therefore, Coffin et al. performed a prospective randomised multicentre study to compare the impact of a preoperative 6-month intragastric balloon treatment (IGB) with standard medical care (SMC) in super-obese patients before undergoing laparoscopic gastric bypass [122]. The primary end point was the proportion of patients requiring a stay at the intensive care for >24 h and secondary end points were weight change, operation time, duration of hospital stay and perioperative complications. They calculated a need of randomisation of 314 patients (157 in each group). Due to insufficient enrolment the study had to be stopped after the inclusion of only 115 patients (BMI 54.3 ± 8.7 kg/m^2), of which 55 underwent IGB insertion. The proportion of patients who stayed in ICU >24 h was similar in both groups, mean operation time was similar and both groups had a similar hospitalisation stay. At 6 months, weight loss in BMI units was significantly greater in the IGB group (2.8 kg/m^2) than in the SMC group (0.4 kg/m^2), mainly occurring in the first 3 months, but the weight loss at 6 months post-operatively was not different anymore. Three severe complications occurred during IGB removal. Five patients had one or more surgical complications, all in the IGB group. Although conclusions may not be well founded because of insufficient numbers, the authors concluded that it is true that IGB insertion before gastric bypass induced weight loss but it did not improve the perioperative outcomes or affect post-operative weight loss.

Conclusions

It is evident that in the preoperative work-up of patients the rather vague guidelines by the authority associations ask for a close cooperation of both gastroenterologist and surgeon. The guidelines leave the decision of a preoperative endoscopy and GI work-up to the surgeons. However, from the patient's point of view a bariatric intervention is an elective procedure with weighing risks against benefits and it is often the last step on a long path of futile weight loss attempts. It is also a decision taken for life time at a relative young age, and this puts a heavy responsibility on the shoulders of the multidisciplinary team. Both surgeons and gastroenterologists should be aware of the fact that obesity is associated with oesophageal motility disturbances and with gastro-oesophageal reflux promoting circumstances. These conditions are often asymptomatic in the obese preoperatively and may become symptomatic after certain types of surgery. Also, the fact that gastro-oesophageal symptoms resolve after an operation does not necessarily signify an improvement as the development of Barrett's epithelium as an adaptation to acid reflux may obscure this premalignant and adverse complication of GORD. Therefore, the statement by the guidelines to evaluate patients with clinically significant gastrointestinal symptoms may withhold investigations for some who urgently needed such a detailed analysis. The two meta-analyses that investigated the yield of endoscopies only considered changes in surgical timing or type of procedure and the necessity of medical interventions preoperatively and concluded that routine endoscopy is not indicated and that a selective approach may be considered based on patients symptoms, risk factors and type of procedure planned. And although most surgeons voted against a sleeve gastrectomy in patients with a Barrett's oesophagus, they did not perform the endoscopy needed to establish this condition. On the other hand, follow-up of a Barrett's oesophagus is easy after a sleeve gastrectomy and after a RYGB. But when it comes to severe dysplasia or even malignancy and endoscopic procedures such as thermal ablation or endoscopic mucosal resection or endoscopic submucosal dissection are not possible or not available, a gastric pull up and a gastric tube reconstruction may be a true surgical challenge. The fear of missing a cancer is not a real problem in low incidence areas and as such not a true indication for a preoperative endoscopy, but this may be different in Asian countries. Similarly, the discussion of histopathological examination of every sleeve specimen is not settled yet, but a macroscopic inspection and a more detailed microscopic examination of suspected areas are probably a feasible compromise. Another point of disagreement is the need of preoperative weight loss, often required by insurance companies, but here the surgeon and gastroenterologist should defy this pressure and should do what they feel comfortable with which will also depend on personal experience, the type and degree of obese referrals, and the volume of operations already having performed.

References

1. Sauerland S, Angrisani L, Belachew M, Chevallier JM, Favretti F, Finer N, et al. Obesity surgery: evidence-based guidelines of the European Association for Endoscopic Surgery (EAES). Surg Endosc. 2005;19:200–21.
2. Ghassemian AJ, MacDonald KG, Cunningham PG, Swanson M, Brown BM, Morris PG, et al. The workup for bariatric surgery does not require a routine upper gastrointestinal series. Obes Surg. 1997;7:16–8.
3. Mechanick JI, Kushner RF, Sugerman HJ, Gonzalez-Campoy JM, Collazo-Clavell ML, Guven S, et al. American Association of Clinical Endocrinologists, The Obesity Society, and American Society for Metabolic & Bariatric Surgery Medical Guidelines for Clinical Practice for the perioperative nutritional, metabolic, and nonsurgical support of the bariatric surgery patient. Surg Obes Relat Dis. 2008;4(5 Suppl):S109–84.
4. Mechanick JI, Youdim A, Jones DB, Garvey WT, Hurley DL, McMahon MM, et al. Clinical practice guidelines for the perioperative nutritional, metabolic, and nonsurgical support of the bariatric surgery patient—2013 update: cosponsored by American Association of Clinical Endocrinologists, the Obesity Society, and American Society for Metabolic & bariatric surgery. Obesity. 2013;21:S1–S27.
5. Fried M, Hainer V, Basdevant A, Buchwald H, Deitel M, Finer N, et al. Interdisciplinary European guidelines in surgery for severe obesity. Obes Facts. 2008;1:52–9.
6. Fried M, Yumuk V, Oppert J-M, Scopinaro N, Torres AJ, Weiner R, et al. Interdisciplinary European guidelines on metabolic and bariatric surgery. Obes Facts. 2013;6:449–68.
7. Korenkov M, Sauerland S, Shah S, Junginger T. Is routine preoperative upper endoscopy in gastric banding patients really necessary? Obes Surg. 2006;16:45–7.
8. Mong C, Van Dam J, Morton J, Gerson L, Curet M, Banerjee S. Preoperative endoscopic screening for laparoscopic roux-en-y gastric bypass has a low yield for anatomic findings. Obes Surg. 2008;18:1067–73.
9. Küper MA, Kratt T, Kramer KM, Zdichavsky M, Schneider JH, Glatzle J, et al. Effort, safety, and findings of routine preoperative endoscopic evaluation of morbidly obese patients undergoing bariatric surgery. Surg Endosc. 2010;24:1996–2001.
10. Carabotti M, Avallone M, Cereatti F, Paganini A, Greco F, Scirocco A, et al. Usefulness of upper gastrointestinal symptoms as a driver to prescribe gastroscopy in obese patients candidate to bariatric surgery. A prospective study. Obes Surg. 2016;26:1075–80.
11. Rosenthal RJ, for the International Sleeve Gastrectomy Expert Panel. International sleeve Gastrectomy expert panel consensus statement: best practice guidelines based on experience of 12,000 cases. Surg Obes Relat Dis. 2012;8:8–19.
12. Gagner M, Hutchinson C, Rosenthal R. Fifth international consensus conference: current status of sleeve gastrectomy. Surg Obes Relat Dis. 2016;12:750–6.
13. Evans JA, Muthusamy VR, Acosta RD, Bruining DH, Chandrasekhara V, Chathadi KV, et al. The role of endoscopy in the bariatric surgery patient. Gastrointest Endosc. 2015;81:1063–72.
14. Anderson MA, Gan SI, Fanelli RD, Baron TH, Banerjee S, Cash BD, et al. ASGE standards of practice committee. Role of endoscopy in the bariatric surgery patient. Gastrointest Endosc. 2008;68:1–10.
15. Mohammed R, Fei P, Phu J, Asai M, Antanavicius G. Efficiency of preoperative esophagogastroduodenoscopy in identifying operable hiatal hernia for bariatric surgery patients. Surg Obes Relat Dis. 2017;13:287–90.
16. Verset D, Houben J-J, Gay F, Elcheroth J, Bourgeois V, van Gossum A. The place of upper gastrointestinal tract endoscopy before and after vertical banded gastroplasty for morbid obesity. Dig Dis Sci. 1997;42:2333–7.
17. Papavramidis ST, Theocharidis AJ, Zaraboukas TG, Christoforidou BP, Kessissoglou II, Aidonopoulos AP. Upper gastrointestinal endoscopic and histologic findings before and after vertical banded gastroplasty. Surg Endosc. 1996;10:825–30.

18. Sharaf RN, Weinshel EH, Bini EJ, Rosenberg J, Sherman A, Ren CJ. Endoscopy plays an important preoperative role in bariatric surgery. Obes Surg. 2004;14:1367–72.
19. Azagury D, Dumonceau JM, Morel P, Chassot G, Huber O. Preoperative work-up in asymptomatic patients undergoing roux-en-y gastric bypass: is endoscopy mandatory? Obes Surg. 2006;16:1304–11.
20. Ng JY, Cheng AKS, Kim G, Kong LWC, Soe KT, Lomanto D, et al. Is elective gastroscopy prior to bariatric surgery in an Asian cohort worthwhile? Obes Surg. 2016;26:2156–60.
21. Lee J, Wong SK-H, Liu SY-W, Ng EK-W. Is preoperative upper gastrointestinal endoscopy in obese patients undergoing bariatric surgery mandatory? An Asian perspective. Obes Surg. 2017;27:44–50.
22. Ben-Menachem T, Decker GA, Early DS, Evans J, Fanelli RD, Fisher DA, et al. Adverse events of upper GI endoscopy. ASGE standards of practice committee. Gastrointest Endosc. 2012;76:707–18.
23. McVay T, Fang JC, Taylor l AA, Williams W, Presson AP, Al-Dulaimi R, et al. Safety analysis of bariatric patients undergoing outpatient upper endoscopy with non-anesthesia administered propofol sedation. Obes Surg. 2017;27:1501–7.
24. Hori Y, SAGES Guidelines Committee. Granting of privilege for gastrointestinal endoscopy. Surg Endosc. 2008;2(2):1349–52.
25. Asfaha S, Alqahtani S, Hilsden RJ, MacLean AR, Beck PL. Assessment of endoscopic training of general surgery residents in a north American health region. Gastrointest Endosc. 2008;68:1056–62.
26. Gill RS, Whitlock KA, Mohamed R, Sarkhosh K, Birch DW, Karmall S. The role of upper gastrointestinal endoscopy in treating postoperative complications in bariatric surgery. J Interv Gastroenterol. 2012;2:37–41.
27. Vassiliou MC, Dunkin BJ, Fried GM, Mellinger JD, Trus T, Kaneva P, et al. Fundamentals of endoscopic surgery: creation and validation of the hands-on test. Surg Endosc. 2014;28:704–11.
28. Parikh M, Liu J, Vieira D, Tzimas D, Horwitz D, Antony A, et al. Preoperative endoscopy prior to bariatric surgery: a systematic review and meta-analysis of the literature. Obes Surg. 2016;26:2961–6.
29. Bennett S, Gostimir M, Shorr R, Mallick R, Mamazza J, Neville A. The role of routine preoperative upper endoscopy in bariatric surgery: a systematic review and meta-analysis. Surg Obes Relat Dis. 2016;12:1116–25.
30. Schirmer B, Erenoglu C, Miller A. Flexible endoscopy in the management of patients undergoing roux-en-y gastric bypass. Obes Surg. 2002;12:634–8.
31. Fernandes SR, Meireles LC, Carrilho-Ribeiro L, Velosa J. The role of routine upper gastrointestinal endoscopy before bariatric surgery. Obes Surg. 2016;26:2105–10.
32. Zanotti D, Elkalaawy M, Hashemi M, Jenkinson A, Adamo M. Current status of preoperative oesophago-gastro-duodenoscopy (OGD) in bariatric NHS units—a BOMSS survey. Obes Surg. 2016;26:2257–62.
33. Scozzari G, Trapani R, Toppino M, Morino M. Esophagogastric cancer after bariatric surgery: systematic review of the literature. Surg Obes Relat Dis. 2013;9:133–42.
34. Safaan T, Bashah M, El Ansari W, Karam M. Histopathological changes in laparoscopic sleeve gastrectomy specimens: prevalence, risk factors, and value of routine histopathological examination. Obes Surg. 2017;27:1741–9.
35. Almazeedi S, Al-Sabah S, Al-Mulla A, Al-Murad A, Al-Mossawi A, Al-Enezi K, et al. Gastric histopathologies in patients undergoing laparoscopic sleeve gastrectomies. Obes Surg. 2013;23:314–9.
36. Clapp B. Histopathologic findings in the resected specimen of a sleeve gastrectomy. J Soc Laparoendosc Surg. 2015;19:e2013.00259.
37. Raess PW, Baird-Howella M, Aggarwal R, Williams NN, Furth EE. Vertical sleeve gastrectomy specimens have a high prevalence of unexpected histopathologic findings requiring additional clinical management. Surg Obes Relat Dis. 2015;11:1020–4.

38. Ohanessian SE, Rogers AM, Karamchandan DM. Spectrum of gastric histopathologies in severely obese American patients undergoing sleeve gastrectomy. Obes Surg. 2016;26:595–602.
39. Lauti M, Gormack SE, Thomas JM, Morrow JJ, Rahman H, MacCormick AD. What does the excised stomach from sleeve gastrectomy tell us? Obes Surg. 2016;26:839–42.
40. AbdulGaffar B, Raman K, Khamas A, AlBradi E. Should we abandon routine microscopic examination in bariatric sleeve specimens? Obes Surg. 2016;26:105–10.
41. Vaz Safatle-Ribeiro AV, Kuga R, Iriya K, Ribeiro U Jr, Faintuch J, Ishida RK, et al. What to expect in the excluded stomach mucosa after vertical banded roux-en-y gastric bypass for morbid obesity. J Gastrointest Surg. 2007;11:133–7.
42. Ovrebo KK, Hatlebakk JG, Viste A, Bassoe HH, Svanis K. Gastroesophageal reflux in morbidly obese patients treated with gastric banding or vertical banded gastroplasty. Ann Surg. 1998;228:51–8.
43. Di Francesco V, Baggio E, Mastromauro M, Zoico E, Stefenelli N, Zamboni M, et al. Obesity and gastro-esophageal acid reflux: physiopathological mechanisms and role of gastric bariatric surgery. Obes Surg. 2004;14:1095–102.
44. Deitel M, Khanna RK, Hagen J, Ilves R. Vertical banded gastroplasty as an antireflux procedure. Am J Surg. 1998;155:512–6.
45. Naslund E, Granstrom L, Melcher A, Stockveld D, Backman L. Gastroesophageal reflux before and after vertical banded gastroplasty in the treatment of obesity. Eur J Surg. 1996;162:303–6.
46. Dixon JB, O'Brien PE. Gastroesophageal reflux in obesity: the effect of lap-band placement. Obes Surg. 1999;9:527–31.
47. Deitel M, Gagner M, Erickson AL, Crosby RD. Third international summit: current status of sleeve gastrectomy. Surg Obes Relat Dis. 2011;7:749–59.
48. Bragghetto I, Lanzarini E, Korn O, Valladares H, Molina JC, Hendriquez A. Manometric changes of the lower esophageal sphincter after sleeve gastrectomy in obese patients. Obes Surg. 2010;20:357–62.
49. Himpens J, Dobbeleir J, Peeters G. Long-term results of laparoscopic sleeve gastrectomy for obesity. Ann Surg. 2010;252:319–24.
50. Jaffin BW, Knoepflmacher P, Greenstein R. High prevalence of asymptomatic esophageal motility disorders among morbidly obese patients. Obes Surg. 1999;9:390–5.
51. Greenstein RJ, Nissan A, Jaffin B. Esophageal anatomy and function in laparoscopic gastric restrictive bariatric surgery: implications for patient selection. Obes Surg. 1998;8:199–206.
52. Suter M, Dorta G, Giusti V, Calmes JM. Gastro-esophageal reflux and esophageal motility disorders in morbidly obese patients. Obes Surg. 2004;14:959–66.
53. Verma S, Sharma D, Kanwar P, Sohn W, Mohanty SR, Tortolani AJ, et al. Prevalence of Helicobacter pylori infection in bariatric patients: a histologic assessment. Surg Obes Relat Dis. 2013;9:679–85.
54. Cordeiro F. H. pylori and gastroplasty in the treatment of morbid obesity. Am J Gastroenterol. 2001;96:605–6.
55. Huang JQ, Sridhar S, Chen Y, Hunt RH. Meta-analysis of the relationship between Helicibacter pylori and gastric cancer. Gastroenterology. 1998;114:1169–79.
56. Eslick GD, Lim LL, Byles JA, Xia HH, Talley NJ. Association of Helicobacter pylori infection with gastric carcinoma: a meta-analysis. Am J Gastroenterol. 1999;94:2373–9.
57. Papasavas PK, Gagné DJ, Donnelly PE, Salgado J, Urbandt JE, Burton KK, et al. Prevalence of helicobacter pylori infection and value of preoperative testing and treatment in patients undergoing laparoscopic roux-en-Y gastric bypass. Surg Obes Relat Dis. 2008;4:383–8.
58. Rasmussen JJ, Fuller W, Ali MR. Marginal ulceration after laparoscopic gastric bypass: an analysis of predisposing factors in 260 patients. Surg Endosc. 2007;21:1090–4.
59. Gisbert JP, Blanco M, Pajares JM. Effects of helicobacter pylori eradication on histologic lesions of gastric mucosa: an 18-month follow-up study. Rev Clin Esp. 2000;9:480–4.
60. Loewen M, Giovanni J, Barba C. Screening endoscopy before bariatric surgery: a series of 448 patients. Surg Obes Relat Dis. 2008;4:709–14.

61. Yang C-S, Lee W-J, Wang H-H, Huang S-P, Lin J-T, Wu M-S. The influence of helicobacter pylori infection on the development of gastric ulcer in symptomatic patients after bariatric surgery. Obes Surg. 2006;16:735–9.
62. Marano BJ. Endoscopy after roux-en-y gastric bypass: a community hospital experience. Obes Surg. 2005;15:342–5.
63. Lee JK, Van Dam J, Morton JM, Curet MJ, Banerjee S. Endoscopy is accurate, safe, and effective in the assessment and management of complications following gastric bypass surgery. Am J Gastroenterol. 2009;104:575–82.
64. Hartin CW Jr, ReMine DS, Lucktong TA. Preoperative bariatric screening and treatment of helicobacter pylori. Surg Endosc. 2009;23:2531–4.
65. Almazeedi S, Al-Sabah S, Alshammari D, Alqinai S, Al-Mulla A, Al-Murad A, et al. The impact of helicobacter pylori on the complications of laparoscopic sleeve gastrectomy. Obes Surg. 2014;24:412–5.
66. Albawardi A, Almaarzooqi S, Torab FC. Helicobacter pylori in sleeve gastrectomies: prevalence and rate of complications. Int J Clin Exp Med. 2013;6:40–3.
67. Rossetti G, Moccia F, Marra T, Buonomo M, Pascotto B, Pezzullo A, et al. Does Helicobacter pylori infection have influence on outcomes of laparoscopic sleeve gastrectomy for morbid obesity? Int J Surg. 2014;12 Suppl 1:S68–71.
68. Malfertheiner P, Megraud F, O'Morain C, Bazzoli F, El-Omar E, Graham D, et al. Current concepts in the management of Helicobacter pylori infection: the Maastricht III consensus report. Gut. 2007;56:772–81.
69. Hong D, Khajanchee YS, Pereira N, Lockhart B, Patterson EJ, Swanstrom LL. Manometric abnormalities and gastroesophageal reflux disease in the morbidly obese. Obes Surg. 2004;14:744–9.
70. Valezi AC, Mardiros Herbella FA, Mali Junior J, de Almeida Menezes M. Esophageal motility after laparoscopic roux-en-y gastric bypass: the manometry should be preoperative examination routine? Obes Surg. 2012;22:1050–4.
71. Korenkov M, Köhler L, Yücel N, Grass G, Sauerland S, Lempa M, et al. Esophageal motility and reflux symptoms before and after bariatric surgery. Obes Surg. 2002;12:72–6.
72. Bueter M, Thalheimer A, le Roux CW, Wierlemann A, Seyfried F, Fein M. Upper gastrointestinal investigations before gastric banding. Surg Endosc. 2010;24:1025–30.
73. Klaus A, Weiss H. Is preoperative manometry in restrictive bariatric procedures necessary? Obes Surg. 2008;18:1039–42.
74. Melissas J, Koukouraki S, Askoxylakis J, Stathaki M, Daskalakis M, Perisinakis K, et al. Sleeve gastrectomy: a restrictive procedure? Obes Surg. 2007;17:57–62.
75. Rosemar A, Angerås U, Rosengren A. Body mass index and diverticular disease: a 28-year follow-up study in men. Dis Colon Rect. 2008;51:450–5.
76. Strate LL, Liu YL, Aldoori WH, Syngal GEL. Obesity increases the risks of diverticulitis and diverticular bleeding. Gastroenterology. 2009;136:115–22.
77. Yamada E, Ohkubo H, Higurashi T, Sakai E, Endo H, Takahashi H, et al. Visceral obesity as a risk factor for left-sided diverticulitis in Japan: a multicenter retrospective study. Gut Liver. 2013;7:532–8.
78. Blain A, Cattan S, Beaugerie L, Carbonnel F, Gendre JP, Cosnes J. Crohn's disease clinical course and severity in obese patients. Clin Nutr. 2002;21:51–7.
79. Steeda H, Walsh S, Reynold N. A brief report of the epidemiology of obesity in the inflammatory bowel disease population of Tayside, Scotland. Obes Facts. 2009;2:370–2.
80. Moran GW, MD DM-F, Kaplan GG, Panaccione R, Ghosh S. The increasing weight of Crohn's disease subjects in clinical trials: a hypothesis-generating time-trend analysis. Inflamm Bowel Dis. 2013;19:2949–56.
81. Stabroth-Akil D, Leifeld L, Pfützer R, Morgenstern J, Kruis W. The effect of body weight on the severity and clinical course of ulcerative colitis. Int J Color Dis. 2015;30:237–42.
82. Flores A, Burstein E, Cipher DJ, Feagins LA. Obesity in inflammatory bowel disease: a marker of less severe disease. Dig Dis Sci. 2015;60:2436–45.
83. Seminerio JL, Koutroubakis IE, Ramos-Rivers C, Hashash JG, Dudekula A, Regueiro M, et al. Impact of obesity on the management and clinical course of patients with inflammatory bowel disease. Inflamm Bowel Dis. 2015;21:2857–63.

84. Chan SS, Luben R, Olsen A, Tjonneland A, Kaaks R, Teucher B, et al. Body mass index and the risk for Crohn's disease and ulcerative colitis: data from a European prospective cohort study (the IBD in EPIC study). Am J Gastroenterol. 2013;108:575–82.
85. Khalili H, Ananthakrishnan AN, Konijeti GG, Higuchi LM, Fuchs CS, Richter JM, et al. Measures of obesity and risk of Crohn's disease and ulcerative colitis. Inflamm Bowel Dis. 2015;21:361–8.
86. Mendall MA, Gunasekera AV, John BJ, Kumar D. Is obesity a risk factor for Crohn's disease? Dig Dis Sci. 2011;56:837–44.
87. Hass DJ, Brensinger CM, Lewis JD, Lichtenstein GR. The impact of increased body mass index on the clinical course of Crohn's disease. Clin Gastroenterol Hepatol. 2006;4:482–8.
88. Kiran RP, Remzi FH, Fazio VW, Lavery IC, Church JM, Strong SA, et al. Complications and functional results after ileoanal pouch formation in obese patients. J Gastrointest Surg. 2008;12:668–74.
89. Bhalme M, Sharma A, Keld R, Willert R, Campbell S. Does weight-adjusted anti-tumour necrosis factor treatment favour obese patients with Crohn's disease? Eur J Gastroenterol Hepat. 2013;25:543–9.
90. Harper JW, Sinanan MN, Zisman TL. Increased body mass index is associated with earlier time to loss of response to infliximab in patients with inflammatory bowel disease. Inflamm Bowel Dis. 2013;19:2118–24.
91. Bultman E, de Haar C, van Liere-Baron A, Verhoog N, West RL, Kuipers EJ, et al. Predictors of dose escalation of adalimumab in a prospective cohort of Crohn's disease patients. Aliment Pharmacol Ther. 2012;35:335–41.
92. Holtmann MH, Krummenauer F, Claas C, Kremeyer K, Lorenz D, Rainer O, et al. Significant differences between Crohn's disease and ulcerative colitis regarding the impact of body mass index and initial disease activity on responsiveness to azathioprine: results from a European multicenter study in 1,176 patients. Dig Dis Sci. 2010;55:1066–78.
93. GonÇalves P, Magro F, Martel F. Metabolic inflammation in inflammatory bowel disease: crosstalk between adipose tissue and bowel. Inflamm Bowel Dis. 2015;21:453–67.
94. Paeschke A, Erbena U, Kredela LI, Kühla AA, Siegmunda B. Role of visceral fat in colonic inflammation: from Crohn's disease to diverticulitis. Curr Opin Gastroenterol. 2017;33: 53–8.
95. Korelitz BI, Sonpal N, Schneider J, Swaminath A, Felder J, Roslin M, et al. Obesity/bariatric surgery and Crohn's disease. J Clin Gastroenterol. 2018;52(1):50–4. https://doi.org/10.1097/MCG.0000000000000765.
96. Arrese M, Cabrera D, Kalergis AM, Feldstein AE. Innate immunity and inflammation in NAFLD/NASH. Dig Dis Sci. 2016;61:1294–303.
97. Buning C, von Kraft C, Hermsdorf M, Gentz E, Wirth EK, Valentini L, et al. Visceral adipose tissue in patients with Crohn's disease correlates with disease activity, inflammatory markers, and outcome. Inflamm Bowel Dis. 2015;21:2590–7.
98. Shoar S, Hoseini SS, Naderan M, Mahmoodzadeh H, Ying Man F, Shoar N, et al. Bariatric surgery in morbidly obese patients with inflammatory bowel disease: a systematic review. Surg Obes Relat Dis. 2017;13(4):652–9. https://doi.org/10.1016/j.soard.23016.
99. Bernstein GR, Pickett-Blakely O. De novo inflammatory bowel disease after bariatric surgery: a case series and literature review. Dig Dis Sci. 2017;62:817–20.
100. Tewksbury C, Williams NN, Dumon KR, Sarwer DB. Preoperative medical weight management in bariatric surgery: a review and reconsideration. Obes Surg. 2017;27:208–14.
101. National Institutes of Health. Clinical guidelines on the identification, evaluation, and treatment of overweight and obesity in adults—the evidence report. National Institutes of Health. Obes Res. 1998;6 Suppl 2:51S–209S.
102. Jensen MD, Ryan DH, Apovian CM, Ard JD, Comuzzie AG, Donato KA, et al. 2013 AHA/ACC/TOS guideline for the management of overweight and obesity in adults: a report of the American College of Cardiology/American Heart Association Task Force on Practice Guidelines and the Obesity Society. J Am Coll Cardiol. 2014;63:2985–3023.
103. Gibbons LM, Sarwer DB, Crerand CE, Fabricatore AN, Kuehnel RH, Lipschutz PE, et al. Previous weight loss experiences of bariatric surgery candidates: how much have patients dieted prior to surgery? Obesity. 2006;14 Suppl:70S–6S.

104. National Institutes of Health. Gastrointestinal surgery for obesity: National Institutes of Health Consensus Development Conference Statement. Am J Clin Nutr. 1992;55:615S–9S.
105. Buchwald H. Bariatric surgery for morbid obesity: health implications for patients, health professionals, and third-party payers. J Am Coll Surg. 2005;200:593–604.
106. Brethauer SA. ASMBS Position statement on preoperative supervised weight loss requirements. Surg Obes Relat Dis. 2011;7:257–60.
107. Lau DC, Douketis JD, Morrison KM, Hramiak IM, Sharma AM, Ur E, et al. Canadian clinical practice guidelines on the management and prevention of obesity in adults and children [summary]. Can Med Assoc J. 2007;2006:S1–13.
108. Baldry EL, Leeder PC, Idris R. IR. Pre-operative dietary restriction for patients undergoing bariatric surgery in the UK: observational study of current practice and dietary effects. Obes Surg. 2014;24:416–21.
109. Tarnoff M, Kaplan LM, Shikora S. An evidence-based assessment of preoperative weight loss in bariatric surgery. Obes Surg. 2008;18:1059–61.
110. Livhits M, Mercado C, Yermilov I, Parikh JA, Dutson E, Amir Mehran A, et al. Does weight loss immediately before bariatric surgery improve outcomes: a systematic review. Surg Obes Relat Dis. 2009;5:713–21.
111. Cassie S, Menezes C, Birch DW, Shi X, Karmali S. Effect of preoperative weight loss in bariatric surgical patients: a systematic review. Surg Obes Relat Dis. 2011;7:760–8.
112. Ochner CN, Dambkowski CL, Yeomans BL, Teixeira J, Pi-Sunyer FX. Pre-bariatric surgery weight loss requirements and the effect of preoperative weight loss on postoperative outcome. Int J Obes. 2012;36:1380–7.
113. Gerber P, Anderin C, Thorell A. Weight loss prior to bariatric surgery: an updated review of the literature. Scand J Surg. 2014;104:33–9.
114. Livhits M, Mercado C, Yermilov I, Parikh JA, Dutson E, Mehran A, et al. Preoperative predictors of weight loss following bariatric surgery: systematic review. Obes Surg. 2012;22:70–89.
115. Anderin C, Gustafsson UO, Heijbel N, Thorell A. Weight loss prior bariatric surgery and postoperative complications. Data from Scandinavian Obesity Register (SOReg). Ann Surg. 2015;261:903–13.
116. Gerber P, Anderin C, Gustafsson UO, Thorell A. Weight loss before gastric bypass and postoperative weight change: data from the Scandinavian Obesity Registry (SOReg). Surg Obes Relat Dis. 2016;12:556–62.
117. Colles SL, Dixon JB, Marks P, Strauss BJ, O'Brien PE. Preoperative weight loss with a very-low-energy diet: quantitation of changes in liver and abdominal fat by serial imaging. Am J Clin Nutr. 2006;84:304–11.
118. Ross LJ, Wallin S, Osland EJ, Ashraf Memon M. Commercial very low energy meal replacements for preoperative weight loss in obese patients: a systematic review. Obes Surg. 2016;26:1343–51.
119. Andersen T, Gluud C, Franzmann M-B, Christoffersen P. Hepatic effects of dietary weight loss in morbidly obese subjects. J Hepatol. 1991;12:224–9.
120. Poirier P, Cornier MA, Mazzone T, Stiles S, Cummings S, Klein S, et al. American Heart Association obesity Committee of the Council on Nutrition, Physical Activity, And Metabolism. Bariatric surgery and cardiovascular risk factors: a scientific statement from the American Heart Association. Circulation. 2011;123:1683–701.
121. Rejane Marcon E, Baglioni S, Bittencourt L, Lopes CLN, Neumann CR, Trindade MRM. What is the best treatment before bariatric surgery? Exercise, exercise and group therapy, or conventional waiting: a randomized controlled trial. Obes Surg. 2017;27:763–73.
122. Coffin B, Maunoury V, Pattou F, Hébuterne X, Schneider S, Coupaye M, et al. Impact of intragastric balloon before laparoscopic gastric bypass on patients with super obesity: a randomized multicenter study. Obes Surg. 2017;27:902–9.

When the Surgeon Needs the Endoscopist in Rescuing Bariatric Surgery: Intraoperative and Early Post-operative Period

5

Contents

E. M. H. Mathus-Vliegen, J. Dargent, *Bariatric Therapy*,
https://doi.org/10.1007/978-3-319-90074-2_5

Abbreviations

AACE	American Association of Clinical Endocrinologists
APC	Argon plasma coagulation
ASGE	American Society for Gastrointestinal Endoscopy
ASMBS	American Society for Metabolic and Bariatric Surgery
BMI	Body mass index
BOLD	Bariatric Outcomes Longitudinal Database
BPD	Biliopancreatic diversion
BPD-DS	Biliopancreatic diversion with duodenal switch
CI	Confidence interval
COM	Centres of excellence
CT	Computed tomography
DBE	Double-balloon enteroscopy
EAES	European Association of Endoscopic Surgery
EASO	European Association for the Study of Obesity
EBMT	Endoscopic bariatric and metabolic therapy
EBT	Endoscopic bariatric therapy
EEA	End-to-end anastomosis
EID	Endoscopic internal drainage
ERCP	Endoscopic retrograde cholangiopancreaticography
Fr	French
GI	Gastrointestinal
GJ	Gastrojejunal
GIA	Gastointestinal anastomis
IFSO-EC	International Federation for the Surgery of Obesity-European Chapter
IOP	Incisionless Operating Platform
LABS	Longitudinal assessment of bariatric surgery
LA(S)GB	Laparoscopic adjustable (silicone) gastric banding
LB	LapBand
LRYGB	Laparoscopic Roux-en-Y gastric bypass
MBSC	Michigan Bariatric Surgery Collaborative
NSET	Non-stent endoscopic treatment
NSQIP	National Surgical Quality Improvement Program
OMTF	Obesity Management Task Force
OS-MRS	Obesity Surgery Mortality Risk Score
OTSC	Over-the-scope-clip
RBC	Red blood cell
RCT	Randomised clinical trial
ROSE	Restorative Obesity Surgery Endolumenal
RYGB	Roux-en-Y Gastric bypass
SAGES	Society of American Gastrointestinal and Endoscopic Surgeons
SB	Swedish band
SEMS	Self-expandable metallic stents
SEPS	Self-expandable plastic stents
SG	Sleeve gastrectomy
SIRS	Systemic inflammatory response syndrome

TOS	The Obesity Society
VAC	Vacuum-assisted closure
VBG	Vertical banded gastroplasty

5.1 Introduction

Endoscopy may be of help during the operation when unexpected findings are in need of a proper diagnosis but most of the endoscopic procedures will be performed to guarantee a safe and airtight anastomosis or staple line. It will depend on the country and local customs and facilities whether the surgeon himself/herself performs the intraoperative endoscopy or whether he/she can call upon an endoscopist to assist in the procedure. Endoscopy in the post-operative period will be performed for clinical reasons, either as an emergency or electively to evaluate symptoms. In the case of positive findings that lend themselves to endoscopic treatment, the endoscopist may come to rescue the bariatric surgery.

5.2 Intraoperative Endoscopy

The American Society of Metabolic and Bariatric Surgery (ASMBS) Clinical Issues Committee issued a guideline on the prevention and detection of gastrointestinal (GI) leaks after a gastric bypass in 2009 which stated that the vast majority of GI leaks occur in the absence of technical errors and no high-quality evidence exists that intraoperative techniques are able to eliminate or substantially decrease the incidence of leaks as a complication of gastric bypass [1]. This was confirmed by a very recent review by Ghosh et al. in 2016 [2]. Yet, intraoperative endoscopy may not only be helpful to detect staple-line leaks, narrowing of the lumen or anastomosis, and bleeding, but also be preventive for post-operative leaks, strictures and haemorrhages by an intraoperative intervention and subsequent checking of the result of this intervention. Intraoperative leak testing has been used successfully to detect procedure-related leaks that occur before the patient leaves the operating room when tissues are still amenable to repair [2]. Multiple techniques are utilised to identify potential anastomotic leaks. Intraoperatively, these include the injection of methylene blue dye or air via a nasogastric or an orogastric tube or an air test by the use of endoscopy. Post-operatively, the injection of methylene blue dye via a nasogastric or an orogastric tube and its retrieval via an intra-abdominal drain, sampling of the drain fluid for (salivary) amylase, upper GI series or computed tomography (CT) scan, and clinical signs and symptoms are used to identify leaks. In contrast to endoscopy, the evaluation of the patency of the anastomosis and stigmata of early bleeding would not be possible with these techniques. Intraoperative leak tests have been discussed mainly in the laparoscopic gastric bypass and the laparoscopic gastric sleeve procedure and are probably most relevant in the laparoscopic gastric bypass [3].

In the *gastric bypass*, the gastrojejunostomy is created using a circular staple and the posterior staple line is not well amenable to visual inspection. In contrast, in the gastric sleeve the staple line is constructed with a linear staple and both anterior and posterior staple lines are readily visible. Having the choice between the methylene blue test and the air test, there is a slight preference for the air test [3, 4]. If there is an inadequate staple line or anastomosis, blue dye will leak out of the anastomosis and can be easily identified by the surgeon. However, following the repair of the anastomotic leak, the surgeon is unable to use methylene blue again as the field is contaminated with blue dye, which is not the case when using air [4]. In case the endoscopic air test is being performed, the endoscope has to be advanced posterior to the endotracheal tube. Occasionally a jaw thrust manoeuvre provided by the anaesthesiologist is required to assist in advancement of the endoscope and sometimes, in case of persistent difficulty with insertion of the endoscope, superior laryngoscopy is helpful [5]. The instrument is introduced under digital control across the upper oesophageal sphincter. In a gastric bypass procedure the proximal pouch is examined and the endoscope is negotiated across the anastomosis to assess the calibre of the stoma and pouch and to exclude a bleeding source. The endoscope is pulled back into the gastric pouch, and the Roux limb is clamped, followed by insufflation with air via the endoscope (pressure-controlled and carbon dioxide insufflation are both feasible) and submerging the gastrojejunostomy in sterile normal saline.

Bubbles escaping from the anastomosis after the endoscopic insufflation with air indicate an anastomotic leak [5] (Fig. 5.1). In case of a leak the endoscope is left in position and the procedure repeated after repair or reinforcement of the gastrojejunostomy suture line. When finished, the jejunum has to be accessed again and to be desufflated making sure that no substantial amount of air is left [5].

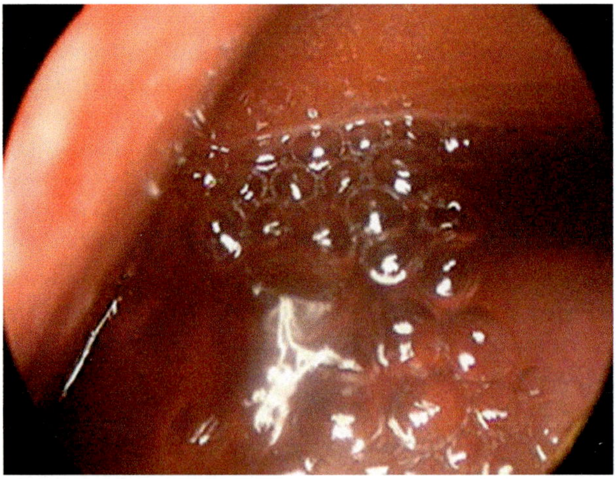

Fig. 5.1 During intraoperative endoscopy the endoscope is introduced and in a gastric bypass procedure the proximal pouch is examined, the calibre of the stoma and pouch is assessed and a bleeding source is excluded. Thereafter, the endoscope is pulled back into the gastric pouch, and the Roux limb is clamped, followed by insufflation with air via the endoscope and submerging the gastrojejunostomy in sterile normal saline. Bubbles escaping from the anastomosis after the endoscopic insufflation with air indicate an anastomotic leak. Reprinted from Obes Surg 2011; 21: 1530–1534, Cingi A, Yavuz Y. Intraoperative endoscopic assessment of the pouch and anastomosis during laparoscopic Roux-en-Y gastric bypass with permission from Springer

In the *sleeve gastrectomy* procedure, some surgeons use the endoscope instead of the 32–36 Fr bougie and at the end of the surgery the endoscope is pulled back into the oesophagus and a diagnostic procedure well into the duodenum is performed looking for bleeding or an obstruction because of a twist or a too narrow sleeve tube [6]. Back into the oesophagus a leak test is performed with a clamp on the pylorus while the entire sleeve is immersed in saline. Sometimes, the introduction across the upper oesophageal sphincter is difficult and performing an endoscopy in the supine position may give problems in the orientation [7].

5.2.1 Detection of Leaks After Roux-En-Y Gastric Bypass (RYGB)

Alasfar and Chand reported 11 (3.7%) leaks in 290 patients which were identified by endoscopy intraoperatively, all but one were located at the gastrojejunal (GJ) anastomosis site [8]. Intraoperative pouch bleeding occurred in ten cases (3.45%). They also assessed the role of intraoperative endoscopy in managing GJ leaks and bleedings. The anastomoses were revised and corrected and upper GI series performed on day 1 did not identify subsequent leaks. In six of the ten bleedings, a significant bleeding from a blood vessel was visible endoscopically, and suturing was performed under direct endoscopic visualisation. The source could not be identified in the other four cases, but they resolved without further intervention. Alaedeen et al. compared retrospectively 200 RYGB cases in which methylene blue was used with 200 RYGB cases in which intraoperative endoscopy was used [9]. On post-operative day 1 all underwent a contrast study of the upper GI tract to identify potential anastomotic leaks. The anastomotic leak rate of 0.4% with intraoperative endoscopy was significantly lower than the anastomotic leak rate of 4% after the use of methylene blue. Sekhar et al. found 56 (56/340, 16.4%) intraoperative leaks which were repaired without a positive leak after the operation [10]. Age >40 years increased the risk of intraoperative leakage by a factor of 2.3 (OR 2.3 (95% Confidence Interval (CI) 1.2/4.6)). There was no influence of body mass index (BMI), length of stay, procedural length, level and gender of the assistant. There was a trend towards more leakage in the GIA group (gastrointestinal anastomosis, linear stapler 22 mm and handsewn, 18%) versus the EEA (end-to-end anastomosis, circular stapler 21 mm, 12%) [10]. Fernandez et al. analysed the risk factors for morbidity in over 3200 patients and found weight, hypertension, type of bypass (in the order revision > open > laparoscopic) and gastrojejunal anastomosis leak to be independent risk factors for post-operative morbidity and male gender, age, diabetes and sleep apnoea to be independent risk factors for developing a leak [11]. The leak-associated mortality was 17% and leakage was an independent risk factor for death. Ramanathan et al. used endoscopy and methylene blue and discovered a 10% leak by endoscopy in 182 patients with a consistently negative methylene blue test in 61 patients [12]. Haddad et al. and Al Hadad et al. reported quite similar results in 2308 and 392 patients, respectively [5, 7]. Haddad et al. found 80 leaks which were transient and not repaired in 34 and true leaks needing repair in 46 with only 2 new post-operative leaks and 2 persistent leaks in the 46 previously repaired subjects [5]. They also discovered 2 very tight anastomoses which were reconstructed and 25 (1.2%) developed a stricture post-operatively, requiring endoscopic dilations. Al Haddad et al. discovered six positive leaks intraoperatively and two new post-operative leaks in the 336 subjects with negative intraoperative tests [7]. One stenosis was discovered intraoperatively and three newly developed a stenosis post-operatively. Both authors had a 100% positive predictive value of the air test to detect a leak and a negative predictive test of 99.9% and 99.4%, respectively. Moreover, the unexpected finding of a stenosis was reported by both. In Hadad's study an important finding was a technically impossible introduction rate of 0.1% (three patients) and an iatrogenic injury rate of 0.1% (three subjects, two tears in the oesophagus and one in the gastric pouch) [5]. So, by using intraoperative endoscopy the post-operative morbidity was 1.3% and would have been 3.2% without endoscopy, a reduction by more than 50%. The low iatrogenic injury rate reported in both studies is important as excessive traction to the operative field or high air pressure used during the endoscopy has been quoted to result in an increased risk for bleeding or leak [3, 13].

Nelson et al. performed a retrospective study in 105 gastric bypass patients, patients having first an identification of staple-line leaks by using a saline submersion technique via a nasogastric tube, and then followed by an intraoperative methylene blue challenge test [14]. These tests were followed on post-operative day 1 by routine upper GI studies and a methylene blue challenge test via the mouth with detection of methylene blue in the tube. No patient was positive for leakage intraoperatively or on post-operative day 1; however, 4 (3.8%) developed a staple-line leak on post-operative day 2 or 3. The reasons for this finding were discussed and may be due to tissue oedema with a communication not wide enough to allow passage of fluid until the postsurgical swelling decreases. Another reason might be the attempt by the body to wall off any infection of fluid collection. The third reason may be ischaemia that takes time to develop and perforate.

5.2.2 Detection of Leaks After Sleeve Gastrectomy (SG)

The data available for sleeve gastrectomy relate to leakage and stenosis. A systematic review and meta-analysis by Parikh et al. evaluated 112 studies encompassing 9991 patients and found that intraoperative leak testing was performed in 6717 patients (67%) and 62 studies (55%) [15]. Aurora et al. [16] found similar results in a systematic review of 29 publications including 4888 patients, with performance of a leak test documented in 15 studies (52%). Sakran et al. [17] analysed 2834 cases and found that 33 of the 44 patients who developed post-operative leaks had been tested intraoperatively using methylene blue dye ($n = 25$) or air ($n = 8$). Only one leak was detected, suggesting that the dye test may be of limited predictive value. Out of these 44 leaks two patients had a bleed from the staple line that was sealed by suturing and four cases had a stapler misfire that was oversewn. They concluded that routine intraoperative leak testing is superfluous for the prevention of post-operative leaks, and that selective testing of patients with specific types of intraoperative complications such as stapler misfire may be more appropriate. In contrast, a study of 712 patients by Wahby et al. supported the routine use of methylene blue intraoperatively as intraoperative testing detected a leakage in 28 cases (3.93%) that were repaired by oversewing [18]. No additional leaks were detected using upper GI contrast after 24–48 h suggesting that the value of subsequent early post-operative upper GI series is limited. Nimeri et al. discovered no positive leaks during endoscopy in 310 sleeve gastrectomy patients and one (0.3%) leak after surgery with upper GI series and CT being negative [6]. There were 10 (3.2%) cases of stenosis at the incisura, treated by removing the oversewing sutures and after the operation no stenosis recurred. A positive predictive value to detect a stenosis of 100% and a negative predictive value of 100% were present. Bingham et al. have concerns about the utility, reliability and safety of the intraoperative leak test in laparoscopic sleeve gastrectomy [3]. No leak test was positive and 13 (2.4%) had a post-operative leak without a positive leak test. Sensitivity and positive predictive value were 0%. There was a non-significant trend of more leaks after a routine leak test versus no test (2.6% vs. 0%). They suggested that an intraoperative leak test may weaken the staple line and increase the risk of a post-operative leak by the sheer stress on the staple line and instrumentation with a small risk of iatrogenic injury. Taken together, these studies demonstrate that detection and repair of intraoperative leaks, which may be mechanical in origin and due to technical issues with staple-line integrity, are of value. However, they have no impact on the development of later, post-operative leaks which may be related to ischaemia. Ghosh et al. reviewed 12 articles on sleeve gastrectomies [2]. Intraoperative leaks were reported in three studies, and bleeds were reported in four studies, with an incidence of up to 3.93% for leaks and 4.07% for bleeds. A panel of 24 surgical centres performing over 12,000 cases of sleeve gastrectomies reported a leak rate of 1.06% and 48% of them agreed with the statement that one should routinely perform an intraoperative leak test without defining the method [19].

A much simpler test to discover a potential staple-line defect – although not frequently reported – is to inflate the carefully extracted stomach with air using a regular syringe until it is well filled [20]. Submersion under water could highlight a potential defect of the stapling line [20].

5.3 Post-operative Endoscopy

5.3.1 Routine Post-operative Investigation by Radiology and Endoscopy

Not only the use of routine preoperative investigations as discussed earlier in Chap. 4 but also the use of routine post-operative investigations have heavily been debated.

Proponents of routinely upper GI series are Toppino et al. who argued that it detected post-operative complications and modified the clinical approach in 8.2% and Serafini et al. who concluded that early detection resulted in less morbidly and shorter hospitalisation [21, 22]. Singh et al. warned that in their routine upper GI series, 8 of 10 studies reporting a leak were falsely positive and Kolakowski et al. reported false-positive studies in 4 of the 12 leaks [23, 24]. They stated that the intraoperative leak test using air insufflation may be more effective than early upper GI series in laparoscopic gastric bypass. Upper GI series may also be falsely negative and Madan et al. reported positive and negative predictive values for upper GI series of 67% and 99%, respectively, in 245 patients with Roux-en-Y gastric bypass (RYGB) [25]. A white blood cell count of >10.5 had a negative predictive value of 100%. Leaks can also be demonstrated by assessing the drain fluid amylase (salivary amylase) level, with a high sensitivity and specificity [26].

Others cite the low sensitivity of 43% and poor positive predictive value of 27–60% for leaks and reported excellent results with a selective approach in only symptomatic patients [23, 27, 28]. A gastrointestinal leak is difficult to recognise because clinical findings in obese patients are often subtle and physical exam rarely shows abdominal tenderness. Persistent tachycardia and tachypnoea are the most common early signs. Low-grade fever and abdominal pain radiating to the back, chest and left shoulder can also be early symptoms [27]. The combination of fever (>38.6 °C), tachycardia (>100/min) and tachypnoea (>20/min) was the most specific indicator of a leak [24]. Nausea and vomiting were the most specific indicators of delayed gastric emptying and gastric outlet obstruction [24]. Raman et al. showed that routine upper GI series on day 1 had a 100% sensitivity and 92.9% specificity for major findings such as an anastomotic leak, complete obstruction of the gastrojejunostomy and communications with the gastric remnant [29]. In one patient, the upper GI series was equivocal for a leak. The clinical condition of the patients prompted a return to the operating room where no leak was found. The post-operative CT revealed a pulmonary embolus. It should be noticed that in their series 82% of upper GI series (399/487) were negative for serious complications [29]. Carter and colleagues found a low sensitivity of 43% of detecting leaks or predicting stricture formation by performing routine upper GI series [30]. White et al. analysed >500 cases and found a questionable sensitivity of routine upper GI series and an almost 100% sensitivity with selective use; they abandoned the routine use of upper GI series and only performed upper GI studies selectively [31]. Yet, quite recently, in 2012, Leslie et al. advocated the use of routine GI series because of a far greater sensitivity of upper GI series when compared with that of clinical signs [32]. In that same year, Aurora et al. published their systemic analysis of 4888 sleeve gastrectomy (SG) patients and they concluded that because most leaks from SG occur late after patient discharge, routine contrast studies on post-operative day 1 have a very low yield of detecting leaks [16].

Indeed, Sethi et al. [33] confirmed in a report of 1762 SGs that all patients were discharged home in a good clinical condition, with the leak being diagnosed several days after surgery. They also demonstrated that the sensitivity of the routine post-operative radiological upper GI series was 10.5% and the specificity was 100%, whereas these figures were 89% and 80%, respectively, for the clinical criteria of fever, systemic inflammatory response syndrome (SIRS) criteria and pain score ≥9 [33]. One or more clinical criteria were present in 89% of patients with leaks in contrast to 20% in the control group without leaks and although not significant clinical symptoms were more conspicuous in those with early compared to those with late/delayed leaks. So, routine post-operative UGI series seems not to be the ideal technique to screen all patients for leaks.

A systemic review evaluated the sensitivity and specificity of upper GI series in detecting anastomotic leaks from data obtained from 19 studies involving 10,139 patients [34]. The index technique was a post-operative upper GI contrast study, with CT scan or follow-up surgery used as the reference. Two studies analysed patients who underwent gastric band, gastric sleeve or Roux-en-Y bypass procedures. Three studies were limited to bands and 12 to gastric bypasses and 2 studies did not mention the type of operation. Nine studies were prospective and ten retrospective. Upper GI series had an overall sensitivity of 54–56% and a specificity of 99–100% for detecting an anastomotic leak within 2 days of bariatric surgery. Positive and negative predictive values were 67% and 98%, respectively. The authors discussed extensively their contradictive findings: the overall sensitivity of 54% called into question the extent to which one might confidently rely on a negative pronouncement from upper GI series [34]. On the other hand, the negative predictive value was nearly 100%, from which it should follow that a negative result was almost certain to be correct. This contradiction was thought to be driven in part by the preponderance of "true negative" results (98% overall) in their sample, because in many of the papers patients with a negative contrast study, who were not specifically noted to be false negatives, were assumed to be true negatives. Moreover, they could not confidently make a distinction between patients coded as negative because the imaging failed to identify the leaking anastomosis at the time of the upper GI series and patients coded as negative because they developed an anastomotic leak at some point far later in time, after the series was conducted [34].

Nowadays, computer tomography (CT) is the first choice in evaluating a symptomatic patient but has the disadvantage of a weight limit for the tabletop and a size limit for the aperture of the scanner [27]. In patients with clinical suspicion of complications the selective use of CT has an almost 100% sensitivity and specificity [27, 35]. Bingham et al. investigated 619 radiographic "leak tests" which were selectively performed and which consisted of an upper GI series always followed by an abdominal CT scan [35]. Both were retrospectively reinterpreted by radiologists who were blinded to the outcome. CT was found to have a sensitivity of 95% and a specificity of 100% in diagnosing post-operative leaks, while upper GI studies demonstrated a sensitivity of 79.4% and a specificity of 95%. CT scan had a positive predictive value of 100% and a negative predictive value of 97.1%, compared with upper GI series which had a positive predictive value of 90% and a negative predictive value of 89.1% [35]. Abdominal CT has the advantage to detect other acute abdominal processes and the ability to evaluate the more distal jejunojejunostomy. Upper GI series may be more precise than CT in delineating the magnitude and anatomic origin of an anastomotic leak and it may therefore be useful in guiding management decisions. Contrast upper GI series can be used when CT is technically impossible. It may still be wise to perform a post-operative GI series during a surgeon's learning curve, in complex cases and after revision surgery [24].

How does radiology perform in comparison with endoscopy? In the period 1998–2005 1079 patients received a RYGB and were included in a prospectively maintained database [36]. In a retrospective analysis 76 (7%) had upper GI symptoms. Thirty-six underwent upper GI series with an overall diagnostic yield of 69.4%. Three of the marginal ulcers and 6 of the 12 anastomotic strictures found by endoscopy were missed. Sensitivity and specificity of upper GI series compared to upper GI endoscopy for aetiological findings were 64% and 85%, respectively [36].

The 88 surgeons with an average experience of 2229 sleeve gastrectomies per surgeon, present at the third international summit on sleeve gastrectomy, reflected the usual procedure: a total of 65.1% ordered an upper GI series either post-operatively day 1 or selectively and 74.6% have been performing upper GI series or endoscopy in follow-up, either as a 1-year routine or for symptoms of reflux, dysphagia or weight regain [37]. Yearly routine upper GI endoscopy has been advocated by some. Csendes et al. stressed the missing of reliable data in many studies and the lack of information on the true incidence of complications [38]. They argued that the collection of reliable data would require a scheduled routine endoscopic follow-up to investigate the incidence of abnormal findings [38]. They performed endoscopies as a routine 1 and 17 months after surgery. At 1 month they detected 112 patients having strictures (varying from 54% with a lumen being 7–9 mm wide and described as mild to 22% being <4 mm described as severe) with complaints in only 29% of the moderate and severe strictures [38]. None of the guidelines has discussed the need of routine post-operative investigations [39–41].

5.3.2 Endoscopy for the Evaluation of Symptoms Post-operatively

The most common indication for endoscopy in bariatric surgical patients is the evaluation of gastrointestinal symptoms because many of the complications and side effects of bariatric procedures are gastrointestinal in origin or related to surgically induced alterations in the gastrointestinal tract [42, 43].

5.3.2.1 Information on Gastric Bypass, Gastric Banding, Vertical Banded Gastroplasty and Biliopancreatic Diversion

Monteforte and Turkelson reviewed 3568 restrictive procedures and 3626 gastric bypasses [44]. They reported vomiting in 8.5% of restrictive and 2.6% of bypass procedures whereas dumping was present in 0.28% and 14.6%, respectively. In restrictive procedures the four major complications included gastric pouch/stoma dilation (2.4%), stoma stenosis/gastric outlet obstruction (2.2%), staple-line failure (1.5%) and stomach erosion/ulcer (1.2%; 0.56% of these were band erosions). The figures for gastric bypass were 0.47%, 2.7%, 5.9% and 1.2% (with 0.06% band erosions), respectively.

Chapman et al. studied more in detail the complications of laparoscopic adjustable gastric banding (LAGB) in 64 studies and those of Roux-en-Y gastric bypass (RYGB) and vertical banded gastroplasty (VBG) in 57 studies [45] (Table 5.1).

Table 5.1 Specific complications across 64 studies reporting complications for laparoscopic adjustable gastric banding (LAGB) and 57 studies reporting complications for Roux-en-Y gastric bypass (RYGB) and vertical banded gastroplasty (VBG) [45]

Complications	LAGB *N* = 8504		VBG *N* = 3849		RYGB *N* = 9413	
	N	%	*N*	%	*N*	%
Mortality	13	0.22	22	0.77	91	0.98
Mortality median %	–	10.7	–	23.6	–	27.4
Stoma stenosis	10	0.12	76	1.97	448	4.76
Marginal ulcer/ulcer	1	0.01	5	0.13	386	4.10
Gastrogastric fistula	–	–	53	1.38	24	0.25
Staple-line disruption	–	–	113	2.94	229	2.43
Occluded/kinked stoma	12	0.14	69	1.79	11	0.12
Displacement of band	138	1.62	–	–	–	–
Band erosion	50	0.59	10	0.26	6	0.06
Small-bowel obstruction	–	–	1	0.03	99	1.05
Clinical failure	–	–	66	1.71	3	0.03
Enlarged stoma	–	–	31	0.81	2	0.02
Infection band	31	0.36	2	0.05	–	–
Tubing problems	68	0.8	–	–	–	–
Port rotation/movement	74	0.84	–	–	–	–
Dilation	338	3.97	12	0.31	–	–
Cholelithiasis	16	0.19	6	0.16	164	1.74

Only the most prevalent gastrointestinal complications are mentioned in number and proportions

They realised that the reported rates were underestimated as not every study would have reported all complications. The most common complications related to LAGB were pouch dilation, displacement of the band, port rotation/port movement, tubing problems and band erosion and for VBG these were staple-line disruption, stoma stenosis, occluded or kinked stoma, failure to lose weight, gastrogastric fistula, enlarged stoma and band erosion. The most common complications associated with RYGB were stenosis of the pouch outlet, marginal ulcer or ulcer disease, staple-line disruption, gallstones and small-bowel obstruction. Vomiting and food intolerance showed broad ranges of occurrence with rates varying from 0% up to 60% in LAGB, from 0.8% up to 76.5% after VBG and from 4.7% to 68.8% for RYGB. Maggard et al. evaluated the prevalence of complications in a meta-analysis of 128 studies [46]. They reported anastomotic leaks in 2.2% of RYGB, 1.0% of VBG and 1.8% of biliopancreatic diversion (BPD). Anastomotic/stomal stenosis was present in 4.6% of RYBG and 6% of VBG. Gastrointestinal symptoms were reported as adverse events in 16.9% of RYGB, 17.5% of VBG, 7.8% of LAGB and 37.7% of BPD patients. Reflux was reported by 10.9% of RYGB, 2.2% of VBG and 4.7% of LAGB patients. Reoperations were more common in patients who had laparoscopic procedures.

5.3.2.2 Information on Sleeve Gastrectomy

There are no meta-analyses available comparing the established operations with newer types such as the sleeve gastrectomy, mini gastric bypass or gastric plication.

Meta-analysis which compared sleeve gastrectomy (SG) with LAGB, RYGB and gastric plication either did not investigate gastrointestinal symptoms and complications [47–49] or mentioned no differences between the groups without any further specification [50]. Brethauer et al. reviewed 36 studies with 2570 patients and divided their review according to the initial application of the sleeve gastrectomy in high-risk patients as a staged procedure and as the first step in the biliopancreatic diversion with duodenal switch [51, 52]. The latter involved 13 studies ($n = 821$), which were compared with the use of the sleeve gastrectomy as a stand-alone procedure after 2006 in 24 studies ($n = 1749$) [51]. Overall, there was a complication rate of 0–24% and a rate of 0–15.3% for studies reporting over more than 100 subjects with a low mortality of 0.19% (Table 5.2). When these two groups were compared, only leaks were significantly higher in the group of sleeve gastrectomy as a primary operation, presumably explained by the fact that most of the early SGs were performed by bariatric surgeons who already had had extensive experience in performing the laparoscopic duodenal switch and gastric bypass procedures. Trastulli et al. performed a systematic review of 15 RCTs involving 1191 patients [53]. The sleeve gastrectomy, performed in 795 patients, was compared with any other bariatric procedure. No mortality and a mean complication rate of 9.2% (range 0–18.7%) were found. Rates for leak, bleeding, need of reoperation and stricture were 1.9%, 3.6%, 1.6% and 0.6%, respectively. Also, the review by Kehagias et al. reported a complication rate varying from 0% to 18% with a 30-day mortality between 0% and 0.4% [54]. The most frequent complication they mentioned was the post-operative haemorrhage occurring in up to 18% of cases with an average of 3.6% and the second most frequent complication was a gastric leak varying between 0% and 3.7%. Li et al. performed a meta-analysis of 32 studies comparing SG with RYGB in 6526 patients and reported the complications in 13 studies, involving 3604 patients [55].

Table 5.2 Comparison of complications according to the application of sleeve gastrectomy in high-risk patients or in patients as a staged approach versus sleeve gastrectomy as a primary procedure [51, 52]

	High-risk patients/staged approach	Primary procedure
Number of studies (number of patients)	13 (821)	24 (1749)
Preoperative BMI range (mean) kg/m^2	49.1–69.0 (60.0)	37.2–54.5 (46.6)
Post-operative BMI range (mean) kg/m^2	36.4–53.0 (44.9)	26.0–39.8 (32.2)
Follow-up months/years	4 months to 5 years	3 months to 3 years
Per cent excess weight loss range (mean)	33.0–61.4% (46.9)	36.0–85.0% (60.4)
Complication rate all studies % range (mean)	0–23.8% (9.4%)	0–21.7% (6.2%)
Complication rate in studies with $n > 100$ patients % range	3.3–15.3%	0–14.1%
Leaks n/N (%)	8/686 (1.2%)	45/1681 (2.7%), p 0.02
Bleeding n/N (%)	11/686 (1.6%)	17/1681 (1.0%)
Strictures n/N (%)	6/686 (0.9%)	9/1681 (0.5%)
Mortality n/N (%)	2/821 (0.24%)	3/1749 (0.17%)

BMI body mass index

Table 5.3 Complications in sleeve gastrectomy versus gastric bypass. Total number of complications was 159/1645 (9.7%) in sleeve gastrectomy versus 389/1959 (19.8%) in Roux-en-Y gastric bypass (RYGB) (odds ratio 1.96 (95% confidence interval 1.26/3.04)), but only gastrointestinal complications, as retrieved from studies in the meta-analysis, are mentioned here [55]

Complications	Sleeve *N* (%)	RYGB *N* (%)
Fistula	2 (0.12)	7 (0.35)
Perforation	0 (0)	2 (0.10)
Occlusion/volvulus/torsion	2 (0.12)	46 (2.3)
Stenosis	3 (0.18)	57 (2.9)
Bleeding	12 (0.73)	48 (2.5)
Leak	15 (0.91)	13 (0.60)
Abscess	5 (0.30)	17 (0.87)
Marginal ulcer	0 (0)	3 (0.15)
Gallstones	31 (1.9)	34 (1.7)
Pancreatitis	2 (0.12)	0 (0)

The overall complication rate was twice as high for RYGB (OR 1.96 (95% Confidence Interval (CI) 1.26/3.04)) compared with SG. Besides an almost 2% of gallstone development, the main complications in the sleeve gastrectomy concerned leaks, bleeding and abscess formation (Table 5.3).

5.3.2.3 Information from Daily Practice Care on Sleeve Gastrectomy and Gastric Bypass

For daily practice, data derived from a large personal experience or from large data sets may be more relevant. Alvarenga et al. investigated in 1020 sleeve patients the overall 30-day mortality rate, which was zero, and the early post-operative complications within 30 days of surgery, which included a leak in 0.1% ($n = 1$), stricture in 0.1% ($n = 1$), vomiting in 23% ($n = 234$), dehydration in 19% ($n = 194$), prolonged ileus in 18% (183) and self-limited bleeding in 3% ($n = 30$) [56]. Long-term morbidity included a stricture in 0.49% ($n = 5$) and GORD in 6% ($n = 61$).

Large data sets provided data from the USA, Sweden, Germany and Europe [57–62]. The Bariatric Outcomes Longitudinal Database is a large cohort study from Bariatric Centres of Excellence across the USA. Their analysis of 36,254 patients who underwent a RYGB (92% laparoscopic) demonstrated a 1.38% rate of adverse events at 30 days post-RYGB, the most common complications being anastomotic leak (0.42%), renal failure (0.31%), respiratory failure (0.27%) and death (0.12%) [57]. The Michigan Bariatric Surgery Collaborative (MBSC) is a consortium of 29 Michigan hospitals and 75 surgeons performing bariatric surgery [58]. Any hospital that performs at least 25 bariatric procedures per year is eligible to participate in the MBSC. Out of a 25,469 patients undergoing bariatric surgery, 14,850 (58%) underwent gastric bypass (1092 via an open approach), 8015 (31%) laparoscopic adjustable gastric band, 2279 (9%) sleeve gastrectomy and 325 (1%) biliopancreatic diversion with duodenal switch. The majority of operations (95%) were performed laparoscopically although 70% of the BPD operations were done in an open procedure. Rates of individual complications but restricted to the GI tract by procedure are listed in Table 5.4. As can be seen, 1245 patients (4.9%) experienced at least 1 minor complication, 644 patients (2.5%) experienced at least 1 serious complication and 23 patients (0.1%) died after bariatric surgery. Rates of at least one serious

Table 5.4 Data from the Michigan bariatric surgery collaborative with mentioned gastrointestinal complications [58]

Complications	Overall $N = 25{,}469$	LAGB $N = 8015$	RYGB open $N = 1092$	LRYGB $N = 13{,}758$	SG $N = 2279$	BPD $N = 325$
Minor[a]						
Anastomotic stricture	281 (1.1)	0	13 (1.2)	249 (1.8)	15 (0.7)	4 (1.2)
Bleeding	335 (1.3)	11 (0.1)	24 (2.2)	281 (2.0)	16 (0.7)	3 (0.9)
≥1 minor complication	1245 (4.9)	109 (1.4)	102 (9.3)	932 (6.8)	75 (3.3)	27 (8.3)
Serious[b]						
Abdominal abscess	116 (0.5)	7 (0.1)	5 (0.5)	69 (0.5)	21 (0.9)	14 (4.3)
Leak	151 (0.6)	0	7 (0.6)	109 (0.8)	22 (1.0)	13 (4.0)
Bowel obstruction	111(0.4)	1 (0.01)	1 (0.1)	105 (0.8)	3 (0.1)	1 (0.3)
Bleeding	118 (0.5)	3 (0.04)	13 (1.2)	94 (0.7)	7 (0.3)	1 (0.3)
Band-related	–	47 (0.4)	–	–	–	–
Death	23 (0.1)	3 (0.04)	5 (0.5)	5 (0.5)	2 (0.1)	1 (0.3)
≥1 major complication	644 (2.5)	75 (0.9)	40 (3.7)	40 (3.7)	53(2.3)	26 (8.0)

LAGB laparoscopic adjustable gastric banding, *RYGB* Roux-en-Y gastric bypass, *LRYGB* laparoscopic Roux-en-Y gastric bypass, *SG* sleeve gastrectomy, *BPD* biliopancreatic diversion

[a]Minor complications also included (but not mentioned here) wound infections, pneumonia, urinary tract infection and *C. difficile* infection. Minor bleeding: requiring transfusion of ≤4 units red blood cell packages

[b]Serious complications also included (but not mentioned here) renal and respiratory failure, severe wound infection and myocardial infection. Serious bleeding: requiring transfusion of >4 units red blood cell packages, endoscopy, reoperation or splenectomy. Band-related complications required reoperation and included reoperation for band slippage, outlet obstruction, gastric/oesophageal perforation and port-site infection

complication varied substantially across procedures, ranging from 0.9% with adjustable gastric banding to 8% with the duodenal switch procedure.

The Longitudinal Assessment of Bariatric Surgery reported the outcomes of 5882 patients (73% RYGB of which 88% laparoscopic and 27% LAGB) [59]. Thirty-day major surgical complication rate was 4.1% and mortality was reported at 0.3%, being 0.04% for adjustable gastric banding and 0.5% for open gastric bypass.

The Scandinavian Obesity Surgery Registry reported the 30-day complications (8.7%) of 25,038 laparoscopic RYGB in 44 accredited centres in Sweden [60]. The most common complications were bleeding (2.1%), leaks or abscesses (1.8%) and small-bowel obstruction (1%).

The German Bariatric Surgery Registry contained data from 11,840 patients who from January 2005 until December 2013 underwent SG as primary procedure for morbid obesity [61]. Intraoperative complications occurred in 1.8% [61]. Injuries of the spleen (0.40%), liver (0.11%) and bleeding (0.11%) were the most frequent events. During post-operative hospitalisation 5.9% of all patients developed general complications. Surgical complications were observed in 4.5% of cases and consisted of leakage (1.5%), stenosis (0.1%), ileus (0.1%), sepsis (0.7%), peritonitis (0.7%) and wound infection (0.7%). The 30-day mortality within the study period was 0.25%.

Even more impressive are the detailed data derived from the International Bariatric Registry with preoperative and post-operative data of all patients operated in institutions participating in the Centres of Excellence (COM) programme of the International Federation of Surgeons in Obesity—the European Chapter (IFSO-EC) [62]. They published data from 37 institutions with 6413 sleeves and 10,622 RYGBs performed as primary procedures with at least a 12-month follow-up (Table 5.5). The 30-day mortality was one subject in each group, 0.016% in the SG, and 0.009% in the RYGB group. Early complication rates were significantly lower for the SG group (2.1%) than for the RYGB (3.02%), mainly explained by a higher rate of leaks in RYGB. The 30-day readmission rate was similar; however, the number of

Table 5.5 Complications as reported by 33 institutes after sleeve gastrectomy or Roux-en-Y gastric bypass (RYGB), as 30-day complication rates, ≤30 day and >30 day readmission rates [62]

Post-operative 30-day complications		
Complications	Sleeve *N* (%)	RYGB *N* (%)
General	13 (0.20)	45 (0.42)
Bleeding	77 (1.20)	108 (1.02)
Leak	10 (0.15)	40 (0.38), *p* 0.01
Intra-abdominal abscess	3 (0.05)	6(0.06)
Wound infection	3 (0.05)	6 (0.06)
Wound dehiscence	3 (0.05)	3 (0.03)
Intestinal obstruction	0 (0)	7 (0.07)
Stricture	2 (0.03)	7 (0.07)
Vomiting	3 (0.05)	12 (0.11)
Other	22 (0.34)	85 (0.80)
Total	136 (2.12)	319 (3.02), *p* 0.0006
Mortality	1 (0.016)	1 (0.009)

≤30-day readmission rates		
Reason	Sleeve *N* (%)	RYGB *N* (%)
General	6 (0.09)	10 (0.09)
Bleeding	4 (0.07)	24 (0.23)
Leak	17 (0.27)	21 (0.20)
Intra-abdominal abscess	19 (0.30)	10 (0.09), *p* 0.004
Wound infection	4 (0.06)	10 (0.09)
Wound dehiscence	0 (0)	2 (0.02)
Obstruction	4 (0.06)	12 (0.11)
Stricture	1 (0.02)	6 (0.06)
Ulcer	2 (0.03)	10 (0.09)
Vomiting	12 (0.18)	23 (0.22)
Other	34 (0.53)	79 (0.74)
Total	103 (1.61)	207 (1.94)
Reoperation	78/103 (75.7)	104/206 (50.5), $p < 0.0001$

(continued)

Table 5.5 (continued)

>30-day readmission rates		
Reason	Sleeve *N* (%)	RYGB *N* (%)
GORD	2 (0.03)	4 (0.04)
Ulcer	2 (0.03)	36 (0.34), p 0.0001
Stricture	4 (0.06)	2 (0.02)
Vomiting	8 (0.12)	23 (0.22)
Protein malnutrition	2 (0.03)	5 (0.05)
Liver failure	1 (0.01)	0 (0)
Incisional hernia	5 (0.07)	12 (0.11)
Obstruction	12 (0.18)	63 (0.59), p 0.0002
Other	31 (0.46)	206 (1.93), $p < 0.001$
Total	67 (0.99)	351 (3.30), $p < 0.001$
Reoperation	61/34 (55.8)	223/351 (62.5)

abscesses and need of reoperation were higher in the SG group. Long-term outcomes favoured the sleeve gastrectomy with significantly more admissions, marginal ulcers and obstructions seen in the gastric bypass group.

Data from surveys at two conferences on sleeve gastrectomy are also available [37, 63]. Complications after SG were reported by the 88 surgeons who attended the third International Summit [37]. They reported an overall mortality of 0.3%, a 2.2–2.4% leak rate with a leak-related mortality of 0.1%, a stricture rate of 0.5–0.6% and a bleeding rate of 0.7%. Symptoms of GORD occurred in 6.8% of patients post-operatively. The fifth International Consensus Conference gathered 120 experienced bariatric surgeons, performing almost a thousand bariatric operations/year and also 103 general bariatric surgeons [63]. The expert surgeons completed the expert survey, and mentioned strictures in 2.1%, leaks in 2.4%, conversion because of weight loss failure in 4.7% and conversion because of GORD in 2.9%. The general bariatric surgeons audience reported significantly lower stricture and leak rates.

To summarise: With increased use of laparoscopy and other advancements in surgical techniques, the overall mortality rate of bariatric surgery is <0.2% [64]. Yet, approximately 4–10% of patients present for complications within the first 30 days after surgery and 9–25% present for evaluation of late complications.

So, it is evident that gastrointestinal symptoms and complications may require the active involvement of a gastroenterologist or endoscopist. But what do the guidelines advise?

5.3.2.4 Guidelines

Guidelines agree with Grade C and moderate level of evidence that persistent and severe GI symptoms (nausea, vomiting, abdominal pain, diarrhoea and constipation) warrant evaluation [40, 41]. While endoscopy is mentioned as a first-line diagnostic study with consultation with the surgeon in the immediate post-operative period by American guidelines, the European guidelines consider both endoscopy and CT as the first diagnostic/therapeutic option in order to evaluate intestinal diseases, bacterial overgrowth, ulcer disease, anastomotic problems, obstruction due to foreign body, etc. The American guidelines prefer endoscopy for GI symptoms suggestive of stricture or foreign body (staple, suture) as it can be both diagnostic and therapeutic (Grade C) [40]. Furthermore they mention that evaluation can also include *Helicobacter pylori* testing as a contributor to persistent GI symptoms (Grade D) and that ultrasound should be used to evaluate patients with right upper quadrant pain for cholecystitis (Grade D) [40].

5.4 Frequency and Predictors of Complaints and Complications in the Post-operative Period

Gastroenterologists may take advantage of the knowledge which complaints and lesions might to be expected and also which circumstances and conditions may predict any abnormal finding. They should be aware of the type of patient who is at increased risk of perioperative complications. Factors that have been found to contribute to increased mortality include patient-related characteristics such as advanced age, male gender, preoperative weight and coexisting conditions, and procedure-related factors such as lack of adequate experience on the part of the surgeon or the hospital, anastomotic leak and operation type (laparoscopy < laparotomy < revision surgery) [11, 65–76]. Risk factors that most frequently correlate with increased risk of complications are advanced age, male gender, presence of diabetes and sleep apnoea, but also surgeon and hospital inexperience [11, 66–70].

5.4.1 Mortality and Morbidity Risk Calculators

Risk assessment and stratification is an important component of all surgical decisions. Therefore, surgeons have always tried to predict post-operative mortality and morbidity which they also may use to inform patients more in depth regarding their decision-making. Moreover, modification of modifiable risk factors before surgery may improve perioperative patient care. Risk calculators to assess an individual's post-operative mortality and/or morbidity may be of help. The discriminative ability of the proposed models is reflected in the c-statistic. The c-statistic ranges from 0.5 to 1.0, where a value of 1.0 represents perfect discrimination of cases from non-cases and a value of 0.5 suggests discrimination that is no better than chance. Generally, an absolute cut-off value of 0.70 is thought to be needed for good discrimination and all risk calculators mentioned below were – with values between 0.67 and 0.69 – just below the cut-off value of 0.70, indicating that other factors such as surgeon experience, technical proficiency and variation in technique may also influence the outcome of surgery.

5.4.1.1 Gastric Bypass

DeMaria et al. constructed an Obesity Surgery Mortality Risk Score (OS-MRS) based on data from 2075 consecutive patients undergoing a primary gastric bypass [74]. Preoperative factors were determined that correlated with a 90-day mortality (all deaths and deaths related to a complication of the bariatric surgery). Post-operative complications were not examined. Multivariate analysis discovered four independent variables that correlated with mortality, including body mass index $\geq$50 kg/m^2, male gender, hypertension and a novel variable pulmonary embolus risk, that included previous thrombosis, pulmonary embolus, inferior vena cava filter, right-heart failure, pulmonary hypertension and obesity hypoventilation. A fifth variable, patient age $\geq$45 years, significant on univariate analysis, was added to the scoring system because of its significance in other studies. Presence or absence was coded by 1 or 0 points, resulting in an overall score of 0–5 points for each patient. The factors were grouped into three risk classes. The mortality rate among the three risk classes was significantly different: class A (0–1 points) had a low risk (0.31%); class B (2–3 points) an intermediate risk (1.90%); and class C (4–5 points) a high risk of mortality (7.56%) [74].

Subsequently, this Obesity Surgery Mortality Risk Score (OS-MRS) was validated in prospectively collected data from 4431 consecutive patients undergoing a primary gastric bypass at four bariatric institutions [75]. The findings were remarkably similar: the mortality rate for 2164 class A patients was 0.2%, for 2142 class B patients was 1.1% and for 125 class C patients was 2.4%. Three-quarters of all deaths occurred within 30 days of surgery and the most common cause of death was pulmonary embolism (30%) followed by cardiac cause (27%), and gastrointestinal leak (21%). The simplicity of the test made it applicable to clinical use. It also helped to guide class C patients, either by using low-risk procedures like laparoscopic sleeve gastrectomy or gastric band only or by using staged/sequential approaches in which a low-risk operation is done first to reduce weight and improve comorbidities followed by subsequent revision to a more durable or effective operation. Out of the risk factors comprising the OS-MRS, only a few factors can be changed such as reducing the preoperative BMI, whereas the effects of an improved blood pressure regulation or optimal coagulation status are largely unknown [75]. Finally, a systematic review of six studies evaluating the OS-MRS in 9382 patients confirmed that OS-MRS stratified the mortality risk in the three risk classification subgroups of patients: there were 13 deaths among 4912 (0.26%) class A patients, 55 deaths among 4124 (1.33%) class B patients and 15 deaths among 346 (4.34%) class C patients [76].

Although the OS-MRS score was developed for analysing mortality after bariatric surgery and more specifically after gastric bypass surgery, the score has been inappropriately used to analyse morbidity. Indeed, both in a personal series and in a review of the literature, the OS-MRS score failed to predict post-operative complications after bariatric surgery [77].

Five years later Maciejewski et al. developed and validated a risk stratification model of composite adverse events related to Roux-en-Y gastric bypass (RYGB) surgery, using one of the largest cohorts of bariatric surgery patients in the world: the Bariatric Outcomes Longitudinal Database (BOLD) registry [78]. There were 36,254 patients who had undergone a primary RYGB, who were at least 90 days past the date of surgery, and this sample of 36,254 was randomly divided into a 50% testing sample and a 50% validation sample (each 18,127 patients). The composite adverse event outcome included 17 endpoints, varying from death and organ failures to anastomotic leakage, sepsis, systemic inflammatory response syndrome and intraoperative bleeding requiring blood transfusions. The rates of composite adverse events at 30 days (1.38%) and at 90 days (1.48%) were both low [78], and substantially lower than the 30-day adverse event rate for gastric bypass in contemporary multicentre studies which ranges between 3.3% and 4.8%, suggesting that adverse events are substantially underreported in BOLD [71, 79, 80]. The most common serious adverse events at 90 days were anastomotic leak (0.42%), renal failure (0.31%), respiratory failure (0.27%) and death (0.12%). The final risk stratification model for 90-day composite adverse events included 12 covariates, including age 40–64 years, age ≥65 years, male gender, BMI 50–59.9 kg/m^2, BMI ≥ 60 kg/m^2, obesity hypoventilation syndrome, back pain, diabetes, pulmonary hypertension, ischaemic heart disease, functional impairment related to ambulation and ASA class 4 or 5. Out of these 12 predictors the most significant were age ≥65 years (OR = 2.44), obesity hypoventilation syndrome (OR = 2.12), functional impairment (OR = 2.01), pulmonary hypertension (OR = 1.94) and BMI ≥60 kg/m^2 (OR = 1.91). The remaining risk factors had ORs between 1.42 and 1.72 and the lowest OR was for a BMI 50–59.9 kg/m^2 (OR 1.25).

5.4.1.2 Bariatric Surgery Excluding Sleeve Gastrectomy

To evaluate more in a broader sense the perioperative safety, the Longitudinal Assessment of Bariatric Surgery (LABS) consortium defined a composite endpoint of a 30-day major adverse outcome, which included death; venous thromboembolism; percutaneous, endoscopic or operative re-intervention; and failure to be discharged from the hospital [79]. The type of procedure (open and laparoscopic Roux-en-Y gastric bypass, as compared with laparoscopic adjustable gastric banding), extremes of body mass index (i.e. >53 kg/m^2), an inability to walk 200 ft., a history of deep-vein thrombosis or venous thromboembolism, and a history of obstructive sleep apnoea were significantly associated with the composite endpoint, whereas age, sex, race, ethnic group and other coexisting conditions were not [79]. The most commonly occurring components of the endpoint were abdominal reoperation (2.6%) and endoscopic intervention (1.1%). The LABS consortium data provide a continuous risk scale rather than stratifying patients into discrete classes as in OS-MRS which is less simple, less easy and less fast. The LABS score already included some morbidity data but still there was a need for a morbidity risk scale.

Gupta et al. developed a morbidity risk calculator by using prospective multicentre National Surgical Quality Improvement Program (NSQIP) data from 2007 and validated the risk calculator with the NSQIP 2008 data set [80]. It should be noted that the NSQIP prospectively collects data on more than 150 variables, including demographic variables, comorbidities, laboratory values and 30-day post-operative mortality and morbidity outcomes for patients undergoing major surgical procedures. It lacks specificity with regard to bariatric-specific comorbidities (such as sleep apnoea) and outcomes (anastomotic leaks). For the 30-day morbidity score 17 post-operative complications were considered including deep-wound infection, organ-space infection, pneumonia, reintubation, being on the ventilator >48 h, pulmonary embolus, deep venous thrombosis, renal insufficiency, acute renal failure, stroke, coma, cardiac arrest, myocardial infarction, transfusion with more than four units within 72 h, sepsis, septic shock and return to the operating room. The reference procedure was the VBG and the reference BMI was a BMI > 60 kg/m^2. They found several risk factors associated with increased post-operative morbidity such as recent (within 6 months) myocardial infarction or recent (last month) angina, dependent functional status, stroke, bleeding disorder, hypertension, BMI and type of surgery. Patients with a BMI of 35–44.9 and >60 kg/m^2 had a higher risk than patients with a BMI 45–60 kg/m^2 and each operation had a different estimate that had to be entered in the equation. The presence or absence of disease has to be filled in by 1 or 0, and there are three classes for BMI and six classes for the types of bariatric procedures. A Web-based calculator is needed, which is easy to use and the final result is a post-operative morbidity probability percentage. The calculator can be downloaded from http://www.surgicalriskcalculator.com/bariatric-surgery-risk-calculator [80]. Hopefully, in the near future the risk score can be more refined and made more bariatric surgery specific because bowel obstruction, gastrointestinal bleed and anastomotic/stoma stenosis are not included. Anastomotic leaks are not specifically mentioned as such but are represented by the term "organ-space infection".

A year later the same authors also provided a mortality calculator [81]. They used the same data set as used for the morbidity risk calculator for construction and validation and the same 17 items. Seven factors were associated with increased post-operative mortality and were entered into the equation: higher age, BMI class, dyspnoea at rest, previous percutaneous coronary intervention, history of peripheral vascular disease requiring revascularisation or amputation, and chronic corticosteroid use. The type of bariatric surgery was forced into the multivariable analysis. The reference group for bariatric surgery was biliopancreatic diversion with duodenal switch (BPD-DS), for BMI class it was BMI > 60 kg/m^2, and for dyspnoea it was dyspnoea at rest. Value of 1 (present) or 0 (absent) has to be given for comorbidities, 0–2 for the level of dyspnoea, 1–3 for BMI class (class I, 45 kg/m^2, class II, 45–60 kg/m^2, class III, >60 kg/m^2), and 1–6 for type of bariatric procedure [81]. The mortality calculator appeared to have a high discriminative and predictive ability and has the advantage over the other existing validated Obesity Surgery Mortality Risk Score that it is applicable to all bariatric interventions with the exception of the sleeve and to both the open and laparoscopic approach. The calculator can be downloaded from http://www.surgicalriskcalculator.com/bariatric-surgery-risk-calculator.

5.4.1.3 Sleeve Gastrectomy

Two recent risk calculators looked into sleeve gastrectomies as one of the operations in the whole spectrum of bariatric surgery or into sleeve gastrectomies more specifically. Finks et al. used the data from the Michigan Bariatric Surgery Collaborative (MBSC) from 25,469 patients undergoing primary, non-revision bariatric surgery between June 2006 and December 2010 [58]. They categorised 30-day complications according to severity as nonlife-threatening (grade 1, for instance anastomotic strictures requiring endoscopic dilation, bleeding requiring blood transfusion of ≤4 units), potentially life-threatening (grade 2, for instance abscess, bleeding, leaks, bowel obstruction, requiring reoperation or invasive interventions) or life-threatening complications associated with permanent residual disability or death (grade 3, such as cardiac, renal or pulmonary failure or death). The most significant risk factor was procedure type. Compared with adjustable gastric band which was the reference group, duodenal switch carried the highest risk for serious complications (odds ratio [OR] 9.68), followed by laparoscopic (OR 3.58) and open (OR 3.51) gastric bypass, and finally sleeve gastrectomy (OR 2.46). Significant patient-related risk factors had odds ratios varying between 1.20 and 1.90 and in descending order of risk included previous history of venous thromboembolism, mobility limitations, coronary artery disease, age over 50 years, pulmonary disease, male gender and smoking history. The risk prediction equation was based on the coefficients from the final regression model. A user-friendly version of this risk calculator is available on the MBSC website at https://www.michiganbsc.org. On the basis of this risk prediction model, 92% of patients had a predicted risk of serious complications less than 5%. The predicted risk for serious complications varied between 5% and 10% for 7% of patients and was greater than 10% in 1% of patients. Interestingly, mobility limitations per se have not been previously associated with morbidity from bariatric surgery but were associated with mortality in the 30-day adverse outcome including death in the LAGS risk calculator and also in the Turner's risk calculator based on the National Surgical Quality Improvement Program (NSQIP) which identified age, BMI, serum albumin and functional status as significant predictors [82]. Body mass index, a commonly reported risk factor in other risk predictor instruments, was not associated with risk for serious complications in the current risk calculator.

Aminian et al. retrieved cases of primary sleeve gastrectomy from the National Surgical Quality Improvement Program (NSQIP) data set at year 2012 ($n = 5871$) to develop a model and cases from 2011 ($n = 3130$) to examine the validity of the model [83]. The primary outcome was a 30-day post-operative composite of adverse events, which was defined as presence of any of 14 serious adverse events. These adverse events were not bariatric specific and included organ/space surgical site infection, stroke, coma, myocardial infarction, cardiac arrest, acute renal failure, deep-vein thrombosis, pulmonary embolism, reintubation, failure to wean from mechanical ventilation, sepsis, septic shock, need for transfusion and death. Thirty-day post-operative mortality was 0.5% and composite adverse event rate was 2.4%. The final model retained 7 risk factors out of 52 examined baseline variables and included a history of congestive heart failure, chronic steroid use, male gender, diabetes, high BMI, elevated preoperative serum bilirubin and low preoperative haematocrit levels. Congestive heart failure (OR 6.23) followed by chronic steroid use (OR 5.0) displayed the strongest independent associations with the probability of adverse events after SG. A user-friendly version of the risk calculator is accessible at http://www.r-calc.com under the bariatric surgery tab.

From the mentioned risk calculators there are some modifiable factors evident such as preoperative BMI, immobility and functional status, and smoking, i.e. factors that can be improved by preoperative weight loss and a preoperative physical conditioning and rehabilitation programme. Comorbid conditions such as hypertension, diabetes and sleep apnoea may call for a better control in the preoperative period, and patients at high risk for venous thromboembolism and pulmonary embolism could be treated with a more aggressive preoperative chemoprophylaxis regimen. The type of the procedure may be tailored to the risk of the patient with the lowest risk operation with the best outcome done first.

5.4.2 Frequency and Predictors of Complaints and Complications in the Post-operative Period According to the Type of Bariatric Surgery

Each type of surgery may have its own spectrum of complaints and complications and for a gastroenterologist it is important to know which complaints are most frequent and which findings at endoscopy, if present at all, may prevail. Although currently Roux-en-Y gastric bypass and sleeve gastrectomy are the most frequently performed operations, they may still encounter patients with vertical banded gastroplasty, mostly performed about 30 years ago, and gastric banding which was in vogue over the last 20 years but abandoned in most countries at present.

5.4.2.1 Vertical Banded Gastroplasty (VBG)

While all patients in the preoperative period in preparation of a VBG had a routine endoscopy, after the operation endoscopy was performed as indicated clinically in the presence of symptoms of recurrent vomiting, epigastric pain, pyrosis, inadequate weight loss, anaemia or complications after vertical banded gastroplasty [84]. This was the case in 55/159 patients (34.6%) who complained mainly of vomiting (70%), gastro-oesophageal reflux (17%) and epigastric pain (3%). In the majority, in 92% of cases, one or more significant lesions were found [84].

5.4.2.2 Laparoscopic Adjustable Gastric Banding (LAGB)

When evaluating the literature on gastric banding one should realise three facts: firstly that the band was approved by the FDA for use in the USA only in June 2001, whereas it was available in Europe since the mid-1990s; secondly that in contrast to the use of gastric bands elsewhere in the world with a fairly unfavourable tenor, reports from Australia with a very meticulous follow-up are mostly positive; and finally that the surgical technique changed from the perigastric approach to the pars flaccida technique [85, 86]. This is also reflected in the reported complications after LAGB that differ substantially between Europe and the USA [85, 87, 88]. The two US clinical trials under FDA protocol starting in 1995 and 1999 used the perigastric method. The FDA-monitored study shows relatively high rates for some complications which may also be attributed to the relatively few number of procedures performed by each surgeon and their lack of experience with adjustments of the band [87]. The most frequently occurring complications associated with the gastric band included gastric prolapse/band slippage/pouch dilation (Europe 2.2–7.8%, USA 3.1–24%), band erosion (Europe 0.4–1.9%, USA 0.2–1.0%), gastric perforation (Europe 0.1–0.5%, USA 1.5%), oesophageal dilation (Europe 0.2%, USA 6–10%) and access port problems (Europe 0.1–11%, USA 2.3–15%) [87, 88]. Many of the problems such as gastric prolapse and pouch dilation were related to the surgical technique and more often seen with the perigastric technique (13.3%) than the currently recommended pars flaccida technique (1.8%) [86, 89, 90]. Also, gastric band erosion, observed in 3.8% of patients having undergone the perigastric technique, is seen less frequent when the pars flaccida technique is used for placement [90].

Also, the design of the original band (Lapband) changed over time and new types of bands became available. In contrast to the high-pressure/low-volume band (Lapband), the Swedish band was a low-pressure/high-volume band. Two reviews compared the Swedish band (SB) and the Lapband (LB) [91, 92]. Both reviews did not see a difference in weight loss outcomes and in improvements of comorbidities. Early (SB 0.1%, LB 0.2%) and late (SB 0.2% and LB 0.1%) mortalities were similar. Complications differed: conversions (3.2% vs. 1.7%), late band leakage (2.7% vs. 1.1%) and early slippage (1.0% vs. 0.2%) were higher in the Swedish band but late reoperations (14.3% vs. 1.2%) and late band slippage/migration (7.0% vs. 1.6%) were higher in the Lapband group. However, none of the eight reviewed studies were randomised and the two bands were used in different time periods and no parallel groups were available [91, 92].

5.4.2.3 Roux-en-Y Gastric Bypass (RYGB)

Following gastric bypass, approximately 20–30% of patients have upper GI symptoms that prompt endoscopy, and of those 70% were found to have an abnormality related to their surgery [93, 94]. Common findings include marginal ulcer (27–52%), stomal stenosis (4–19%) and staple-line dehiscence (4–16%) [93, 94]. A total of 226 patients out of 1001 RYGB patients (23%) had an endoscopy to evaluate upper GI symptoms [95]. The most common finding was a normal postsurgical anatomy ($n = 99$; 44%). The remaining 127 patients presented with relevant abnormalities. Mainly marginal ulcers ($n = 81$; 36%), stomal stenosis (not able to pass a 9.8 mm endoscope; $n = 29$; 13%) and staple-line dehiscence ($n = 8$; 4%) were found. Other findings were oesophagitis in seven and a non-marginal ulcer in six. Factors that increased significantly the risk of marginal ulcers following surgery include smoking (adjusted OR 30.6 (6.4/146)) and NSAID use (adjusted OR 11.5 (4.8/28)). PPI therapy was protective against marginal ulcers (adjusted OR 0.33 (0.11/0.97)) [95]. Prophylactic PPI therapy therefore was advised for the first 12 months of surgery because a significant majority (91%) of marginal ulcers presented within 12 months and the median time for diagnosis of 2 months. Presentation with complaints more than 6 months after surgery was associated with a lower likelihood of stomal ulceration and stenosis (OR 0.04 and 0.25, respectively). Both NSAIDs (OR 12.1 (1.1/90.1)) and smoking (OR 20.9 (1.1/411)) were associated with the finding of staple-line dehiscence. Surprisingly, the risk of stomal stenosis was not affected by PPI use or by the surgical technique [95].

1079 RYGB patients, operated in the period 1998–2005 and included in a prospectively maintained database, were retrospectively analysed [36]. Seventy-six (7%) had gastrointestinal symptoms: dysphagia in 41 (53.9%), nausea/vomiting in 37 (48.7%), abdominal pain (19, 25%) and haematemesis (1, 1.3%). Endoscopy showed normal anatomy in 24 (31.6%), anastomotic stricture (defined by resistance to passage of the 9.6 cm endoscope) in 40 (52.6%), marginal ulcer in 12 (15.8%), sutures causing obstruction in 3 (4%) and a gastrogastric fistula in 2 (2.6%). Patients with abnormal findings presented at a mean of 110 days whereas those with normal findings presented after 347 days. Age, gender, ethnicity, BMI and type of surgery (open, laparotomy, robotic) were not related to the finding of endoscopic lesions, but patients with abnormal findings reported significantly more dysphagia (67.3% vs. 25%) and patients with normal findings had more abdominal pain (45.8% vs. 15.4%) [36].

5.4.2.4 Sleeve Gastrectomy (SG)

Stroh et al. investigated the rate of leaks and predictive factors for the occurrence of leaks in sleeve gastrectomy [61]. Between 2005 and 2013 the staple-line leak rate decreased from 6.5% to 1.4%. Male sex, higher body mass index, concomitant sleep apnoea, conversion to laparotomy, longer operation time, a combination of buttresses and oversewing compared with using either buttresses or oversewing alone, and the occurrence of intraoperative complications were associated with a significantly higher leakage rate. On multivariable analysis, operation time and year of procedure had a significant impact on the staple-line leakage rate. A higher number of leaks were observed within the first years of study participation, signifying an important effect of a learning curve. The leakage risk decreased each year by an OR of 0.78 (0.71/0.86). The second important factor was the presence of intraoperative complications, which increases the risk of leakage by 2.27 (2.12/7.44). This study demonstrated that there are factors that increase the risk of leakage. This would enable the bariatric team to define risk groups, select patients more carefully and offer closer follow-up during the post-operative course with early recognition and adequate treatment.

5.4.2.5 Role of *Helicobacter pylori*

The role of *Helicobacter pylori* has been discussed at length in Chap. 4. To summarise the findings: three studies reported an increased risk of marginal ulcer development [96–98] and five studies did not find a role for *Helicobacter pylori* in the gastric bypass patient [36, 94, 99–101]. As to the risk of perforation, Hartin et al. found a trend of decreased symptoms, less need for endoscopy, less marginal ulcer formation, less bleedings and less perforations in patients being negative for *Helicobacter pylori* [102]. As to the sleeve gastrectomy, five studies could not find a predictive role for the presence of *Helicobacter pylori* in developing complications [103–107].

So, the kind of complaints may help in the diagnosis but also the timing of occurrence: patients with symptoms less than 3 months after surgery are more likely to have abnormal findings on endoscopy, being mainly anastomotic strictures. Marginal ulcers appeared more likely after 3 months after surgery.

5.5 Description of Surgical Procedure and Herewith Associated Normal Endoscopic Findings

Endoscopy is justified after bariatric surgery:

- For the follow-up of symptomatic patients.
- For analysis of the causes of failure of bariatric surgery.
- To identify and treat complications [108, 109].

The endoscopist should carefully read the reason for referral to the endoscopy unit, review the formal operative notes on the altered gastric anatomy and the extent of resection and length of surgically created intestinal limbs, review the perioperative and post-operative records and review all available post-operative abdominal imaging studies [41, 109–111]. He/she should also discuss the bariatric operation with the patient's surgeon, and all these requirements are more easily fulfilled when the endoscopist is part of the bariatric team. He/she should then select the most appropriate type of endoscope and accessories needed, which will depend on the indication for the endoscopy. He/she should recognise that specially designed accessories may be necessary and that in case of an early post-operative endoscopy with leaks or fresh anastomosis carbon dioxide insufflation may be useful [41, 109–111]. Endoscopists should consider the appropriate sedation and analgesia plan and the need of performing the endoscopy while the patient is intubated. They should also choose the appropriate venue for the procedure (i.e. endoscopy suite vs. operating room).

5.5.1 Choice of the Endoscope

A standard endoscope can be used to evaluate patients following VBG, LAGB, SG and gastric pouch or proximal Roux limb in patients with RYGB. When after a RYGB the jejunojejunostomy has to be examined, a paediatric colonoscope or an enteroscope may be needed depending on the length of the Roux limb. Retrograde evaluation of the biliopancreatic limb or bypassed stomach can be accomplished with a paediatric colonoscope or an enteroscope. Methods for deep small-bowel enteroscopy include double-balloon enteroscopy, single-balloon enteroscopy, spiral tube enteroscopy and ShameLock technology [112]. Balloon-assisted enteroscopy uses balloons attached to an overtube with (double balloon) or without a balloon (single balloon) at the tip of the enteroscope. The balloons anchor the enteroscope and overtube as the enteroscope is advanced through the small bowel. With spiral tube enteroscopy a spiral tube is placed over the enteroscope. As the spiral is rotated the small bowel is ruled onto the overtube, advancing the enteroscope through the small bowel. The use of a ShameLock enteroscopy guide, a novel overtube device with a unique lockable on-demand feature, initially designed to prevent loop formation during colonoscopy, has also been used to facilitate intubation of the bypassed stomach. All these methods for deep small-bowel enteroscopy facilitate the performance of an ERCP. In exceptional cases a double-channel endoscope is needed.

5.5.2 Endoscopic Armamentarium

Depending on the skills of the endoscopist tools for endoscopic interventions are indispensable [113]. For the injection of saline, epinephrine and various glue agents conventional sclerosing needles are needed. Sometimes, in the case of fibrin glue, a double-channel catheter is needed. An endoscopic scissor and graspers are needed to remove suture material. Endoclips of any kind, thermic coagulation catheters (mono- or bipolar) and haemospray® catheter (Cook Medical, Winston-Salem, NC, USA) may be useful in haemostasis. Partially or fully covered self-expandable metallic stents (SEMS) and self-expandable plastic stents (SEPS) may be introduced to treat leaks or refractory strictures. The endoscope may also be mounted externally with larger bear claw clips (Over-the-Scope-Clip [OTSC®], Ovesco, Tübingen, Germany). To remove eroded bands a gastric band cutter device or a Soehendra Biliary Mechanical Lithotriptor (Wilson-Cook Medical Inc., Winston-Salem, NC, USA) is helpful. In case of leakage, different kinds of endosponges® (Braun AG, Melsungen, Germany) are inserted into the gastrointestinal lumen through a plastic overtube.

The endoscopist should also not be surprised to find no abnormalities at all in up to 45% of cases despite sometime severe symptomatology [36, 93–95, 97]. For instance, vomiting has been reported in 30% of operated patients and might be due to various causes such as non-compliance with the requested eating behaviour with an inadequate volume, insufficient mastication and a too rapid food intake, besides clinical causes such as cholelithiasis, obstruction by a food bolus, stricture of the anastomosis, internal hernia and adhesions. Weight gain after bariatric surgery may be related to non-compliance with the diet with consuming high-calorie liquids or snacking between meals and will not always be explained by surgical complications.

Parameters that are predictive of abnormal endoscopic findings include the symptoms reported, time since surgery and patient-related risk factors and exposures. Symptoms that have been associated with abnormal endoscopic findings are dysphagia, nausea, vomiting and signs of upper GI bleeding such as haematemesis and melaena. In general the longer the interval since surgery, the greater the likelihood of a patient having a normal endoscopy with the possible exception of patients with a staple-line dehiscence who frequently present later in the post-operative course. Huang et al. [93] demonstrated that of 49 symptomatic patients, 85% of those presenting within the first 6 months had abnormal endoscopic findings compared with 47% of patients evaluated after 6 months. Patient-related factors are the use of NSAIDs, smoking and alcohol use.

5.5.3 Endoscopy and Surgically Induced Altered Anatomy

The endoscopic view after bariatric surgery will vary according to the surgical technique used [42, 43, 114].

5.5.3.1 Roux-en-Y Gastric Bypass (RYGB) [42, 43, 109, 110, 114]

RYGB involves an upper 30 mL gastric pouch performed by transverse stapling or complete division between fundus and bypassed stomach with a gastrojejunal anastomosis on a Roux-en-Y limb. Most recent techniques create the gastric pouch along the lesser curve with complete separation from the bypassed stomach. Endoscopically, the Roux-en-Y gastric bypass consists of a small gastric pouch that extends just 5–7 cm from the Z-line and is emptying via a stoma, measuring 10–12 mm in diameter, into the jejunum. Surgically speaking, the

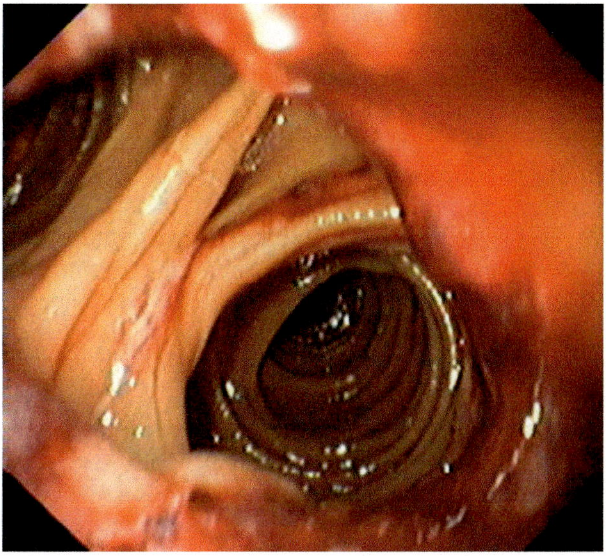

Fig. 5.2 The normal endoscopic view of a Roux-en-Y gastric bypass, consisting of a small gastric pouch that extends just 5–7 cm from the Z-line. The pouch empties via a stoma, measuring 10–12 mm in diameter, into the jejunum. The gastrojejunostomy is an end-to-side anastomosis and it gives the endoscopist a double-barrel view when examined through the gastric lumen. Reprinted from Obes Surg 2011; 21: 1530–1534, Cingi A, Yavuz Y. Intraoperative endoscopic assessment of the pouch and anastomosis during laparoscopic Roux-en-Y gastric bypass with permission from Springer

gastrojejunostomy is an end-to-side anastomosis, connecting the end of the gastric pouch to the side of the jejunum. It gives the endoscopist a double-barrel view when examined through the gastric lumen (Fig. 5.2). There is typically a short (1–2 cm) blind limb of jejunum just distal to the gastrojejunostomy in addition to the Roux limb. The gastric pouch is small, so minimal air should be inflated and the short blind limb of thin-walled jejunum may be perforated easily by too much pressure by the endoscope or by wires and balloons used in case of dilation [93, 97]. Also, the gastric pouch is too small to permit safe retroflexion. For the construction of the gastrojejunostomy, a 21 or a 25 mm circular stapler or linear stapler, with additional suturing or stapling at the entry point of the linear staple to close this side, is used and staples can be recognised. Approximately 50% of bariatric surgeons use hand-sewn anastomoses with absorbable sutures, which retain their tensile strength for about 4–6 weeks after surgery. The gastric remnant, duodenum and part of the jejunum are outside the normal food circulation (biliopancreatic limb) and are connected distally to the jejunum via a jejunojejunostomy. Normally, the jejunojejunal anastomosis can be reached by a standard endoscope with a Roux limb of 75 cm. In severe obesity the limb may be extended to 150 cm and then the jejunojejunal anastomosis can only be reached by enteroscopy with either a double balloon, single balloon or spiral enteroscopy. This holds also true when access to the stomach is needed via the jejunojejunostomy and the biliopancreatic limb. Surgeons find it useful to have data on the pouch length and width, stoma size, visible suture material and length of the blind limb. The endoscopist should examine the gastric pouch, suture line and jejunal mucosa for fistula and ulcerations. The blind limb should be small; when excessively long it may be a cause of postprandial pain. The Roux limb should be examined in patients with nausea and vomiting to evaluate for evidence of obstructions which can occur with adhesions or internal hernias. Gastrogastric fistulisation may enable to inspect the excluded stomach. In the bypassed stomach usually gastritis (erosive, erythematous, atrophic or haemorrhagic) – partly due to biliary reflux – can be seen even in patients with a normal preoperative endoscopy. Its significance is uncertain [115].

5.5.3.2 Variations of the Gastric Bypass

Endoscopists should be aware of variations such as the gastric plication and the omega loop gastric bypass, known under many other names such as the omega loop bypass, the mini gastric bypass or the one-anastomosis gastric bypass. In the gastric plication the lumen of the stomach has a tubular form with disturbance of the normal fold pattern of the lesser and greater curve by the plication, performed by the surgeon. In the mini gastric bypass, the endoscopic view is a Billroth II resection alike, with a very small gastric remnant, and the efferent loop in front of the endoscope. The afferent limb can often be negotiated to investigate the proximal duodenum and distal stomach, although it may need some effort to enter the afferent loop. There exists also a banded gastric bypass which makes no difference for the endoscopic procedure and endoscopic view itself but the endoscopist should carefully inspect the inner side of the stomach for signs of band erosion.

5.5.3.3 Sleeve Gastrectomy (SG) [42, 43, 109, 110, 114]

Sleeve gastrectomy, also known as longitudinal or vertical gastrectomy, was initially used in the super-obese (BMI $\geq$ 50 kg/m^2) as the first step of a staged operation of the biliopancreatic diversion with duodenal switch (BPD-DS), to reduce weight to a safer level before undergoing a more complex surgery such as biliopancreatic diversion or gastric bypass [2]. The resulting weight loss and resolution of comorbidities obtained with laparoscopic sleeve gastrectomy were comparable to laparoscopic Roux-en-Y gastric bypass. So, the sleeve gastrectomy became an appealing alternative as a simpler, safer procedure and is a stand-alone operation since 2006. In the gastric sleeve, the stomach is a calibrated tube-like structure (around a 32–36 Fr tube) without the usual findings of a fundic pouch (Fig. 5.3). The pylorus and the duodenum are intact. A long staple line along the greater curvature is visible. The stapled gastric remnant is removed. The staple line should be carefully inspected for defects and ulcerations and retroflexion is relatively contraindicated.

5.5.3.4 Gastric Plication

In gastric plication the stomach is folded or imbricated along the greater curvature. At endoscopy the gastric folds created by the plication are visible and identical to the folds seen after fundoplication for gastro-oesophageal reflux disease.

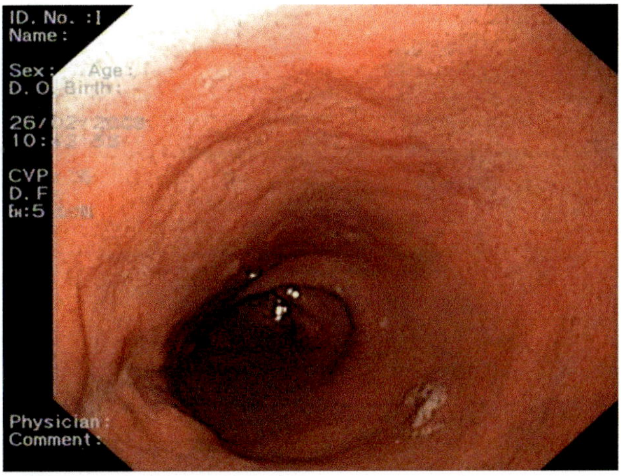

Fig. 5.3 The normal endoscopic view of a gastric sleeve, a tube-like structure without the usual findings of a fundic pouch with intact pylorus and duodenum. A long staple line along the greater curvature is visible

5.5.3.5 Biliopancreatic Diversion (BPD) and Biliopancreatic Diversion with Duodenal Switch (BPD-DS) [42, 43, 109, 110, 114]

Biliopancreatic diversion involves a distal gastrectomy. The ileum is divided 250 cm proximal to the ileocecal valve and the distal ileum (alimentary limb) is anastomosed to the remaining stomach. The jejunum and proximal ileal segment (biliopancreatic limb) are anastomosed to the terminal ileum (common limb) 50 cm proximal to the ileocaecal valve. Upon endoscopy a large (200 mL) gastric remnant is present, which is anastomosed end-to-side to the ileum giving a double-barrel view when examined through the gastric lumen. In the biliopancreatic diversion with duodenal switch the stomach is resected as described above (sleeve gastrectomy) and looks like a tube-like structure without the usual findings of a gastric fundus, the pylorus is intact and the duodenum is stapled end-to-end to the ileum. The biliopancreatic limb is anastomosed to the ileum 100 cm proximal to the ileocaecal valve resulting in a longer common limb. In both versions of the BPD, the biliopancreatic limb is out of the reach of the normal endoscope.

5.5.3.6 Laparoscopic Adjustable Gastric Banding (LAGB) [42, 43, 109, 110, 114]

The stomach is banded using an inflatable band close to the cardia, leaving a tiny upper pouch (<25 mL) and a narrow outlet. The band is connected by a thin tube to a reservoir in the rectus sheath which by injecting saline might tighten the band by inflating a balloon located circumferentially on the inner side of the band. In case of a "virtual" pouch, no pouch at all can be visualised. Two operative techniques have been used: initially the perigastric technique and later the pars flaccida technique. The endoscopic appearance is that of an elongated cardia. When the pouch volume is 15–60 mL, there is a visible separation between the impression made by the band and the cardia. The distance between the cardia and the band is usually less than 3 cm. Sometimes some resistance can be met upon introduction of the endoscope through the annular ring of the band lying on the outside of the stomach. In

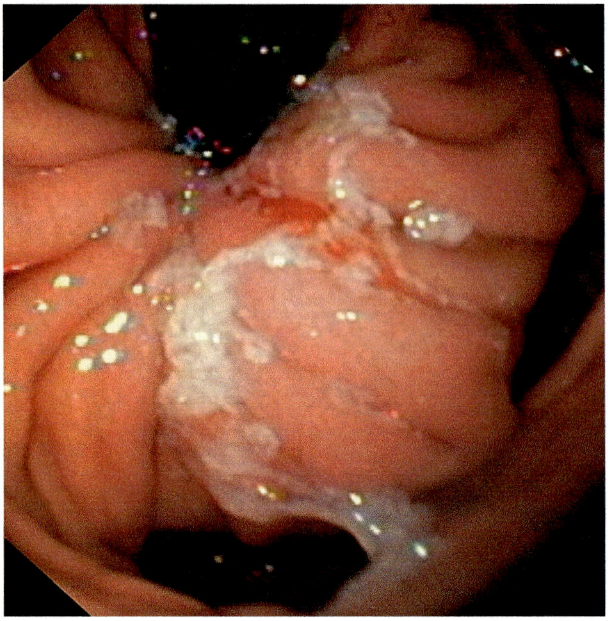

Fig. 5.4 The normal endoscopic view of a gastric band. Upon entering the stomach there is a very small pouch and upon introduction of the endoscope through the annular ring of the band a resistance may be felt. In retroflexion the band produces an outbulging rosette encircling the endoscope

retroflexion the band produces an outbulging rosette encircling the endoscope (Fig. 5.4). The endoscopist should assess the presence of pouch dilation or band slippage by measuring the length of the pouch from the gastro-oesophageal junction to the impression of the band. The presence of band erosion is usually best observed in a retroflex position.

5.5.3.7 Vertical Banded Gastroplasty (VBG) [42, 43, 83, 116–118]

The Mason VBG involves a transgastric window made 6–8 cm below the His angle by a circular 25 mm stapler, followed by the placement of a linear stapler to create the pouch. The narrow outlet is surrounded by a non-distensible collar to avoid enlargement. Complete division between the pouch and fundus has been performed in order to prevent late disruption of the vertical staple line. A normal appearance in VBG consisted of a clean gastric channel along the lesser curvature, 6–8 cm long, with a rosette at 46.6 cm from the incisors. Usually, the stoma, that gives access to the distal part of the stomach, is 11–12 mm wide and 1–2 cm long, and lies on the lesser curvature of the stomach, 8–10 cm distal to the oesophagogastric junction. An 11 mm endoscope should be able to pass snugly without difficulty into the distal stomach and the duodenum. The outlet of the VBG is formed by a calibrated channel (around a 32 Fr tube) and externally restricted to a 5.0 cm outlet by an annular Marlex mesh band 1.5 cm high. The internal diameter may vary due to the inherent thickness of the gastric wall and the amount of stomach wall puckered by the annular mesh band. Retroflexion of the tip of the endoscope in the distal stomach allows inspection of the caudal aspect of the staple-line partition and the remainder of the gastric fundus. As the endoscope passes the gastro-oesophageal junction, the gastric channel should be clearly in view directly ahead of the end of the endoscope. It should not be necessary to angle the endoscope in any way to find the opening. When such is the case, the channel is angulated. The staple line should be carefully inspected for staple-line dehiscence and the stoma for narrowing and band erosion.

5.6 Emergencies and Endoscopic Findings and Therapy in the Early (<6 Weeks) Post-operative Period

In the immediate post-operative period procedure-specific complications needing emergency treatment are gastrointestinal perforations; suture or anastomotic leaks or bleedings; and gastrointestinal obstruction [43, 114, 119].

In the immediate post-operative period it is unusual for patients to need endoscopy unless a diagnosis is uncertain, but more importantly, in certain conditions endoscopic assistance and treatment may be an indispensable tool to salvage the surgical intervention or to manage the emergency when other measures have failed. When proceeded with caution, concerns about the barotrauma and the anastomotic tightness and integrity by endoscopy are unfounded and the low risk could be minimised further by the insufflation of carbon dioxide (CO_2) instead of ambient air during endoscopy [113]. In most cases, a stable and firm anastomosis by stapling has been performed and in case of a handsewn anastomosis, absorbable sutures retain their tensile strength for about 4–6 weeks after surgery [114].

5.7 Gastrointestinal Perforations

Oesophageal perforation as a complication of gastric banding, sleeve gastrectomy or gastric bypass can occur during nasogastric intubation, introduction of the nasogastric calibrator in case of gastric banding, the retrogastric and the retro-oesophageal passage with "Goldfinger" or thermal injury of the oesophagus during the dissection [120]. Perforation usually causes acute mediastinitis, which is associated with a high morbidity and mortality. Early detection is essential. Indicative clinical signs and symptoms are respiratory distress, chest pain, dysphagia, fever, tachycardia, crepitus and oedema of the head and neck. On X-ray, mediastinal widening, pleural effusion, mediastinal or subcutaneous emphysema and/or pneumoperitoneum can be seen. Diagnosis can be confirmed with contrast oesophagography or with a CT scan. Although oesophagoscopy has a high sensitivity and specificity, it may enlarge the oesophageal defect and is not recommended. Since the condition is life threatening, the treatment should be urgent reoperation. Gastric perforation is a complication specifically associated with gastric banding. When not recognised intraoperatively, abdominal pain and sepsis with symptoms like fever, tachycardia, oliguria, hypotension and tachypnoea are noticed in the early post-operative period. The Cleveland Clinic Florida reported immediate post-operative complications such as oesophageal perforation and gastric perforation, each in 0.6% after 152 LAGB, with no mortality [121]. Immediate surgical revision often including band removal is necessary.

5.8 Leaks and Fistulas

Gastrointestinal leaks and fistulas are feared complications of many abdominal procedures resulting in poor nutrition, skin irritation and breakdown, infection, sepsis, multi-organ failure and even death [122]. Both pulmonary embolism and anastomotic leaks are the leading cause of death after bariatric surgery, and patients with a symptomatic leak requiring re-intervention have a mortality rate of 6–16% but also carry a high morbidity rate [123–126].

An anastomotic leak can be defined as a disruption at a surgical anastomosis or a defect in a suture line, resulting in extraluminal drainage of GI contents into a contained cavity or an abscess with or without evidence of extravasation of contrast medium on radiologic evaluation [127, 128]. A leakage can be classified based on the time of onset, clinical presentation, site of leak, radiological appearance and/or a mix of these factors. Leaks after sleeve gastrectomy are classified, depending on the time between the operation and the development of a leak, into acute (post-operative days 1–7), early (post-operative weeks 1–6), late (post-operative weeks 6–12) and chronic leaks (more than 12 weeks after SG) [19]. In addition, gastrointestinal leaks, in general, are classified according to severity into three types (A, B and C). Type A leaks are leaks with a micro-perforation without clinical or radiographic signs of a leak. Type B leaks are leaks without clinical signs but with a leak seen on radiographic studies, and type C leaks are those with both clinical and radiographic signs [129]. By clinical presentation and extent of dissemination, type I or subclinical leakage is defined as a well-localised leak without dissemination into the pleural or abdominal cavity and without systemic clinical manifestations, and usually they are easy to treat medically [2, 130]. Type II leakage is defined as a leak which disseminates into abdominal or pleural cavity, with consequent severe and systemic clinical manifestations. These classifications are important to guide the appropriate management strategy.

A fistula is an abnormal non-anatomical communication between two luminal structures or two epithelialised surfaces. Examples are a gastrogastric fistula, an abnormal communication between the surgically created functional gastric pouch and the excluded gastric remnant after RYGB, a complication that occurs when the gastric pouch is created in continuity with the remnant stomach or only partially transected [131], and a gastrocutaneous fistula, an abnormal communication between the stomach and the outside of the body surface allowing the passage of secretions to the exterior [132]. Leaks in contact with the diaphragm can evolve into a subphrenic abscess and into a gastrobronchial fistula, a rare but serious complication that is extraordinarily difficult to manage and sometimes require a total gastrectomy and thoracotomy with inferior lobectomy [133].

5.8.1 Pathophysiology of Leaks and Predisposing Factors for a Leak

Before discussing the appropriate management of leaks, gastroenterologists may take advantage of knowing the pathophysiology of their genesis and also the measures surgeons can take to prevent their development.

Leaks develop when the intraluminal pressure exceeds tissue or suture line resistance. Leaks can be due to either mechanical or ischaemic causes [11]. Mechanical aspects are related to stapler misfiring or stapler malfunction, suture or staple seepage or direct tissue injury, for instance by instrumentation and electrocautery. Also an optimal stapling procedure with adequate time for tissue compression and preventing production of excessive tensile strength is emphasised. Tissue ischaemia, distal obstruction and haematoma may cause a leak. Leaks after mechanical causes appear early, within 2 days of surgery, whereas ischaemic leaks occur later, starting from the 5th–sixth days after surgery.

Factors predisposing for a leak are important and can be divided into technical, procedure-related and patient-related factors.

5.8.1.1 Gastric Bypass Leaks

After RYGB the most common site of leaks is the gastrojejunal anastomosis (68%), due to the single blood supply to the gastric pouch, followed by the gastric pouch staple line (10%) and jejunojejunal anastomosis (5%). An additional 14% involve multiple sites [134]. Incidence of leaks is highest in divided RYGB. When the pouch and excluded stomach are contiguous, the risk of a chronic gastrogastric fistula is highest. The incidence of leaks after bariatric surgery is 1.7–2.6% after open RYGB and 2.1–5.2% after laparoscopic RYGB [110, 134]. The higher incidence after a laparoscopic gastric bypass can be explained by the fact that laparoscopy produces a smaller amount of inflammation and fewer adhesions and may have less ability to contain the leak than an open procedure. After RYGB the mortality is 9% after a leak at the gastrojejunal anastomosis but much higher (40%) after a leak at the jejunojejunal anastomosis [122]. Mortality is also higher in patients with leaks after open RYGB than after laparoscopic RYGB. In addition, leaks result in a sixfold increase in hospital stay [124, 135].

Risks of leak after gastric bypass may be increased in patients with impaired wound healing, infection, diabetes, hypertension, sleep apnoea, age >55 years, male gender and previous surgery [11, 134, 136]. Masoomi et al. analysed data of 226,452 patients after open and laparoscopic RYGB and factors associated with a higher risk of GI leak were open gastric bypass (OR 4.85), congestive heart failure (OR 3.04), chronic renal failure (OR 2.38), older age than 50 (OR 1.82), Medicare payer (OR 1.54), male sex (OR 1.50) and chronic lung disease (OR 1.21) [137].

5.8.1.2 Sleeve Gastrectomy Leaks

In patients with SG most (87.5%) leaks occur in the proximal third of the stomach near the gastro-oesophageal junction at the former angle of His where the staple line meets the gastro-oesophageal junction. In this area the gastric muscular layer is anatomically thinner than in the remainder distal third [16]. There is a lengthy staple line. Other factors that may increase the risk of leaks are ischaemia and elevated intragastric pressure and relative dysmotility. Ischaemia may be associated with ligation of the short gastric arteries. Saber et al. studied the gastric wall perfusion by CT scans [138]. They demonstrated that the gastric wall perfusion is significantly decreased at the level of the gastric fundus and angle of His compared with the perfusion at other gastric points. Gastric perfusion at all the points studied was inversely related to the BMI [138]. There is nearly a twofold increase of intragastric pressures following sleeve gastrectomy [139]. Mid-gastric strictures at the incisura angularis and twisted sleeves create a "hourglass model" of the sleeve with different pressure zones in the upper and lower parts and these strictures increase the intragastric sleeve pressure even further, favouring dilation of the upper portion and leaks at angle of His [130, 140]. Intragastric pressure has been shown to increase further with coughing and with vomiting, thereby clarifying the possible relation between post-operative vomiting and a leak. However, prophylactic decompression via a nasogastric tube did not improve leak rates in a randomised study, raising the question if indeed the increased intragastric pressure is a factor in its aetiology [141]. The leak incidence is 2.2–2.4% and the leak-associated mortality is 0.11% [15, 16]. Most leaks will occur after discharge as a late event: 50% occurred more than 10 days post-operatively, between 11 and 31 days [16, 17].

Many factors can predispose to leakage after SG which are either technically related or patient related. As far as the risk of leaks in sleeve gastrectomy is concerned, technical and procedure-related factors have been more widely discussed than patient-related factors. Many studies acknowledge the experience of the surgeon [2]. In sleeve gastrectomy, the bougie size, staple height and reinforcement of the staple line determine the risk of leaks. A recent meta-analysis of Parikh et al. including 198 leaks in 8922 patients supports the use of ≥40 Fr bougies to decrease the leak rates without affecting weight loss up to 36 months [15]. In an earlier review of 115 leaks in 4888 sleeve patients, Aurora et al. also found a lower leak rate of 0.6% with the use of a 40 Fr or higher bougie size compared with a leak rate of 2.8% with the use of smaller sizes [16]. In their study the staple height and use of buttressing material to reinforce the staple line did not affect the leak rate. Yet, others emphasise the adequate choice of staple heights for the different parts of the stomach according to the gastric wall thickness which varies by sex and location [130]. Staple-line bleeding is considered a direct predisposing factor for leakage after sleeve gastrectomy [130]. Reinforcement of the long staple line in sleeve gastrectomy has been proposed to reduce the risk of leaks and bleeding. Both oversewing and use of different synthetic or biologic buttress materials are current practice. The majority of surgeons present at the international sleeve consensus expert panels practiced reinforcement and all panellists agreed with the statement that reinforcement may definitively minimise haemorrhage, although historically it was aimed at leak prevention [19]. Several meta-analyses and systematic reviews tried to solve the issue of staple-line reinforcement. Choi et al. found reinforcement to result in a lower bleeding rate but 1 year later Knapps et al. did not find a difference between the groups [142, 143]. The systematic review by Gagner et al. and the meta-analysis by Shikora and Mahoney agreed that absorbable buttress applied on the staple line seemed to offer a safer and more effective control of staple-line leaks and bleeding [144, 145]. Buttressing materials are expensive and unfortunately the cheapest option of oversewing the staple line did not show any advantage compared with the control group with respect to leak and haemorrhage [144, 145].

The principles whereby surgeons can reduce the risk of a leak after sleeve gastrectomy are summarised in a beautiful overview by Iossa et al. [130]. They based their technical recommendations to avoid leaks after sleeve gastrectomy on the available evidence and expert consensus. These recommendations with evidence levels (EL) encompassed the following:

1. Use a bougie size ≥40 Fr, EL:1.
2. Begin the gastric transection 5–6 cm from the pylorus, EL:2–3.
3. Use appropriate cartridge colours – referring to the height of the staples – from antrum to fundus, EL:1.
4. Reinforce the staple line with buttress material, EL:1.
5. Follow a proper staple line.
6. Remove the crotch staples, EL:4.
7. Maintain proper traction on the stomach before firing.
8. Stay away from the angle of His at least 1 cm, EL:1.
9. Check the bleeding from the staple line.
10. Perform an intraoperative methylene blue test, EL:4 [130].

Patient-related factors predisposing to anastomotic or suture line leaks in sleeve gastrectomy have been investigated and from several studies patients with factors such as male gender, age above 45–55 years, presence of supermorbid obesity (BMI >48 or >50 kg/m^2), presence of comorbid conditions, especially diabetes and hypertension, and sleep apnoea, and those undergoing revision surgery are at increased risk for anastomotic leak and death [16, 125, 146–148].

5.8.1.3 Biliopancreatic Diversion (BPD) with or Without Duodenal Switch Leaks

For leaks related to the sleeve gastrectomy see the discussion above. A leak after a duodenal switch is typically at the duodenal-ileal staple line.

5.8.2 Symptoms and General Treatment

Subtle signs such as unexplained tachycardia, tachypnoea, dyspnoea, increased fluid requirements, fever and left shoulder pain, and the patient's feeling of impending doom are frequently the only warning of an intra-abdominal leak and may be confused with pulmonary embolism, which is the second most common cause of perioperative mortality [122, 149]. A left pleural effusion may point to a left subphrenic abscess which is almost always caused by a gastric leak. A systemic inflammatory response syndrome (SIRS), septic shock, increased levels of C-reactive protein and a raised white blood cell count may also be present [111]. The combination of fever, tachycardia and tachypnoea was identified as a significant predictor of an anastomotic leak; it was the most specific indicator with a high positive predictive value [24]. Similarly, Arteaga-González et al. found that clinical variables significantly related to post-operative leaks were heart rate over 100 beats/min (other studies report a heart rate of >120 beats/min), leukocytes over 15,000/mm^3 and systolic arterial pressure below 100 mmHg [147]. However, in patients with a clinical suspicion of leakage, 7.7% of abdominal CT scans returned false negative, versus 28.6% for oral methylene blue and 33.3% for upper gastrointestinal swallow with Gastrografin [147]. So, abdominal examination may not be helpful, a contrast study with Gastrografin may be non-diagnostic and CT scans often cannot accommodate the size or weight of the patient. CT scanning has the advantage that besides demonstrating the leak itself, it can also show the presence of intra-abdominal collections, which are in general indirect signs of leaks. The low sensitivity and specificity of routine radiological investigations have been discussed earlier.

The timing, size and exact location of the leak; the viability of the surrounding tissues; and the clinical evaluation of the patient largely determine the treatment [138, 150, 151]. The major clinical factors affecting the prognosis of patients with anastomotic leaks are the interval from perforation to the intervention and the size of the dehiscence [152]. The most efficient treatment for gastrointestinal leaks remains controversial and the management of leaks still lacks a universally accepted algorithm. The large number of alternative techniques reported from different centres around the world means that the existing approaches to this challenging complication remain inadequate or extremely difficult to implement. Some authors suggest aggressive therapy with surgical reoperation, while others recommend conservative treatment with broad-spectrum antibiotics, adequate drainage, nasogastric tubes and adequate nutrition support.

An urgent operation is justified if the patient remains hemodynamically instable or appears to be deteriorating, if the index of suspicion of a leak is high or if a leak is detected in order to control the source of sepsis [149]. When a leak is diagnosed early and the site of the leak, the viability of the surrounding tissue and the clinical status of the patient allows for a primary closure, a laparoscopy with intent to suture the defect in combination with adequate drainage is performed. However, when attempting to suture, sutures may be applied to tissues affected by a severe inflammatory process. This may result in a low ability to maintain the margins of the leak closed and to obtain healing of the leak [16, 153]. Surgical revision, due to surrounding inflammation and ischaemic edges, is often unsuccessful and burdened with high post-operative complications [154]. If an exploratory laparoscopy is performed, it should be done for debridement and drainage of the leak and to wash out the infected fluids.

Surgical management is associated with a high mortality (up to 10%), a high morbidity (up to 50%) and a high conversion rate to open surgery (up to 48%). As a result, management has been moved towards conservative supportive care with aggressive fluid resuscitation, medical treatment of sepsis, endoscopic or radiological drainage of collections, antimicrobial therapy, artificial nutrition, nil per mouth and endoscopic treatment. Non-operative and endoscopic therapies should be attempted only in haemodynamically stable patients. Early/intermediate leaks have the best prognosis and heal spontaneously after drainage, antimicrobials, nil per mouth and nutritional support within 5 weeks in 90% of patients [155]. In series with late leaks non-operative strategies had lower rates of success, varying between 40% and 80%.

5.8.3 Non-operative Endoscopic Treatment

Several overriding principles apply to all patients undergoing non-operative endoscopic strategies, excellently summarised by Willingham and Buscaglia [156]. First, care should be delivered by a team that will typically involve advanced endoscopy, surgery, interventional radiology and nutrition. Second, definition and delineation of the site of the leak often by contrast radiology studies are critical. Third, if a fluid collection or cavity exists, adequate percutaneous drainage should be considered first. Fourth, careful evaluation of the quality and viability of the tissue surrounding the leak is critical in determining which endoscopic closure technique is best applied. Fifth, the main goal of endoscopic therapy is the interruption of the flow of luminal contents across the defect and several methods are available such as stent placement, clipping, tissue adhesives and endoscopic suturing. Sixth, the adequacy of the closure should be checked, both at the time of the procedure after the closure and in follow-up to confirm adequate continued sealing [156]. Also, local components that may exacerbate or maintain the leakage such as a distal obstruction or non-resorbable material located in the leak area should be managed by dilation of a distal stenosis in case of a proximal blown-out and removal of suture material with endoscopic scissors and grasping forceps [132].

Most of the studies reporting their results used the same definitions [127, 157]. Primary closure was defined as sealing of the leak diagnosed both endoscopically and radiologically after a single endoscopic procedure. Secondary closure was defined as sealing of the leak after further endoscopic procedures. Failure was defined as persistence of the leak after the last endoscopic procedure and when a decision has been made for no further endoscopic attempts.

Endoscopic management of leaks and fistulas knows two different and to some extent opposing approaches:

(a) The occlusion of or bypassing the leak and fistula and in this respect stents, clips, endoscopic suturing devices or tissue sealants are different options, used solely or in combination; in these cases adequate drainage of the leak is achieved by surgery or radiology.
(b) Drainage of leaks without the use of stents by endoscopic internal drainage (EID), vacuum-assisted drainage, etc.

5.8.3.1 The Occlusion of Leaks and Fistulas

Endoscopic Stents

The major advantages of stent placement are the immediate control of leaks, protection of the gastrojejunostomy and oesophageal and gastric wall during mucosal healing, possibility of early oral feeding and prevention of stricture formation [150]. They also shield the site of leakage from oesophagogastric secretions, thereby preventing further contamination. Stents do not reduce the total time to cure the leak but make their care easier as patients can tolerate oral feeding and antibiotics and can be treated on an outpatient basis [111]. Stents may reduce the time to cure in complex fistulae, in very large leaks, and in cases of high leaks. Stenting should always be combined with external drainage to prevent the formation of a closed-off abscess or cavity [158]. Covered or partially covered self-expandable metal stents (SEMSs) and self-expandable plastic stents (SEPSs) have been used. Examples of stents are self-expandable plastic stent (SEPS) (Polyflex stent, Boston Scientific

Corp, Natick, MA, USA), partially covered nitinol stents (Ultraflex stent, Boston Scientific Corporation, Natick, MA, USA) and fully covered nitinol stents (Niti-S™ oesophageal stent, Taewoong Medical, South Korea; Hanarostent, M.I.Tech Co. Ltd., Seoul, South Korea). The Polyflex stent is the most commonly used SEPS, made of polyester, fully covered with silicone, and with a flared proximal end to prevent migration. The advantages over a SEMS are the soft material which provides secure and efficient force to close the leakage, and the fully covered silicone membrane which prevents tissue ingrowth and thus facilitates its removal. The disadvantages of SEPS placement are a complicated loading and delivery device and a high stent migration rate [159]. Fully covered stents migrate easily because of the smooth outer surface and because of a reduced anchoring ability and the absence of an obstructive lesion to keep the stent in place, whereas partially covered stents are kept in place by the ingrowth of tissue in the meshes of the uncovered parts of the stent. The stent material influences the extent of tissue hyperplasia, with metal or Nitinol® stents causing more hypertrophy than plastic stents. Depending on the system, stent deployment may begin proximally or distally. In addition, until recently, most commercially available covered stents are not deployed by using through-the-scope delivery catheters [156]. Therefore, stent placement is usually performed over a wire under fluoroscopic guidance. Recently, endoscopic stent anchoring with clips or sutures by using the Apollo OverStitch device (Apollo Endosurgery, Austin, TX) have been employed resulting in less migration rates [156]. One study showed a positive predictive value of non-migration after placement of a clip to be 87% [160, 161]. Sharaiha and colleagues reported on 37 patients treated with oesophageal stents, 17 of whom received adjunctive suturing [162]. Stent migration was 11% in the group who received suturing versus a 55% migration rate in the group who did not receive suturing ($p = 0.04$).

A method to simplify stent removal is to remove the stent from the distal end by inverting the stent in itself, or by insertion of a temporary stent to induce superficial necrosis of the excessive granulation tissue and thereby release the original stent. Eisendrath et al. treated 21 patients endoscopically by partially covered nitinol self-expanding metal stents (SEMSs) which are soft and most effective for closure of fistulas, especially in the absence of associated strictures [163]. Development of tissue hyperplasia at both ends minimises the risk of migration and increases water tightness. On the other hand, hyperplasia makes removal difficult. Placement of self-expanding plastic stents (SEPSs) inside SEMSs can induce pressure necrosis of the ingrown tissue (Fig. 5.5). The stents can be removed together 7–10 days later. SEMS insertion led to 62% (13/21) primary closure. Secondary closure by complementary endoscopic treatments of sealant, tissue adhesives and plugs led to four secondary closures, with a total success rate of 81% (17/21) [163]. After stent insertion, 30% of the patients reported transient thoracic pain probably related to an inflammatory reaction due to expansion of the stent. The unsuccessful patients died. Tissue ingrowth in the stent can also be ablated by argon plasma coagulation (APC) at standard power settings, thereby exposing the underlying metal meshes of the uncovered portions of the stent [156, 164]. Dedicated stents for treating leaks should decrease the migration frequency and dedicated instruments for stent removal might

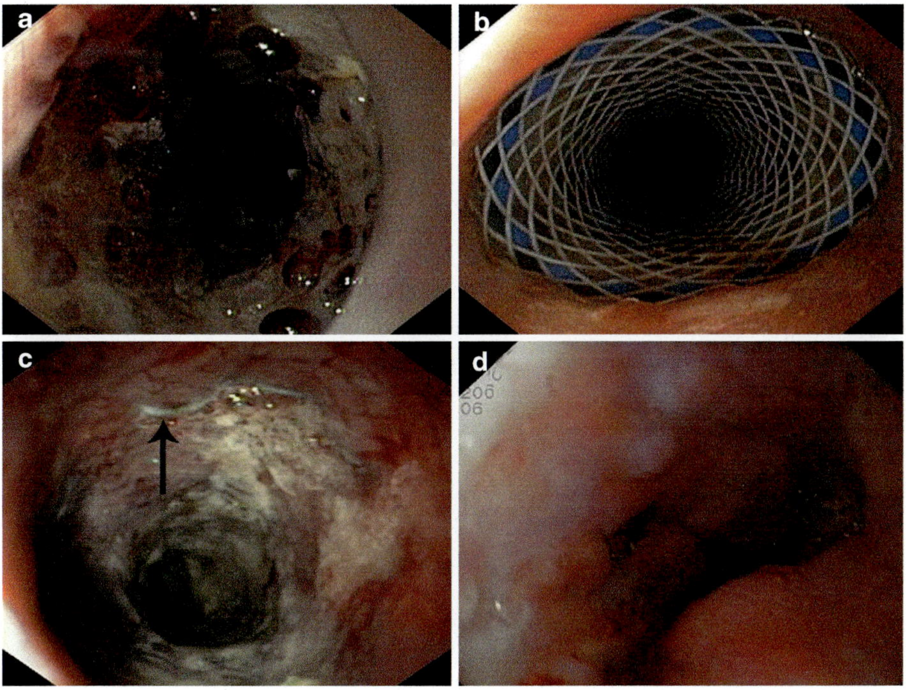

Fig. 5.5 (**a**) A partially covered nitinol self-expanding metal stent (SEMS) is placed to seal the leakage with the development of tissue hyperplasia at both ends. (**b**) Placement of plastic stent to induce necrosis of hyperplastic tissue by radial forces. (**c**) Disappearance of proximal hyperplasia and visibility of the proximal polypropylene drawstring attached to the SEM stent to allow for collapse of the stent. (**d**) Aspect of proximal part after removal of both stents. Reprinted from Gastrointest Endosc 2011; 73: 890–899, Swinnen J, Eisendrath P, Rigaux J, Kahegeshe L, Lemmers A, Le Moine O, et al. Self-expandable metal stents for the treatment of benign upper GI leaks and perforations, with permission from Elsevier

further decrease the risk of bowel damage during stent removal. Recent development of wider and longer stents, including additional anti-migratory mechanisms, resulted in the Taewoong Niti-S™ Beta stent (24 mm wide, 150–200 mm long, double anti-migratory cuffed stent with a 32 mm wide proximal flared end) and the Taewoong Niti-S™ Megastent (24 mm wide, 230 mm long, with two 32 mm wide flared ends) (Fig. 5.6).

In RYGB leaks at the gastrojejunal anastomosis are suitable for stent therapy. In SG, gastric leaks at the proximal and mid-aspect are the only leaks suited to endoscopic treatment with a stent. A distal leak is not amenable as the stent would be too small and would not provide appropriate sealing of the defect but this may change in the near future by the above-mentioned recent developments in stent design [165].

Most of the studies with stents are retrospective and have no comparison group. Only one study could be found that compared using stents or non-stent therapy after total gastrectomy for leaks of 2 cm or smaller [152]. Covered self-expanding

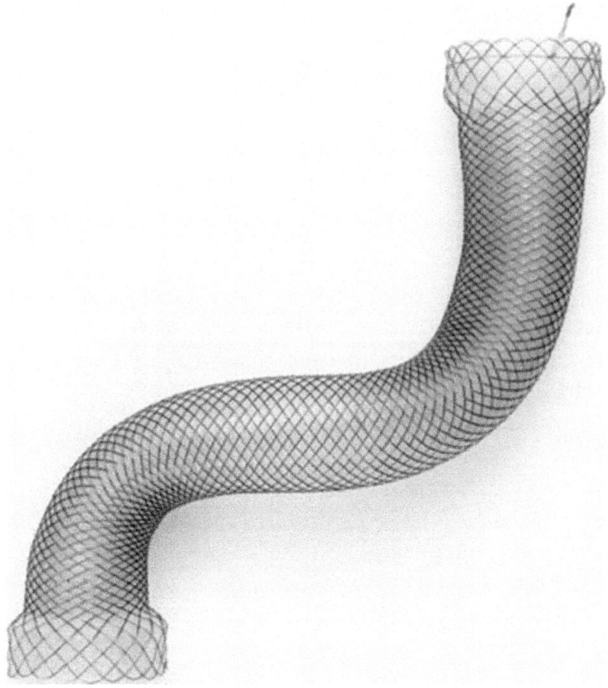

Fig. 5.6 One example of a Megastent (Taewoong Medical, Seoul, Korea) specially adapted for bariatric surgery. The ultra-large stent has an s-configuration of fully covered nitinol mesh with significant flexibility despite the large diameter and with cuffed ends. Reprinted from Obes Surg 2016; 26: 941–948, Shehab HM, Hakky SM, Gawdat KA. An endoscopic strategy combining mega stents and over-the-scope clips for the management of post-bariatric surgery leaks and fistulas (with video), with permission from Springer

metal stents (Choo stent, M.I.Tech, Seoul, South Korea, or Niti-S stent (Taewoong Medical, Seoul, South Korea)) to seal anastomotic leaks were compared with non-stent therapy consisting of endoclip, a detachable snare, a tissue adhesive or fibrin sealant (2–4 mL). As far as the size of the dehiscence is concerned the authors thought that for a leak <2 cm and <70% of the circumference endoscopic treatment should be feasible. Twenty-seven patients underwent endoscopic treatment, 13 with SEMS (16 SEMS sessions) and 14 were treated by non-stent endoscopic treatment (NSET) (21 NSET sessions) [151]. The successful sealing rate at the first attempt was significantly higher with SEMS (80.0%) than with NSET (28.6%). The successful sealing after multiple treatments was not significantly different: 80% with SEMS and 64.3% with NSET. Complications were absent in the NSET group and occurred in 5/13 (38.5%) of the SEMS group with migration in four, malpositioning in one and tissue overgrowth in one. So, SEMS is superior to NSET because of the higher primary closure and lower number of endoscopic sessions per patient.

Many authors have reported on the use of stents in leaks, often without a further detailed discussion of the type of leak and the type of operation (RYGB or SG) associated with the leak [17, 153, 157, 158, 165–175]. The emerging picture from these studies is a leak closure rate of about 75%, with a more favourable outcome in case of a shorter time between diagnosis of leakage and stent insertion and a smaller luminal opening diameter [152, 160, 171, 172, 175], with the most unfavourable results in chronic leaks and fistulas. A reoperation was of no need in the vast majority of the cases. Also, a fairly high migration rate varying from 25 to 40% is reported which is lowered by using partially covered stents and which is also lower when the easy repositioning of the stents is not included in the overall migration rate. For instance, Southwell et al. reported a primary stent migration rate of 48%; however, after adjusting for minor migrations which were easily corrected with repositioning of the stents, this rate was reduced to 19% [153]. Swinnen et al. reported a significantly lower spontaneous stent migration rate of 11% by using partially covered self-expanding metal stents [175]. In case of migration, a second stent can be "nested" in the migrated stent. Moreover, the fate of migrated stents was studied. In the largest series of 70 migrated stents, being 8% of stents in 888 patients, only 3 stents (4%) required surgical removal [176]. Some studies report that patients complain of symptoms of nausea, dysphagia and mild transient retrosternal discomfort during stent treatment, and sometimes endoscopic dilation is needed after stent removal because of symptomatic stenosis [163, 175]. Eubanks et al. reported a retrospective study of stents used for acute post-operative leaks (11, within 1 month), chronic gastrocutaneous fistula (2, >1 month) and anastomotic strictures [166]. Thirty-four silicone-covered stents (23 polyester and 11 metal with anti-migration struts) were used. Both RYGB and SG operations were included. Immediate symptomatic relief occurred in 90% (91% in cases with leaks, 100% with fistulas, 84% with strictures) and oral feeding was started in 79% immediately after stenting. In three patients (each in one group) the use of stents was unsuccessful. Migration of stents occurred in 58% of 34 stents and repositioning of the stent was needed in 42% of cases. Migration was mostly minimal but three stents were removed surgically after distal small-bowel migration. One migrated and passed per rectum. Despite the anti-migration struts in the metal stents, the migration rate was similar in both groups.

A meta-analysis by Puli et al. in 2012, including 7 studies and 67 patients, showed that successful leak closure using oesophageal stents is obtained in 87.8% of cases with radiographic confirmation after stent removal [177]. Both SEPSs and SEMSs were used in the seven included studies. Stents were left in place for 4–8 weeks and were successfully extracted in 91.6% of cases. Overall stent migration was noted in 16.9%. Re-stenting was needed in four of seven studies and the need for revision surgery caused by failure of endoscopic leak closure was only 9%. Moreover, no stent-related mortality was reported. SEMSs were generally well tolerated with reported symptoms of nausea, dysphagia and mild transient retrosternal discomfort. In 2015, Murino et al. reported the largest series from one institution in 91 patients (36 RYGB, 55 SG) [172]. Partially covered nitinol stents were used which was successful in 74 patients (81%) with primary closure after 1 stent in 36 patients (39%) and secondary closure after 2 or more stents in 38 (42%). Among the 17 patients with SEMS failure (in 4 out of 36 RYGB (11%) and 13 of the 55 SG (23%)), 6 patients were ultimately healed by internal drainage of the leakage and a fistula plug. Endoscopic treatment failed in 11 patients (12%) in whom a surgical rescue was attempted, with success in 8. Of these 8 patients, 6 underwent total gastrectomy. In multivariate analysis, gender and delay between surgery and SEMS placement were independent predictive factors of endoscopic success. The type of bariatric surgery did not influence the leak closure. Twenty-seven SEMS-related complications occurred in 23 (22%) patients: 5 haemorrhages, 2 perforations (1 died, resulting in an overall mortality of 1%), 7 SEMS migrations (1 into the small bowel needing surgery) and 13 oesophageal strictures.

Swinnen et al. studied in detail the feasibility of SEMS removal in 88 patients with 153 partially covered SEMSs using the technique of stent removal as discussed earlier by Eisendrath et al. [163, 175]. Of the 88 patients, 76 patients were available for analysis and 73 (96.1%) had successful SEMS removal and per stent 132/134 (97.8%) successful stent removal [174]. Immediate closure of the perforation had a success rate of 100% compared to 50% when SEMSs were inserted more than 1 month later. The results of leak closure were quite impressive; leaks closed in 78% of cases after a first attempt and in 84% after two or more attempts. Closure in non-infectious patients produced better results (100%) than in chronic leaks (40%) or in infectious patients (75.9%). Minor complications (dysphagia, hyperplasia, rupture of stent coating) occurred in 21% and major complications (bleeding, perforation, tracheal compression) in 6% of patients.

Healing of leaks after sleeve gastrectomy is impeded by the high-pressure system produced by the restricted expansibility of the sleeve, sometimes aggravated by a stricture or stenosis at the incisura angularis or by the presence of delayed gastric emptying. A non-surgical option would be an endoscopic pylorus dilation to decrease intragastric pressure to facilitate fistula healing. Van de Vrande et al. performed endoscopic stent placement followed by pylorus dilation in two cases [151]. Southwell et al. utilised additional distal sleeve dilations with balloon dilators such as controlled radial expansion (CRE) balloons 15–20 mm (Boston Scientific Corp, Natick, MA, USA) and Rigiflex II achalasia dilators 30–35 mm (Boston Scientific Corp, Natick, MA, USA) or pyloric Botox injections in some cases to reduce distal pressure and improve clearance of food [153].

A very recent and new approach is the development of ultra-large expandable stents specifically tailored for bariatric surgery leaks [153, 157]. These Megastents (Taewoong Medical, Seoul, South Korea) are fully covered metallic stents with a specific design supposed to minimise migration and to better conform to the anatomy of a gastric sleeve. The wider diameter also provides sufficient radial force to cause dilation of possible stenosis, an important factor in delaying the leak closure [153]. Shehab et al. used these stents in 22 patients with post-bariatric surgery leaks; 13 (59%) had a sleeve gastrectomy while 9 (41%) had a RYGB [157]. To insert such an ultra-long stent, a metal guidewire was placed beyond the third duodenal part in cases of sleeve gastrectomy or beyond the first jejunal loop in cases of RYGB. After removal of the endoscope the stent was inserted and deployed over the wire under fluoroscopic guidance. All stents had a shaft diameter of 28 mm with 36 mm flared ends. The choice of the length of the stent (18 or 23 cm) depended on the aim to place the upper edge of the stent in the lower or mid-oesophagus but at least 5 cm above the site of leak, while the lower edge was situated in the duodenal bulb or just before the pyloric ring in cases of sleeve gastrectomy, and proximal to the first jejunal loop in cases of gastric bypass. Primary closure (after one endoscopic procedure) was achieved in 13 patients (59%) and in a total of 18 patients after multiple endoscopic procedures (82%). An average of 1.4 stents and 2.8 endoscopic procedures were required per patient. Stent migration occurred in four patients (18%), and all were retrieved endoscopically. It is impossible for the stent to slide around the duodenal curvature in SG or to pass beyond the first jejunal loop in RYGB. Complaints of retrosternal pain and vomiting were frequent in 20 patients (91%) which necessitates early removal in 1 patient. Complications consisted of bleeding in two patients (9%), a perforation of the jejunum in one patient (5%) caused by compression of the distal end of the stent 5 days after the insertion and treated by inserting a longer stent that bypassed the level of the perforation, and an oesophageal stricture in one patient (5%). Two mortalities were encountered, and one of them was stent related: a fatal bleeding caused by erosion of the duodenum by the distal end of the stent.

De Moura et al. reported the use of such a modified stent in a case of extreme stenting after gastric bypass surgery [167]. Endoscopy showed disruption of nearly the entire staple line at the gastric pouch. The stent was placed between the gastro-oesophageal junction and the alimentary jejunal limb. After 31 days, the stent had migrated and was removed endoscopically. Total closure of the fistula was reported 30 days afterwards. The gastric remnant leak was treated with vacuum-sponge dressings.

There is presently no standardisation of the type, length and diameter, or the number of the stents to be used [178]. Although there is agreement about the placement of stents as early as possible, the optimal timing for stent removal is unknown, and in most studies it ranges from 22 to 88 days after insertion. In addition, one should remember that the use of endoscopic stents for benign disease is an off-label use of these stents. Whereas stents can bridge large leaks and fistulas and should be used for a dehiscence ranging between 30% and 70% of the lumen circumference, other endoscopic modalities such as clips, suturing and tissue sealants have a more limited tissue-bridging capacity and are the best therapeutic options for small defects. Larger disruptions should be treated surgically [150]. Van de Vrande et al. reported that in 9 (28.1%) of the 32 patients in whom a proximal leak after sleeve gastrectomy developed, the leak was not responsive to treatment. A chronic fistula that persisted beyond 4 months developed [151]. They decided to place a Roux limb on the defect by laparoscopy and showed a success rate of 100% with a mean time for the chronic fistula to heal of 12.5 ± 10.2 days.

Endoscopic Clips and Over-the-Scope Clips (OTSCs)

Endoscopic clips have also been used to close leaks and fistulas. Clips are used to approximate the tissue surrounding the defect to effect closure [111]. The clip should be deployed perpendicularly to the long axis of the defect. If needed multiple clips can be placed sequentially starting at either edge of the defect and meeting at the centre. The successful application of clips is determined by the quality of the tissue surrounding the fistula or leak. An endoscopic examination before the attempted closure is frequently indicated. If the tissue is weak, friable, inflamed or necrotic, the clip may incise the mucosa without bringing the edges into approximation [150, 156]. Similarly, in the presence of indurated tissue, fibrotic changes or scarring at the fistula site the tissue cannot be aspirated and grasped by the clips. For well-epithelialised fistulae, some authors have suggested that ablating the tissue edges of the fistula orifice with Gold Probe cauterisation or argon plasma coagulation, or abrading them with the cytology brush, to create raw surfaces and to induce granulation before an attempt at closing the fistula, may result in a more resilient seal and may help the defect to heal [179].

There are several through-the-scope metal clips and delivery systems available [150]. Endoscopic clips are composed of two stainless steel ribbons (with various lengths and shapes as needed); they differ in the width of the opening span with a range of 90° to 135° angle, and the possibility for rotation and clip reopening, allowing for flexibility in securing the desired amount of tissue. The clips are available in preloaded and reloadable forms. One of the frequently used through-the-scope metal clips is the Resolution clip (Boston Scientific Corp, Natick, MA, USA). Clips typically slough off after a period of 2–4 weeks. In general, through-the-scope clips can close luminal defects <2 cm in size, often by the application of several clips or by a combined technique using an Endoloop and through-the-scope clips. To enhance successful clip application, gentle suction should be applied before clip closing so that the edges of the defect are reversed and approximated and more tissue is captured by the clip arms [150].

A fundamentally different clip is the Over-The-Scope Clip (OTSC, Ovesco Endoscopy AG, Tübingen, Germany), commonly known as the "bear claw". This is a nitinol-based metal clip that is packaged on a transparent plastic cap that fits over the tip of the endoscope. Caps are available in three different sizes (11, 12 and 14 mm) and there are two different depths of caps for grasping more or less tissue during approximation [150]. The clips are available in three sizes adapted to the cap sizes and three different clips can be chosen: the clip with blunt teeth for less traumatic compression of fresh lesions, spiked teeth for rather thick and fibrotic tissue, and long and sharp teeth to close the perforation or fistula of the bowel wall. The assembly and deployment system are very similar to the system used for variceal banding. The cap is mounted on the tip of the endoscope and a thread is guided through the working channel of the endoscope outwards by the thread retriever. The thread is attached to a wheel-operated deployment device inserted into access port of the working channel of the endoscope. The region of interest is suctioned into the cap, and the clip is closed and released by tightening the thread with the hand wheel. To facilitate the approximation of the edges, especially when the tissue is indurated, two dedicated accessories, the OTSC Twin Grasper and the OTSC Anchor, are available. As is the case with variceal banding, the insertion of an endoscope with preloaded clips may be difficult because the mounted OTSC system increases the diameter of the endoscope. Rogalski et al. suggest to perform an endoscopy with a transparent distal attachment without the clip and to attempt to aspirate or grasp the edges of the defect into the cap [150]. If the tissue cannot be aspirated or grasped with any of the two additional accessories into the cap, there is a little chance of the defect being effectively closed by the OTSC system. Care must be taken to ensure that both edges are within the cap; clips improperly deployed onto the edge of a lesion may make subsequent attempts at closure more challenging [156]. The

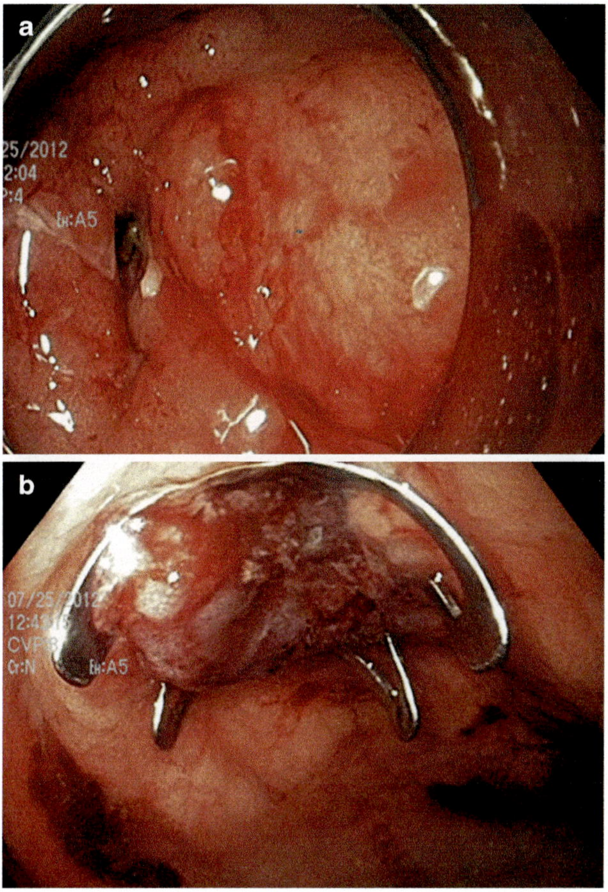

Fig. 5.7 (**a**) Full-thickness gastric defect. (**b**). Successful deployment of the over-the-scope clip (OTSC) and complete closure of the defect. Reprinted from Gastrointest Endosc 2014; 80: 610–622, Haito-Chavez Y, Law JK, Kratt T, Arezzo A, Verra M, Morino M, et al. International multicenter experience with an over-the-scope clipping device for endoscopic management of GI defects (with video), with permission from Elsevier

advantage of OTSC over the through-the-scope clips is their ability to grasp larger amounts of tissue and to achieve full-thickness closure due to a greater compressive force. A single application of the OTSC can provide full-thickness closure of open defects up to 2–3 cm (Fig. 5.7).

There are few data specifically addressing bariatric patients. Most of the studies report on surgical patients in general and on the closure of perforations, leaks and fistula, and data on long-term fistula closure are scant. Mercky et al. reported that 19 of the 30 patients had a gastric fistula after laparoscopic sleeve gastrectomy and the overall success rate of using the OTSC system was 71% [180]. A retrospective review of 47 patients who underwent OTSC placement to close chronic fistulas demonstrated a high initial technical success rate (42/47 patients, 89%), which was defined by a lack of contrast extravasation immediately after OTSC placement [181]. At a median of 39 days, a recurrent fistula, defined by the recurrence of symptoms and/or re-demonstration of the fistula by the presence of contrast extravasation after initial success, occurred in 19/41 (46%) patients. Only 25/47 (53%) patients followed for a median duration of 178 days demonstrated long-term clinical success. Winder et al. identified 22 patients with 28 defects (22 fistulae and 6 leaks) and 54.5% were related to a bariatric procedure [128]. The majority of defects involved the upper GI tract (82%) and had been present for >30 days (50%). Median number of attempts at endoscopic closure required in the leak group was 2.5, while the median number in successfully treated fistulae was 1. In two patients, a distal obstruction or stricture was found which was subsequently stented or balloon dilated and in six patients a suture was uncovered and extracted. Overall success rate was 82% (100% for leaks and 76% for fistulae) at a median follow-up of 4.7 months.

Recently, a multicentre international review by Haito-Chavez et al. studied 188 patients with acute perforations, leaks and fistulae who were treated with the OTSC system [127]. Reliable data were present in 161 patients. Ten patients suffered from a technical failure (one with a perforation, three with a leak and six with a fistula). Among 151 patients who underwent successful OTSC placement, 140 (92.7%) achieved immediate clinical success, and 11 (7.3%) were clinical failures. Long-term success was achieved in 60.2% of patients during a median follow-up of 146 days and long-term closure rates were achieved in 90% of perforations, 73.3% of leaks and 42.9% of fistulas. In univariate analysis, there were three statistically significant predictors for long-term success: (1) type of defect (perforations and leaks as compared with fistulae), (2) primary therapy versus rescue therapy and (3) chronicity of defects (≤30 days vs. >30 days). In multivariate analysis the type of defect (fistula, leak or perforation) was the only prognostic factor for failure, with fistula being the hardest to treat.

The determinants of long-term failure have been previously described. These include epithelialisation of the tract, friability and inflammation at the opening of the tract, presence of foreign bodies, presence of untreated infection, nutritional status of the patient, and distal obstruction or stenosis [182–184]. Shehab et al. certified these reasons for clip failure to be present in the typical scenario encountered in a post-sleeve gastrectomy leak: the friability of tissues, tissue ischaemia, presence of infection and persistence of distal stenosis forming a high-pressure zone at the site of leakage [157]. In contrast to clips inserted through the endoscope, the OTSC clip can perform full-thickness apposition with closure rates of 72–91% in case series of gastrointestinal perforations and fistulas [185–187].

Endoscopic Suturing

Endoscopic suturing of leaks creates plications of adjacent mucosa which are closed over the defect. Abrasion or ablating the defect may promote healing and may facilitate the adhesion of flanking plications [111]. Several operating systems have been reported such as the StomaphyX suturing system, the Apollo OverStitch, the incisionless operating platform (IOP, ROSE: Restorative Obesity Surgery Endoluminally) and the Bard EndoCinch system of which the OverStitch Endoscopic Suturing System (Apollo Endosurgery, Austin, TX, USA) and the incisionless operating platform (IOP, USGI Medical, San Clemente, CA, USA) are currently the only systems approved by the FDA in 2006 for clinical use in tissue approximation by the FDA (see Chap. 2). These suturing devices are complex systems that require high manual skills, additional training and considerable expertise on the part of the endoscopist

[111, 188]. However, suturing systems approximate the tissues by full-thickness stitches and may be capable of closing larger defects. The same concerns regarding the quality of the tissue surrounding the area of leak as mentioned above with endoscopic clipping also apply with endoscopic suturing [156]. The tissue must be sufficiently healthy and strong to hold the sutures. The edges may not tear or incise when the sutures are cinched and when the edges are pulled towards apposition. The OverStitch Endoscopic Suturing System device requires a double-channel therapeutic endoscope [150]. The main parts of the system are the end cap, needle driver handle and an anchor exchange catheter. The end cap is mounted on the distal tip of the endoscope. The tissue approximation and suture placement may be facilitated by a tissue-retracting helix device or grasping forceps. During the procedure, these additional assists can be inserted through the working channel of the endoscope. The OverStitch Endoscopic Suturing System allows interrupted or continuous stitches without needing to remove the device. Both absorbable and non-absorbable sutures are available. Absorbable suture such as polydioxanone provides tissue support for the first 60 days after implantation and is fully absorbed after 183–238 days, properties that are conducive for treatment of anastomotic leaks. The Restorative Obesity Surgery Endolumenal (ROSE) procedure is done perorally with the Incisionless Operating Platform (IOP), a stable platform with 4 working ports, which is steerable in four directions with a 360-degree rotation and has a 73 cm insertion length. One channel allows a 4.9 mm endoscope for endoscopic visualization. Three channels are for the 3 specialised instruments: the g-Prox Endoscopic Grasper with 33 mm stainless steel jaws, for grasping, mobilising and approximating full-thickness (serosa-to-serosa) tissue folds and to cut the suture, the g-Lix Tissue Grasper, a helix, to grasp tissue and pull it into the jaws of the g-Prox, and the g-Cath Suture Anchor Delivery system, a catheter system that penetrates the target tissue with a needle at its distal tip, installs a pair of preloaded tissue anchors and cinches the anchored tissue fold. The sutures are snow-shoe-shaped. The device can be reloaded in vivo [64].

Endoscopic suturing has been used to close both acute perforations and chronic fistulas. Cai et al. reported the first case series of full-thickness endoscopic suturing of post-sleeve staple-line leaks and suggested that suturing alone may be sufficient in treating small leaks; however, large leaks may require adjunctive stenting [189]. Fernandez-Esparrach et al. compared endoscopic suturing (EndoCinch; C. R. Bard Inc., Murray Hill, NJ, USA) with endoscopic clipping for the management of gastrogastric fistulae after Roux-en-Y gastric bypass [190]. There were 95 patients; 24 received endoscopic clipping and 71 received endoscopic suturing. They reported an initial success rate of 95% with durable success in only 35% as 65% showed reopening of the fistula site. One bleed and one perforation occurred [190]. The size of the fistula determined the long-term closure. None of the larger fistulae (initial size >20 mm) remained closed and one-third with a fistula size ≤10 mm achieved long-term closure [190, 191].

Tissue Sealants

Several sealants are available to close fistulas and leaks. Fibrin glue or sealant is a kit that contains freeze-dried fibrinogen, fibrinolysis-inhibiting solution aprotinin, thrombin and calcium chloride. Fibrin glue has haemostatic and tissue-adhesive capabilities. Fibrin also provides a matrix and co-stimulatory molecules to enhance wound healing although their effectiveness may be tempered in the degrading acidic environment of the stomach [155]. These substances are mixed as two components, a sealer and a thrombin solution, which are kept in two separate syringes. Mixing at the double-lumen catheter tip leads to rapid coagulation and a mechanically stable fibrin clot formation that adheres to the wound surface and achieves sealing of the tissue [192]. The larger lumen of the catheter should be reserved for the more viscous component. One should be careful with the catheter because the sealant may leak out the side holes of the catheter and may damage the endoscope channel [156]. Once the target mucosa has been de-epithelialised by a cytology brush or APC at low-power settings to promote a reactive inflammatory response around the opening, the fibrin can be applied and a plug then forms. Multiple sessions may be needed. Treatment of leaks and gastrobronchial and gastrocutaneous fistulas have been reported [192–194]. Reported sealing rates vary between 36.5% with fibrin alone and 55.7% with fibrin together with additional endoscopic therapies to sealing rates of 86.6% of fistulas after a mean of 2.5 sessions in 16 days [195, 196]. Patients with fistulas without infection and with a low output have higher cure rates.

Cyanoacrylate (N-butyl-2-cyanoacrylate; Histoacryl, B. Braun, Melsingen, Germany) polymerises after contact with moisture, causing tissue necrosis and an inflammatory response. It is not affected by gastric or pancreatic enzymes. It has been used as monotherapy to close GI fistulas in three cases [197]. Lee et al. compared the safety and efficacy of endoscopic therapy (including the use of tissue sealants in 14 of the 20 patients) with surgical methods [123]. Endoscopic therapy resulted in a very high technical success rate (95%) and lower frequency of leakage at the end of the study, compared to surgical treatment (17.5% vs. 58.3%).

Vicryl mesh plugs or soft-tissue grafting material such as SurgiSIS (Cook Inc., West Lafayette, IN, USA) may be used before glue injection or in combination with clips and stent placement [156]. SurgiSIS strips consist of acellular fibrogenic matrix from the porcine small intestinal submucosa that stimulates proliferation and formation of fibroblasts in the region of wounds. Endoscopic insertion of strips of SurgiSIS has been shown to be successful in the closure of 71% and 92% refractory oesophagogastric fistulas and in 80% of refractory gastrocutaneous fistulas [198–200]. More easy is the use of SurgiSIS anal fistula plugs to treat enterocutaneous fistula. Toussaint et al. described an elegant method and could demonstrate an overall success rate of 80% after 1–2 procedures [201].

New Developments

A novel device developed for the occlusion of atrial septal defects (the Amplatzer Septal Occluder (AGA Medical Group, Plymouth, MN, USA)) has also been used off-label to close gastrointestinal fistula [64, 150]. Kumbhari and colleagues reported its use to treat gastric anastomotic leaks after sleeve gastrectomy [202]. The device is a self-expandable double umbrella-shaped Nitinol® mesh covered by polyester, connected by a short waist that has various diameters. First, the size of the defect should be measured, for instance by inflating a balloon under fluoroscopic guidance. Then a guidewire is endoscopically placed through the leak and the occluder is delivered via a 12 Fr deployment catheter inserted over the guidewire under direct visualisation by passing the endoscope alongside the occluder. The device remains in place permanently and should be used as a salvage therapy in cases of persistent leaks.

5.8.3.2 The Drainage of Leaks

The drainage of leaks without further interventions of stenting, clips, tissue sealants, etc. can be achieved by endoscopy alone or by a cooperation between endoscopist and surgeon in the operating room.

Endoscopic Drainage Via Pigtails (Endoscopic Internal Drainage (EID))

Pequignot et al. reported the first experience with pigtail drains inserted through the fistulous orifice in leaks after SG [203]. They always performed surgery in early-onset leaks ($n = 14$) with systemic inflammation; endoscopic treatment was mainly restricted to delayed-onset leaks ($n = 11$) with pulmonary symptoms and intra-abdominal abscesses. They changed their treatment from covered stents, clips and *n*-butyl-2-cyanoacrylate glue to endoscopically placed double-pigtail drains in delayed-onset leaks. These pigtails were removed after 6 weeks. This resulted in a lower median number of endoscopies (2 vs. 5.5), a shorter healing period (62 vs. 129 days) and a success rate of 82% (9 out of 11). Donatelli et al. treated 67 patients presenting with a leak following sleeve gastrectomy with deployment of double-pigtail plastic stents (Advanix®, Boston Scientific®, MA, USA) across the orifice of the leak, positioning one end inside the collection to be drained and the other end in the sleeved stomach [154] (Fig. 5.8). Stents were changed every 4–6 weeks until complete fistula healing. According to the leak size, stents varying from 1 to 10 Fr in size were inserted. A nasojejunal feeding tube was left in place in the third part of the duodenum if necessary. Leaks were diagnosed at an average time interval of 52.2 days (after 3.7 days for the 26 acute leaks, 16 days for the 32 early leaks, 61.7 days for 3 late leaks and 450.3 days for 6 chronic leaks) from surgery. The endoscopic internal drainage (EID) procedure was carried out 60.5 days (range, 4–1460 days) after sleeve gastrectomy surgery. The aim of EID was to internally drain the collection and at the same time to promote leak healing. Double-pigtail stents were successfully delivered in 66 out of 67 patients (98.5%). Fifty patients (50/64, 78.2%) were cured by EID after a mean time of 57.5 days and an average of 3.14 endoscopic sessions. There were five documented failures (7.8%): two patients were successfully cured by *n*-butyl-2-cyanoacrylate glue and the other three patients were definitively treated by total gastrectomy. There were two mortalities not related to EID. Nine were still under treatment and six patients developed late stenosis which needed dilations with an achalasia balloon (Rigiflex, Boston Scientific, MA, USA) up to 40 mm (Fig. 5.9). The authors proposed EID to be considered as primary management for both early and late leaks if no diffuse peritonitis or multi-organ failure is present. The technique seems to have several advantages including low cost, good tolerance and absence of stent-induced complications. The disadvantages include the use of parenteral or nasojejunal feeding for several weeks rather than oral feeding and an incidence of stricture formation in six patients (9%).

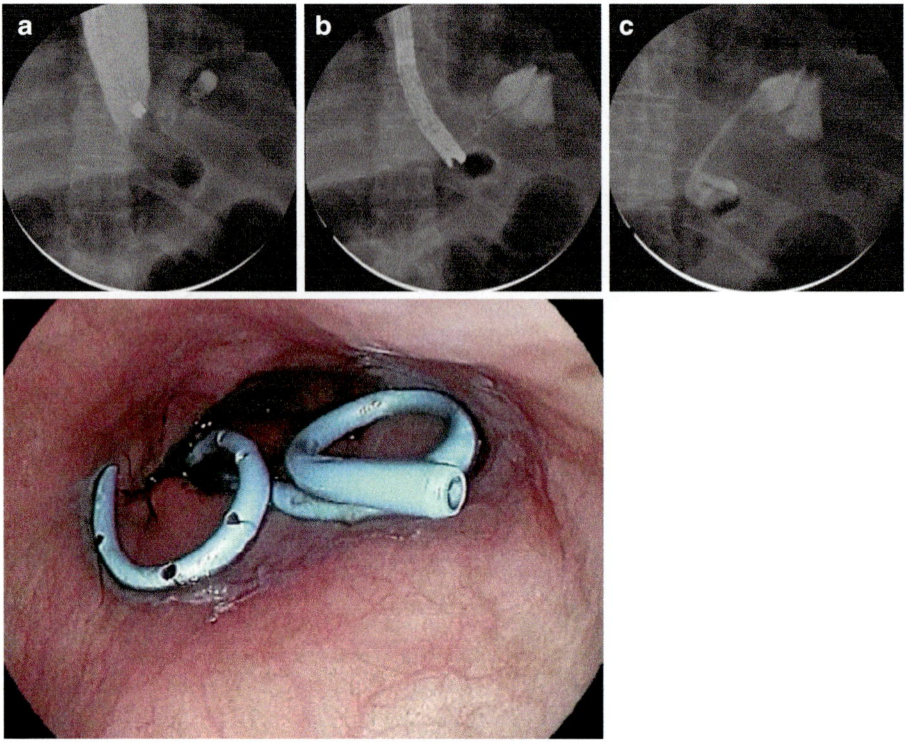

Fig. 5.8 (**a**) Left figure: Opacification of gastric leak linked with perigastric collection; in the middle: Insertion of a guidewire into the collection; and right figure: Deployment of double-pigtail stent and achievement of endoscopic internal drainage (EID), demonstrated by contrast medium in the stomach. Reprinted from Obes Surg 2015; 25: 1293–1301, Donatelli G, Dumont J-L, Cereatti F, Ferretti S, Vergeau BM, Tuszynski T, et al. Treatment of leaks following sleeve gastrectomy by endoscopic internal drainage (EID), with permission from Springer. (**b**) Two double pigtail stents placed through the leak. Reprinted from Obes Surg 2017; 27:1335–1337, Debs T, Petrucciani N, Kassir R, Vanbiervliet G, Ben Amor I, Myx Staccini A, et al. Migration of an endoscopic double pigtail drain into the abdominal wall placed as a treatment of a fistula post revisional bariatric surgery, with permission from Springer

Complications include ulceration of the viscera at the tip of the drain and bleeding [154] and occasionally pigtail migration which were reported twice invading the spleen and once into the abdominal wall [203–206].

Recently, Soufron proposed a combination of laparoscopic and endoscopic approach as a rendezvous procedure, in order to insert a pigtail drain in the gastric tube and the peritoneal cavity [207]. His series of two patients had favourable results and healing of fistula on the 30th and 41st post-operative days.

Endoscopic Drainage Via Endoluminal Vacuum Therapy

The vacuum-assisted closure (VAC) system is a new minimally invasive treatment used successfully to treat anastomotic leaks [208]. Since its introduction in the 1990s, the number of indications for the VAC system has steadily increased. Initial reports

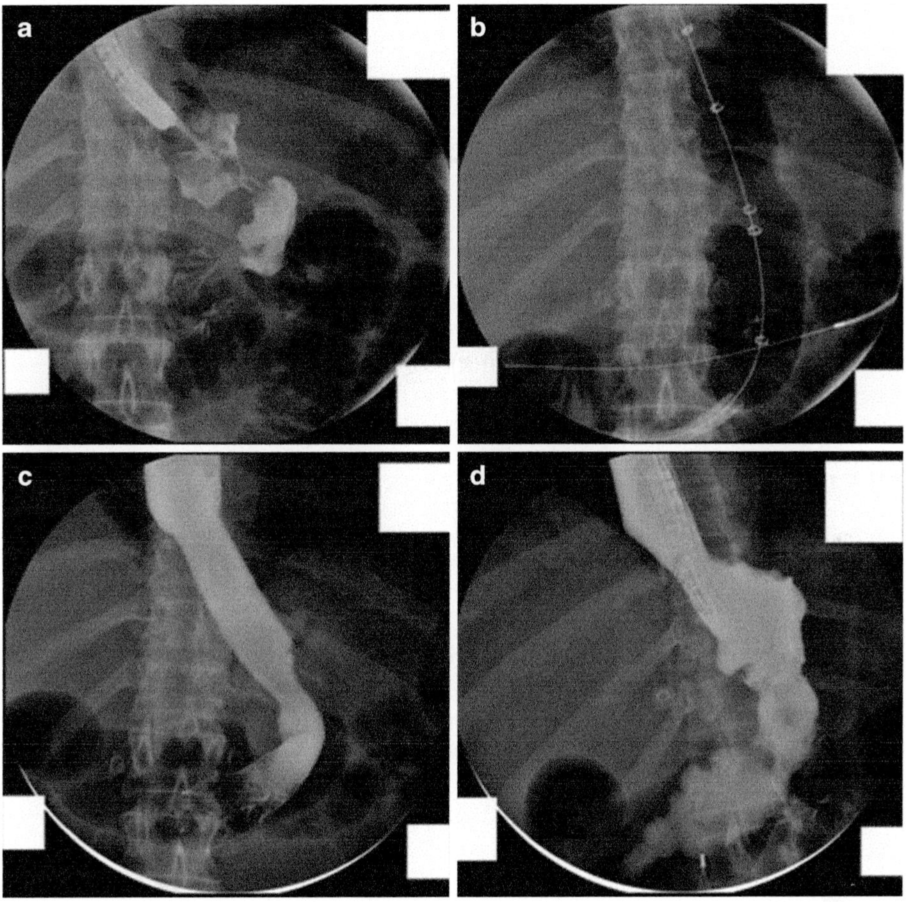

Fig. 5.9 (**a**) Endoscopic internal drainage treatment for dehiscence of gastric staple line resulting in gastric stenosis. (**b**) Pneumatic dilation using Rigiflex® Balloon up to 40 mm. (**c**) Fully covered self-expandable metal stent (SEMS) to treat the refractory stenosis. (**d**) Complete resolution of the refractory stenosis after 5 weeks of SEMS. Reprinted from Obes Surg 2015; 25: 1293–1301, Donatelli G, Dumont J-L, Cereatti F, Ferretti S, Vergeau BM, Tuszynski T, et al. Treatment of leaks following sleeve gastrectomy by endoscopic internal drainage (EID), with permission from Springer

have shown good results for endoscopically placed VAC systems in the treatment of leakage of rectal anastomoses [209, 210]. Negative pressure is applied to the wound with a vacuum-sealed open-pored polyurethane foam sponge, resulting in drainage of wound secretion, improved blood flow, reduction of oedema, promotion of granulation and consecutive wound closure (Fig. 5.10). The system of the sponge (VAC® Granu-Foam™, pore size 400–600 µm; KCI® – Kinetic Concepts Inc., TX, USA, and Wiesbaden, Germany) and the suction tube which after placement is connected to a wound drainage system can be self-made or ready-to-use sets can be purchased (Endo-Sponge system, B. Braun, Melsungen, Germany). First, an endoscopy is performed to estimate the size of the leak cavity. If the defect entrance is not wide

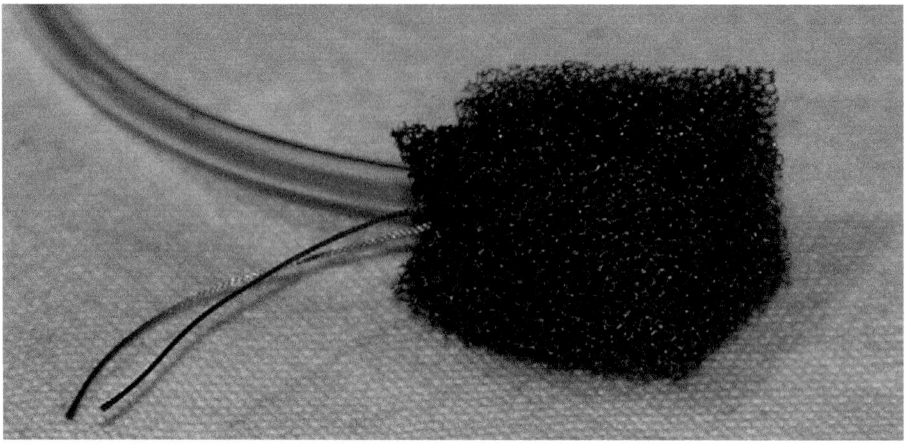

Fig. 5.10 Endoscopic vacuum-assisted closure sponge fixed to a nasoduodenal tube. Reprinted from Gastrointest Endoscopy 2010; 71: 382–386: Management of major postsurgical gastroesophageal intrathoracic leaks with an endoscopic vacuum-assisted closure system. Wedemeyer J, Brangewitz M, Kubicka S, Jackobs S, Winkler M, Neipp M, et al., with permission from Elsevier.

enough to accommodate the endoscope, the opening must be dilated. The sponge is cut into shape according to the wound size and wound geometry as estimated by the endoscopist. The sponge must be smaller than the wound cavity to promote collapse and subsequent closure. For placement of the sponge and the tube two methods can be used. In the first method, the endoscope and an overtube are inserted into the leak cavity. After removal of the endoscope, the sponge is placed into position through the overtube using a pusher and released. In the second method, the sponge drainage system is dragged alongside the endoscope and placed appropriately. Continuous suction of 100–125 mmHg is generated by a vacuum pump connected to the drainage tube. One disadvantage is the need to change the sponge every 3–5 days, until the wound cavity has healed. To remove the sponge, suction must be discontinued and it is advisable to flush the tube with 0.9% saline solution to dissolve the granulation tissue from the pores of the sponge prior to removal. Seven studies between 2010 and 2013 have reported the results in 101 patients with upper digestive leaks of whom 88 had a post-operative leak and 13 had a perforation [208]. None of the patients included in these studies did suffer from any intervention-related complication. The overall success of closing the leaks by the VAC system in these patients was 76/84 (90%; with success rates varying over the studies between 84% and 100%). The main complication associated with endoluminal vacuum therapy is a stenosis after completed therapy due to scarring. Such post-treatment stenosis occurred in 8/69 (12%). As yet, evidence in bariatrics is limited [172, 211].

Endoscopic Drainage and Debridement

Endoscopic transluminal necrosectomy is done for the treatment of organised pancreatic necrosis and pseudocyst clearance. After a leak, the percutaneous drainage alone may not be effective due to the thick solid material. The success of endoscopic percutaneous or transluminal drainage and debridement of post-operative infected collections following bariatric surgery has been reported by Lemmers et al. [212]. They reported the results of drainage and debridement in nine cases; three patients were treated by percutaneous endoscopic debridement of abscesses and six patients were treated by transluminal endoscopic drainage, debridement and necrosectomy, either as a first-line option or after failure of improvement after endoscopic treatment. Resolution of collections was seen in seven out of nine patients, but two required further surgery. In eight of the nine patients, final closure of the fistula was achieved with SEMS, fistula plugs or clips. The number of sessions required ranged from 1 to 3. Most of the severely affected patients had rapid improvement of their haemodynamic and respiratory conditions. In eight of the nine patients, the authors were able to close the fistula by stent, fistula plugs or a macroclip.

Multimodality therapy employs a combination of a nasocystic catheter, transluminal endoscopic debridement and copious saline lavage solutions as done with pancreatic pseudocysts, followed by stenting and after removal of the stent closure of the hole by endoclips or filling the hole with injectable glue [160]. In 27 anastomotic fistula, 25 leaks after SG and 2 leaks after RYGB, a 100% success was obtained after a median of 4.4 endoscopies in a mean of 86 days, even though 93% had fistulas larger than 10 mm and 53% had multiple or complex fistulas.

Endoscopic Drainage Via a T-Tube in a Cooperation Between Endoscopist and Surgeon

El Hassan et al. performed laparoscopy for early type (within 7 days) and type C leaks after sleeve gastrectomy [178]. During laparoscopy an intraoperative endoscopy was done to delineate the leak. If the leak was large, a T-tube was placed inside the leak for decompression and for a conversion into a controlled fistula. However, if no large hole was found or if the leak was not clearly identifiable, only wide drainage of the abdomen with two closed suction drains was done without attempting to place sutures. In every patient a jejunostomy tube was inserted for jejunostomy tube feeding and they received nil per mouth. All leaks healed after an initial period of hospital stay, followed by an outpatient period with a time of healing of 3–6 weeks.

Treatment of Leaks Through a One–Step Intervention in a Cooperation Between Endoscopist and Surgeon

Patients with gastric sleeve leaks were treated in a one-step intervention, with the aim to achieve three objectives: a prolonged decompression of the gastric sleeve tube through a laparoscopically endoscopically placed gastrostomy tube, a laparoscopically placed feeding jejunostomy and external drainage [213]. During laparoscopy an endoscope was cautiously introduced, the perforation was identified and the endoscope was advanced distally into the sleeve till the antrum under laparoscopic and endoscopic vision. In the healthy anterior wall of the antrum tissue a tiny gastrotomy of about 3 mm was made by the operating surgeon, just big enough to allow the endoscopist to pass a polypectomy snare to grasp an 18 Fr tube. This tube was inserted from the outside through a right upper quadrant port, which later formed the exit site of the gastrostomy. After checking the adequate position of the tube, the endoscope was withdrawn and the gastrotomy site was then secured by the surgeon with a purse-string suture. The

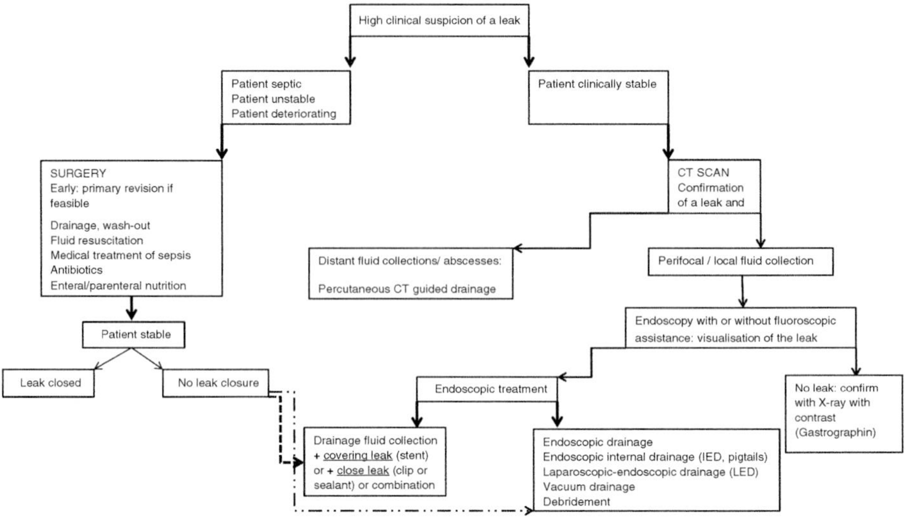

Fig. 5.11 Algorithm, proposed for the treatments of leaks, taking into consideration the condition of the patient and the available treatment options

gastrostomy tube was connected to a vacuum system for drainage of the perforation and for gastric decompression. Six out of seven leaks healed and one patient with a large rent was managed by a Roux-en-Y fistulojejunostomy.

In case of a leak in a haemodynamically stable patient there are many endoscopic options and the treatment of choice depends on the skills of the endoscopist and the preferences of the surgeon. Sometimes, a rendez-vous procedure of both endoscopist and surgeon is needed. To help in the decision which treatment is preferable, guidelines might be useful. One should, however, realise that guidelines may be rendered out of date by the very rapid developments. To guide both gastroenterologists and surgeon in the decision-making, an algorithm is proposed in Fig. 5.11.

5.8.4 Guidelines

The 2008 ASGE/ASMBS/SAGES guidelines state that there is little role for an endoscopy in the presence of known leaks or fistulas in the early post-operative period because air insufflation may have potentially detrimental effects in the presence of leaks and fragile anastomoses [214]. The recommendation for the endoscopist is to consider contrast radiography as an initial diagnostic test and only if the patient is clinically stable there is uncertainty of the diagnosis, or if there is a planned endoscopic intervention, an endoscopy can be considered [214]. In the updated 2015 version they recommend water-soluble radiography rather than endoscopy as the initial investigation in patients suspected of having a leak or fistula (moderate level of evidence) [41]. The guidelines recommend endoscopy as a first-line diagnostic study in patients with abdominal pain, nausea or vomiting but only after consultation with the surgeon (moderate level of evidence). Endoscopic management in fistulas and leaks in consultation with a bariatric surgeon is suggested (very low level of evidence) [41].

Surgical intervention with drainage, oversewing or surgical revision is discussed in two guidelines (EAES and IFSO-EC/ EASO/OMTF [39, 215]). One guideline gives no recommendation at all (AACE/TOS/ASMBS [40]). In the sleeve summit, the use of glue, clips and endoscopic dilation is mentioned with the use of stents in persisting leaks [37]. In the best practice recommendations by Rosenthal et al. surgeons agreed in 86% that an unstable patient with a contained or uncontained leak requires immediate operation and in 90% that a patient with tachycardia and fever with normal findings on upper GI studies also needs immediate reoperation or re-intervention [19]. The use of a stent is a valid option for an acute proximal leak (93% agreement) for which conservative treatment had failed (95% consensus) [19]. The fifth International Consensus on Sleeve Gastrectomy in 2016 mentioned that when acute leaks occur within 7 days, two algorithms prevail: stenting endoscopically or fluoroscopically with percutaneous drainage of surrounding abscesses, or laparoscopy with drainage, feeding jejunostomy and careful observation [63].

5.9 Gastrointestinal Bleeding

Bleeding in the patient after bariatric surgery may be acute and early (<30 days) or chronic and late (≥30 days) and then may present as iron-deficiency anaemia [19]. Acute post-operative bleeding is accompanied with signs of hypovolaemia, such as an increase in heart rate > 20 beats per minute or a decrease in systolic blood pressure >20 mmHg, and/or a significant drop in haemoglobin (>2 g/dL; >0.3 mmol/L). An early GI bleeding typically presents within 48 h after surgery. The bleeding can be extraluminal and can be a result of blood vessel injury, visceral injury (spleen, liver), mesenteric injury or from dissection planes or sites of trocar entry. Intraluminal bleeding is more easily diagnosed because besides the symptoms of hypovolaemic shock, specific signs such as haematemesis, haematochezia and/or melaena are present. Intraluminal bleeding presents with either haematemesis (from the gastrojejunostomy bleed in RYGB, from the long staple line in sleeve gastrectomy, or duodenoileal anastomosis bleed after BPD with duodenal switch) or melaena/haematochezia (from the already named sites but also from the jejunojejunostomy bleed after RYGB, gastric remnant or duodenum bleed after RYGB, or ileoileal anastomosis bleed after BPD) [159]. It can even present as a small-bowel obstruction caused by a clot [159]. Upper GI bleeding occurs more often after RYGB than after LAGB, SG or VBG and death as a consequence of bleeding is uncommon [216, 217]. Bleeding is rare (0.1%) in patients undergoing LAGB; it varies between 1% and 3% after a sleeve gastrectomy and between 1.9% and 4.4% after RYGB [2, 111, 214].

A meta-analysis reported a rate of bleeding after gastric bypass of 1.9% [218]. When in the analysis open versus laparoscopic RYGB was compared, it was noted that the frequency of GI tract haemorrhage was significantly higher in the laparoscopic series [218]. Another study reported a bleeding in 3.2% [219]. However, bleeding was extraluminal in 50% and higher in the laparoscopic group than in the open group (5.1% vs. 2.4%). Dick et al. reported early post-operative (≤30 days) bleedings in 26 (3.3%) of 776 RYGB patients with tachycardia in 46%, melaena in 32% and haematemesis in 18% [220]. Of the 26 bleeding patients, 8 (31%) required operation, 6 had a bleeding identified at the jejunojejunostomy and 2 at the gastrojejunostomy site. One patient bleeding from the jejunojejunostomy died (3.8%). Heneghan et al. reported a bleeding in 42 (0.94%) of 466 patients after a gastric bypass [221]. In 30 (71%) the bleeding occurred early in the post-operative period (<30 days, usually at a mean of 3.2 days) and even 13 bleedings occurred within 24 h after the procedure. Early bleeding was predominantly intra-abdominal in 16 (53.5%) and in only 10 (33.3%) related to the staple line. Late post-operative bleeding in 12 was secondary to marginal ulceration in 10 and twice being intra-abdominal.

Although endoscopy is often used as a first-line modality for investigation of the source of acute bleedings and the efficacy of endoscopy for treatment of bleeding ulcers has been proven by a meta-analysis of randomised controlled trials, the case for the bariatric patient is not so evident [222]. Standard endoscopy is able to reach the gastrojejunostomy anastomosis and carbon dioxide insufflation is favoured over air insufflation to minimise the risk of perforation [64, 217]. However, endoscopic management for early bleeds with the use of several endoscopic therapies, including thermal therapies (heater probe, mono and bipolar electrocoagulation, argon plasma coagulation), injections with epinephrine and various sclerosants, clips and fibrin glue, carries the risk of perforation at the staple line and dehiscence of immature anastomoses [64, 217, 222]. These risks may be enhanced by combination therapy (epinephrine used in combination with a second therapy such as bipolar electrocoagulation, injectable sclerosants or clips) shown to be a superior approach in high-risk bleeding ulcers when compared to epinephrine as a single agent [223]. These dangers are even greater when forces are applied to the gastrointestinal tract during balloon-assisted or spiral-assisted enteroscopy, required to access the excluded gastric remnant or Roux limb in altered RYGB anatomy [64, 119]. Even though ischaemia and necrosis are theoretically possible with the injection of diluted adrenaline or sclerosant and the use of the heater probe, only a few cases describing this phenomenon following endoscopic haemostasis of bleeding gastric ulcers have been published, but deep ulceration and perforation are extremely rare [224, 225]. The application of argon plasma coagulation (APC) once resulted in a perforation, presumably caused by heat conduction by the surgical staples resulting in a transmural burn and perforation of the jejunojejunal anastomosis [226]. Therefore, the endoscopist should proceed with caution when application of APC is required with the presence of surgical clips in near proximity to the lesion.

In contrast to the acute bleeding situation in an average patient where endoscopy should be performed to both diagnose and treat the bleeding source which is often an ulcer or oesophageal/gastric varices, in the bariatric patient the approach might be different. Conservative treatment and observation is the first approach and indeed up to 30–63% of cases only require blood transfusion and bleedings seem to be self-limited [217, 227, 228]. Endoscopy is considered in the early period when patients have proven bleeding with haematemesis or melaena and the bleeding is refractory to supportive therapy [217]. However, when post-operative bleeding is severe and associated with haemodynamic instability, surgical re-exploration may be required with oversewing the staple line. In the literature, there is a wide range between 6 and 85% of reported therapeutic endoscopy interventions. Other diagnostic modalities are radiologic tests such as CT angiography, Tc-99 m RBC bleeding scan or invasive angiography, modalities that apart from invasive angiography with embolisation do not treat the bleeding. This holds also true for the diagnostic video capsule endoscopy that has been used to identify small-bowel lesions in patients with normal anatomy but is not at all useful for bleedings in the bypassed stomach and afferent limb in Roux-en-Y gastric bypass.

In a retrospective study Jamil et al. identified 933 patients that underwent RYGB over a 5-year study period [227]. Thirty patients presented with signs of upper GI bleeding. Of the 30 patients that bled, 14 bled once, 13 had two and 3 patients had three bleeding episodes, for a total of 49 bleeding episodes. The majority of these bleedings were manifested by haematemesis (36 episodes (73%)). Upper GI endoscopy performed in 27 of these 30 patients identified the bleeding site at the gastrojejunostomy staple line. Endoscopic findings revealed active oozing in 13 (48%) patients, a visible bleeding vessel in 7 (26%) patients and an adherent clot in 7 (26%) patients. Endoscopic intervention was needed in 24 (89%) and consisted of epinephrine with heater probe (at 15–30 Joules) in 14, epinephrine alone in 3, heater probe alone in 4 and endoclips in 2 combined with the other methods. One patient required all three methods [227]. Sixteen patients experienced a second bleeding episode following a mean of 38 h after the first endoscopy and five required a repeat endoscopy. Oozing from the gastrojejunostomy site was present in four and red streaks in one. Heater probe and epinephrine were used in four and epinephrine only in one. Three patients had a third discrete bleeding episode 4 h after the second endoscopy with no significant haemodynamic changes and without endoscopy. None of the patients required operation. Complications were one massive aspiration and death and one perforation in a patient treated with epinephrine, heater probe and clip placement [227]. The bleeding in a small gastric pouch with a limited gastric reservoir puts the patient at higher risk of aspiration. So, bleeding patients are best managed in the operating room with the patient being intubated. This gives also the opportunity to proceed directly to surgical intervention should endoscopy therapy fail. A prospective study by Fernández-Esparrach et al. reported results of upper GI bleedings in 22 of 381 RYGB patients (5.8%) [229]. Sixteen were managed with conservative measures without procedural intervention. Six patients required endoscopic intervention and were managed with epinephrine injections either as a single therapy or in combination with polidocanol. In Heneghan's study, during a 10-year period 466 patients underwent a gastric bypass and 42 (0.94%) experienced a bleeding complication [221]. In 30 (71%) the bleeding occurred early in the post-operative period (<30 days, usually at a mean of 3.2 days) and of these, 13 occurred within 24 h after the procedure. Half of the patients underwent endoscopy but in no case endoluminal treatment was considered appropriate. Early bleeding was predominantly intra-abdominal in 16 (53.5%) and required operative intervention in 13 (43%). Late post-operative bleeding in 12 was mainly intraluminal (10/12) and due to marginal ulcers and warranted surgical intervention in 4 (33%). The overall operative intervention rate was 38.1% and one patient needed embolisation. Rabl et al. published a retrospective review of 722 patients with a haemorrhage in 19 (2.6%) patients within 2 weeks after surgery [228]. Six had endoscopy and five were treated successfully by epinephrine and clipping.

So, endoscopic management of intraluminal bleeding by adrenaline injection, electrocoagulation or haemostatic endoclips is successful and safe, with low failure rates. This treatment can be repeated [227, 229]. In case of failure of coagulation therapy, the application of topical haemostatic agents such as haemostatic powder (haemospray, Cook Medical, Winston-Salem, NC, USA) is a newly available treatment option, particularly for lesions that span extended surface areas. As yet, there is no data describing their use after bariatric surgery [230]. The use of tranexamic acid, 1 g given after induction, which is a relatively inexpensive drug known to reduce bleeding, was investigated in a prospective randomised study [231]. Twenty-five patients were each allocated to the control and treatment arms. The tranexamic acid group required significantly less haemostatic stitches for staple-line bleeding, incurred less intraoperative blood loss and had quicker operating times. There has been a lot of discussion whether in sleeve gastrectomy reinforcement of the long staple line with oversewing or buttressing materials may prevent staple-line bleeding. A meta-analysis published by Shikora et al. revealed that the incidence of bleeding was dependent on the reinforcement method [145]. In 33 studies where a running suture was used for reinforcement, the bleeding rate was 2.41%, while in 25 studies without staple reinforcement, the bleeding rate was 4.94%.

A predictive model for haemorrhagic complications after bariatric surgery might be of great help. Janik et al. performed a retrospective analysis of 522 patients after primary SG [232]. The rate of haemorrhagic complications was 4% (21/522). A total of 12 variables were examined; four were associated with risk of haemorrhagic complications. Protective factors for haemorrhagic complications were the absence of a history of obstructive sleep apnoea and an absence of hypertension; however, a low level of expertise in bariatric surgery and no staple-line reinforcement were associated with higher risk of haemorrhagic complications. Among the four variables, a history of obstructive sleep apnoea and the lack of staple-line reinforcement showed the strongest independent associations with the probability of post-sleeve haemorrhagic complications. The data were put into a regression formula and the authors developed a risk calculator named SLEEVE BLEED which is available at http://www.r-calc.com.

Late (more than 30 days post-operatively) intraluminal bleeding is classically caused by a marginal ulcer. Sometimes the bleeding is not manifest and the investigation of obscure GI bleeding or iron-deficiency anaemia is challenging in surgically altered anatomy, particularly in those operations (gastric bypass and biliopancreatic diversion) where potential bleeding sites such as distal anastomotic sites and excluded stomach might not be accessible with conventional endoscopy. The American Society for Gastrointestinal Endoscopy placed their recommendation for deep enteroscopy as the initial diagnostic evaluation in post-bariatric surgery patients with obscure GI bleeding in the lowest evidence of experts' opinion [233]. Currently, there is only one case series by Skinner et al. focused on the efficacy of double-balloon enteroscopy (DBE) to successfully identify and treat lesions responsible for obscure GI bleeding in the bypassed stomach [226]. They performed DBE 17 times in 12 patients with altered anatomy, 6 of them having a gastric bypass. Nine cases had overt bleeding and three had occult bleeding. In 10 of the 12 patients, the bleeding site could be identified with DBE. In nine, the bleeding site was at the anastomosis and once in the afferent limb. The stomach was found to be normal in nine of ten patients (90%), including five of six with gastric bypass. Endoscopic treatment was applied in eight patients, four patients required repeat endoscopy due to bleeding recurrence and there was one perforation requiring emergent surgery [226]. Finally, access to the excluded portion of the stomach and/or Roux limb can be facilitated through laparoscopic endoscopy via a surgically created gastrostomy, when traditional endoscopic techniques fail [41, 234].

5.9.1 Guidelines

Similar as is the case with leaks and fistula, there are no detailed guidelines on how to proceed in post-bariatric haemorrhages. The European Association of Endoscopic Surgery (EAES) guideline of 2005 suggests that bleeding from staple lines with minor or major blood loss should be treated conservatively [215]. The 2008 ASGE/ASMBS/SAGES guidelines state that patients with signs or symptoms of acute or chronic bleeding should be evaluated with an endoscopy without, however, mentioning the timing and eventual institution of treatment [214]. The updated 2015 ASGE/ASMBS/SAGES guidelines mention that endoscopic diagnosis and treatment are indicated, sometimes requiring the use of a colonoscope or device-assisted enteroscope [41]. The American Society for Gastrointestinal Endoscopy recommends deep enteroscopy as the initial diagnostic evaluation in post-bariatric surgery patients with obscure GI bleeding [234]. When traditional approaches of the excluded stomach and/or the Roux limb are unsuccessful a surgically created gastrostomy may allow access but again without giving a time limit [41]. No advice at all is given by two guidelines (AACE/TOS/ASMBS and IFSO-EC/EASO/OMTF [39, 40]) and also the sleeve summits and conferences give no indication of when and how to deal with haemorrhages [19, 37, 63].

5.10 Acute Gastrointestinal Obstruction

5.10.1 Gastric Obstruction

Gastric outlet obstruction at the site of the gastric band in LAGB or at the gastrojejunal anastomosis in RYGB can be caused by tissue oedema. In the early postoperative period oedematous, non-mechanical obstruction is common and resolves with time and with the use of supportive measures (nasogastric tube decompression, antacids, liquid/soft diet, meat tenderisers, or metoclopramide) [43]. In this situation, there always exists a potential for aspiration pneumonia and stomach ischaemia. Acute stomal obstruction can occur in up to 14% of patients after gastric banding and is usually caused by inclusion of excess perigastric fat, use of bands with a too small band diameter for the thickness of the tissue or significant tissue oedema. Patients present with persistent nausea, vomiting and inability to tolerate oral food intake or even their own saliva. Upper GI series with contrast demonstrate no passage through the band. When the acute stomal obstruction does not subside, revision or removal of the band is required. The use of larger diameter bands may help to reduce the incidence of acute postoperative obstruction [43].

The incidence of symptomatic anastomotic stenosis after RYGB peaks 3–4 weeks after surgery and patients who develop obstruction somewhat later, 6 to 12 weeks post-surgery, may have had subclinical leaks leading to peristomal inflammation and fibrosis [113]. If conservative treatment fails early balloon dilation to a maximum of 12 mm may temporarily relieve the dysphagia. Strictures in sleeve gastrectomy may also occur early in the evolution (<6 weeks). Stenosis and strictures in RYGB and SG may be treated endoscopically [41]. Sometimes, an unusual approach is needed [108]. A complete stenosis on the third post-operative day after gastric bypass surgery was treated by a combined endoscopic and laparoscopic approach, whereby the surgeon punctured the jejunal loop and the endoscopist passed a guidewire to perform pneumatic dilation. After successful dilation, the puncture site was closed by the surgeon.

Gastric remnant distension following gastric bypass surgery is a rare but potentially lethal complication resulting from distal mechanical obstruction at the jejunojejunostomy or paralytic ileus [235, 236]. Iatrogenic injury to vagal fibres along the lesser curvature may further contribute by impairment of gastric emptying. Progressive distension by large volumes of acid, bile and pancreas secretions can ultimately lead to rupture, massive spillage of gastric contents and severe peritonitis. Clinically, the patients present with symptoms of abdominal and shoulder pain, hiccups, abdominal distension, tachycardia and tachypnoea. On X-ray a large gastric air bubble can be seen. Treatment consists of emergent operative decompression or percutaneous drainage. Patients at risk for this complication are elderly superobese patients, patients with diabetic gastropathy and patients having revision surgery. One might consider the construction of a gastrostomy in these cases.

5.10.2 Small-Bowel Obstruction

Also acute small-bowel obstruction can be life threatening and represents a surgical emergency.

Small-bowel obstruction may mostly be due to internal hernias, but can also be caused by trocar site hernia, intussusception, adhesions, stricture, kinking or blood clots. An obstruction will result in a closed-loop obstruction that can be rapidly fatal if not recognised and decompressed. Symptoms of obstruction that persist, acidosis, a rise of lactate and signs of an acute abdomen should prompt an exploration.

Internal hernia is widely recognised as the most frequent cause of small-bowel obstruction in bariatric patients. Long-term follow-up of patients after LRYGB reveals that internal hernia becomes the most common complication over time, with an incidence ranging from 1 to 9%. There are three classic locations: a mesenteric defect at the jejunojejunostomy, a defect in the transverse mesocolon in patients with a retrocolic Roux limb and a Petersen hernia: a space between the transverse mesocolon and the Roux limb mesentery. Herniation of the small intestine through one of the mesenteric defects can cause small-bowel obstruction. All three mesentery defects should be closed in order to avoid internal hernias with non-absorbable sutures. Some surgeons have pointed out that there is no higher incidence of internal hernia without closure of mesenterics defects and that after weight loss and loss of intra-abdominal fat defects will reappear. The majority of internal hernias occur through the transverse mesocolon defect. The use of an antecolic Roux limb can, in theory, reduce the risk of internal hernia formation. This can be explained by the fact that a retrocolic approach creates all three mesenteric defects, whereas the antecolic approach creates only two mesenteric defects: one at the jejunojejunostomy and a Petersen defect. Indeed, a recent meta-analysis found that the use of an antecolic Roux limb as opposed to a retrocolic limb was associated with lower rates of post-operative internal hernias (1.3% vs. 2.3%) [237]. Small-bowel obstruction after open bariatric surgery has been reported to be in the range of 1–5%. After laparoscopic bypass a recent review reported an overall incidence of 3.6% [238]. In the meta-analysis by Podnos et al. early bowel obstruction was not reported in any of the open bypass studies but in 1.7% in laparoscopic gastric bypass procedures [218]. So, while this complication was relatively rare during the era of open RYGB, it is more frequent following laparoscopic RYGB. Some groups have suggested that the reduced bowel manipulation and peritoneal irritation with the laparoscopic approach caused fewer post-operative adhesions, resulting in reduced fixation of the Roux limb and less scarring to help close mesenteric defects. Internal hernias are notoriously difficult to diagnose, especially when they do not present as an urgency and when small-bowel loops are intermittently endangered. A CT scan is the imaging modality of choice and up to 14 signs have been described but sensitivity and specificity varied substantially per sign and per radiologist. Ideally, a CT scan should be done immediately when the patient presents with symptoms. Lockhart et al. compared the results of three radiologists using seven signs on CT scan [239]. They found an individual sensitivity between 0 and 83% and a specificity of 67–100%, and an overall score of 56–78% sensitivity and overall score of 78–89% specificity. In Table 5.6 data on sensitivity and specificity of CT scans are summarised [239–242].

Table 5.6 Sensitivity and specificity of CT scans for the detection of internal hernias

Author	Year	No. of signs used	No. of patients	No. (%) of internal hernias	% Sensitivity	% Specificity
Yu [240]	2004	?	890	3 (0.3)	66.6	100
Lockhart [239]	2007	7	501	18 (3.5)	56–78	78–89
Guabusbanam [241]	2009	8	835	13 (1.6)	33.3	100
Iannuccilli [242]	2009	8	768	9 (1.2)	11–100	70–90

Martin et al. analysed the 2006–2007 inpatient samples and had 9505 admissions for small-bowel obstruction in bariatric patients versus 54,342 in non-bariatric patients [238]. Surgery was performed in 62% of bariatric patients versus 28% in non-bariatric patients and bariatric patients were also taken earlier into the operating room (after 1 vs. 3.3 days).

Besides oedema at the gastroenterostomy after gastric bypass, signs of early post-operative obstruction may concern the jejunal Roux limb [114]. The Roux limb is brought to the upper abdomen in an antecolic in front of the transverse colon or retrocolic fashion in the transverse mesocolon. An antecolic configuration of the Roux limb has been demonstrated to lead to fewer internal hernias and small-bowel obstruction than a retrocolic approach. When the tunnel is too small or the sutures needed to fixate the limb to the tunnel edges to prevent migration are placed too tightly, obstruction will result. Obstruction can also be caused by a rotation of the limb inadvertently performed at surgery. At endoscopy a normal-appearing gastrojejunostomy is recognised with a proximally dilated jejunum, to the point where it traverses the mesentery [41, 114]. Also, the rotational stricture may be visible. Both need surgical correction.

As has already been mentioned, endoscopy is sometimes needed to diagnose the outlet obstruction in case of a too tight band or oedema or a stenosis or stricture in case of a gastric bypass or sleeve gastrectomy. Sometimes indications for an endoscopy are rather unusual [94]: the surgeons asked twice for an endoscopy with a peculiar indication: once in case of a distal obstruction of the biliopancreatic limb. A colonoscope was used and the obstruction at the level of the jejunojejunostomy was identified without a possibility to relieve it by endoscopic treatment. In the second case, an abscess cavity suspicious of a perforation could not be identified by GI radiography and by endoscopy the correct diagnosis of a perforation was made. This emphasises once more that mutual understanding and a good cooperation between bariatric surgeon and endoscopist are mandatory.

5.10.3 Guidelines

The AACE/TOS/ASMBS guidelines just state in general that persistent and severe GI symptoms (nausea, vomiting, abdominal pain, diarrhoea and constipation) warrant evaluation (Grade C, level of evidence 3) [40]. Endoscopy may be the preferred procedure for GI symptoms suggestive of stricture or foreign body (staple, suture) as it can be both diagnostic and therapeutic (Grade C, level of evidence 3) [40]. The 2015 ASGE/ASMBS/SAGES guidelines recommend endoscopy as a first-line diagnostic study in patients with abdominal pain, nausea or vomiting but only after consultation with the surgeon (moderate level of evidence) [41]. The IFSO-EC/EASO/OMTF guideline has a general statement that in case severe symptoms are present and persistent such as nausea, vomiting, abdominal pain and change in stools, endoscopy or CT may be considered as the first diagnostic/therapeutic option [39]. The fifth International Conference on Sleeve Gastrectomy in 2016 mentioned that strictures early in the evolution (<6 weeks) may be treated endoscopically [63].

None of the guidelines went into detail on diagnosis or treatment of above-mentioned gastrointestinal obstructions.

Conclusion

Intraoperative endoscopy, apart from using it as a leak test, offers additional information on intraluminal bleeding and narrowing of the lumen/anastomosis which may be relevant in gastric bypass surgery and even more so in sleeve gastrectomy. Routine radiology and endoscopic investigations on the days following surgery have a low sensitivity and a poor positive predictive value to detect leaks and only a high degree of suspicion and careful monitoring of symptoms should warrant further investigations. Moreover, leaks mostly occur after discharge when the patient is already home. The indication and need for an endoscopy in the early days after the operation is a matter of intensive discussion between surgeon and endoscopist, who both have to take into consideration the haemodynamic status of the patient and the diagnostic gain and therapeutic options offered by the endoscopic examination. An emergency endoscopy and an endoscopy in the early post-operative period (<6 weeks) are safe when performed by a skilled and experienced endoscopist, who has knowledge of the changed anatomy and who inspects cautiously, without too much force and pressure and with the use of carbon dioxide instead of room air, the entire mucosa, anastomosis and staple line for signs of leaks, bleeding or obstruction. The therapeutic options in leaks should be taken into deliberation by both specialists and approaches may vary according to the aim, subdivided into whether the occlusion of leaks and fistulas should be aimed at by endoscopic stents, clips, suturing and/or sealants, with adequate drainage of collections, or whether merely drainage of leaks by pigtails, endoluminal vacuum therapy, drainage and debridement, and/or rendez-vous procedures of endoscopist and surgeon should be the choice. The same applies to the options available to achieve haemostasis in case of bleeding such as thermal therapies (heater probe, mono- and bipolar electrocoagulation, argon plasma coagulation), injections with epinephrine and various sclerosants, haemostatic clips and fibrin glue. In gastrointestinal obstruction, the role of endoscopy is less obvious and if present will be mostly of diagnostic purpose.

References

1. The ASMBS Clinical Issues Committee. ASMBS guideline on the prevention and detection of GI leak after gastric bypass including the role of imaging and surgical exploration. Surg Obes Relat Dis. 2009;5:293–6.
2. Ghosh SK, Roy S, Chekan E, Fegelman EJ. A narrative of intraoperative staple line leaks and bleeds during bariatric surgery. Obes Surg. 2016;26:1601–6.
3. Bingham J, Lallemand M, Barron M, Kuckelman J, Carter DOP, Blair K, et al. Routine intraoperative leak testing for sleeve gastrectomy: is the leak test full of hot air? Am J Surg. 2016;211:943–7.

4. Gill RS, Whitlock KA, Mohamed R, Sarkhosh K, Birch DW, Karmall S. The role of upper gastrointestinal endoscopy in treating postoperative complications in bariatric surgery. J Interv Gastroenterol. 2012;2:37–41.
5. Haddad A, Tapazoglou N, Singh K, Averbach A. Role of intraoperative esophagogastroenteroscopy in minimizing gastrojejunostomy-related morbidity:experience with 2311 laparoscopic gastric bypasses with linear stapler anastomosis. Obes Surg. 2012;22:1928–33.
6. Nimeri A, Maasher A, Salim E, Ibrahim M, Al Hadad M. The use of intraoperative endoscopy may decrease postoperative stenosis in laparoscopic sleeve gastrectomy. Obes Surg. 2016;26:1398–401.
7. Al Hadad M, Dehni N, Elamin D, Ibrahim M, Ghabra S, Nimeri A. Intraoperative endoscopy decreases postoperative complications in laparoscopic roux-en-Y gastric bypass. Obes Surg. 2015;25:1711–5.
8. Alasfar F, Chand B. Intraoperative endoscopy for laparoscopic roux-en-Y gastric bypass: leak test and beyond. Surg Laparosc Endosc Percutan Tech. 2010;20:424–7.
9. Alaedeen D, Madan AK, Ro CY, Khan KA, Martinez JM, Tichansky DS. Intraoperative endoscopy and leaks after laparoscopic roux-en-Y gastric bypass. Am Surg. 2009;75:485–8.
10. Sekhar N, Torquati A, Lufti R, Richards WO. Endoscopic evaluation of the gastrojejunostomy in laparoscopic gastric bypass. Surg Endosc. 2006;20:199–201.
11. Fernandez AZ, DeMaria EJ, Tichansky DS, Kellum JM, Wolfe LG, Meador J, et al. Experience with over 3,000 open and laparoscopic bariatric procedures. Surg Endosc. 2004;18:193–7.
12. Ramanathan R, Ikramuddin D, Gourash W, Schauer P. The value of intraoperative endoscopy during laparoscopic Roux-en-Y gastric bypass for morbid obesity. Surg Endosc. 2000;14(suppl 1):S212; (abstract).
13. Cingi A, Yavuz Y. Intraoperative endoscopic assessment of the pouch and anastomosis during laparoscopic Roux-en-Y gastric bypass. Obes Surg. 2011;21:1530–4.
14. Nelson L, Moon RC, Teixeira AF, Jawad MA. Methylene blue or upper GI, which is more effective for detecting leaks in gastric bypass patients? Surg Laparosc Endosc Percutan Tech. 2015;25:451–4.
15. Parikh M, Issa R, McCrillis A, Saunders JK, Ude-Welcome A, Gagner M. Surgical strategies that may decrease leak after laparoscopic sleeve gastrectomy: a systematic review and meta-analysis of 9991 cases. Ann Surg. 2013;257:231–7.
16. Aurora AR, Khaitan L, Saber AA. Sleeve gastrectomy and the risk of leak: a systematic analysis of 4,888 patients. Surg Endosc. 2012;26:1509–15.
17. Sakran N, Goitein D, Raziel A, Keidar A, Beglaibter N, Grinbaum R, et al. Gastric leaks after sleeve gastrectomy: a multicenter experience with 2834 patients. Surg Endosc. 2013;27:240–5.
18. Wahby M, Salama AF, Elezaby AF, Belgrami F, AbdEllatif ME, El-Kaffas HF, et al. Is routine postoperative gastrografin study needed after laparoscopic sleeve gastrectomy? Experience of 712 cases. Obes Surg. 2013;23:1711–7.
19. Rosenthal RJ, for the International Sleeve Gastrectomy Expert Panel. International sleeve Gastrectomy expert panel consensus statement: best practice guidelines based on experience of 12,000 cases. Surg Obes Relat Dis. 2012;8:8–19.
20. Kassir R, Blanc P, Gugenheim J, Lointier P, Bachir E, Ben Amor I, et al. Performing sleeve gastrectomy. Int J Surg. 2015;13:131–2.
21. Toppino M, Cesarani F, Comba A, Denegri F, Mistrangelo M, Gandini G, et al. The role of early radiological studies after gastric bariatric surgery. Obes Surg. 2001;11:447–54.
22. Serafini F, Anderson W, Ghassemi P, Poklepovic J, Murr MM. The utility of contrast studies and drains in the management of patients after Roux-en-Y gastric bypass. Obes Surg. 2002;12:34–8.
23. Singh R, Fisher BL. Sensitivity and specificity of postoperative upper GI series following gastric bypass. Obes Surg. 2003;13:73–5.
24. Kolakowski S Jr, Kirkland ML, Schuricht AL. Routine postoperative upper gastrointestinal series after Roux-en-y gastric bypass determination of whether it is necessary. Arch Surg. 2007;142:930–4.

25. Madan AK, Stocklein HH, Ternovits CA, Tichansky DS, Philips JC. Predictive value of upper gastrointestinal studies versus clinical signs for gastrointestinal leaks after laparoscopic gastric bypass. Surg Endosc. 2007;21:194–6.
26. Maher J, Bakhos W, Nahmias N, Wolfe LG, Meador JG, Baugh N, et al. Drain amylase levels are an adjunct in detection of gastrojejunostomy leaks after Roux-en-Y gastric bypass. J Am Coll Surg. 2009;208:881–6.
27. Lyass S, Khalili TM, Cunneen S, Fujita F, Otsuka K, Chopra R, et al. Radiological studies after laparoscopic Roux-en-Y gastric bypass: routine or selective? Am Surg. 2004;70:918–21.
28. Katasani VG, Leeth RR, Tishler DS, Leath TD, Roy BP, Canon CL, et al. Water-soluble upper GI based on clinical findings is reliable to detect anastomotic leaks after laparoscopic gastric bypass. Am Surg. 2005;71:916–8.
29. Raman R, Raman B, Raman P, Rossiter S, Curet MJ, Mindelzun R, et al. Abnormal findings on routine upper GI series following laparoscopic Roux-en-y gastric bypass. Obes Surg. 2007;17:311–6.
30. Carter JT, Tafreshian S, Campos GM, Tiwari U, Herbella F, Cello JP, et al. Routine upper GI series after gastric bypass does not reliably identify anastomotic leaks or predict stricture formation. Surg Endosc. 2007;21:2172–7.
31. White S, Han SH, Lewis C, Patel K, McEvoy B, Kadell B, et al. Selective approach to use of upper gastroesophageal imaging study after laparoscopic Roux-en-Y gastric bypass. Surg Obes Relat Dis. 2008;4:122–5.
32. Leslie DB, Dorman RB, Anderson J, Serrott FJ, Kellogg TA, Buchwald H, et al. Routine upper gastrointestinal imaging is superior to clinical signs for detecting gastrojejunal leak after laparoscopic Roux-en-Y gastric bypass. J Am Coll Surg. 2012;214:208–13.
33. Sethi M, Magrath M, Somoza E, Parikh M, Saunders J, Ude-Welcome A, et al. The utility of radiological upper gastrointestinal series and clinical indicators in detecting leaks after laparoscopic sleeve gastrectomy: a case-controlled study. Surg Endosc. 2016;30:2266–75.
34. Mbadiwe T, Prevatt E, Duerinckx A, Cornwell E III, Fullum T, Davis B. Assessing the value of routine upper gastrointestinal contrast studies following bariatric surgery: a systematic review and meta-analysis. Am J Surg. 2015;209:616–22.
35. Bingham J, Shawhan R, Parker R, Wigboldy J, Sohn V. Computed tomography scan versus upper gastrointestinal fluoroscopy for diagnosis of staple line leak following bariatric surgery. Am J Surg. 2015;209:810–4.
36. Lee JK, Van Dam J, Morton JM, Curet MJ, Banerjee S. Endoscopy is accurate, safe, and effective in the assessment and management of complications following gastric bypass surgery. Am J Gastroenterol. 2009;104:575–82.
37. Deitel M, Gagner M, Erickson AL, Crosby RD. Third international summit: current status of sleeve gastrectomy. Surg Obes Relat Dis. 2011;7:749–59.
38. Csendes A, Burgos AM, Burdiles P. Incidence of anastomotic strictures after gastric bypass: a prospective consecutive routine endoscopic study 1 month and 17 months after surgery in 441 patients with morbid obesity. Obes Surg. 2009;19:269–73.
39. Fried M, Yumuk V, Oppert J-M, Scopinaro N, Torres AJ, Weiner R, et al. Interdisciplinary European guidelines on metabolic and bariatric surgery. Obes Facts. 2013;6:449–68.
40. Mechanick JI, Youdim A, Jones DB, Garvey WT, Hurley DL, McMahon MM, et al. Clinical practice guidelines for the perioperative nutritional, metabolic, and nonsurgical support of the bariatric surgery patient—2013 update: cosponsored by American Association of Clinical Endocrinologists, the Obesity Society, and American Society for Metabolic & Bariatric Surgery. Obesity. 2013;21:S1–S27.
41. Evans JA, Muthusamy VR, Acosta RD, Bruining DH, Chandrasekhara V, Chathadi KV, et al. The role of endoscopy in the bariatric surgery patient. Gastrointest Endosc. 2015;81:1063–72.
42. Mathus-Vliegen EMH. The role of endoscopy in bariatric surgery. Best Pract Res Clin Gastroenterol. 2008;22:839–65.
43. Mathus-Vliegen EMH. The cooperation between endoscopists and surgeons in treating complications of bariatric surgery. Best Pract Res Clin Gastroenterol. 2014;28:703–25.

44. Monteforte MJ, Turkelson CM. Bariatric surgery for morbid obesity. Obes Surg. 2000;10:391–401.
45. Chapman AE, Kiroff G, Game P, Foster B, O'Brien P, Ham J, et al. Laparoscopic adjustable gastric banding in the treatment of obesity: a systematic literature review. Surgery. 2004;135:326–51.
46. Maggard MA, Shugarman LR, Suttorp M, Maglione M, Sugerman HJ, Livingston EH, et al. Meta-analysis: surgical treatment of obesity. Ann Intern Med. 2005;142:547–59.
47. Wang S, Li P, Sun XF, Ye NY, Xu ZK, Wang D. Comparison between laparoscopic sleeve gastrectomy and laparoscopic adjustable gastric banding for morbid obesity: a meta-analysis. Obes Surg. 2013;23:980–6.
48. Yang X, Yang G, Wang W, Chen G, Yang H. A meta-analysis: to compare the clinical results between gastric bypass and sleeve gastrectomy for the obese patients. Obes Surg. 2013;23:1001–10.
49. Shoar S, Saber AA. Long-term and midterm outcomes of laparoscopic sleeve gastrectomy versus Roux-en-Y gastric bypass: a systematic review and meta-analysis of comparative studies. Surg Obes Relat Dis. 2017;13:170–80.
50. Ye Q, Chen Y, Zhan X, Wang Y, Zhu J. Comparison of laparoscopic sleeve gastrectomy and laparoscopic greater curvature plication regarding efficacy and safety: a meta-analysis. Obes Surg. 2017;27:1358–64.
51. Brethauer SA, Hammel JP, Schauer PR. Systematic review of sleeve gastrectomy as staging and primary bariatric procedure. Surg Obes Relat Dis. 2009;5:469–75.
52. Brethauer SA. Sleeve gastrectomy. Surg Clin N Am. 2011;91:1265–79.
53. Trastulli S, Desiderio J, Guarino S, Cirocchi R, Scalercio V, Noya G, et al. Laparoscopic sleeve gastrectomy compared with other bariatric surgical procedures: a systematic review of randomized trials. Surg Obes Relat Dis. 2013;9:816–30.
54. Kehagias I, Zygomalas A, Karavias D, Karamanakos S. Sleeve gastrectomy: have we finally found the holy grail of bariatric surgery? A review of the literature. Eur Rev Med Pharmacol Sci. 2016;20:4930–42.
55. Li J-F, Lai D-D, Lin Z-H, Jiang T-Y, Zhang A-M, Dai J-F. Comparison of the long-term results of Roux-en-Y gastric bypass and sleeve gastrectomy for morbid obesity: a systematic review and meta-analysis of randomized and nonrandomized trials. Surg Laparosc Endosc Percutan Tech. 2014;24:1–11.
56. Alvarenga ES, Lo Menzo E, Szomstein S, Rosenthal RJ. Safety and efficacy of 1020 consecutive laparoscopic sleeve gastrectomies performed as a primary treatment modality for morbid obesity. A single-center experience from the metabolic and bariatric surgical accreditation quality and improvement program. Surg Endosc. 2016;30:2673–8.
57. DeMaria EJ, Pate V, Warthen M, Winegar DA. Baseline data from American Society for Metabolic and Bariatric Surgery-designated Bariatric Surgery Centers of excellence using the bariatric outcomes longitudinal database. Surg Obes Relat Dis. 2010;6:347–55.
58. Finks JF, Kole KL, Yenumula PR, English WJ, Krause KR, Carlin AM, et al. Predicting risk for serious complications with bariatric surgery results from the Michigan Bariatric Surgery Collaborative. Ann Surg. 2011;254:633–40.
59. Greenstein AJ, Wahed AS, Adeniji A, Courcoulas AP, Dakin G, Flum DR, et al. Prevalence of adverse intraoperative events during obesity surgery and their sequelae. J Am Coll Surg. 2012;215:271–7.
60. Stenberg E, Szabo E, Agren G, Näslund E, Boman L, Bykind A, et al. Early complications after laparoscopic gastric bypass surgery: results from the Scandinavian obesity surgery registry. Ann Surg. 2014;260:1040–7.
61. Stroh C, Köckerling F, Volker L, Frank B, Wolff S, Knoll C, et al. Results of more than 11,800 sleeve gastrectomies data analysis of the German bariatric surgery registry. Ann Surg. 2016;263:949–55.
62. Melissas J, Stavroulakis K, Tzikoulis V, Peristeri A, Papadakis JA, Pazouki A, et al. Sleeve gastrectomy versus Roux-en-Y gastric bypass. Data from IFSO-European chapter Center of Excellence program. Obes Surg. 2017;27:847–55.

63. Gagner M, Hutchinson C, Rosenthal R. Fifth international consensus conference: current status of sleeve gastrectomy. Surg Obes Relat Dis. 2016;12:750–6.
64. Cai JX, Schweitzer MA, Kumbhari V. Endoscopic management of bariatric surgery complications. Surg Laparosc Endosc Percutan Tech. 2016;26:93–101.
65. Flum DR, Dellinger EP. Impact of gastric bypass operation on survival: a population-based analysis. J Am Coll Surg. 2004;199:543–51.
66. Courcoulas A, Schuchert M, Gatti G, Luketich J. The relationship of surgeon and hospital volume to outcome after gastric bypass surgery in Pennsylvania: a 3-year summary. Surgery. 2003;134:613–21.
67. Liu JH, Zingmond D, Etzioni DA, O'Connell JB, Maggard MA, Livingston EH, et al. Characterizing the performance and outcomes of obesity surgery in California. Am Surg. 2003;69:823–8.
68. Livingston EH. Procedure incidence and in-hospital complication rates of bariatric surgery in the United States. Am J Surg. 2004;188:105–10.
69. Moreno P, Alastrue A, Rull M, Formiguera X, Casas D, Boix J, et al. Band erosion in patients who have undergone vertical banded gastroplasty: incidence and technical solutions. Arch Surg. 1998;133:189–93.
70. Fernandez AZ Jr, Demaria EJ, Tichansky DS, Kellum JM, Wolfe LG, Meador J, et al. Multivariate analysis of risk factors for death following gastric bypass for treatment of morbid obesity. Ann Surg. 2004;239:698–702.
71. Flum DR, Salem L, Elrod JA, Dellinger EP, Cheadle A, Chan L. Early mortality among Medicare beneficiaries undergoing bariatric surgical procedures. JAMA. 2005;294:1903–8.
72. Poulose BK, Griffin MR, Moore DE, Zhu Y, Smalley W, Richards WO, et al. Risk factors for post-operative mortality in bariatric surgery. J Surg Res. 2005;127:1–7.
73. Omalu BI, Ives DG, Buhari AM, Lindner JL, Schauer PR, Wecht CH, et al. Death rates and causes of death after bariatric surgery for Pennsylvania residents, 1995 to 2004. Arch Surg. 2007;142:923–8.
74. DeMaria EJ, Portenier D, Wolfe L. Obesity surgery mortality risk score: proposal for a clinically useful score to predict mortality risk in patients undergoing gastric bypass. Surg Obes Relat Dis. 2007;3:134–40.
75. DeMaria EJ, Murr M, Byrne TK, Blackstone R, Grant JP, Budak A, et al. Validation of the obesity surgery mortality risk score in a multicenter study proves it stratifies mortality risk in patients undergoing gastric bypass for morbid obesity. Ann Surg. 2007;246:578–82.
76. Thomas H, Agrawal S. Systematic review of obesity surgery mortality risk score-preoperative risk stratification in bariatric surgery. Obes Surg. 2012;22:1135–40.
77. García-García ML, Martín-Lorenzo JG, Lirón-Ruiz R, Torralba-Martínez JA, García-López JA, Aguayo-Albasini JL. Failure of the obesity surgery mortality risk score (OS-MRS) to predict postoperative complications after bariatric surgery. A single-center series and systematic review. Obes Surg. 2017;27:1423–9.
78. Maciejewski ML, Winegar DA, Farley JF, Wolfe BM, DeMaria EJ. Risk stratification of serious adverse events after gastric bypass in the bariatric outcomes longitudinal database. Surg Obes Relat Dis. 2012;8:671–8.
79. LABS. The Longitudinal Assessment of Bariatric Surgery (LABS) Consortium. Perioperative safety in the longitudinal assessment of bariatric surgery. N Engl J Med. 2009;361:445–54.
80. Gupta PK, Franck C, Miller WJ, Gupta H, Forse RA. Development and validation of a bariatric surgery morbidity risk calculator using the prospective multicenter NSQIP dataset. J Am Coll Surg. 2011;212:301–9.
81. Ramanan B, Gupta PK, Gupta H, Fang X, Forse RA. Development and validation of a bariatric surgery mortality risk calculator. J Am Coll Surg. 2012;214:892–900.
82. Turner PL, Saager L, Dalton J, Abd-Elsayed A, Roberman D, Melara P, et al. Nomogram for predicting surgical complications in bariatric surgery patients. Obes Surg. 2011;21:655–62.
83. Aminian A, Brethauer SA, Sharafkhah M, Schauer PR. Development of a sleeve gastrectomy risk calculator. Surg Obes Relat Dis. 2015;11:758–64.

84. Verset D, Houben J-J, Gay F, Elcheroth J, Bourgeois V, van Gossum A. The place of upper gastrointestinal tract endoscopy before and after vertical banded gastroplasty for morbid obesity. Dig Dis Sci. 1997;42:2333–7.
85. Rubenstein RB. Laparoscopic adjustable gastric banding at a U.S. center with up to 3-year follow-up. Obes Surg. 2002;12:380–4.
86. O'Brien PE, MacDonald L, Anderson M, Brennan L, Brown WA. Long-term outcomes after bariatric surgery: fifteen-year follow-up of adjustable gastric banding and a systematic review of the bariatric surgical literature. Ann Surg. 2013;257:87–94.
87. Spivak H, Favretti F. Avoiding postoperative complications with the LAP-BAND system. Am J Surg. 2002;184(suppl 2):31S–7S.
88. DeMaria EJ, Jamal MK. Laparoscopic adjustable gastric banding: evolving clinical experience. Surg Clin North Am. 2005;85:773–87, vii.
89. O'Brien PE, McPhail T, Chaston TB, Dixon JB. Systematic review of medium-term weight loss after bariatric operations. Obes Surg. 2006;16:1032–40.
90. Singhal R, Bryant C, Kitchen M, Khan KS, Deeks J, Guo B, et al. Band slippage and erosion after laparoscopic gastric banding: a meta-analysis. Surg Endosc. 2010;24:2980–6.
91. Fried M, Miller K, Kormanova K. Literature review of comparative studies of complications with Swedish band and lap-band. Obes Surg. 2004;14:256–60.
92. Fielding GA, Pattyn P, Horber F, Steffen R, Potoczna N. Bariatric surgery using the Swedish adjustable gastric band (ASGB) or lap-band (LB): a systematic review of the literature and meta-analysis. Obes Surg. 2005;15:962; (abstract).
93. Huang CS, Forse RA, Jacobson BC, Farraye FA. Endoscopic findings and their clinical correlations in patients with symptoms after gastric bypass surgery. Gastrointest Endosc. 2003;58:859–66.
94. Marano BJ Jr. Endoscopy after Roux-en-Y gastric bypass: a community hospital experience. Obes Surg. 2005;15:342–5.
95. Wilson JA, Romagnuolo J, Byrne TK, Morgan K, Wilson FA. Predictors of endoscopic findings after Roux-en-Y gastric bypass. Am J Gastroenterol. 2006;101:2194–9.
96. Rasmussen JJ, Fuller W, Ali MR. Marginal ulceration after laparoscopic gastric bypass: an analysis of predisposing factors in 260 patients. Surg Endosc. 2007;21:1090–4.
97. Schirmer B, Erenoglu C, Miller A. Flexible endoscopy in the management of patients undergoing Roux-en-y gastric bypass. Obes Surg. 2002;12:634–8.
98. Fernandes SR, Meireles LC, Carrilho-Ribeiro L, Velosa J. The role of routine upper gastrointestinal endoscopy before bariatric surgery. Obes Surg. 2016;26:2105–10.
99. Papasavas PK, Gagné DJ, Donnelly PE, Salgado J, Urbandt JE, Burton KK, et al. Prevalence of Helicobacter pylori infection and value of preoperative testing and treatment in patients undergoing laparoscopic Roux-en-Y gastric bypass. Surg Obes Relat Dis. 2008;4:383–8.
100. Loewen M, Giovanni J, Barba C. Screening endoscopy before bariatric surgery: a series of 448 patients. Surg Obes Relat Dis. 2008;4:709–14.
101. Yang C-S, Lee W-J, Wang H-H, Huang S-P, Lin J-T, Wu M-S. The influence of Helicobacter pylori infection on the development of gastric ulcer in symptomatic patients after bariatric surgery. Obes Surg. 2006;16:735–9.
102. Hartin CW Jr, ReMine DS, Lucktong TA. Preoperative bariatric screening and treatment of Helicobacter pylori. Surg Endosc. 2009;23:2531–4.
103. Almazeedi S, Al-Sabah S, Al-Mulla A, Al-Murad A, Al-Mossawi A, Al-Enezi K, et al. Gastric histopathologies in patients undergoing laparoscopic sleeve gastrectomies. Obes Surg. 2013;23:314–9.
104. Lauti M, Gormack SE, Thomas JM, Morrow JJ, Rahman H, MacCormick AD. What does the excised stomach from sleeve gastrectomy tell us? Obes Surg. 2016;26:839–42.
105. Almazeedi S, Al-Sabah S, Alshammari D, Alqinai S, Al-Mulla A, Al-Murad A, et al. The impact of Helicobacter pylori on the complications of laparoscopic sleeve gastrectomy. Obes Surg. 2014;24:412–5.
106. Albawardi A, Almaarzooqi S, Torab FC. Helicobacter pylori in sleeve gastrectomies: prevalence and rate of complications. Int J Clin Exp Med. 2013;6:40–3.

107. Rossetti G, Moccia F, Marra T, Buonomo M, Pascotto B, Pezzullo A, et al. Does Helicobacter pylori infection have influence on outcomes of laparoscopic sleeve gastrectomy for morbid obesity? Int J Surg. 2014;12(suppl 1):S68–71.
108. Weber J, Azagra-Goergen M, Strock P, Azagra J. Endoscopy after bariatric surgery. Acta Endosc. 2007;37:27–37.
109. Stellato TA, Crouse C, Hallowell PT. Bariatric surgery: creating new challenges for the endoscopist. Gastrointest Endosc. 2003;57:86–94.
110. Huang CS, Farraye FA. Endoscopy in the bariatric surgical patient. Gastroenterol Clin N Am. 2005;34:151–66.
111. Kumar N, Thompson CC. Endoscopic management of complications after gastrointestinal weight loss surgery. Clin Gastroenterol Hepatol. 2013;11:343–53.
112. Pai RD, Carr-Locke DL, Thompson CC. Endoscopic evaluation of the defunctionalized stomach by using ShapeLock technology (with video). Gastrointest Endosc. 2007;66:578–81.
113. Valli PV, Gubler C. Review article including treatment algorithm: endoscopic treatment of luminal complications after bariatric surgery. Clin Obes. 2017;7:115–22.
114. Wetter A. Role of endoscopy after Roux-en-Y gastric bypass surgery. Gastrointest Endosc. 2007;66:1253–5.
115. Safatle-Ribeiro AV, Kuga R, Iriya K, Ribeiro U Jr, Faintuch J, Ishida RK, et al. What to expect in the excluded stomach mucosa after vertical banded Roux-en-y gastric bypass for morbid obesity? J Gastrointest Surg. 2007;11:133–7.
116. Strodel WE, Knol JA, Eckhauser FE. Endoscopy of the partitioned stomach. Ann Surg. 1984;200:582–6.
117. Freeman JB. The use of endoscopy after gastric partitioning for morbid obesity. Gastroenterol Clin N Am. 1987;16:339–47.
118. Deitel M, Bendago M. Endoscopy of vertical banded gastroplasty. Am Surg. 1989;55:287–90.
119. Campanile FC, Boru CE, Rizzello M, Puzziello A, Copaescu C, Cavallaro G, et al. Acute complications after laparoscopic bariatric procedures: update for the general surgeon. Langenbeck's Arch Surg. 2013;398:669–86.
120. Car Peterko A, Kirac I, Gaurina A, Diklić D, Bekavac-Bešlin M. Diagnosis and management of acute and early complications of/after bariatric surgery. Dig Dis. 2012;30:178–81.
121. Rosenthal RJ, Szomstein S, Kennedy CI, Soto FC, Zundel N. Laparoscopic surgery for morbid obesity: 1001 consecutive bariatric operations performed at the bariatric institute, Cleveland Clinic Florida. Obes Surg. 2006;16:119–24.
122. Byrne TK. Complications of surgery for obesity. Surg Clin North Am. 2001;81:1181, viii.
123. Lee S, Ahn JY, Jung HY, Lee JH, Choi KS, Kim DH, et al. Clinical outcomes of endoscopic and surgical management for postoperative upper gastrointestinal leakage. Surg Endosc. 2013;27:4232–40.
124. Almahmeed T, Gonzalez R, Nelson LG, Haines K, Gallagher SF, Murr MM. Morbidity of anastomotic leaks in patients undergoing Roux-en-Y gastric bypass. Arch Surg. 2007;142:954–7.
125. Samuel I, Mason EE, Renquist KE, Huang YH, Zimmerman MB, Jamal M. Bariatric surgery trends: an 18-year report from the international bariatric surgery registry. Am J Surg. 2006;192:657–62.
126. Mejia AF, Bolanos E, Chaux CF, Unigarro I. Endoscopic treatment of gastrocutaneous fistula following gastric bypass for obesity. Obes Surg. 2007;17:544–6.
127. Haito-Chavez Y, Law JK, Kratt T, Arezzo A, Verra M, Morino M, et al. International multicenter experience with an over-the-scope clipping device for endoscopic management of GI defects (with video). Gastrointest Endosc. 2014;80:610–22.
128. Winder JS, Kulaylat AN, Schubart JR, Hal HM, Pauli EM. Management of non-acute gastrointestinal defects using the over-the-scope clips (OTSCs): a retrospective single-institution experience. Surg Endosc. 2016;30:2251–8.
129. Welsch T, Von Frankenberg M, Schmidt J, Büchler MW. Diagnosis and definition of anastomotic leakage from the surgeon's perspective. Chirurg. 2011;82:48–55.
130. Iossa A, Abdelgawad M, Watkins BM, Silecchia G. Leaks after laparoscopic sleeve gastrectomy: overview of pathogenesis and risk factors. Langenbeck's Arch Surg. 2016;401:757–66.

131. Flicker MS, Lautz DB, Thompson CC. Endoscopic management of gastrogastric fistulae does not increase complications at bariatric revision surgery. J Gastrointest Surg. 2011;15:1736–42.
132. Vilallonga R, Himpens J, Bosch B, van de Vrande S, Bafort J. Role of percutaneous glue treatment after persisting leak after laparoscopic sleeve gastrectomy. Obes Surg. 2016;26:1378–83.
133. Guillaud A, Moszkowicz D, Nedelcu M, Caballero-Caballero A, Rebibo L, Reche F, et al. Gastrobronchial fistula: a serious complication of sleeve gastrectomy. Results of a French multicentric study. Obes Surg. 2015;25:2352–9.
134. Ballesta C, Berindoague R, Cabrera M, Palau M, Gonzales M. Management of anastomotic leaks after laparoscopic Roux-en-Y gastric bypass. Obes Surg. 2008;18:623–30.
135. Morales MP, Miedema BW, Scott JS, de la Torre RA. Management of postsurgical leaks in the bariatric patient. Gastrointest Endosc Clin N Am. 2011;21:295–304.
136. Livingston EH, Huerta S, Arthur D, Lee S, De Shields S, Heber D. Male gender is a predictor of morbidity and age a predictor of mortality for patients undergoing gastric bypass surgery. Ann Surg. 2002;236:576–82.
137. Masoomi H, Kim H, Reavis KM, Mills S, Stamos MJ, Nguyen NT. Analysis of factors predictive of gastrointestinal tract leak in laparoscopic and open gastric bypass. Arch Surg. 2011;146:1048–51.
138. Saber AA, Azar N, Dekal M, Abdelbaki TN. Computed tomographic scan mapping of gastric wall perfusion and clinical implications. Am J Surg. 2015;209:999–1006.
139. Moszkowicz D, Arienzo R, Khettab I, Rahmi G, Zinzindohoue F, Berger A, et al. Sleeve gastrectomy severe complications: is it always a reasonable surgical option? Obes Surg. 2013;23:676–86.
140. Yehoshua RT, Eidelman LA, Stein M, Fichman S, Mazor A, Chen J, et al. Laparoscopic sleeve gastrectomy--volume and pressure assessment. Obes Surg. 2008;18:1083–8.
141. Rossetti G, Fei L, Docimo L, Del Genio G, Micanti F, Belfiore A, et al. Is nasogastric decompression useful in prevention of leaks after laparoscopic sleeve gastrectomy? A randomized trial. J Investig Surg. 2014;27:234–9.
142. Choi YY, Bae J, Hur KY, Choi D, Kim YJ. Reinforcing the staple line during laparoscopic sleeve gastrectomy: does it have advantages? A meta-analysis. Obes Surg. 2012;22:1206–13.
143. Knapps J, Ghanem M, Clements J, Merchant AM. A systematic review of staple-line reinforcement in laparoscopic sleeve gastrectomy. JSLS. 2013;17:390–9.
144. Gagner M, Buchwald JN. Comparison of laparoscopic sleeve gastrectomy leak rates in four staple-line reinforcement options: a systematic review. Surg Obes Relat Dis. 2014;10:713–23.
145. Shikora SA, Mahoney CB. Clinical benefit of gastric staple line reinforcement (SLR) in gastrointestinal surgery: a meta-analysis. Obes Surg. 2015;25:1133–41.
146. Sturm R. Increases in morbid obesity in the USA: 2000–2005. Public Health. 2007;121:492–6.
147. Arteaga-González I, Martín-Malagón A, Martín-Pérez J, Carrillo-Pallarés A. Usefulness of clinical signs and diagnostic tests for suspected leaks in bariatric surgery. Obes Surg. 2015;25:1680–4.
148. Benedix F, Benedix DD, Knoll C, Weiner R, Bruns C, Manger T, et al. Are there risk factors that increase the rate of staple line leakage in patients undergoing primary sleeve gastrectomy for morbid obesity? Obes Surg. 2014;24:1610–6.
149. Livingston EH. Complications of bariatric surgery. Surg Clin North Am. 2005;85:853–68, vii.
150. Rogalski P, Daniluk J, Baniukiewicz A, Wroblewski E, Dabrowski A. Endoscopic management of gastrointestinal perforations, leaks and fistulas. World J Gastroenterol. 2015;21:10542–52.
151. van de Vrande S, Himpens J, ElMourad H, Debaerdemaeker R, Leman G. Management of chronic proximal fistulas after sleeve gastrectomy by laparoscopic Roux-limb placement. Surg Obes Relat Dis. 2013;9:856–61.
152. Shim CN, Kim H-I, Hyung WJ, Noh SH, Song MK, Kang DR, et al. Self-expanding metal stents or nonstent endoscopic therapy: which is better for anastomotic leaks after total gastrectomy? Surg Endosc. 2014;28:833–40.
153. Southwell T, Lim TH, Ogra R. Endoscopic therapy for treatment of staple line leaks post-laparoscopic sleeve gastrectomy (LSG): experience from a large bariatric surgery centre in New Zealand. Obes Surg. 2016;26:1155–62.

154. Donatelli G, Dumont J-L, Cereatti F, Ferretti S, Vergeau BM, Tuszynski T, et al. Treatment of leaks following sleeve gastrectomy by endoscopic internal drainage (EID). Obes Surg. 2015;25:1293–301.
155. Bhayani NH, Swanstrom LL. Endoscopic therapies for leaks and fistulas after bariatric surgery. Surg Innov. 2014;21:90–7.
156. Willingham FF, Buscaglia JM. Endoscopic management of gastrointestinal leaks and fistulae. Clin Gastroenterol Hepatol. 2015;13:1714–21.
157. Shehab HM, Hakky SM, Gawdat KA. An endoscopic strategy combining mega stents and over-the-scope clips for the management of post-bariatric surgery leaks and fistulas (with video). Obes Surg. 2016;26:941–8.
158. Freedman J, Jonas E, Naslund E, Nilsson H, Marsk R, Stockeld D. Treatment of leaking gastrojejunostomy after gastric bypass surgery with special emphasis on stenting. Surg Obes Relat Dis. 2013;9:554–8.
159. Malli CP, Sioulas AD, Emmanouil T, Dimitriadis GD, Triantafyllou K. Endoscopy after bariatric surgery. Ann Gastroenterol. 2016;29:249–57.
160. Bege T, Emungania O, Vitton V, Ah-Soune P, Nocca D, Noel P, et al. An endoscopic strategy for management of anastomotic complications from bariatric surgery: a prospective study. Gastrointest Endosc. 2011;73:238–44.
161. Vanbiervliet G, Filippi J, Karimdjee BS, Venissac N, Iannelli A, Rahili A, et al. The role of clips in preventing migration of fully covered metallic esophageal stents: a pilot comparative study. Surg Endosc. 2012;26:53–9.
162. Sharaiha RZ, Kumta NA, Doukides TP, Vasco E, Gonda TA, Widmer JL, et al. Esophageal stenting with sutures: time to redefine our standards? J Clin Gastroenterol. 2015;49: e57–60.
163. Eisendrath P, Cremer M, Himpens J, Cadiere GB, Le Moine O, Deviere J. Endotherapy including temporary stenting of fistulas of the upper gastrointestinal tract after laparoscopic bariatric surgery. Endoscopy. 2007;39:625–30.
164. Musquer N, Letessier E, Le Rhun M, Coron E. Endoscopic removal of a migrating polyester band using argon plasma coagulation. Clin Res Hepatol Gastroenterol. 2013;37:e89–e91.
165. Nguyen NT, Nguyen XM, Dholakia C. The use of endoscopic stent in management of leaks after sleeve gastrectomy. Obes Surg. 2010;20:1289–92.
166. Eubanks S, Edwards CA, Fearing NM, Ramaswamy A, de la Torre RA, Thaler KJ, et al. Use of endoscopic stents to treat anastomotic complications after bariatric surgery. J Am Coll Surg. 2008;206:935–9.
167. de Moura EGH, Galvao-Neto MP, Ramos AC, de Moura ETH, Galvao TD, de Moura DTH, et al. Extreme bariatric endoscopy: stenting to reconnect the pouch to the gastrojejunostomy after a Roux-en-Y gastric bypass. Surg Endosc. 2012;26:1481–4.
168. El Mourad H, Himpens J, Verhofstadt J. Stent treatment for fistula after obesity surgery: results in 47 consecutive patients. Surg Endosc. 2013;27:808–16.
169. Simon F, Siciliano I, Gillet A, Castel B, Coffin B, Msika S. Gastric leak after laparoscopic sleeve gastrectomy: early covered self-expandable stent reduces healing time. Obes Surg. 2013;23:687–92.
170. Alazmi W, Al-Sabah S, Ali DA, Almazeedi S. Treating sleeve gastrectomy leak with endoscopic stenting: the Kuwaiti experience and review of the literature. Surg Endosc. 2014;28:3425–8.
171. El Hajj II, Imperiale TF, Rex DK, Ballard D, Kesler KA, Birdas TJ, et al. Treatment of esophageal leaks, fistulae, and perforations with temporary stents: evaluation of efficacy, adverse events, and factors associate with successful outcomes. Gastrointest Endosc. 2014;79:589–98.
172. Murino A, Arvanitakis M, Le Moine O, Blero D, Devière J, Eisendrath P. Effectiveness of endoscopic management using self-expandable metal stents in a large cohort of patients with post-bariatric leaks. Obes Surg. 2015;25:1569–76.
173. Quezada N, Maiz C, Daroch D, Funke R, Sharp A, Boza C, et al. Effect of early use of covered self-expandable endoscopic stent on the treatment of postoperative stapler line leaks. Obes Surg. 2015;25:1816–21.

174. Chang J, Sharma G, Boules M, Brethauer S, Rodriguez J, Kroh M. Endoscopic stents in the management of anastomotic complications after foregut surgery: new applications and techniques. Surg Obes Relat Dis. 2016;12:1372–81.
175. Swinnen J, Eisendrath P, Rigaux J, Kahegeshe L, Lemmers A, Le Moine O, et al. Self-expandable metal stents for the treatment of benign upper GI leaks and perforations. Gastrointest Endosc. 2011;73:890–9.
176. Ko HK, Song HY, Shin JH, Lee GH, Jung HY, Park SI. Fate of migrated esophageal and gastroduodenal stents: experience in 70 patients. J Vasc Interv Radiol. 2007;18:725–32.
177. Puli SR, Spofford IS, Thompson CC. Use of self-expandable stents in the treatment of bariatric surgery leaks: a systematic review and meta-analysis. Gastrointest Endosc. 2012;75:287–93.
178. El Hassan E, Mohamed A, Ibrahim M, Margarita M, Al Hadad M, Nimeri AA. Single-stage operative management of laparoscopic sleeve gastrectomy leaks without endoscopic stent placement. Obes Surg. 2013;23:722–6.
179. Felsher J, Farres H, Chand B, Farver C, Ponsky J. Mucosal apposition in endoscopic suturing. Gastrointest Endosc. 2003;58:867–70.
180. Mercky P, Gonzalez JM, Aimore Bonin E, Emungania O, Brunet J, Grimaud J-C, et al. Usefulness of over-the-scope clipping system for closing digestive fistulas. Dig Endosc. 2015;27:18–24.
181. Law R, Wong Kee Song LM, Irani S, Baron TH. Immediate technical and delayed clinical outcome of fistula closure using an over-the-scope clip device. Surg Endosc. 2015;29:1781–6.
182. Csendes A, Braghetto I, Leon P, Burgos AM. Management of leaks after laparoscopic sleeve gastrectomy in patients with obesity. J Gastrointest Surg. 2010;14:1343–8.
183. von Renteln D, Denzer UW, Schachschal G, Anders M, Groth S, Rosch T. Endoscopic closure of GI fistulae by using an over-the-scope clip (with videos). Gastrointest Endosc. 2010;72:1289–96.
184. Zolotarevsky E, Kwon Y, Bains M, Schattner M. Esophagobronchial fistula closure using a novel endoscopic over-the-scope-clip. Ann Thorac Surg. 2012;94:e69–e70.
185. Parodi A, Repici A, Pedroni A. Endoscopic management of GI perforations with a new over-the-scope clip device. Gastrointest Endosc. 2010;72:881–6.
186. Surace M, Mercky P, Demarquay JF, Gonzalez JM, Dumas R, Ah-Soune P, et al. Endoscopic management of GI fistulae with the over-the-scope clip system (with video). Gastrointest Endosc. 2011;74:1416–9.
187. Manta R, Manno M, Bertani H, Barbera C, Pigo F, Mirante V, et al. Endoscopic treatment of gastrointestinal fistulas using an over-the-scope clip (OTSC) device: case series from a tertiary referral center. Endoscopy. 2011;43:545–8.
188. Dakin GF, Eid G, Mikami D, Prior A, Chand B. Endoluminal revision of gastric bypass for weight regain—a systematic review. Surg Obes Relat Dis. 2013;9:335–42.
189. Cai JX, Khashab MA, Okolo PI, Kalloo AN, Khumbhari V. Full-thickness endoscopic suturing of staple-line leaks following laparoscopic sleeve gastrectomy. Endoscopy. 2014;46(Suppl 1):E623–4.
190. Fernandez-Esparrach G, Lautz DB, Thompson CC. Endoscopic repair of gastrogastric fistula after Roux-en-Y gastric bypass: a less-invasive approach. Surg Obes Relat Dis. 2010;6:282–8.
191. Spaun GO, Martinec DV, Kennedy TJ, Swanström LL. Endoscopic closure of gastrogastric fistulas by using a tissue apposition system (with videos). Gastrointest Endosc. 2010;71:606–11.
192. Brolin RE, Lin JM. Treatment of gastric leaks after Roux-en-Y gastric bypass: a paradigm shift. Surg Obes Relat Dis. 2013;9:229–33.
193. Rebibo L, Dhahri A, Berna P, Yzet T, Verhaeghe P, Regimbeau JM. Management of gastrobronchial fistula after laparoscopic sleeve gastrectomy. Surg Obes Relat Dis. 2014;10:460–7.
194. Papavramidis TS, Kotzampassi K, Kotidis E, Eleftheriadis EE, Papavramidis ST. Endoscopic fibrin sealing of gastrocutaneous fistulas after sleeve gastrectomy and biliopancreatic diversion with duodenal switch. J Gastroenterol Hepatol. 2008;23:1802–5.

195. Rabago LR, Ventosa N, Castro JL, Marco J, Herrera N, Gea F. Endoscopic treatment of postoperative fistulas resistant to conservative management using biological fibrin glue. Endoscopy. 2002;34:632–8.
196. Lippert E, Klebl FH, Schweller F, Ott C, Gelbmann CM, Scholmerich J, et al. Fibrin glue in the endoscopic treatment of fistulae and anastomotic leakages of the gastrointestinal tract. Int J Color Dis. 2011;26:303–11.
197. Lee YC, Na HG, Suh JH, Park I-S, Chung KY, Kim NK. Three cases of fistulae arising from gastrointestinal tract treated with endoscopic injection of Histoacryl. Endoscopy. 2001;33:184–6.
198. Maluf-Filho F, Moura E, Sakai P, Garrido A, Ishioka S, Gana-Rodrigues J, et al. Endoscopic treatment of esophagogastric fistulae with an acellular matrix. Gastrointest Endosc. 2004;59:P151; (abstract).
199. Raju GS, Thompson C, Zwischenberger JB. Emerging endoscopic options in the management of esophageal leaks (videos). Gastrointest Endosc. 2005;62:278–86.
200. Maluf-Filho F, Hondo F, Halwan B, de Lima MS, Giordano-Nappi JH, Sakai P. Endoscopic treatment of Roux-en-Y gastric bypass-related gastrocutaneous fistulas using a novel biomaterial. Surg Endosc. 2009;23:1541–5.
201. Toussaint E, Eisendrath P, Kwan V, Dugardeyn S, Devière J, Le Moine O. Endoscopic treatment of postoperative enterocutaneous fistulas after bariatric surgery with the use of a fistula plug: report of five cases. Endoscopy. 2009;41:560–3.
202. Kumbhari V, Storm AC, Saxena P, Okolo PI. Closure of a persistent gastric leak using a cardiac septal occluder. Endoscopy. 2014;46(suppl 1):E147–8.
203. Pequignot A, Fuks D, Verhaeghe P, Dhahri A, Brehant O, Bartoli E, et al. Is there a place for pigtail drains in the management of gastric leaks after laparoscopic sleeve gastrectomy? Obes Surg. 2012;22:712–20.
204. Donatelli G, Airinei G, Poupardin E, Tuszynski T, Wind P, Benamouzig R, et al. Double-pigtail stent migration invading the spleen: rare potentially fatal complication of endoscopic internal drainage for sleeve gastrectomy leak. Endoscopy. 2016;48(Suppl 1):E74–5.
205. Genser L, Pattou F, Caiazzo R. Splenic abscess with portal venous gas caused by intrasplenic migration of an endoscopic double pigtail drain as a treatment of post-sleeve gastrectomy fistula. Surg Obes Relat Dis. 2016;12:e1–e3.
206. Debs T, Petrucciani N, Kassir R, Vanbiervliet G, Ben Amor I, Myx Staccini A, et al. Migration of an endoscopic double pigtail drain into the abdominal wall placed as a treatment of a fistula post revisional bariatric surgery. Obes Surg 2017; 27:1335–1337.
207. Soufron J. Leak or fistula after sleeve gastrectomy: treatment with pigtail drain by the rendezvous technique. Obes Surg. 2015;25:1979–80.
208. Mennigen R, Senninger N, Laukoetter MG. Novel treatment options for perforations of the upper gastrointestinal tract: endoscopic vacuum therapy and over-the-scope clips. World J Gastroenterol. 2014;20:7767–76.
209. Glitsch A, von Bernstorff W, Seltrecht U, Partecke I, Paul H, Heidecke CD. Endoscopic transanal vacuum-assisted rectal drainage (ETVARD): an optimized therapy for major leaks from extraperitoneal rectal anastomoses. Endoscopy. 2008;40:192–9.
210. Weidenhagen R, Gruetzner KU, Wiecken T, Spelsberg F, Jauch KW. Endoscopic vacuum-assisted closure of anastomotic leakage following anterior resection of the rectum: a new method. Surg Endosc. 2008;22:1818–25.
211. Seyfried F, Reimer S, Miras AD, Kenn W, Germer C-T, Scheurlen M, et al. Successful treatment of a gastric leak after bariatric surgery using endoluminal vacuum therapy. Endoscopy. 2013;45(Suppl 2):E267–8.
212. Lemmers A, Tan DMY, Ibrahim M, Loi P, De Backer D, Closset J, et al. Transluminal or percutaneous endoscopic drainage and debridement of abscesses after bariatric surgery: a case series. Obes Surg. 2015;25:2190–9.
213. Zachariah PJ, Lee W-J, Ser K-H, Chen J-C, Tsou J-J. Laparo-endoscopic gastrostomy (LEG) decompression: a novel one-time method of management of gastric leaks following sleeve gastrectomy. Obes Surg. 2015;25:2213–8.

214. Anderson MA, Gan SI, Fanelli RD, Baron TH, Banerjee S, Cash BD, et al. ASGE standards of practice committee. Role of endoscopy in the bariatric surgery patient. Gastrointest Endosc. 2008;68:1–10.
215. Sauerland S, Angrisani L, Belachew M, Chevallier JM, Favretti F, Finer N, et al. Obesity surgery: evidence-based guidelines of the European Association for Endoscopic Surgery (EAES). Surg Endosc. 2005;19:200–21.
216. Morino M, Toppino M, Forestieri P, Angrisani L, Allaix ME, Scopinaro N. Mortality after bariatric surgery: analysis of 13,871 morbidly obese patients from a national registry. Ann Surg. 2007;246:1002–7.
217. Ferreira LE, Song LM, Baron TH. Management of acute postoperative hemorrhage in the bariatric patient. Gastrointest Endosc Clin N Am. 2011;21:287–94.
218. Podnos YD, Jimenez JC, Wilson SE, Stevens CM, Nguyen NT. Complications after laparoscopic gastric bypass: a review of 3464 cases. Arch Surg. 2003;138:957–61.
219. Bakhos C, Alkhoury F, Kyriakides T, Reinhold R, Nadzam G. Early postoperative hemorrhage after open and laparoscopic Roux-en-y gastric bypass. Obes Surg. 2009;19:153–7.
220. Dick A, Byrne TK, Baker M, Budak A, Morgan K. Gastrointestinal bleeding after gastric bypass surgery: nuisance or catastrophe? Surg Obes Relat Dis. 2010;6:643–7.
221. Heneghan HM, Meron-Eldar S, Yenumula P, Rogula T, Brethauer SA, Schauer PR. Incidence and management of bleeding complications after gastric bypass surgery in the morbidly obese. Surg Obes Relat Dis. 2012;8:729–35.
222. Laine L, McQuaid KR. Endoscopic therapy for bleeding ulcers: an evidence-based approach based on meta-analyses of randomized controlled trials. Clin Gastroenterol Hepatol. 2009;7:33–47.
223. Marmo R, Rotondano G, Piscopo R, Bianco MA, D'Angella R, Cipolletta L. Dual therapy versus monotherapy in the endoscopic treatment of high-risk bleeding ulcers: a meta-analysis of controlled trials. Am J Gastroenterol. 2007;102:279–89.
224. Molina-Infante J, Fernandez-Bermejo M, Vinagre-Rodriguez G. Severe gastric ischemia after combined sclerotherapy for bleeding gastric ulcer. Endoscopy. 2011;43(Suppl 2):E191; (abstract).
225. Kim SY, Han SH, Kim KH, Kim SO, Han SY, Lee S-W, et al. Gastric ischemia after epinephrine injection in a patient with liver cirrhosis. World J Gastroenterol. 2013;19:411–4.
226. Skinner M, Peter S, Wilcox CM, Mönkemüller K. Diagnostic and therapeutic utility of double-balloon enteroscopy for obscure GI bleeding in patients with surgically altered upper GI anatomy. Gastrointest Endosc. 2014;80:181–6.
227. Jamil LH, Krause KR, Chengelis DL, Jury RP, Jackson CM, Cannon ME, et al. Endoscopic management of early upper gastrointestinal hemorrhage following laparoscopic Roux-en-Y gastric bypass. Am J Gastroenterol. 2008;103:86–91.
228. Rabl C, Peeva S, Prado K, James AW, Rogers SJ, Posselt A, et al. Early and late abdominal bleeding after Roux-en-Y gastric bypass: sources and tailored therapeutic strategies. Obes Surg. 2011;21:413–20.
229. Fernández-Esparrach G, Bordas JM, Pellisé M, Gimeno-García AZ, Lacy A, Delgado S, et al. Endoscopic management of early GI hemorrhage after laparoscopic gastric bypass. Gastrointest Endosc. 2008;67:552–5.
230. Parsi MA, Jang S. Hemospray for diffuse anastomotic bleeding. Gastrointest Endosc. 2014;80:1170.
231. Chakravartty S, Sarma DR, Chang A, Patel AG. Staple line bleeding in sleeve gastrectomy—a simple and cost-effective solution. Obes Surg. 2016;26:1422–8.
232. Janik MR, Walędziak M, Brągoszewski J, Kwiatkowski A, Paśnik K. Prediction model for hemorrhagic complications after laparoscopic sleeve gastrectomy: development of SLEEVE BLEED calculator. Obes Surg. 2017;27:968–72.
233. Fisher L, Lee Krinsky M, Anderson MA, Appalaneni V, Banerjee S, Ben-Menachem T, et al. The role of endoscopy in the management of obscure GI bleeding. Gastrointest Endosc. 2010;72:471–9.

234. Issa H, Al-Saif O, Al-Momen S, Bseiso B, Al-Salem A. Bleeding duodenal ulcer after Roux-en-Y gastric bypass surgery: the value of laparoscopic gastroduodenoscopy. Ann Saudi Med. 2010;30:67–9.
235. Gagner M, Gentileschi P, de Csepel J, Kini S, Patterson E, Inabnet WB, et al. Laparoscopic reoperative bariatric surgery: experience from 27 consecutive patients. Obes Surg. 2002;12:254–60.
236. Papasavas PK, Yeaney WW, Caushaj PF, Keenam RJ, Landreneau RJ, Gagné DJ. Perforation in the bypassed stomach following laparoscopic Roux-en-Y gastric bypass. Obes Surg. 2003;13:797–9.
237. Al Harakeh AB, Kallies KJ, Borgert AJ, Kothari SN. Bowel obstruction rates in antecolic/antegastric versus retrocolic/retrogastric Roux limb gastric bypasss: a meta-analysis. Surg Obes Relat Dis. 2016;12:194–8.
238. Martin MJ, Beekley AC, Sebesta JA. Bowel obstruction in bariatric and nonbariatric patients: major differences in management strategies and outcome. Surg Obes Relat Dis. 2011;7:263–9.
239. Lockhart ME, Tessler FN, Canon CL, Smith JK, Larrison MC, Fineberg NS, et al. Internal hernia after gastric bypass: sensitivity and specificity of seven CT signs with surgical correlation and controls. AJR Am J Roentgenol. 2007;188:745–50.
240. Yu J, Turner MA, Cho SR, Fulcher AS, DeMaria EJ, Kellum JM, et al. Normal anatomy and complications after gastric bypass surgery: helical CT findings. Radiology. 2004;231:753–60.
241. Gunabushanam G, Shankar S, Czerniach DR, Kelly JJ, Perugini RA. Small-bowel obstruction after laparoscopic Roux-en-Y gastric bypass surgery. J Comput Assist Tomogr. 2009;33:369–75.
242. Iannuccilli JD, Grand D, Murphy BL, Evangelista P, Roye GD, Mayo-Smith W. Sensitivity and specificity of eight CT signs in the preoperative diagnosis of internal mesenteric hernia following Roux-en-Y gastric bypass surgery. Clin Radiol. 2009;64:373–80.

When the Surgeon Needs the Endoscopist in Rescuing Bariatric Surgery: Intermediate and Late Post-operative Period

6

Contents

E. M. H. Mathus-Vliegen, J. Dargent, *Bariatric Therapy*,
https://doi.org/10.1007/978-3-319-90074-2_6

Abbreviations

3D	3-Dimensional
AACE	American Association of Clinical Endocrinologists
AE	Adverse event
APC	Argon plasma coagulation
ARMS	Anti-reflux mucosectomy
ASGE	American Society for Gastrointestinal Endoscopy
ASMBS	American Society for Metabolic and Bariatric Surgery
BAROS	Bariatric analysis and reporting system
BEA-ERCP	Balloon enteroscope-assisted ERCP
BEL	Best evidence level
BMI	Body mass index
BOLD	Bariatric Outcomes Longitudinal Database
BPD	Biliopancreatic diversion
BPD-DS	biliopancreatic diversion with duodenal switch
CBD	Common bile duct
CRE	Controlled radial expansion
CT	Computed tomography
DBE	Double-balloon-assisted enteroscopy
DBE-ERCP	Double-balloon-assisted enteroscopy ERCP
ERCP	Endoscopic retrograde cholangiopancreaticography
ESD	Endoscopic submucosal dissection
EUS	Endoscopic ultrasound
EUS-CP	Endoscopic ultrasound-guided cholangiopancreatography
EWL	Excess weight loss
FDA	Food and Drug Administration
GI	Gastrointestinal
Fr	French

GIP	Glucose-dependent insulinotropic polypeptide/gastric inhibitory peptide
GJA	Gastrojejunal anastomosis
GLP-1	Glucagon-like peptide-1
GORD	Gastro-oesophageal reflux disease
H. pylori	*Helicobacter pylori*
Hp	*Helicobacter pylori*
IOP	Incisionless operating platform
ITT	Intention-to-treat
LA-ERCP	Laparoscopy-assisted ERCP
LA(S)GB	Laparoscopic adjustable (silicone) gastric banding
LATG-RV	Laparoscopic transgastric rendez-vous
LOS	Lower oesophageal sphincter
LRYGB	Laparoscopic Roux-en-Y gastric bypass
MRCP	Magnetic resonance cholangiopancreaticography
MRI	Magnetic resonance imaging
MU	Marginal ulcer
Nd:YAG	Neodymium:yttrium aluminium garnet
NOTES	Natural orifice transluminal endoscopic surgery
NSAID	Non-steroidal anti-inflammatory drug
OD	Outer diameter
OR	Odds ratio
OTSC	Over-the-scope clip
PATENT	Percutaneous-assisted transprosthetic endoscopic therapy
PBH	Postbariatric hypoglycaemia
PEG	Percutaneous endoscopic gastrostomy
PPI	Proton pump inhibitor
PTC	Percutaneous transhepatic cholangiography
PYY	Peptide YY
QoE	Quality of the evidence
ROSE	Restorative obesity surgery endoluminally
RYGB	Roux-en-Y gastric bypass
SAE	Serious adverse event
SAGES	Society of Gastrointestinal and Endoscopic Surgeons
SBE	Single-balloon enteroscopy
SB-ERCP	Single-balloon enteroscopy ERCP
SEMS	Self-expandable metal stent
SEPS	Self-expandable plastic stent
SG	Sleeve gastrectomy
SOAE	Spiral-overtube-assisted enteroscopy
SOAE-ERCP	Spiral-overtube-assisted enteroscopic ERCP
TAS	Tissue apposition system
TOS	The Obesity Society
TPN	Total parenteral nutrition
TTS	Through-the-scope
UDCA	Ursodeoxycholic acid
VIP	Vasoactive intestinal peptide

6.1 Introduction

Immediate and early post-operative symptoms within 2 weeks after surgery often indicate an emergency problem. Although complaints in the intermediate (between 2 and 6 weeks after surgery) and late (more than 6 weeks after surgery) are mostly not an emergency, exceptions to this rule occur such as a late anastomotic or staple-line leak after sleeve gastrectomy (SG), Roux-en-Y gastric bypass (RYGB) and biliopancreatic diversion (BPD) with or without duodenal switch (BPD-DS) and internal herniation after RYGB and BPD/BPD-DS. A gastrointestinal bleed can occur in any (bariatric) patient. Also, bariatric surgery can evoke new emergencies such as complications of gallstones and bile duct stones due to (rapid) weight loss in every post-bariatric patient and can cause more specific procedure-related problems such as gastric prolapse and band erosion after laparoscopic adjustable gastric banding (LAGB). A very recent report on the largest group of patients ever reported put the results, both beneficial and adverse, into perspective [1]. The effectiveness of bariatric surgery in the USA was analysed from the 4-year data from the Bariatric Surgery Center of Excellence Data File. The adverse and serious adverse events, 1-year weight loss and 1-year comorbidity resolution were investigated in 130,796 patients, of whom 57,094 patients underwent LAGB, 5942 patients SG, 66,324 patients RYGB and 1436 patients BPD-DS. Adverse events (AEs) and serious adverse events (SAEs) were recorded at 30 days and 1 year. The data are given in Table 6.1. At 30 days, the adverse events were lowest for LAGB at 3.5%, and increased progressively with increasing complexity of the bariatric operation to 8.0% for SG, 11.8% for RYGB and 20.3% for BPD-DS. At 1 year, the AE rates were 6.5% for LAGB, 10.0% for SG, 18.0% for RYGB and 27.5% for BPD-DS. Serious adverse events for LAGB at 30 days were 0.2% and increased to 0.8% for SG, 1.4% for RYGB and 3.6% for BPD-DS. At 1 year, SAE rates were 0.3%for LAGB, 0.9% for SG, 1.6% for RYGB and 4.6% for BPD-DS. Rates of bleedings and leaks were reported separately and are shown in Table 6.1 with an increase with increasing complexity of the surgical intervention. As to the resolution of comorbidities and weight loss the trend was in the reverse way. The authors concluded in saying that the more complex the operation the greater the number of adverse and serious adverse events, but also the greater the weight loss and comorbidity resolution.

6.2 Symptomatology and Differential Diagnosis

Patients can present a variety of symptoms with even a greater variety of differential diagnoses and herewith associated different therapeutic approaches [2–12]. The type of surgery and the time since surgery are important determinants of complaints and abnormalities. In general the longer the interval since surgery, the greater the likelihood of patients having a normal endoscopy.

Table 6.1 Comparative effectiveness of primary bariatric operations in the USA [1]

	LAGB $N = 57,094$	SG $N = 5942$	RYGB $N = 66,324$	BPD-DS $N = 1436$
Kg change at 1-year mean (SD)	20.1 (11.9)	38.2 (15.5)	44.2 (14.8)	56.9 (19.4)
Kg matched with LAGB change at 1-year mean (SE)	Reference	16.1 (0.71)‡	26.0 (0.09)‡	38.2 (0.77)‡
BMI change at 1-year mean (SD)	7.2 (4.3)	13.6 (5.2)	15.8 (5.0)	19.9 (6.1)
BMI matched with LAGB change mean (SE)	Reference	5.7 (0.06)‡	9.3 (0.03)‡	10.6 (0.15)‡
30-days (%)				
Adverse event (%)	3.5	8.04	11.77	20.26
Serious adverse event (%)	0.23	0.81	1.35	3.63
Bleed (%)	0.10	0.63	1.38	0.99
Leak (%)	0.01	0.14	0.36	0.89
1-year (%)				
Adverse event (%)	6.5	10.03	17.99	27.52
Serious adverse event (%)	0.3	0.93	1.58	4.60
Bleed (%)	0.10	0.67	1.46	1.00
Leak (%)	0.01	0.24	0.43	1.18
30-day OR[a]				
Adverse event 30 days	Reference	2.42 (2.27, 2.58)‡	3.65 (3.51, 3.80)‡	7.22 (6.53, 7.98)‡
Serious adverse event 30 days	Reference	3.60 (2.90, 4.47)‡	5.43 (4.75, 6.21)‡	17.91 (14.17, 22.64)‡
Bleed 30 days	Reference	6.45 (4.87, 8.54)‡	12.24 (9.86, 15.21)‡	9.41 (5.80, 15.25)‡
Leak 30 days	Reference	20.08 (8.21, 49.09)‡	46.67 (21.02, 103.62)‡	Unreported due to small *n*
1-year OR[a]				
Adverse event 1 year	Reference	1.61 (1.52, 1.70)‡	3.15 (3.06, 3.25)‡	5.69 (5.21, 6.22)‡
Serious adverse event 1 year	Reference	3.22 (2.64, 3.92)‡	4.92 (4.38, 5.54)‡	17.47 (14.19, 21.52)‡
Bleed 1 year	Reference	6.70 (5.11, 8.78)‡	12.67 (10.25, 15.65)‡	9.29 (5.90, 14.63)‡
Leak 1 year	Reference	33.37 (14.12, 78.82)‡	58.87 (26.50, 130.81)‡	Unreported due to small *n*
1-year OR[a]				
Gastro-oesophageal reflux disease	Reference	0.87 (0.79, 0.95)**	1.53 (1.48, 1.58)‡	1.20 (0.95, 1.52)
Hypertension	Reference	1.93 (1.79, 2.08)‡	3.08 (2.98, 3.18)‡	3.82 (3.21, 4.55)‡
Musculoskeletal disease	Reference	1.15 (1.03, 1.29)*	1.78 (1.71, 1.86)‡	1.63 (1.23, 2.16)***
Obstructive sleep apnoea syndrome	Reference	1.98 (1.78, 2.19)‡	3.19 (3.07, 3.32)‡	3.06 (2.39, 3.91)‡
Type 2 diabetes	Reference	2.11 (1.92, 2.31)‡	3.51 (3.39, 3.64)‡	5.62 (4.60, 6.88)‡

*$p < 0.05$; **$p < 0.01$; ***$p < 0.001$; ‡$p < 0.0001$

[a]OR odds ratio with 95% confidence interval

6.2.1 Nausea and Vomiting

Nausea and vomiting are extremely common after bariatric surgery. The history should be taken about the types of foods associated with vomiting, the amount of food eaten, the time over which the food is eaten, the consistency of the food and the extent to which it is chewed and whether liquids were drunk immediately after eating solid food [12]. Certain types of food, such as red meats, dry white parts of poultry and foods that tend to clump together after being chewed, such as fried or scrambled eggs and bread, are sometimes not well tolerated. Another frequent cause of vomiting is overfilling of the pouch by a large volume of food or drinking liquids immediately after eating certain solids. The addition of liquids results in acute overdistension of the pouch which temporarily blocks the outlet. Teaching on eating behaviour such as eating slowly, chewing well, small-volume meals, consuming liquid 30 min after finishing solid foods and avoiding foods that engender difficulty is of primary importance in the prevention of vomiting [13].

Acute onset of vomiting is frequently due to ingestion of something that acts acutely to obstruct the outlet, such as uncooked beans, cherry stones, unpopped popcorn or bezoars. Endoscopy is anticipated to retrieve or push down the obstructing item or to institute treatment to remove the bezoar. In the case of acute and repeated vomiting, such as with a viral gastroenteritis, the resulting oedema and inability to tolerate solid foods may require a liquid diet for 4–7 days. Vomiting can also be associated with gallstones.

Vomiting after restrictive operations. Acute vomiting after LAGB can be related to gastric prolapse or pouch slippage superiorly through the gastric band producing obstruction at the band, a too tightly closed band, a malpositioned band, angulation or kinking of the outlet, erosion of the prosthetic material or the gastric band, or a pouch dilation that "hangs over" and thereby obstructs the stoma. Due to imminent gastric necrosis this signifies a need of early diagnosis and intervention. Vomiting after a sleeve gastrectomy may indicate a stenosis or obstruction at the incisura angularis, requiring dilation or reoperation. Chronic vomiting with stable weight or weight gain may suggest persistent pouch dilation. In case of an inflated gastric band, the band should be deflated. Also, removal or repositioning of the band might be considered.

Vomiting after RYGB and BPD can be due to anastomotic ulceration, anastomotic stenosis, erosion of the band in a banded gastric bypass, obstruction of the Roux limb, or partial or complete obstruction of the small bowel by internal herniation or adhesions. Patients with anastomotic stenosis present with epigastric pain and vomiting of undigested food followed by vomiting of liquids. Many of these cases will require dilation or reoperation. Anastomotic ulceration may be treated with PPIs, sucralfate and eradication of *Helicobacter pylori* when identified. Nausea and vomiting can be symptoms of the dumping syndrome. Dumping is precipitated by ingestion of food and liquids with high sugar content which enters immediately into the small bowel because of the reduced size of the stomach. Symptoms are gastrointestinal (nausea, vomiting, diarrhoea, abdominal cramps) and systemic (hypotension, rapid heartbeat, light-headedness, flushing and syncope), induced by vasoactive hormones. Dumping syndrome can be seen in patients non-compliant with their diet. It is common in the early post-operative period and subsides within 12–18 months after surgery. Prevention includes consumption of small frequent meals, avoidance of foods with high sugar content, eating and drinking slowly, chewing food thoroughly and consuming liquids between and apart from meals.

Delayed gastric emptying, inherently present or after operative injury to the vagus nerves to the stomach, may become manifest as vomiting [14]. Prokinetic drugs may be tried.

Persistent vomiting in the post-operative bariatric patient may lead to dehydration, protein-calorie malnutrition and peripheral neuropathy, or Wernicke's encephalopathy with ataxia and nystagmus, because of a thiamine deficiency. Patients with gastric restriction will restrict their energy and protein intake and will avoid meats in favour of more easily consumed foods. In 20% of cases, protein-calorie malnutrition will develop. Especially gastric bypass patients who avoid meat because of intolerance and milk because of the dumping syndrome are at risk. Administration of thiamine before the administration of glucose or nutrients is important.

6.2.2 Heartburn, Reflux, Epigastric or Retrosternal Pain

These symptoms, suggestive of gastro-oesophageal reflux, are often caused by an excessively tight band, gastric prolapse, pouch dilation, excessive eating with overfilling of the pouch and gastric emptying disturbances in case of restrictive operations, or stenosis of the upper anastomosis in RYGB and BPD and alkaline reflux in the presence of a loop gastric bypass.

6.2.3 Diarrhoea and Constipation

Diarrhoea can be multifactorial, due to the dumping syndrome, lactose intolerance, malabsorption, bacterial overgrowth and infection. Constipation may be due to limited food, fibre and fluid intake in the context of energy restriction or because of complaints. Calcium and iron supplements may contribute.

6.2.4 Abdominal Pain

Abdominal pain has many causes.

In *restrictive surgery* the differential diagnosis includes gastric and duodenal ulcer, oesophagitis, pouch outlet obstruction, gallstones, incisional hernia, an abscess or a perforation at the site of the eroding band. A spontaneous disconnection between tube and port should be suspected in LAGB patients with a gastric band who report acute abdominal pain.

After *gastric bypass surgery*, the afferent loop syndrome sometimes with pancreatitis, efferent limb obstruction, anastomotic ulcer, peptic ulcer in the bypassed stomach or duodenum, pouch outlet obstruction, incisional hernia, gallstones and adhesions should be considered. Traction on sutures or staples may also evoke pain. Removal of foreign material with endoscopic scissors results in immediate improvement or resolution of symptoms in 71–83% of cases [15, 16].

Severe (crampy) abdominal pain and pain out of proportion to physical examination suggest ischaemia by internal herniation or adhesions and warrant further investigation of explorative laparoscopy or laparotomy.

6.2.5 Haematemesis and Melaena

Haematemesis and melaena suggest a gastrointestinal bleeding. In *LAGB and SG* bleeding may come from severe oesophagitis and band deflation and/or intensive medical therapy is indicated.

In *gastric bypass surgery* a haemorrhage may originate from the oesophagus, gastric pouch, bypassed stomach and duodenum, gastrojejunostomy and jejunojejunostomy [17]. Endoscopic accessibility will determine the therapeutic options for haemostasis including epinephrine injection, cauterisation with heater or gold probe, argon plasma coagulation and haemoclipping. Late bleeding is typical due to a marginal ulcer at the gastrojejunal anastomosis or an ulcer in the gastric remnant or duodenum. In case of a lack of access and a significant bleed, angiography should be performed to control bleeding by embolisation.

6.2.6 Inadequate Weight Loss or Weight Gain

In the case of inadequate weight loss or weight regain after initial adequate weight loss, patient-specific (dietary non-compliance, endocrinopathies/metabolic causes, physical inactivity and psychiatric causes) and operation-specific causes should be investigated [18]. Karmali et al. systematically reviewed the existing literature to assess the incidence and definition of weight regain and causative factors associated with weight regain following bariatric surgery [18]. Sixteen studies were included in this analysis: seven case series, five surveys and four non-randomised controlled trials, with a total of 4864 patients for analysis, with a number of patients ranging from 26 to 1845 per study and follow-up ranging from 12 months to 11.4 years post-surgery. They discovered a high degree of variability in assessing weight, making quantitative comparisons difficult. Five studies investigated the non-compliance with diet and besides increased daily caloric intake, poor diet quality and lack of appropriate nutritional follow-up, new dietary patterns with loss of dietary control and grazing behaviours (defined as consumption of smaller amounts of foods over extended periods of time) emerged. Three studies investigated hormonal and metabolic imbalances and found that both increased ghrelin levels and cyclical glucose fluctuations may generate hunger and food temptation a few hours after a meal, leading to frequent snacking or meals and thus potential weight regain. As to mental health, reported in five studies, binge-eating, depression, alcohol and drug use, food urges, presence of an eating disorder, increased impulsive behavioural traits, increased number of psychiatric diagnoses and fewer follow-up visits were associated with weight regain. Inadequate physical activity was identified as a contributing factor for weight regain in one study. Therefore, in patients with weight regain following bariatric surgery, diet (25.3%), physical activity (21.0%) and motivational issues (19.7%) were identified to be the most common reasons [18].

Secondly, surgical causes should be considered which are procedure specific, such as a staple-line disruption with a gastrogastric fistula in VBG and RYGB, an enlarged stoma or pouch dilation in RYGB, pouch distension or band slippage in LAGB, and a neofundus and dilation of the sleeve in SG. Also, erosion of the band will cause a loss of its restrictive function with weight gain after VBG, LAGB and a banded gastric bypass.

6.3 Bariatric Surgery-Specific Endoscopic Findings and Interventions

The bariatric-specific endoscopic findings and interventions will be discussed according to the frequency of performance of operations. Although vertical banded gastroplasty (VBG) is no longer performed but was very popular in the 1980s, many patients still possess this anatomy and so its inherent complications have to be discussed. Complications of less current and not generally accepted operations such as gastric plication and mini gastric bypass/omega-loop bypass will not be discussed but mostly complications and their treatment can be found under the respective headings. The complications are not described in order of incidence, but merely discussed this way for logistic reasons.

6.4 (Laparoscopic) Roux-En-Y Gastric Bypass (RYGB)

Patients who developed gastrointestinal (GI) symptoms after RYGB and who were referred for endoscopic evaluation had normal findings in 25–44% [19–22]. In general, the longer the interval since surgery, the greater the likelihood of patients having a normal endoscopy with the possible exception of patients with a staple-line dehiscence who frequently present later in the post-operative course. Huang et al. demonstrated that 85% of patients presenting with symptoms within the first 6 months had abnormal endoscopic findings compared with 47% of patients evaluated after 6 months [20]. Predictive of a normal endoscopy was presentation with abdominal pain beyond the sixth post-operative month [3]. Patients with abnormal findings presented more with dysphagia and within 3 months and those with normal findings more with abdominal pain and later, after 3 months [23]. Symptoms that have been associated with abnormal endoscopic findings are dysphagia, nausea, vomiting and upper GI bleeding. The most common abnormality was marginal ulcer, present in 27–52%, followed by stomal stenosis in 4–39% [3, 21, 22]. Nausea, vomiting or dysphagia was present in patients with stomal stenosis; the absence of these symptoms ruled out the diagnosis although the predictive value of these symptoms was only 40% [3].

It is also important to realise that a change in the type and frequency of complications is associated with the introduction of laparoscopy. Podnos et al. reviewed 10 laparoscopic gastric bypass studies with 3646 patients and 8 studies with 2771 patients with gastric bypasses done by laparotomy [24]. In the laparoscopic RYGB they found a decrease in wound-related complications such as infection, wound dehiscence and incisional hernia and decreased need for (iatrogenic) splenectomy and a decreased mortality. In contrast, there appeared to be a higher frequency of early and late bowel obstruction, gastrointestinal haemorrhage and stomal stenosis in the laparoscopic group. They also tried to explain their findings and reported the higher early and late post-operative bowel obstruction after laparoscopic RYGB to be related to the technique of construction of the jejunojejunostomy. The early obstruction was related to the use of a circular stapler; the late bowel obstruction was due to not closing the three mesenteric defects: the jejunojejunostomy mesenteric defect, the transverse mesocolon defect and the Petersen hernia defect. The higher frequency of gastrointestinal haemorrhage after LRYGB may be related to the frequent use of a handsewn technique for creation of the gastrojejunostomy, the oversewing of gastric staple line and the use of stapled but non-transected gastric pouch technique in open gastric bypass surgery. The reason for a higher frequency of stomal stenoses after laparoscopic RYGB is unknown but might be related to the higher number of mechanically stapled anastomoses in laparoscopic versus the handsewn in open gastric bypass. This is the more important as on average 2.2% of laparoscopic operations have to be converted to open laparotomy.

6.4.1 Marginal Ulcer

A marginal ulcer (MU) is defined as an ulcer of the jejunal mucosa near the site of the gastrojejunostomy, on the small-bowel site of the anastomosis. The terms marginal, stomal and anastomotic ulcers have been used to describe these ulcers. Marginal ulcers can be early (<12 months) and late (>12 months) with different underlying aetiology and treatment. The risk of marginal ulcers is highest in the first 2–4 months after surgery, after which there is a small but continued risk up to at least 1 year after surgery [4]. Of these marginal ulcers, 83–95% present in the first year and late marginal ulcers 12–48 months after RYBG is reported in a small proportion (1%) of patients [25, 26]. A review of 42 articles with 16,987 patients found marginal ulcers to develop in 787 (4.6%) subjects with a range of 0.6–25% dependent on the length of follow-up [27]. There are few prospective studies with planned endoscopy irrespective of symptomatology. One of those studies by Csendes et al. described the findings on routine endoscopy after RYGB operations and found at 1 month following surgery marginal ulcers in 4.1% of patients after open and 12.3% after laparoscopic surgery, so in 6% overall, with 28% of ulcers occurring in the absence of symptoms [28]. Repeat endoscopy after 17 months identified only one new ulcer and one recurrent ulcer despite PPI treatment. This led to the concept of early and late ulcers with incidence rates of 6% and 0.6%, respectively. A follow-up study of 550 patients undergoing serial endoscopy to assess for late marginal ulcers by the same group found that 1% had a marginal ulcer, with four being identified over 4 years post-operatively [25]. As mentioned earlier, one-quarter of patient will be asymptomatic, but symptoms, when present, are vague and consist of an epigastric burning sensation in 56.8%, nausea and vomiting in 18–58% and dysphagia in 36% [26, 27]. They may also present as an emergency and 5.1% of patients present with bleeding and <1% with a perforation [26, 27]. In their review of 47 studies Carr et al. showed that the mean time to perforation is 12 months [26]. Csendes et al. demonstrated that for late marginal ulcers, symptoms were the typical peptic ulcer pains with a very precise localisation and wake up at night from pain [25].

Many factors have been associated with the development of marginal ulcers and three main categories can be discerned: increased gastric pouch acidity, mucosal disruption and ischaemia.

The introduction of gastric bypass for the treatment of morbid obesity raised concern over its ulcerogenic potential, remindful of the 5–10% occurrence rate, reported with subtotal gastic resections for the treatment of duodenal ulcer [29]. The jejunum has no native protection against gastric acid and after RYGB there is no buffering of acid by pancreatic bicarbonate secretions. The original hypothesis was that if sufficient acid secretion occurred in the excluded stomach, it stays unbuffered by food in the excluded stomach and so it would inhibit the secretion of gastrin, resulting in less acid production in the pouch and thus preventing stomal ulceration [29]. The acid secretion is indeed reduced after gastric bypass because of a small fundic pouch [29]. However, the pouch, stoma and jejunum are bathed in gastric acid after staple-line dehiscence and the formation of a gastrogastric fistula. The bathing of jejunum in acid as a cause of marginal ulcer was investigated by several authors. MacLean et al. documented the lowered incidence of gastrogastric fistula formation and marginal ulcer presence when the gastric bypass in continuity was changed into an isolated gastric bypass [30]. Capella and Capella reported on how this complication may be further avoided by the interposition of a Roux limb between the pouch and the gastric remnant and by a handsewn anastomosis with absorbable sutures [31]. Gilmore et al. demonstrated the importance of the acid pocket when performing a RYGB with a too large gastric pouch of >40 cc compared to a 20 cc pouch [32]. So, pouch orientation and size (large vertically oriented pouch, lesser curvature pouch, pouch length >5 cm, all associated with a greater number of acid-producing cells), staple-line dehiscence and gastrogastric fistula may lead to marginal ulcers through the role of acid [22, 25, 26]. In the late marginal ulcer occurrence, gastric acid within the jejunum has been considered the main mechanism for ulceration [25].

Mucosa disruption is another cause and factors, that increased significantly the risk of marginal ulcers following surgery, included bile reflux, smoking (adjusted odds ratio (OR) 30.6) and NSAID use (adjusted OR 11.5) due to inhibition of cyclo-oxygenase and thereby decreased prostaglandin E2 levels [22]. Pope et al. did not believe in the role of staple-line dehiscence and demonstrated that local, tissue-injury-related factors may be responsible, supported by the finding of prolonged irritation by foreign material such as non-absorbable sutures at the gastrojejunostomy [33]. Absorbable sutures are associated with a significant lower rate of ulceration than non-absorbable sutures and staples, and visible non-absorbable sutures should be extracted when possible [34]. Rasmussen et al. showed remnants of suture material in 7% of marginal ulcer beds but also a twice as high prevalence of *Helicobacter pylori* (Hp) [35]. The role of *H. pylori* in the pathogenesis of marginal ulcer is inconclusive. This inconsistency is partly related to testing for Hp only in selective cases, limited time of follow-up, absent verification of eradication, no information on the time relationship of PPI use and testing for Hp, etc. [26]. In the review on symptomatic marginal ulcers by Coblijn et al. 12 articles tested the presence of Hp and in 10.5% Hp was positive and no relationship with Hp could be found [27]. Csendes et al. prospectively followed and endoscoped 130 RYGB patients for 10 years: 18% of patients had a *H. pylori* infection, and only 6% had marginal ulcers [36]. In a series of 442 patients 16 suffered from marginal ulcers but *H. pylori* was not found to be a risk factor [37]. Four studies have reported that preoperative screening and eradication resulted in reduced marginal ulcer [19, 38, 39]. Conversely, Loewen et al. [40] found that *H. pylori* infection preoperatively was not a risk factor for 37 marginal ulcers in a series of 286 RYGB, with only one patient being positive for *H. pylori*. Both Loewen et al. and Rasmussen et al. suggested that preoperative duodenitis or gastritis was a positive risk for marginal ulcer, whether or not being related to *H. pylori* infection [35, 40]. They received support for their ideas by the findings of D'Hondt et al. in a prospective multicentre study [41]. Preoperatively, D'Hondt et al. tested and eradicated *H. pylori* using repeat endoscopy to confirm eradication and to retreat if needed. A total of 449 patients underwent RYGB with 48 developing ulcers. While they found that the incidence of ulceration was independent of *H. pylori* status, they did find that treating patients with *H. pylori* with PPI therapy led to a reduction in stomal ulcer rates compared to those who did not receive PPI therapy [41]. This protective effect was not seen in *H. pylori*-negative patients. This suggests that preoperative infection results in gastritis leading to increased ulcer risk, which could be reduced by PPI therapy for 1 month after surgery [41].

Ischaemia by tension at the gastrojejunal anastomosis and circular stapling may play a role as well [42]. Azagury et al. investigated 103 patients with marginal ulceration and found visible sutures in 35% and a gastrogastric fistula in 8% [43]. The mean pouch length was 5.6 cm. Associated with marginal ulcer were in univariate analysis: diabetes (OR 2.5), pouch length (OR 1.2) and smoking (OR 2.5), but in multivariate analysis only diabetes remained (OR 5.6) [43]. PPI therapy was protective against marginal ulcers (adjusted OR 0.33) [22].

When marginal ulcers are identified, the pouch must be carefully examined for the presence of anatomical abnormalities, such as gastrogastric fistulae, enlarged pouches or distal strictures. When these are left untreated, medical treatment alone may be unsuccessful. Sometimes upper GI series are needed because they may detect a gastrogastric fistula not seen on prior endoscopy.

Treatment should consist of the modification of patient-related risk factors such as smoking and NSAID use and inhibition of gastric acid secretion and is reported to be successful in treating 68–100% of marginal ulcers [26, 27, 43]. Both NSAID use and smoking play a role in the formation as well as in lesser healing of marginal ulcers [27]. Moreover, smoking is a risk factor for marginal ulcer perforation [27]. Medical treatment consists of PPIs, sucralfate and H_2 antagonists. Thirty-one articles discussed 801 subjects of whom 68% could be sufficiently treated by medication; 23% of patients needed one or more operations because of perforation, dilated pouch, intractable marginal ulcer and gastrogastric fistula [27]. As the tablet form of sucralfate and the capsule form of PPIs might be less effective, soluble PPI (or capsules broken open) and sucralfate solution (four times 1 g) should be taken for 2–6 months [10, 44]. Most centres advocate for indefinite PPI use after development of anastomotic ulcers in RYGB. However, if aspiration of gastric pouch fluid reveals a near-neutral or elevated pH, then acid suppression may be less effective and sucralfate solution is the treatment of choice [45]. In the case of bile reflux, bile acid-binding drugs such as cholestyramine or colestipol should be prescribed. Relapse rates of 8% have been reported [10, 26, 46].

As PPIs appear to be protective, the prophylactic prescription of PPIs has become standard practice although there is disagreement about the duration, varying from 1 month to 2 years post-operatively. PPIs provide significant protection when used with NSAIDs. However, some authors did not find a protective role. Garrido et al. treated 118 morbidly obese subjects who were negative for *H. pylori* and who underwent a Roux-en-Y gastric bypass, followed by esomeprazole treatment for 60 days after surgery [47]. Before surgery and 2 months later an endoscopy was performed. At endoscopy, foreign body material was found in the anastomosis in 12 (10.2%) and a marginal ulcer was observed in 9 (7.6%) subjects, 2 of which had suture material or metallic staple granuloma in the gastrojejunostomy. None of the ulcers was related to the use of non-steroidal anti-inflammatory drugs. The rather high incidence of marginal ulcers within the first 2 months following Roux-en-Y gastric bypass under proton pump inhibition in this study may highlight that action only on the acid peptic factor may be insufficient. Moon and colleagues found that despite the use of routine PPI for 90 days after RYGB, the incidence of marginal ulceration was still remarkable in 59 (2.3%) of a total of 2535 patients [48]. Urgent operation was required in 14 (23.7%) because of perforation (12; 20.3%) or bleeding (2; 3.4%). In total 26 of the 59 (44.1%) needed operation [48]. Conversely, a meta-analysis of 2917 participants showed that patients who received prophylactic PPI experienced significantly less ulceration compared with patients who did not receive PPI prevention (OR 0.50) [49].

Marginal ulcer perforation is a surgical emergency. Marginal ulcer bleeding can be treated endoscopically by injecting epinephrine, by using bipolar haemostasis, or clips. Endoscopic suturing with the OverStitch Endoscopic Suturing System (Apollo Endosurgery, Austin, Texas, USA) has been applied in massive ulcer bleeding and in the treatment of recalcitrant marginal ulcers before to have to resort to surgery [50, 51].

6.4.2 Gastrojejunal/Stomal Stenosis

A stomal stenosis is present if a standard 9.5 mm endoscope cannot traverse the anastomosis, mostly in the presence of symptoms of nausea and vomiting, food intolerance and dysphagia for solids, followed by dysphagia for fluids. Significant weight loss over a short period of time or malnutrition may ensue. Usually abdominal pain is absent, a symptom characteristically present in internal herniation which should always be considered in the differential diagnosis. Stenosis can be identified by contrast radiography, but direct endoscopic visualisation is preferable. It is important to recognise that obstructive symptoms may also result from the Roux limb more distally. In patients with an RYGB, the Roux limb can be delivered to the upper abdomen to connect with the gastric pouch in an antecolic fashion, in front of the transverse colon, or through a retrocolic tunnel created in the transverse mesocolon. Obstructive symptoms can occur when this tunnel is created too tightly or by post-operative stricturing. On endoscopic examination, the gastrojejunal anastomosis will be normal, but the jejunum beyond the anastomosis will be dilated until the point where it traverses the mesentery where the stricture will be seen. Because the risk of perforation is high, dilation in these cases is not advised [52]. Scanty data suggest that, similar to leaks, rates of stenosis can decrease by means of intraoperative endoscopy [53, 54].

The risk of stenosis at the gastrojejunal anastomosis is highest in the first 2–3 months after surgery; thereafter the risk declines dramatically to negligible levels by 8–10 months [55–57]. Rates of 3–5% have been reported after open RYGB and 5–12% after laparoscopic RYGB [10, 24, 28]. In case of stricture formation incited by foreign material or an ulcer, the presentation may be delayed for months or years. Most authors report an incidence between 3 and 27%, but as can be seen in Table 6.2, the incidence ranges from 1.7 to 15.7% in studies that report on dilation and outcomes [23, 55–81]. It is honest to say that there are no true incidence data as routine endoscopies, also in patients without complaints, are not performed. Csendes et al. are the exception to the rule: they performed endoscopies as a routine 1 and 17 months after surgery irrespective of the presence or absence of complaints [28]. At 1 month they detected 112 patients having strictures (in 54% being 7–9 mm reported as mild, in 24% being 5–6 mm reported as moderate and in 22% being <4 mm and severe) with complaints in only 29% of the moderate and severe strictures. This may suggest a considerable underreporting of cases when relying on symptoms. At 17 months all anastomoses, including those with strictures in the past, looked normal.

The aetiology of stomal stenosis and anastomotic stricture is probably multifactorial [22, 42, 55, 64, 66–68, 76, 79, 82–84] and related to

(a) Surgery-technical factors which include the construction of the anastomosis: most commonly with the circular stapler with stenosis in 31% (OR 11.3) compared to 3% with handsewn or 0% with the linear stapler with linear stapling providing a tension-free gastrojejunal anastomosis [42, 68, 71, 79].
(b) Factors promoting local ischaemia such as reinforcement sutures, dissection, tension on the anastomosis with an antecolic, antegastric Roux limb, and the use of 21 mm compared to 25 mm staples [66]: Indeed, Papasavas et al. had an overall incidence of stenosis of 8.9% but when the Roux limb was placed retrocolic and retrogastric the incidence of stenosis was 3.4% but 14.0% when the Roux-en-Y was antecolic and antegastric [85]. The longer antecolic antegastric route may contribute to tension and subsequent stenosis of the gastrojejunal anastomosis.

Table 6.2 Endoscopic therapy of anastomotic strictures after bariatric surgery, only studies involving ≥10 patients are mentioned (modified and updated after Campos et al. [58] and Malli et al. [59])

Author	Country and year	Incidence of stricture (N)	Method dilation[a]	No. of patients	No. of dilations in total (N/patient)	Complications	Success rate (%)
Escalona [60]	Chile; 2007	6.9% (N 769)	SGB	53	71	1 perforation	100
Fernandez-Esparrach [61]	Spain; 2008	5.7% (N 424)	SGB	24	38 (1.6/p)	None	100
Costa [62]	Brazil; 2009	–	SGB/TTS	30	48	None	100
Vance [63]	USA; 2002	–	BU	28	41	None	100
Schwartz [64]	USA; 2004	3.0% (N 1000)	BU/TTS	30	68	4 perforations	73
Sanyal [65]	USA; 1992	10.5% (N 191)	TTS	20	23	None	100
Ahmad [57]	USA; 2003	3.1% (N 450)	TTS	14	23	None	100
Barba [56]	USA; 2003	11.0% (N 218)	TTS	24	33	None	100
Nguyen [66]	USA; 2003	15.7 (N 185)	TTS	29	35	None	100
Go [55]	USA; 2004	6.8% (N 562)	TTS	38	80 (2.1/p)	1 perforation	95
Goitein [67]	USA; 2005	4.9% (N 369)	TTS	18	56 (3.1/p)	1 perforation M	100
Carrodeguas [68]	USA; 2006	7.3% (N 1291)	TTS	94	188	2 perforations	98
Catalano [69]	USA; 2007	–	TTS	26	63	None	100
Peifer [70]	USA; 2007	5.4% (N 801)	TTS	43	56 (1.3/p)	Minor bleeds	98
Takata [71]	USA; 2007	4.0% (N 379)	TTS	15	22 (1.4/p)	None	100
Caro [72]	Argentina; 2008	6.2% (N 1800)	TTS	111	200 (1.8/p)	2 perforations M 1 haematoma	100
Ukleja [73]	USA; 2008	6.0% (N 1012)	TTS	61	128 (2.2/p)	3 perforations M	100
Alasfar [74]	USA; 2009	23.0% (N126)	TTS	29	36	None	100
Dolce [75]	USA; 2009	7.6% (N 196)	TTS	15	20	None	93
Lee [23]	USA; 2009	3.7% (N 1079)	TTS	40	86	None	100
Ryskina [76]	USA; 2010	–	TTS	58	117	None	100
Da Costa [77]	Spain; 2011	7.9% (N 1330)	TTS	105	169 (1.6/p)	3 perforations 1 haemorrhage	100
Espinel [78]	Spain; 2011	4.2% (N 525)	TTS	22	31	1 tear	100
Yimcharoen [79]	USA; 2012	–	TTS	72	165 (2.3/p)	1 perforation-related death	85
Rossi [80]	USA; 2004	17.0% (N 223)	NS	38	61 (1.6/p)	1 severe vomiting	100
Mathew [81]	USA; 2009	6.5% (N 888)	NS	58	125	4 perforations	100

[a] *SGB* Savary-Gilliard bougie, *TTS* through-the-scope balloon, *BU* balloon unspecified, *NS* not specified, *M* micro-perforation, not found at laparoscopy

(c) Factors promoting a local inflammatory response such as excess acid production in a large gastric pouch or due to a gastrogastric fistula, a marginal ulcer, a subclinical leak, reaction to foreign material – such as staples or sutures, but also non-absorbable anastomotic rings or bands in the banded gastric bypass, that may result in erosions, ulceration and stricture formation – an anastomotic leak and ulcerations due to ischaemia or the use of NSAIDs, alcohol or tobacco.

Some authors have published an analysis of preoperative predictors of complications. Perugini et al. identified surgeon's experience, sleep apnoea and hypertension as predictive of complications in general, but cautioned that the factors they discovered may, in fact, "be specific for the complication of gastrojejunal stenosis" [86]. Blackstone and Rivera found preoperative findings associated with stricture risk to be GORD (odds ratio almost a factor 2) and age with younger rather than older age being associated with the risk of stenosis: aged ≤35 years were 2 times at greater risk than those aged 36–45 years and 2.3 times greater at risk than those 46–55 years [87]. They found out to be in error in their assumption that higher rates of central fat distribution in males might place greater tension on the anastomosis predisposing male patients, particularly those with higher BMIs, towards stricture, and also ischaemic effects of diabetes, sleep apnoea and chronic respiratory disease were not contributing.

6.4.2.1 Endoscopic Dilation

Endoscopic dilation of anastomotic stenosis after bariatric surgery is safe, effective and durable [10, 46, 58, 59]. There are multiple options to dilate a stenotic anastomosis, including fluoroscopic guided balloon dilation, dilation with bougies over an endoscopically placed guidewire (Eder-Puestow olives, Savary-Gilliard bougies) and endoscopic guided through-the-scope (TTS) controlled radial expansion (CRE) balloon dilation or outside-the-scope balloon dilation. Most commonly used are the Savary-Gilliard bougies and the CRE balloons, but in bariatric surgery mainly CRE balloons have been used (Bard Endoscopic Technologies, Billerica, MA, USA). Savary-Gilliard dilators (Wilson-Cook, Medical Inc., Winston-Salem, NC, USA) are tapered dilators made of polyvinylchloride; they possess a hollow central channel which allows for insertion over a guidewire. They are available in 1 mm increments from 5 mm in diameter to 20 mm. Each CRE balloon has the capability of dilating to three different sizes (so 8-9-10 mm, 11-12-12.8 mm, 12-13.5-15 mm). The balloons are 8 cm in length. They require an endoscope with a working channel of at least 2.8 mm. A soft guidewire inside the TTS balloon is helpful to direct the balloon in case of a pinpoint stenosis. The guidewire is introduced into the stenosis, paying careful attention that the wire string slips with ease and without resistance through the orifice. Then the balloon is carefully advanced distally and placed across the anastomosis and dilation is accomplished in three blow-up steps (Fig. 6.1). Though there are no comparative studies between both techniques, the Savary-Gilliard bougies have the disadvantage of sometimes a need for radiologic control, the rather long distance from mouth to anastomosis and the repeated introduction of at least three bougies at a time. The advantage is its cost-effectiveness due to its

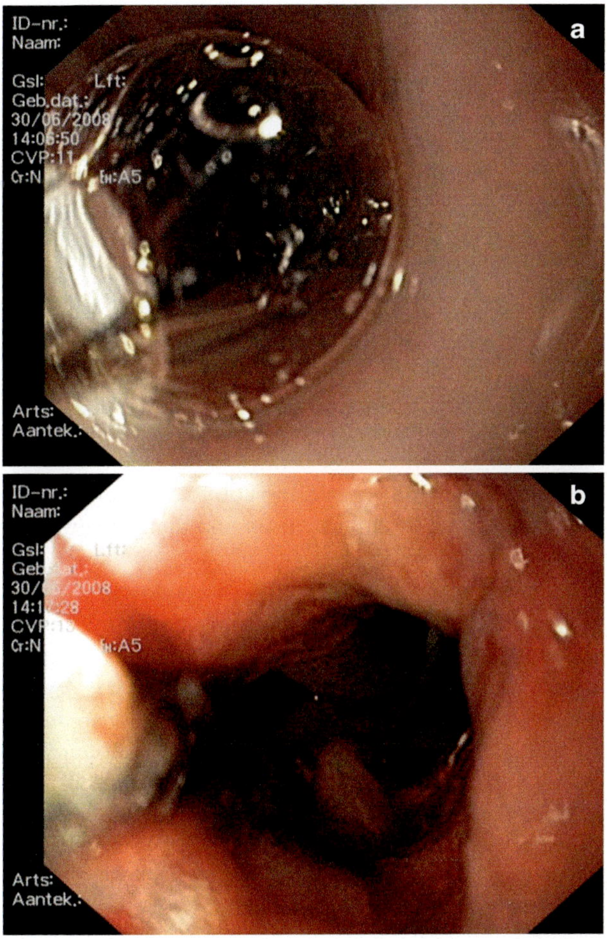

Fig. 6.1 (**a**) Controlled radial expansion (CRE) balloon dilation of a gastrojejunal anastomosis stenosis after gastric bypass; (**b**) endoscopic result after balloon dilation

reusability and the fact of having feedback about the firmness and stenosis resistance during dilation with the first size of the bougie. This may assist in the decision if further dilation with a larger diameter bougie is indicated and safe. A hydrostatic balloon can be gradually inflated with saline solution under direct vision, controlled by a syringe connected to a manometer. The companies that manufacture the devices indicate the pressure in psi that has to be generated for each size of the balloon but without recommending a dilation time. Also, the literature has not established a recommended time for dilation procedures. Most authors dilated for 1 min, but dilation time did not exceed 3 min in any of the studies. The procedure should be stopped if the patient experiences abdominal pain.

Perforation is the greatest concern after endoscopic dilation of strictures. To minimise this risk, the diameter of the initial stricture has traditionally dictated the initial size of the dilator to be used and then the "rule of threes" is followed. Following this rule a stricture, i.e. a stenosis that is felt as a slight resistance at endoscopy, is dilated in no more than three steps (in total 3 mm in diameter) during a single session. This rule was originally described for bougie-type dilators. Controlled data for this rule are not available. Balloon dilations are performed passing a soft guidewire through the anastomosis, then advancing the balloon and positioning the deflated balloon so that the anastomotic stricture is aligned with the balloon's midpoint. The balloons may be inflated with water, saline or water-soluble contrast and kept in place inflated for 1 min before increasing the diameter (1 mm every minute); the choice of the balloon thus determines the finally obtained anastomosis width. Perforation of the anastomosis is related to the size of the balloon and the amount of circular force (in atmospheres) exerted on the stricture, which is related to the initial narrowing and length of the stricture [67]. Perforation of the jejunal Roux limb is related to traumatic manipulation of the guidewire or the tip of the balloon [68].

Dilation is at the earliest safe after 3–4 weeks after the operation although some suggest that dilation after 7 days should be a safe option as well [56, 66, 82]. If endoscopic dilation is performed during the first 3 weeks post-operatively, a smaller balloon (12 mm) should be used and the anastomosis should be dilated at a lower pressure (<2 atmospheres) [66].

In patients with stomal stenosis, endoscopic dilation can be attempted in the absence of ulceration at the stoma. The initial dilation should be only enough to accommodate an endoscope of 9–10 mm for evaluation beyond to ensure that there is no ulceration distal to the stenosis. If there is an ulcer, patients should be placed on an ulcer treatment regime as dilation of the stoma might cause a perforation [57]. In case of exposed sutures these should be removed with endoscopic scissors to achieve successful dilation [10, 15, 16]. The goal stomal diameter after dilation is 10–12 mm, up to a maximum of approximately 15 mm. In almost no case should dilation progress to dilators in excess of 15 mm diameter for fear of disrupting the anastomosis, resulting in leak or in progressive dilation and loss of restrictive function and risk of dumping complaints. Barba et al. recommended that strictures should be dilated to at least 15 mm, realising that dilating to at least 15 mm decreased the chance of symptomatic recurrence [56]. If the scope could traverse the stricture, the latter was dilated to 18 mm. If a patient returned with recurrent symptoms and a stricture, dilation was always performed to 18 mm. This was confirmed by Ahmad et al. [57] who mentioned that nearly 60% of patients had complete symptomatic resolution after a single-balloon dilation session with a 15 mm balloon, suggesting that this size should be used initially, and by Peifer et al. [70], who reported a significant lower rate of repeat endoscopic dilation of strictures dilated to at least 15 mm, when compared to those dilated to 12 mm or less [57, 70]. Campos et al. reviewed the literature between 1988 and 2010 and retrieved 23 articles with 1298 procedures in 760 patients (Table 6.2) [58]. Through-the-scope balloons were used in 16 studies (69.5%) and Savary-Gilliard bougies in 4; in the remainder unspecified balloons were used or the method was not mentioned in detail. Most patients (398/760; 52%) had clinical resolution after a single procedure. The reported complication rate was 2.5% ($n = 19$), perforation being the most common, reported in 14 patients (1.8%) and requiring immediate operation in 2 patients. Other complications were also reported: one oesophageal haematoma, one Mallory-Weiss tear, one case of severe nausea and vomiting, and two cases of severe abdominal pain. Only 2% ($n = 15$) of patients required surgical revision after dilation. Table 6.2 is an extension of their study report with more studies added and studies with <10 subjects being removed [23, 55–81]. An almost 100% success rate in a large number of patients and a few complications of perforations, sometimes only micro-perforations not visible at laparoscopy [60, 72, 73], and bleeding are reported. Clearly, the study by Schwartz et al. is an outlier, and when looking more in detail these authors operated 1000 patients by laparoscopy with the construction of the gastrojejunostomy with a linear stapler [64]. A polyester running suture was used to close the stapler defect and the anastomosis was banded with fascia lata to prevent late enlargement. They used cadaver fascia lata with a 5.4% stenosis rate (11/205), autogenous fascia lata with 2.7% stenosis (21/790) and no stenosis in the only case with bovine pericardium. The cadaver fascia acted as a foreign body in four patients and eroded into the gastroenterostomy causing ulceration and stenosis. They also discussed the perforation in four patients: three of the four occurred at the initial attempt at dilation [64]. The stenotic orifice sizes were 2, 3, 8 and 9 mm at the time of the dilation and a 15 mm TTS balloon was used in all the dilations resulting in perforation. The 15 mm balloon was probably too large for the 2 and 3 mm orifices and perhaps the 8 and 9 mm orifices needed no dilation at all [64].

It is obvious from Table 6.2 that the success rate is high both with Savary-Gilliard bougies and TTS balloons and an overall 1.3–3.1 dilations are needed.

The need for multiple dilations was associated with a smaller initial balloon size [76]. Using a larger balloon in the initial dilation was also associated with a reduced risk of stricture recurrence (OR 0.32). A balloon size of at least 11 mm was associated with a significantly lower odds of stricture recurrence (OR 0.05) [76]. Apart from initial balloon size also the timing appeared to be relevant. Costa et al. discovered that the largest diameter achieved at the first dilation and the longer time from surgery to the appearance of symptoms are predicting factors of the need of one dilation [62]. They explained their unexpected findings by arguing that the earlier the stricture develops, the more difficult is its treatment, and more sessions are needed to obtain a sustained response, perhaps because the fibrous scarring of the anastomosis is not complete until the second to third months after the procedure, keeping its tendency towards the stricture formation after the dilation. In contrast, Yimcharoen et al. found late strictures ≥90 days after RYGB less amenable to balloon dilations than early strictures occurring within 90 days post-operatively [79]. Successful dilations were performed in 98% of the early strictures (within 90 days) whereas only 62% of the late strictures – 63% after 90 days–1 year and 60% after 1 year – resolved with dilation. Ten patients (38%) required surgical revision, compared to only one in the early group. In the early group 23/46 (50%) required >1 dilation, and in both late groups 54 and 60% required >1 dilation, although this was not significant.

There may be a role for steroid injection following balloon dilation but there is no study in bariatric patients. In a multicentre randomised study, 60 untreated patients with a cervical anastomotic stricture after oesophagectomy with gastric tube reconstruction and dysphagia for at least solid food were randomly assigned to groups given saline (controls, $n = 31$) or four quadrant injections of 0.5 mL triamcinolone (40 mg/mL, $n = 29$) into the stricture, followed by Savary dilation to 16 mm in both groups [88]. The proportion of patients that remained dysphagia-free for 6 months was similar (45% of intervention group compared with 36% of controls). Median time to repeat dilation was not different, 108 days (range, 15–180 days) in the corticosteroid group versus 42 days (range, 17–180 days) for controls. Also the number of dilation was equal: a median number of 2 dilations (range, 1–7) was performed in the corticosteroid group versus 3 dilations (range, 1–9) in controls. The only difference was a *Candida* oesophagitis in four patients in the corticosteroid group, but in none of the controls.

6.4.2.2 Endoscopic Stenting

Treatment by stenting might be another option, but results are not easy to abstract from the studies because a variety of indications such as leaks, fistula and strictures are included and sometimes not discussed separately. The technique is similar. The area of leak, stricture or fistula is delineated endoscopically and marked either with a radiopaque marker on the skin or with contrast injected in the mucosa adjacent to the pathology. A flexible guidewire is passed through the endoscope down into the Roux limb. After removal of the endoscope, the stent is positioned over the guidewire across the leak or stricture. Repeat endoscopy is needed to confirm adequate proximal or distal coverage and to assess the need for placement of additional stents. Both nitinol silicone-covered and partially covered stents have been used. Refractory anastomotic strictures were defined as persistent strictures after >2 endoscopic dilations. Out of the 13 patients retrieved from 3 studies with refractory strictures only 5 patients (38%) achieved good results because some of these patients reported considerable pain asking for removal after 7–8 days without tolerating the stent for periods up to at least 8 weeks [89–91]. Migration was the most common complication, 58% in Eubanks's study with no differences between plastic and metallic stents, and migration required laparoscopic removal in two of the patients with strictures [92]. In Iqbal's study the migration rate was as high as 40% and by using longer and multiple overlapping stents their migration rate decreased to 27%, thus being able to approach the migration rate for oesophageal stents (24%) [90]. To prevent migration partially covered stents are also an option, but Wei et al., albeit not having any stent migration, discouraged the use of partially covered stent due to significant mucosal injury and difficulty of subsequent stent removal [91]. The solution of a fully covered stent, placed inside the partially covered stent to induce pressure necrosis of the ingrown tissue followed by removal of both stents, is a costly solution to the problem [93]. Puig and colleagues reported their results of endoscopic stenting in 16 patients with chronic anastomotic strictures (15 at the gastrojejunostomy after RYGB and 1 at the duodenoileal anastomosis after BPD-DS) [94]. Again, only 2 of 16 were successfully treated (12.5%). Of the remaining 14 unhealed strictures, 11 required surgical revision.

Analogous to other benign strictures the use of diathermy to create flaps and argon plasma coagulation to reduce the flaps may be considered, but this technique has not yet been investigated in anastomotic strictures in RYGB [95].

One should always exclude the presence of torsion or angulation of the stoma and marginal ulceration with oedema because in these cases failure of dilation and other methods may be predicted [55]. Similarly, the presence of a band in banded gastric bypass should be considered as a cause of obstructive symptoms (see under the heading of banded gastric bypass).

6.4.3 Internal Hernias

Internal hernias may be life-threatening because of the possibility of strangulation and perforation of bowel loops trapped within the hernia. Internal hernias are notoriously difficult to diagnose clinically or with radiographic imaging. The symptoms are typically episodic and can range from innocuous intermittent, colicky periumbilical pain and nausea to vomiting, anorexia and abdominal distension. Sometimes there is a dramatic acute presentation of peritonitis and septic shock. Often, gastroenterologists are consulted because of the unspecific presentation and sometimes an endoscopy is asked to rule out other causes. A more detailed discussion can be found in Chap. 5.

6.4.4 Gastrointestinal Haemorrhage

Similar to an acute bleeding situation in an average patient, where endoscopy should be performed to both diagnose and treat the bleeding source which is often an ulcer or oesophageal/gastric varices, in the bariatric patient the approach might be different (see also Chap. 5). The oesophagus and gastric pouch are within the reach of a normal endoscope but a usual endoscope is not at all useful for bleedings in the bypassed stomach and afferent limb in Roux-en-Y gastric bypass. Symptomatology may sometimes be helpful as haematemesis points more to a bleeding from the gastrojejunostomy, and melaena/haematochezia more to a bleeding from the jejunojejunostomy, gastric remnant or duodenum. An intraluminal bleeding is classically caused by a marginal ulcer. Sometimes, the bleeding is not manifest and the investigation of obscure GI bleeding or iron-deficiency anaemia is challenging in surgically altered anatomy. Deep enteroscopy by push enteroscopy or overtube-assisted enteroscopies such as double-balloon, single balloon or spiral or rotational enteroscopy are then needed. These will be discussed extensively under the heading problems related to the bypassed stomach and duodenum. Currently, there is only one case series by Skinner et al. that focused on the efficacy of double-balloon enteroscopy (DBE) to successfully identify and treat lesions responsible for obscure GI bleeding in the bypassed stomach [96]. They performed DBE 17 times in 12 patients with altered anatomy, 6 of them having a gastric bypass. Nine cases had overt bleeding and 3 had occult bleeding. In 10 of the 12 patients, the bleeding site could be identified with DBE. In nine, the bleeding site was at the anastomosis and once in the afferent limb. The stomach was found to be normal in nine of ten patients (90%), including five of six with gastric bypass. Endoscopic treatment was applied in eight patients, four patients required repeat endoscopy due to bleeding recurrence and there was one perforation requiring emergent surgery [96]. Treatment options available to achieve haemostasis in case of bleeding are thermal therapies (heater probe, mono- and bipolar electrocoagulation, argon plasma coagulation), injections with epinephrine and various sclerosants, haemostatic clips and fibrin glue. Finally, access to the excluded portion of the stomach and/or Roux limb can be facilitated through laparoscopic endoscopy via a surgically created gastrostomy, when traditional endoscopic techniques fail [97].

6.4.5 Dilation of the Gastrojejunal Anastomosis and the Gastric Pouch and Weight Regain

It is well recognised by bariatric surgeons that a certain weight regain occurs after obesity surgery compared to the lowest weight observed between 18 and 24 months after surgery. This regain mainly occurs between 2 and 5 years after gastric bypass. Studies comparing weight loss failure between 5 and 7 years after surgery, with losses of less than 50% excess weight, reported failure rates of 5–7% [98]. During the same follow-up period higher failure rates have been observed in superobese patients (BMI >50 kg/m^2) ranging from 20 to 33% [99, 100]. A prospective long-term follow-up study up to 60 months in 782 patients with a clear definition of surgical failure – defined as an excess weight loss ≤50% or BMI >35 kg/m^2 for patients with a preoperative BMI <50 kg/m^2 and BMI >40 kg/m^2 for patients with a preoperative BMI >50 kg/m^2 – showed a higher rate of surgical failure in the superobese versus the non-superobese group: 18.8% versus 11.0% [98]. Of those patients who failed, 60% never underwent nutritional follow-up, and 80% never underwent psychological follow-up. Some weight regain was observed in approximately 50% of the patients (46% within 24 months and 63.6% within 48 months) [98].

Studies that tried to find pathophysiological explanations for the inability to keep off the weight in the long term looked at ghrelin secretion with no differences between weight-stable and weight-gaining subjects [101, 102]. However, meal-induced secretion of glucose-dependent insulinotropic polypeptide (GIP) and glucagon-like peptide-1 (GLP-1) was higher in weight-stable and lower in weight-regaining subjects [101].

Other studies looked for anatomic explanations. Sometimes patients are referred for unexplained weight gain or increased volume tolerance, and upon endoscopy a dilated anastomosis or dilated pouch is discovered. Surgeons have long speculated that loss of restriction because of stoma dilation or pouch dilation is a significant contributing factor in failure and weight gain [103]. This has yet to be proven in large controlled trials but there are some recent indications pointing into the direction of stoma dilation. Yimcharoen et al. demonstrated that in 205 RYGB patients who were assessed for weight regain, stoma dilation was the most common anomaly in 58.9% of patients, an enlarged pouch in 28.8%, and both an enlarged pouch and stoma in 12.3% [104]. Abu Dayyeh et al. examined 165 RYGB patients by endoscopy because of symptoms and measured the stoma diameter and pouch length during this investigation [103]. Of these patients, 59% had significant weight regain (≥20% of maximum weight lost after the RYGB) and 41% did not. Gastrojejunal stoma diameter was significantly associated with weight regain after RYGB surgery, but the length of the gastric pouch was not associated with weight regain on both univariate and multivariate analyses. Also, time since surgery and presence of marginal ulcerations on endoscopy were predictive. A gastrojejunal stoma diameter of >15 mm was proposed to be the cut-off value for a dilated gastrojejunal anastomosis. They developed a simple prediction rule for weight regain after RYGB using a 7-point scoring system that includes the gastrojejunal stoma diameter (0 points when <15 mm, 2 points when 15–25 mm and 4 points when ≥25 mm), race (white 2 points, otherwise 0 points) and percentage of maximal body weight lost after RYGB (≤50% 0 points and >50% 1 points). A cut-off score of 4 or more points had a positive predictive value of 75% [103].

Heneghan et al. performed upper endoscopy in 380 patients 5.9 years after RYGB surgery [105]. They divided the patients into two groups: those who had maintained successful weight loss (>50% EWL or a BMI <30 kg/m^2) referred for GI symptoms and those who were referred for weight regain. Pouch and stoma were measured during endoscopy. A stoma >2 cm and a pouch >6 cm in length and >5 cm in width were considered enlarged. In the 175 patients with successful weight loss, the majority (63.4%) had normal pouch and stoma sizes. In contrast, this was the case in only 28.8% of the 205 patients with weight regain. Pouch length, pouch volume and stoma diameter were inversely related to weight loss, but in multivariate analysis only stoma size was independently associated with weight regain. A more recent study again compared 48 patients with weight regain (gaining of ≥20% of maximal weight lost after the RYGB) with 15 patients with no weight regain and showed that a dilated gastrojejunal stoma diameter is a risk factor for weight regain and uncontrolled eating behaviour [103].

When patient-related factors as an explanation for weight regain have been excluded or have been adequately addressed, revision surgery seems the only option. However, many studies have demonstrated a higher risk and higher morbidity after revision bariatric than primary bariatric surgery. For instance, Himpens et al. reported the results of revision surgery in 70 patients with weight regain or insufficient loss of weight more than 2 years after RYGB, of whom 58 patients had adequate follow-up [106]. Although the BMI decreased substantially from 39.1 to 29.6 kg/m^2 in 4 years, the rate of general complications was 20.7%, and the reoperation rate was 7.3%. The overall leak rate was 12.1%; patients suffering from leaks could be treated conservatively or by stent placement. Two patients needed reconversion after distal bypass. The BAROS score for quality of life was 3, which is considered a fair outcome, and the satisfaction index was good in 51.7% of the patients [106]. So, revision may not be the first choice but, unfortunately, the data are sparse in what is the best method to assist in further weight loss after "failed" RYGB.

Less invasive endoscopic treatments are available and should precede the utmost decision of surgical revision. These endoluminal options consist of endoscopic sclerotherapy, endoscopic suturing devices, clips and argon plasma coagulation [107] (Table 6.3). They all aim at reducing the stoma and/or pouch size.

6.4.5.1 Sclerotherapy of the Gastrojejunostomy

Sclerotherapy of the gastrojejunostomy with injections of sodium morrhuate (currently unavailable from commercial sources) was performed using a 25-gauge

Table 6.3 Endoscopic management of dilated gastrojejunal stoma and enlarged gastric pouch after RYGB. Endocinch and Stomaphyx are no longer available instruments

Author	Year	Method	No. of pts	Complications	Success rate (%)[a]	Remarks
Spaulding [108]	2003	Sclerotherapy	20	10% Vomiting	W6 75%	1.3 sessions/pt
Catalano [109]	2005	Sclerotherapy	28	1 Stenosis	W 64%	14.5 mL/session
Spaulding [110]	2007	Sclerotherapy	32	None	W12 90%	56.3% WL, 34.4% WS
Loewen [111]	2008	Sclerotherapy	71	1 Pain	W12 72%	13 mL/session; 49% >1 session/pt
Madan [112]	2010	Sclerotherapy	6	Mild nausea	W 50%	575 sessions; 16 mL/session
Abu Dayyeh [113]	2012	Sclerotherapy	231	14 Bleeds, 6 ulcers	W6 92% W12 78%	
Giurgius [114]	2014	Sclerotherapy	48	None	W 58%	52% >1 session/pt
Schweitzer[115]	2004	EndoCinch[b]	4	None	S: 25% reduced	1 repeat procedure
Thompson [116]	2006	EndoCinch+A	8	None	W 37%	2 stitches; 3 pt twice treated
Thompson [117]	2010	EndoCinch+A	77	1 Gastric tear	W 96% S: 89% <10 mm	4 stitches; NVC throat pain
Fernandez-Esparrach [118]	2010	EndoCinch	6	1 Haematemesis	C 100% S: 68% reduced	2 stitches
Ryou [120]	2009	IOP	5	None	W 100%	None
Mullady [121]	2009	IOP	20	1 Mild bleed, 1 nausea	W 85% S: 65% reduced P: 36% reduced	5 tissue plications; bloating, mild throat pain
Horgan [122]	2010	IOP	116	3 Oesophageal tears intraoper	W 86% S: 50% reduced P: 44% reduced	5.9 tissue plications; 41% pharyngitis, 12% nausea, 11% abdominal pain
Brengman [123]	2010	IOP	8	None	W12 100% S: 50% reduced P: 42% reduced	4.8 anchors
Borao [124]	2010	IOP	21	None	W6 86% S: 53% reduced P: 41% reduced	5.3 anchors; 1 failure

Raman [125]	2011	IOP	37	2 Stenoses	W6 92% S: 52% reduced	None
Gallo [126]	2015	IOP	26	None	W12 81% W24 62% S: 61% reduced P: 50% reduced	4 anchors
Mikami [127]	2010	StomaphyX[b]	39	None	W3 80%	17 H-fasteners; 87% sore throat, 77% epigastric pain
Leitman [128]	2010	StomaphyX	64	1 Bleed, 1 severe vomiting	W3 79% S: 59% reduced	23 H-fasteners; 65% epigastric pain, 50% need of iv drugs for nausea/vomiting
Ong'uti [129]	2013	StomaphyX	27	None	W6 67%	In follow-up weight regain
Goyal [130]	2013	StomaphyX	59	None	S: 46% reduced P: 80% reduced	21 H-fasteners, in follow-up weight regain and dilation
Eid [131]	2014	StomaphyX	45	1 Gastric perforation	W12 22% S: 50% reduced P: 86% reduced	2 bowel obstructions 1 hiatal hernia, 1 abdominal pain,1 vomiting, 1 bloody stools
Galvao Neto [132]	2011	OverStitch	8	1 Stenosis, 3 severe vomiting	W3 100%	100% technically successful
Jirapinyo [133]	2013	OverStitch	25	1 Oesophageal abrasion, 2 art. bleeds intraop., postop. 2 bleeds	W 90% S: 77% reduced	100% technically successful
Gitelis [134]	2015	OverStitch	25	None	W6 91% S: 78% reduced	100% technically successful, 3 sutures, 2 vomiting
Kumar [135]	2016	Overstitch	125	5 bleedings	W12 96% S: 63% reduced	6 abdominal pain, 3 nausea

EndoCinch+A: EndoCinch plus mucosal ablation; IOP: incisionless operating platform: Restorative Obesity Surgery Endoluminal (ROSE) procedure (USGI Medical, San Clemente, CA, USA), OverStitch: OverStitch suturing system (Apollo Endosurgery Inc., Austin, Texas, USA)

art. arterial, *intraop.* intraoperative, *post-op.* post-operative, *pt* patient, *NVC* nausea, vomiting, constipation

[a]Success defined as the % of subjects attaining W weight loss, W3 weight loss at 3 months, W6 weight loss at 6 months, W12 weight loss at 12 months; W24 weight loss at 24 months; success defined as % reduction in stoma size: S; success defined as % reduction in pouch size: P; WS weight stable; iv intravenous

[b]EndoCinch and StomaphyX are no longer available instruments

needle with 1–2 mL per site in blebs. Injection of a too large dose, indicated by dark red or black discoloration and subsequent overt bleeding, should be avoided. On average, a total of 10–30 mL was injected per session. A test dose of the sclerosing agent should be injected at the rim of the anastomosis, and the patient should be monitored for an adverse reaction and blood pressure elevation before further injection. A total of 1–3 injection sessions were performed in an attempt to achieve a stoma diameter of 12 mm or smaller. Parameters of success were weight loss or halted weight regain (Table 6.3) [108–135]. Catalano et al. had the best results with a weight loss of 22 kg in the 64% of successfully treated patients [109]. They selected patients with greater weight regain and used more aggressive sclerotherapy injections (14.5 mL per session) with injection until tissues turned deep purple. This aggressive approach resulted in higher rates of ulcers on repeat endoscopy (36%) which were healed within 8 weeks. Of their patients, 75% required pain medications. One patient experienced a stricture requiring two sessions of dilation [109]. In their experience anastomotic sizes larger than 15 mm did not benefit. Abu Dayyeh et al. treated 231 patients with 575 sclerotherapy sessions [113]. The median number of procedures per patient was two and the average volume of sclerosant per procedure 16 mL. After 8 months a weight loss of 4.5 kg (18% of the weight regained) was seen. At 6 and 12 months weight regain had stabilised in 92% and 78% of the cohort, respectively. Patients who underwent 2–3 sclerotherapy sessions had better weight regain stabilisation than those receiving a single-sclerotherapy session (90% vs. 58% at 12 months). Three patients developed abdominal pain (0.5%) and bleeding was reported in 14 (2.4%) requiring endoscopic clipping in 8. Small ulcerations were found after 6 procedures (1%) and transient diastolic blood pressure increases in 64 (15%). AbuDayyeh et al. also reviewed all published studies till 2012 which dealt with 157 patients with an average follow-up of 12 months [113]. Weight regain stabilised in 83%. The results by Giurgius et al. appear to be a bit more sobering, but in spite of these results they did not abandon the therapy but have become somewhat more aggressive with injection volume, follow-up evaluation and counselling for these patients [114]. Sclerotherapy is an easy and straightforward procedure with few complications. Its effectiveness is limited with moderate weight losses at short-term follow-up of 6–12 months. The effect may be transient in nature, but the procedure can be repeated.

6.4.5.2 Endoscopic Suturing

Endoscopic sutured revision of the dilated gastrojejunal anastomosis (GJA) and gastric pouch has been studied with suturing devices such as the Bard EndoCinch suturing system and the Apollo OverStitch Endoscopic Suturing System, developed from its predecessor the Eagle Claw suturing device (see also Chaps. 2 and 5). Also tissue approximation has been studied with devices such as the StomaphyX, a tissue approximation device which uses H-fasteners that can create full-thickness, serosa-to-serosa, endoluminal plications, and the multichannel incisionless operating platform, which is a modality that allows for endoluminal cutting, sewing, tissue manipulation and creation of tissue plications by anchors [10, 46, 59, 107]. Several factors such as device limitations, procedural complexity and need for specialised technical skills have limited a general adoption. The EndoCinch, StomaphyX and incisionless operating platform (IOP), which are not commercially available, and to a lesser extent the commercially available OverStitch are significantly complex and technically not easily feasible procedures. The many reports with their outcomes in reduction of stoma and pouch sizes and weight loss or halting of weight gain are summarised in Table 6.3.

The EndoCinch Suturing System (Bard Endoscopic Technologies, Billerica, MA, USA)

This suturing system consists of a hollow capsule that is fit onto the end of an endoscope and uses suction to pull tissue into the capsule. A hollow needle is used to pass the suture through the tissue suctioned in the capsule and the suture is then tied with a knot pusher. Several sutures can be placed. Of primary concern is the superficial nature of the bites which are mainly mucosal and submucosal and thus the durability of the plications (Table 6.3) [115–118]. In a multicentre, randomised sham-controlled study (Randomized Evaluation of Endoscopic Suturing Transorally for Anastomotic Outlet Reduction (RESTORe)), patients with inadequate weight loss, weight regain and a dilated stoma were randomly assigned in a 2:1 randomisation ratio to undergo EndoCinch reduction combined with mucosal ablation or sham treatment [117]. The stoma diameter had to be >2 cm and patients with a dilated pouch (length >6 cm and width >5 cm) as well as patients with a short pouch (<1 cm) and a short Roux limb (<30 cm) were excluded. Due to these requirements only 129 of 358 potential candidates could be enrolled in the study. The two most common exclusionary findings were a GJA less than 2 cm in diameter (32.8%) or the presence of a dilated gastric pouch (21.4%). Fifty-two subjects were enrolled in the lead-in phase, and 77 were enrolled in the randomised phase of the programme: 50 in the intervention group and 26 in the sham group instead of the calculated number of 88 and 44, respectively. Technical success, defined as the ability to reduce the GJA to 10 mm or less, was achieved in 89.6% of cases and a mean of four stitches were placed; 96% of the EndoCinch-treated patients achieved weight loss or weight stabilisation compared to 78% in the sham group ($p < 0.019$). The significantly higher weight loss in the intervention group resulted in improved diastolic and systolic blood pressure and improvement of metabolic parameters. After 6 weeks the stoma size was reduced with 39%, and at 6 months with 26%. Positive predictors for the outcome were a greater nadir weight loss and a greater weight regain since, and negative predictors were a high preoperative BMI, greater waist circumference and weight gain later in time post-operatively. Complaints of nausea, vomiting, throat pain and constipation were slightly higher in the sham group (41.4% vs. 37.5%), who had the same endoscopy exam as the intervention group. There was one gastric mucosal tear because the EndoCinch needle ensnared a staple from the anastomotic staple line. After 6 weeks one or more of the plications were visible at endoscopy; after 6 months this was the case in 76%. Fernandez-Esparrach et al. treated six patients with severe dumping thought to be related to a wide stoma; they reduced the gastrojejunal anastomosis from 23 to 8 mm with two stitches with symptom resolution in all for the follow-up duration of 2 years [118]. One patient suffered from haematemesis which was treated endoscopically. Thompson's group was able to compare superficial-thickness with full-thickness sutures in 59 historical patients treated with EndoCinch and 59 newly treated patients with the Apollo OverStitch [119], sequentially matched by gastrojejunal aperture size, then by BMI and then by age. All had dilated gastrojejunal anastomoses >20 mm. Post-intervention gastrojejunal apertures were similar (EndoCinch 6.9 mm vs. OverStitch 7.1 mm). One transfusion-requiring bleeding event occurred in each group. Weight loss was greater at 6 months in the OverStitch group (10.6 kg vs. 4.4 kg in the EndoCinch group; $p < 0.01$) and at 1 year (8.6 kg vs. 2.9 kg in the EndoCinch group; $p < 0.01$). This greater weight loss was attributed to the more accurately placed, more durable sutures, with less tissue compliance and less trauma and inflammation in the OverStitch group. Unfortunately, endoscopic data were not available.

The Incisionless Operating Platform (IOP) (USGI Medical Inc., San Clemente, CA, USA)

The incisionless operating platform has been used extensively in a procedure called ROSE (Restorative Obesity Surgery Endoluminally) for stoma reduction after RYGB (Table 6.3) [120–126]. The incisionless operating platform includes the transport multilumen platform, with one channel for the endoscope and three operating channels, the g-Prox Grasping/tissue approximation device, g-Cath tissue anchor delivery catheter and a variety of tissue graspers. The tissue-grasping device enables large, full-thickness tissue bites. Tissue approximation is feasible at the gastrojejunostomy to reduce the outlet and within the pouch to reduce pouch volume. The largest multicentre study is by Horgan et al. and included 116 patients [122]. At least one anchor was successfully placed in 97% of cases. The four failures were due to anatomic limitations or device malfunction. There were three mild oesophageal tears, all asymptomatic with one requiring a clip as a precaution. The stoma and the pouch diameter and pouch length were reduced by 50 and 44%, respectively. At 6 months 97 patients had lost 6.5 kg, 32% of the weight previously regained. The weight regain was stopped in 88% of patients at 6 months. The 3-month endoscopy confirmed the presence of anchors and tissue folds in 94% of patients ($n = 83$). The most common complaints were pharyngitis in 41%, nausea/vomiting in 12% and abdominal pain in 11%. On a patient level, predictive for the 6 months weight loss outcome was the pre-ROSE BMI (negative) and the % excess weight loss (EWL) after RYGB (positive). On a group level, the number of anchors placed, the % EWL after RYGB, the pre-ROSE pouch length and female age >50 predicted outcome of weight loss at 6 months. A 12-month follow-up showed the weight loss in 73 patients to be 5.9 kg [136]. Of these 73, 73% had no weight gain after the procedure and 70% had weight loss; 33% achieved ≥20% additional EWL. Anchors were present in 61/66 (92%). So, their outcomes after 12 months showed that the results were durable with no long-term adverse events and that stoma repair to a diameter of less than 10 mm was related with greater sustainable weight loss [136]. Adequate visualisation and working space facilitate success, as demonstrated by Mullady et al.: two of the three failures were due to once a long but narrow and tubular pouch with little space and the second had a short and relatively small pouch of 5 cm with less manipulation possibility [121]. Authors advise not to start the first procedure in eccentric stomas and short pouches. Brengman et al. suggest pouch lengths to be greater than or equal to 4 cm to allow adequate room for use of the IOP instrumentation [123]. Gallo et al. reviewed their experience in 26 patients over time. Initially a good result with a 50% reduced pouch and 61% reduced stoma size was seen with a good weight loss [126]. In follow-up, a total of 12 (46%) and 7 (28%) patients underwent an endoscopy at 3 and 12 months post-operatively. The mean pouch length and stoma diameter were still reduced but less than before with 26.5% and 42.9% reduction at 3 months and 10% reduction and 4.7% increase at 12 months, respectively. All anchors were present in 11 (91.6%) at the 3-month and 6 (85.0%) of patients at the 12-month endoscopy [126].

The StomaphyX (Endogastric Solutions Inc., Redmond, WA, USA)
The StomaphyX is a tissue approximation device. It uses H-fasteners that can create full-thickness, serosa-to-serosa, endoluminal plications. It is used over a normal endoscope. The mechanism of action of the StomaphyX is the approximation and immobilisation of two or more serosal surfaces through tissue fastening utilising 7 mm, 3.0 polypropylene H-fasteners. The fastener leads to a desired mild foreign-body reaction without tissue ischaemia. The results are shown in Table 6.3 [127–131]. Mikami et al. treated 39 patients being successful in 80% after 3 months with many complaints of a sore throat (87%) and epigastric pain (77%) in the first days [127]. Leitman et al. treated 64 patients with diverse symptomatology of dumping ($n = 42$), severe GORD ($n = 15$) and weight gain ($n = 7$) [128]. Improved symptoms were observed in 100% of the dumping and 80% of the GORD patients with complete solving of the problem in 71% and 20%, respectively. In 79% of patients weight regain was halted. Apart from one bleeding and one severe vomiting, also here complaints were often: 65% complained of epigastric pain and 50% needed intravenous medication to alleviate nausea and vomiting. Ong'uti et al. treated 27 patients [129]. Of these 27, 3 were lost to follow-up. Eleven subjects had their lowest weight at 1–3 months, 7 at 6 months, 3 at 9 months and 3 at 12 months. Eighteen patients had ≥6-month follow-up and 13 (72%) experienced an increase in weight after achieving their lowest weight after gastric plication. Twelve of the 14 (86%) with 12-month follow-up had regained weight after achieving their lowest weight after the plication [129]. Also, Goyal found that the loss of regained weight decreased over time and was only 1.7 kg and 4.3% EWL after 41 months [130]. Moreover, in 12 patients a repeat endoscopy was performed at an average follow-up of 18 months. These 12 patients had an average pre-procedure stoma size of 21 mm and pouch volume of 119.5 cc that were reduced to 12.3 mm and 24.8 cc, respectively, at the end of the procedure. Eighteen months later, the average stoma and pouch sizes were found to be 22.6 mm and 110.4 cc, respectively [130]. Eid et al. designed a 1-year study with 120 patients in their centre and 30 patients in a second centre to be randomized 2:1 to multiple full-thickness plications within the gastric pouch and stoma using the StomaphyX device with SerosFuse fasteners or a sham endoscopic procedure [131]. The hypothesis was that only 15% of the sham group and at least 50% of the intervention group would achieve a meaningful weight loss, defined as their primary efficacy endpoint (pre- to

post-StomaphyX decrease of ≥15% excess BMI loss and BMI <35 kg/m^2). The study was closed prematurely because preliminary results indicated failure to achieve the primary efficacy endpoint: at month 12 meaningful weight loss was obtained by only 10 of 45 patients (22.2%) after the StomaphyX and by 1 of 29 patients (3.4%) after the sham procedures ($p < 0.01$). StomaphyX successfully reduced pouch and/or stoma size in 53 of 55 treated patients (96.4%) with a median reduction in pouch size of 85.5% and in stoma size of 50.0% [131].

After gastric plication a maximal effective weight loss was seen in the first 6 months, beyond which most patients experienced weight gain. So, apparently, the effect of the StomaphyX is maximally for 6 months and the lack of sustained weight loss might be due to the fasteners not being durable in reducing the size of the pouch and the GJA. A disadvantage is that the device cannot be used in gastric pouches with a large fundus: the endoscope has difficulties in reaching that area because the instrument is too rigid and too large.

The OverStitch Endoscopic Suturing System (Apollo Endosurgery, Inc., Austin, Texas, USA)

The OverStitch Endoscopic Suturing System is developed from its predecessor the Eagle Claw suturing device. It is a cap-based suturing system that mounts onto a double-channel endoscope. A curved needle deploys both running and interrupted, full-thickness sutures under direct view which are secured with a Cinch device. The technique does not rely on suction for tissue acquisition as required by previous devices and appears to allow a greater depth of penetration than other suturing devices. The OverStitch system not only allows placement of sutures around the GJA, which are then tightened to reduce the anastomotic aperture, but is also able to create full-thickness tissue plications in the gastric pouch, which provides further volume reduction. It is currently the only available endoluminal suturing device on the market (Table 6.3) [132–135]. Galvao Neto et al. treated eight patients with pre-procedure stoma size varying from 20 to 40 mm (mean 25 mm) [132]. Seven patients had three stitches applied, reducing the stoma size to 10 mm in diameter. In one patient, the stoma size was reduced to 15 mm. The four patients that were followed for 90 days achieved weight loss from 6 to 8 kg with a 28% loss of regained weight. No post-operative complications were recorded. Jirapinyo et al. treated 25 patients with the OverStitch system and also ablated the tissue at the rim of the anastomosis using argon plasma coagulation [133]. They achieved a technical success, defined as achieving a gastrojejunal anastomosis of less than 12 mm, signifying a 77.3% reduction in GJA size, in all patients. In their series, 91% (21/23), 90% (17/19) and 89% (16/18) of the patients experienced weight loss at 3, 6 and 12 months, respectively. The mean weight loss in successful cases was 11.5 kg (63.8% of weight regain lost), 11.7 kg (69.5% of weight regain lost) and 10.8 kg (56.3% of weight regain lost) at 3, 6 and 12 months, respectively. During the 25 procedures, there were three intra-procedural events: a small oesophageal abrasion from the overtube and two arterial bleeding after stitch placement, which were managed endoscopically. Additionally, there were six post-procedural events: one haematemesis on post-procedural day 1 and one delayed gastrointestinal bleeding, both treated conservatively. Four patients reported post-procedural nausea and emesis, two of whom had severe emesis. One of these four patients revealed a stenosis of the GJA and required balloon dilation [133]. Kumar et al. reviewed their 150 patients with a follow-up of 3 years and had good weight loss results [135]. They could calculate the number needed to treat: the number needed to treat for arrest of weight regain was 1.0 at 6 months, 1.1 at 1 year and 1.2 at 2 and 3 years. The number needed to treat to maintain a weight loss of ≥5 kg was 1.2 at 6 months, 1.5 at 1 year, 1.9 at 2 years and 2.0 at 3 years. The number needed to treat to maintain a weight loss of ≥10 kg was 2.0 at 6 months, 2.3 at 1 year, 2.9 at 2 years and 2.4 at 3 years [135].

6.4.5.3 Endoscopic Clipping

Over-the-scope clips (OTSC) (Ovesco, Tübingen, Germany) are mounted on a transparent applicator cap placed on the tip of an endoscope (see also Chaps. 2 and 5). The assembly and deployment system are very similar to the system used for variceal banding. The cap is mounted on the tip of the endoscope and a thread is guided through the working channel of the endoscope outwards by the thread retriever. The thread is attached to a wheel-operated deployment device inserted into the access port of the working channel of the endoscope. The region of interest is suctioned into the cap, and the nitinol clip (an alloy of nickel and titanium) is closed and released by tightening the thread with the hand wheel. To facilitate the approximation of the edges, especially when the tissue is indurated, two dedicated accessories, the OTSC Twin Grasper and the OTSC Anchor Grasper, are available. The Ovesco Twin Grasper has two jaws that move separately to approximate the edges of the gastrointestinal tract wall before applying suction. The Ovesco Anchor Grasper has three retractable hooks, which facilitate approximation of the margins of the tissue before suctioning. Moreover, according to the characteristics of the tissue, three different clips are available: the clip may have blunt teeth for less traumatic compression of fresh lesions, spiked teeth for rather thick and fibrotic tissue, and long and sharp teeth to close the perforation or fistula of the bowel wall. In 2011 Heylen et al. reported the results in 94 patients with dilated gastrojejunostomy and 10% weight gain [137]. The stoma diameter was reduced from 35 to 8 mm, a reduction of 80%. Five had post-procedural dysphagia; two had to be dilated. Weight loss at 1 year was remarkable and at least 29% of the clips were still attached to the pouch outlet.

6.4.5.4 Argon Plasma Coagulation

Recently, Baretta et al. reported their result in 30 patients that were treated with argon plasma coagulation (APC), in 3 sessions, each 8 weeks apart [138]. APC is a noncontact electrocoagulation method in which radiofrequency energy is applied to the tissue by means of ionised argon gas with a potency of 90 Watts and an argon flow of 2 L/min. The entire circumference of the gastrojejunal anastomosis is treated with a distance from the point of the catheter up to the mucosa of 3–5 mm. The limited depth of tissue penetration of 2–3 mm can be enhanced by a higher power input in watts (90 Watts instead of 70 Watts), which then can affect even the muscular layer of mucosa. The patients lost 15.5 kg of the 19.6 kg of regained weight and the final anastomotic diameter was reduced by 67%. The interval of 6 weeks was prolonged to 8 weeks given the high incidence of anastomotic ulcers observed at the beginning. Severe stenosis (anastomotic diameter less than 3 mm) developed in two patients after the first session of APC. Seven transient ulcerations were noticed in five patients [138].

It is good to realise that most of the above-mentioned methods are either off-label use of medication such as sodium morrhuate or not approved by the FDA. The only techniques approved by the FDA for tissue apposition are the incisionless operating platform and the OverStitch [139]. Moreover, methods have to be standardised [136]. Some investigators used APC to ablate the 5–10 mm mucosa area around the margin of the gastrojejunal anastomosis with settings of 20 Watts [134] or 30 Watts [117, 119, 135], while others wanted also to expose the submucosa and abraded deeper with a cytology brush following the APC ablation [117]. Abidi et al. used a modified endoscopic submucosal dissection (ESD) technique to incise the mucosa surrounding the gastrojejunal anastomosis and to suture directly into the exposed submucosa and muscularis propria [140]. Also, mostly an interrupted stitching technique is used. Kumar et al. proposed a purse-string suture to reinforce the entire margin of the anastomosis against future dilation and to allow a more precise sizing of the final anastomotic aperture, avoiding excessive or insufficient restriction [141]. They proposed either a single- or double-running purse-string suture, which is started at the 11 o'clock position and is continued in a counterclockwise fashion, using a double-lumen endoscope. A dilation balloon is introduced through the second instrumentation channel. The balloon is inflated to a diameter of 8 mm inside the anastomosis. The purse-string suture is then tightened around the balloon and cinched.

If specialised equipment is not available or the endoscopist does not feel comfortable with using this high-tech devices, procedures such as sclerotherapy, over-the-scope clips and argon plasma coagulation are of low cost, easy to use and not dependent on further training of the endoscopist, and they are safe, rapid and associated with minimal side effects and complications. Also, they must know which risks surgeons would accept to incur. In a survey to assess the expectations of 214 bariatric surgeons by the American Society for Metabolic and Bariatric Surgery (ASMBS) Emerging Technologies Committee 76% of physicians were willing to accept the risk equal to or less than a therapeutic endoscopy and 25% of surgeons indicated to expect a 10–20% EWL, 37% a 20–30% EWL, and 23% a 30–40% EWL [142]. A total of 58% of physicians would not recommend endoluminal procedures until efficacy has been established, regardless of the risk [142].

6.4.6 Fistula

A fistula is defined as abnormal communication between two epithelialised surfaces. After bariatric surgery, gastrogastric fistulae, enterocutaneous fistulae and gastrobronchial fistulae may be the result of an anastomotic leak or occur after staple-line dehiscence. An anastomotic leak is a disruption at a surgical anastomosis resulting in a fluid collection with or without evidence of extravasation of contrast medium on radiologic evaluation. As such, the term gastric fistula is misleading, mostly referring to the result after an anastomotic leak, with a track with only one opening. The combination of endoscopy and radiological fluoroscopy is a reasonable option in case of fistulae both for diagnosis and for treatment [143]. The fistula should be intubated with a catheter from the inside by the endoscopist and water-soluble contrast medium should be applied in order to visualise the fistula tract. It is crucial to assess the length and the course of the fistula in order to plan and determine the most likely successful therapeutic course of action [143].

6.4.6.1 Gastrogastric Fistula and Staple-Line Dehiscence

After staple-line failure a leak develops with an abscess which then drains into the distal stomach forming the gastrogastric fistula: a communication between the proximal gastric pouch and the distal gastric remnant. These fistulas are more likely to be "true fistulas" of an inflammatory nature. A gastrogastric fistula may also be a technical complication from the incomplete division of the stomach during the creation of the pouch [144]. Many other putative mechanisms of gastrogastric fistula formation have been mentioned such as mucosal damage due to gastric acid and pepsin, marginal ulceration, perforation of the pouch or the remnant stomach, mucosal erosion from a foreign body or migrating staples, and anastomotic stricture leading to distension and increased pressure within the gastric pouch [145].

Capella and Capella beautifully described their experience in reducing the gastrogastric fistula risk in their banded gastric bypass procedure [31]. In the first 272 cases, they stapled the pouch in continuity which led to an unacceptable rate of staple-line disruption (49%). In the next 217 operations, the gastric segments were stapled and transected and the staple line of the excluded stomach was inverted with a running suture. The incidence of staple-line disruption and gastrogastric fistula fell to 2.6%. In the following 777 patients they transected the stomach, and interposed a limb of jejunum between the pouch and the excluded stomach, and this virtually eliminated the problem of gastrogastric fistula [31]. Some have warned against advocating to divide the stomach rather than stapling in continuity to avoid this complication, because in this situation, when the staple line breaks, the risk is to develop a clinically significant leak rather than a benign gastrogastric fistula [4].

Early symptoms may mimic those of a leak or perforation including fever, tachycardia, abdominal pain, tachypnoea and shoulder pain. Failure to lose weight, epigastric pain due to the exposure of the pouch to acid or presence of a marginal ulcer is a late clinical sign. Barium contrast radiography is the preferred initial study for the detection of staple-line dehiscence [3]. At endoscopy a dehiscence is frequently small and easily overlooked and they may have an endoscopic appearance similar to that of a diverticulum. Large dehiscences are identified easily and may permit passage of the endoscope into the bypassed stomach and duodenum.

Patients with a gastrogastric fistula are usually treated with a 6–8-week course of high-dose PPIs and sucralfate and avoidance of NSAIDs and then undergo repeat endoscopy. This course of medical management has been shown to result in symptom resolution in 37% of patients who experience this complication [146]. Failure to document improvement in gastrogastric fistula after 3 months is an indication for surgical therapy or endoscopic treatment. Similar options as have been discussed previously in leaks and fistulae are applicable (Chap. 5). In most cases a combination of treatments is given, not so much guided by an algorithm or by guidelines, which are not available, but more by the experience and preference of the endoscopist. In many cases argon plasma coagulation or debridement with a biopsy forceps is applied to the mucosa surrounding the opening of the fistula in an attempt to ablate the mucosa before tissue approximation. This was thought to promote fusion of the apposed tissue.

Endoscopic Stenting

There are only a few reports on stenting in fistulas. Yimcharoen et al. treated 18 patients with stents, with an overall failure of 28%; among them there was 1 patient with a gastrogastric fistula and 1 with an enterocutaneous fistula and only the latter closed successfully [89]. Iqbal et al. had 4 patients with fistula among the 26 patients treated with stenting [90]. Overall, stent migration occurred in 40% and treatment failed in 15% of these 26 patients. Three of the four patients had a successful closure. One of these four patients needed a laparoscopy to retrieve the migrated stent [90].

Endoscopic Clipping

Clipping the fistula has been tried with through-the-scope (TTS) endoclips and with the over-the-scope clips (OTSC). Bhardwaj et al. first removed any foreign materials like sutures or staples and then debrided the fistulous margins using a cold biopsy forceps or ablated using argon plasma coagulation (APC) to ensure the exposure of submucosa [145]. The fistula was then repaired with Resolution endoclips (Microvasive Endoscopy, Boston Scientific Corp, Natick, MA, USA), starting at the proximal and distal edges of the fistula, followed by additional clips in the middle. The size of the fistula was small (<20 mm). Immediately after the intervention all eight gastrogastric fistulae were closed but repair has remained successful in only four patients (50%) at 8–46-month follow-up [145]. Both the Natural Orifice Transluminal Endoscopic Surgery (NOTES) studies and clinical studies indicated that the lack of reliability of TTS endoclips for closure is due to various reasons [146, 147]. The largest distance between the tips of a fully open TTS endoclip is about 11 mm, limiting its use to only small defects. Also, due to the small depth of bite with TTS endoclips, one cannot achieve a full-wall-thickness repair. Moreover, simple closure with TTS endoclips may not provide a high enough mean burst pressure in the hollow viscus. In contrast, over-the-scope clips (OTCS) (Ovesco, Tübingen, Germany) can capture a large amount of tissue, deliver a compression force of approximately 8–9 Newton when released and compress the lesions until the wall defects have healed. The clips are available in three sizes and, according to the characteristics of the tissue, a clip with blunt teeth for less traumatic compression of fresh lesions, spiked teeth for rather thick and fibrotic tissue, and long and sharp teeth to close the perforation or fistula of the bowel wall can be chosen [147]. There are no data specifically related to gastrogastric fistula but there are three reports on fistula in general with sometimes bariatric patients included. A retrospective review of 47 patients who underwent OTSC placement to close chronic fistulas demonstrated a high initial technical success rate (42/47 patients, 89%), which was defined by a lack of contrast extravasation immediately after OTSC placement [148]. At a median of 39 days, a recurrent fistula, defined by the recurrence of symptoms and/or re-demonstration of fistula by the presence of contrast extravasation after initial success, occurred in 19/41 (46%) patients. Only 25/47 (53%) patients followed for a median duration of 178 days demonstrated long-term clinical success. Winder et al. identified 22 patients with 28 defects (22 fistulae and 6 leaks) and 54.5% were related to a bariatric procedure [149]. The majority of defects involved the upper GI tract (82%) and had been present for >30 days (50%). In 50% of patients the tissue around the fistula opening was ablated with APC. The success rate was 76% for fistulae at a median follow-up of 4.7 months. The median number of attempts at endoscopic closure in successfully treated fistulae was 1. Finally, a large multicentre international review by Haito-Chavez et al. studied 188 patients with acute perforations, leaks and fistulae who were treated with the OTSC system [150]. Twenty-two patients had bariatric surgery. Fistulae were present in 108 patients. Technical failure occurred ten times with six times in patients with a fistula. The tissue was too fibrotic to be grasped. Immediate post-treatment closure was present in 82.4% of the 91 fistulae and long-term closure after a median of 222 days, only in 42.9% (31/91) [150].

Endoscopic Suturing

The EndoCinch suturing system (Bard Endoscopic technologies, Billerica, MA, USA) was used by Thompson et al. and Fernandez-Esparrach et al. [151, 152]. Thompson et al. achieved complete closure of a gastrogastric communication in six out of eight patients with a combination of endoscopic suturing, haemoclips and argon plasma coagulation [151]. The mean size was 2.1 cm. Three plications and two haemoclips were used. It is important to notice that treatment failed in two patients because of impossible instrument retroflexion. Fernandez-Esparrach et al. compared the endoscopic repair by the endoscopic suturing system in 71 patients or by endoscopic clips in 24 patients using a mean of 2.2 sutures or 3 clips [152]. Also argon plasma coagulation and Tisseel fibrin glue (Baxter, Deerfield, IL, USA) were used: in the EndoCinch group fibrin glue in 59, APC in 63 and clips in 14; in the clip group APC was used in 9 and fibrin glue in 15. The mean size of the gastrogastric fistula was significantly larger in the suturing group (14.5 mm) than in the clip group (7.7 mm). In eight patients, the EndoCinch system could not be applied due to angulation and tissue characteristics. Gastrogastric fistula closure was achieved in 90 (95%) patients but reopening occurred in 59 (65%) after a mean of 177 days. Of these, 28 underwent repeat endoscopic treatment but 20 presented again with a recurrence. Final and durable closure could be achieved in 14/73 (19%) in long-term follow-up of a mean of 395 days. There was no difference in closure as to the methods used (EndoCinch 17% vs. clips 24%) [152]. None of the gastrogastric fistula with initial size >20 mm remained closed in contrast to 10/31 (32%) of those with a size ≤10 mm. Two significant complications were reported: a bleeding treated endoscopically and oesophageal tear and possible oesophageal perforation, treated with clips.

The StomaphyX (Endogastric Solutions Inc., Redmond., WA, USA) was successfully used by Leitman et al. in four gastrogastric fistulae [128]. Raman et al. have reported the closure of three gastrogastric fistula using the incisionless operating platform (IOP) (USGI Medical Inc., San Clemente, CA, USA) [125].

The tissue apposition system (TAS) (Ethicon Endo Surgery, Cincinnati, OH, USA) refers to the use of T-tags or T-anchors similar as those used in the placement of gastrostomies but now adapted for use through the endoscope. The tissue anchor consists of a monofilament, non-resorbable, polypropylene thread fixed to a stainless steel anchor element. The tissue anchor is loaded into the T-tag applier, a hollow needle attached to a plastic sheath with a stylet to eject the T-tag. Before apposition the mucosa surrounding the orifice of a fistula is ablated by using needle-knife cautery, snares and hot/cold biopsy graspers. A T-anchor is placed on one side of the fistula and after removal of the T-tag applier, leaving the thread behind in the instrumentation channel, a newly loaded T-tag applier is introduced and placed on the opposite site. Over the two threads the knotting element, consisting of an implantable polymer, is delivered by a knotting element applier. Four patients with five gastrogastric fistula were treated [153]. The diameter of the fistula was 18.6 mm (range 10–30 mm). The primary closure rate of the gastrogastric fistula after one endoscopic session was 100% (5/5). After 3 months, only the smallest fistula (10 mm) was still completely closed, and after 6 months it opened up as well, thus giving a 20% success rate at 3 and 0% at 6 months.

Flicker et al. wondered whether endoscopic attempts to close gastrogastric fistulas might interfere with subsequent surgery. They reviewed their large series of gastrogastric fistula: 35 cases of whom 22 had attempted endoscopic closure by clips and sutures before surgical revision whereas 13 went directly for surgical revision [154]. In the endoscopy group two minor and seven major complications (40.9%) occurred whereas in the surgery group three minor and three major complications (46.1%) occurred. So, prior attempts to endoscopically close gastrogastric fistulae did not lead to increased surgical complications when surgical revision was indicated.

6.4.6.2 Gastrocutaneous Fistula

Gastrocutaneous fistulas along the vertical staple line of the gastric pouch are usually treated with wound drainage, nutritional support, antibiotics and acid suppression. This may be ineffective in one-third of patients. Eubanks et al. had two patients with a gastrocutaneous fistula in their series of covered stents but only one was treated successfully [92]. Closure with tissue sealants may be attempted. SurgiSIS (Wilson-Cook, Winston-Salem, NC, USA) is an acellular fibrogenic matrix from the porcine small intestinal submucosa that stimulates proliferation and formation of fibroblasts in the region of wounds and stimulates scar formation with minimum inflammatory reaction and no rejection. SurgiSIS is available in strips and in cone-shaped plugs. Strips of SurgiSIS can be placed into the fistula by dragging the strips with a polypectomy snare on the outside of the endoscope into the fistula, or by a rendez-vous procedure where via the endoscope a polypectomy snare is brought outwards through the fistula. After mounting the plug into the snare the snare is moved inwards, thereby pulling the cone into the fistula until it occupies the entire fistulous tract. Maluf-Filho et al. reported a successful closure of the fistula with SurgiSIS, after 1 session in 6, after 2 applications in 11, and 3 applications in 3, so in a total of 20/25 patients (80%) [155]. The gastrocutaneous fistula ranged from 5 to 20 mm in diameter. Using cone-shaped matrix, fistula closure was accomplished after a single session in all patients. This may be related to better deployment and better packing of the fistula using the cone-shaped biomaterial. Toussaint et al. only used SurgiSIS plugs (Cook Biotech Inc., West Lafayette, Indiana, USA) in two patients with RYGB and three patients with sleeve gastrectomy and achieved healing in four of the five (80%) enterocutaneous fistula with a median follow-up of 18 months [156]. They first abraded the fistulous tract under endoscopic and fluoroscopic guidance using a stent pusher with multiple barbs passed over the guidewire to promote better wound healing.

6.4.6.3 Gastrobronchial Fistula

A review on the literature about gastrobronchial fistulas after bariatric surgery produced 11 studies, comprising a total of 36 patients [157]. Of the 36 gastrobronchial fistulae 67% occurred after a sleeve gastrectomy. Most patients, 15 in this review, presented with a gastric leak prior to the diagnosis of gastrobronchial fistula with a long mean period until diagnosis of 7.2 months. Treatment for the gastric leak was given such as a stents, percutaneous drainage or reoperation, but after this initial treatment patients started experiencing symptoms again. Due to its proximity to the respiratory tract, an abdominal infection from an upper gastric leak can result in a subphrenic abscess that may lead to a pulmonary abscess and gastrobronchial fistula. The morbidity rate is high, usually leading to a severe lung infection, and in this series a death occurred before any treatment was instituted [157]. The main presenting symptoms were productive cough (n = 13) and a subphrenic abscess (n = 12). Both endoscopic and surgical treatments have been evaluated. Endoscopic treatment was successful in 18 out of 20 patients (90%), with minimal complications: once a self-limited upper digestive haemorrhage and once a distal migration of stent, which was adjusted endoscopically. In two patients stents and fibrin glue failed and they went for surgery. Surgical treatment was successful in all 17 cases with significant and numerous complication such as 2 fistulas, 4 bleeds with transfusion, 3 infections and 1 intrathoracic anastomotic breakdown.

Part of this series were the ten patients after a gastric bypass and five after a sleeve gastrectomy treated by Campos et al. [158]. The principle of the treatment was the correction of both the distal stricture and high-pressure zone and the anatomic defect near the internal orifice of the fistula. The treatment consisted of a choice and combination of aggressive endoscopic balloon dilation with a 20 mm CRE or 30 mm Rigiflex balloon; stricturotomy with a microknife and subsequent 20 mm balloon dilation; gastric septoplasty to internally drain the abscess; and placement of a self-expandable plastic stent, mainly when the fistula size was >10 mm and/or a distal gastric stenosis was present [158]. The choice of the specific endoscopic intervention and their combination was based on the following variables: type of bariatric surgery, presence of a ring in banded gastric bypass or banded sleeve, location of the gastric stricture, presence of a perigastric abscess, and anatomy of the gastric pouch/sleeve and fistula. A mean of 4.5 endoscopic sessions per patient were needed but led to a 93.3% (14 out of 15) success rate in gastrobronchial fistula closure with an average healing time of 4.4 months, being shorter in the stent group. They continued the dilation every 30 days for a 3-month period, even in the absence of obstructive symptoms, and thus prevented the recurrence of the gastrobronchial fistula. They advised against the use of fibrin glue in this setting because it tends to fail in high intragastric pressure settings. Surgeons criticised the good results of Campos et al. by referring to the high number of gastric bypass cases in their study which are known to dry up more easily after a leak compared with sleeve gastrectomy leaks [159].

6.4.7 Banded Gastric Bypass

In gastric bypass surgery, there is no consensus on whether the placement of a silastic ring or band is beneficial or not. The ring seems to be related to long-term weight loss maintenance. Capella and Capella argued that especially from the third year after surgery when the dumping phenomenon disappears, the band becomes important [31]. After this time the pouch dilates, restriction at the anastomosis is no longer present and patients are able to ingest large amounts of food. They realised that restriction of the pouch at the level of the anastomosis with foreign material might result in intraluminal migration of the band, usually called band erosion. In their experience the incidence of band migration was very small when the band is placed over intact serosa, not stitched to the stomach and placed 1.5 cm proximal to the anastomosis. Band erosion and intractable vomiting may result from the presence of a band.

6.4.7.1 Band Erosion

Band erosion is a complication that may be caused by a too tightly placed band resulting in necrosis and erosion, suturing the band to the stomach, covering the band with the stomach, and infection [160]. The best diagnostic test of band erosion is endoscopic evaluation. Band erosion can be managed expectantly, by endoscopic band removal or by open surgical intervention. Endoscopic band removal is the treatment of choice, 16 bands were removed without a bleeding or a leak, 8 had spontaneous extrusion of the band and 26 had surgical revision [160]. Placement of a self-expanding metal-covered stent may facilitate band migration into the stomach and subsequent removal [161].

6.4.7.2 (Intractable) Vomiting

Vomiting may occur as a consequence of ring slippage, which can lead to gastric pouch outlet stenosis, but vomiting may also occur even when there is no gastric stenosis, due to the presence of the prosthesis, often requiring prosthesis removal. The study by Schwartz et al., referred to earlier, demonstrated the poor results of balloon dilation in patients who had their anastomosis banded with fascia lata to prevent late enlargement [64]. Stenosis occurred in 3.2% and balloon dilation was successful in only 62.5% with a perforation in four patients. The inexperience of the surgeon, the too aggressive dilation scheme and the foreign body material contributed to this disastrous outcome. Ferraz et al. included 63 patients presenting with more than four vomiting episodes per week in a prospective study [162]. Proven by upper digestive endoscopy vomiting was not related to gastric pouch outlet stenosis or ring slippage and a standard 9.8 mm endoscope could pass easily. Patients with a ring other than a silastic ring were excluded. Endoscopic dilation with an achalasia balloon was performed with the idea that this would promote either rupture or stretching of the thread running inside the silastic ring and thereby resolving patient's symptoms. The ring area in the gastric pouch was dilated up to 30 mm, using a Rigiflex® balloon (Boston Scientific, Natick, MA, USA), which was gradually inflated (maximum 20 psi) using a manometer (Figs. 6.2 and 6.3). When thread rupture or symptom resolution was not obtained after the first session, the procedure was subsequently repeated every other week up to four sessions, until symptoms resolved. Patients who still showed four or more vomiting episodes after four sessions were considered treatment failures and referred to surgery. Symptom improvement was reached in 61 cases: 59 (93.6%) demonstrated complete improvement and 2 (3.2%) had partial improvement. The two patients who failed to achieve improvement were referred for surgical ring removal by laparotomy. Four dilation sessions were performed in 12 patients (19%), three in 14 (22.2%), two in 24 (38%) and one in 13 (20.6%). Complications occurred in 9.5%, including three cases of bleeding and treated with adrenaline solution injection, two intragastric ring erosions treated by endoscopic removal using scissors and foreign-body forceps, and one pneumoperitoneum, observed clinically. The case of pneumoperitoneum and three cases of bleeding might have been avoided by firmly holding the balloon catheter in place as these complications were due to distal balloon slippage [162]. On the other hand, endoscopist should be aware that sometimes endoscopic findings are in discrepancy with the severity of complaints of patients. This was emphasised by Swain et al. who discussed the fate of six of their patients [163]. They suffered from nausea, vomiting, regurgitation and dysphagia to solids and liquids for a mean duration of 29 months. Previously, the patients had undergone multiple upper endoscopies (mean 4.2, range 3–6) and dilations (mean 1.3, range 1–2), without substantial relief of their symptoms. One patient also underwent multiple injections of Botox (Allergan, Irvine, CA, USA) without success. The endoscopist described the gastrojejunostomy as patent and of a normal size in five, with one showing a patent but narrowed anastomosis. However, in these cases, endoscopy is deceptive in judging the stomal size, because the endoscope can be pushed through the band area. Laparoscopic removal of the band of the banded gastric bypass relieved the symptoms immediately and appeared to be safe [163].

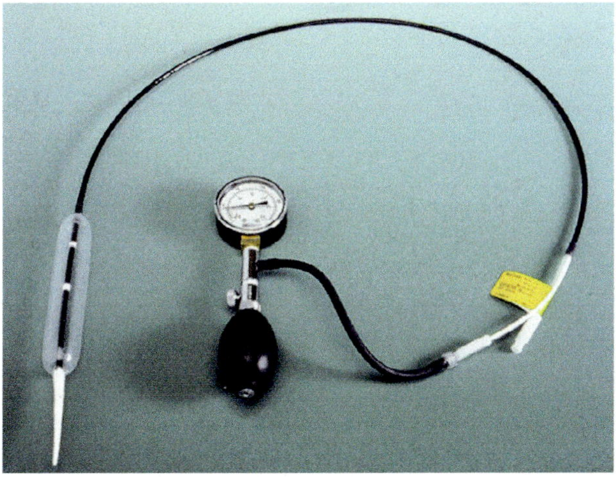

Fig. 6.2 Rigiflex achalasia balloon (Boston Scientific, Natick, MA, USA), which can be gradually inflated using a manometer. Reprinted from Surg Endosc 2017 DOI https://doi.org/10.1007/s00464-016-5385-9.247, Al Sabah S, Al Haddad E, Siddiqui F. Endoscopic management of post-laparoscopic sleeve gastrectomy stenosis, with permission from Springer

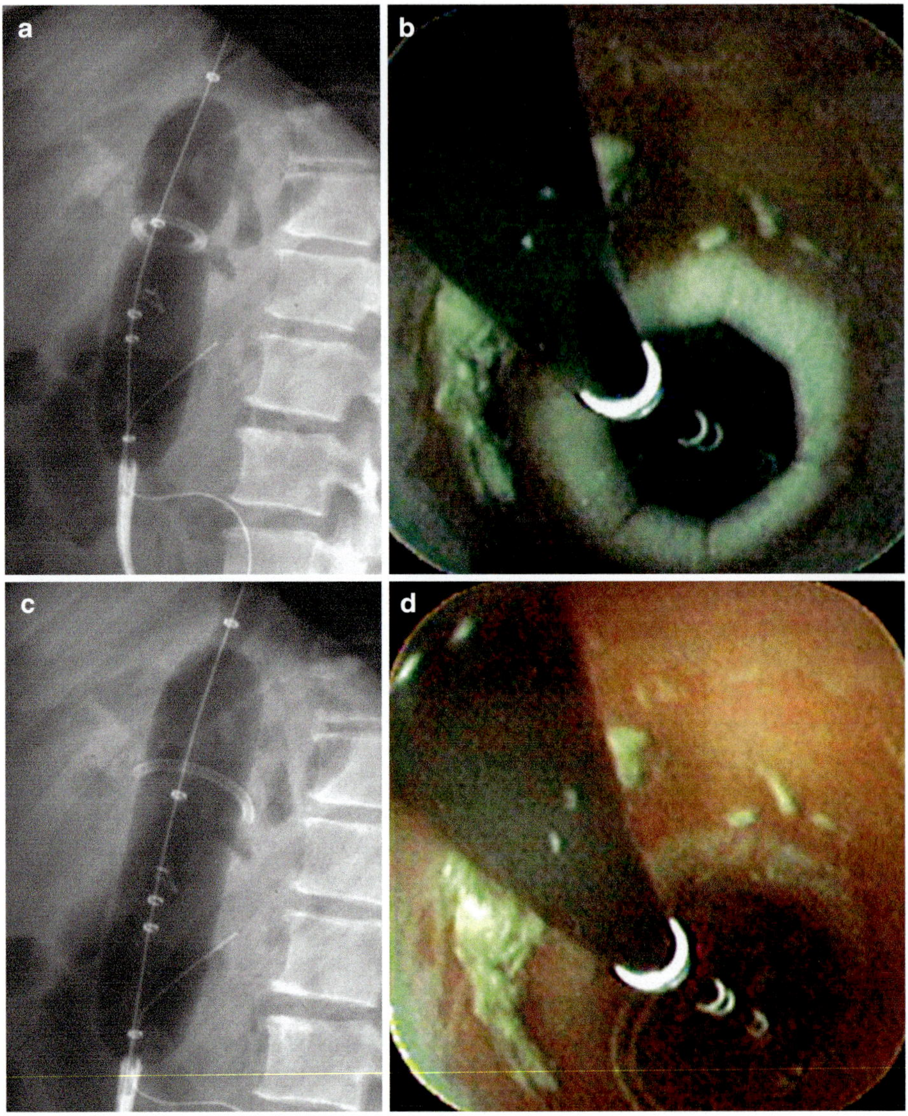

Fig. 6.3 (**a** and **b**) X-ray and endoscopic view of inflated Rigiflex balloon with compression by gastric band. (**c** and **d**) X-ray and endoscopic view evidencing the opening of the band after a few minutes of Rigiflex balloon dilation. Reprinted from Obes Surg 2013; 23: 959–964165, Ferraz A, Campos J, Dib V, Silva LB, de Paula PS, Gordejuela A, et al. Food intolerance after banded gastric bypass without stenosis: aggressive endoscopic dilation avoids reoperation, with permission from Springer.

6.4.8 Phytobezoar

Gastric bezoars are conglomerate masses of food or foreign matter in the stomach, and when formed from plant fibres such as cellulose, hemicellulose, lignin and fruit tannin, these are called phytobezoars [164, 165]. Patients with a gastric bypass are prone to develop phytobezoars due to poor mechanical breakdown of ingested solids that serve as a nidus for the formation of phytobezoars in the stomach, and related to the surgical bypass of the gastric antrum and body, the parts of the stomach responsible for breaking down ingested solids. Furthermore, hypoacidity, reduced gastric motility through the neuropeptide changes after the RYGB, i.e. GLP-1 and PYY, the relatively restricting gastroenterostomy together with a small gastric pouch may contribute. Also, poor mastication and intake of high-fibre and tannin-rich foods and especially persimmon and citrus piths are important as these can be addressed in trying to prevent this complication. Affected individuals may be asymptomatic or may present with a variety of symptoms, including epigastric pain, bloating, nausea, vomiting, early satiety, dysphagia, weight loss and upper gastrointestinal bleeding [164, 165]. Complications are gastritis, gastric ulcer, gastric perforation and small-intestine obstruction. Diagnosis is suggested with an upper gastrointestinal barium studies or computed tomography (CT) and confirmed with endoscopy. Barium studies show phytobezoars as mobile round to ovoid masses in the stomach that float in the barium pool and have a mottled appearance due to trapping of barium in the interstices of the lesion [166]. In their review of the literature Ben-Porat et al. found 15 cases of phytobezoar formation in the stomach [165]. Treatment options of gastric pouch bezoars include endoscopic fragmentation by waterjet fragmentation or lithotripsy by waterjet fragmentation or lithotripsy and removal, chemical enzyme therapy by papain, an enzyme extracted from the *Carica papaya* plant, also known as meat tenderiser, or surgery. Bezoars at the jejunojejunostomy or in other small-bowel locations require surgical intervention.

6.4.9 Dumping

As a result of the changed anatomy after surgery, ingested food immediately "dumps" into the jejunum facilitated by fluid ingestion during the meal. An estimated 45–75% of patients with gastric bypass may suffer from symptoms related to dumping [167–169]. There are two distinct forms of dumping with different symptomatology and pathophysiology: early dumping and late dumping which is also named post-bariatric hypoglycaemia (PBH) (Fig. 6.4). Early dumping begins within 30 min following a meal and symptoms are attributable to bowel distention, gastrointestinal hormone hypersecretion and autonomic dysregulation. Because of the sudden entry of high-voluminous, hyperosmolar and undigested food in the small bowel, an osmotic fluid shift from the intravascular compartment to the intestinal lumen results in gastrointestinal and vasomotor symptoms. Gastrointestinal symptoms are the result of bowel distension and increased contractility and consist of epigastric pain and fullness, nausea, vomiting, bloating, cramps, borborygmi and diarrhoea. Vasomotor symptoms such as the need to lie down, light-headedness, palpitations, hypotension, tachycardia, fatigue, dizziness, sweating, headache and flushing are the result of a reduction in plasma volume and a sympathetic compensatory reaction. The increased release of multiple gastrointestinal hormones and peptides, such as the vasoactive agents neurotensin, bradykinin, serotonin, substance P and vasoactive intestinal peptide [VIP]; the incretins gastric inhibitory polypeptide or glucose-dependent insulinotropic polypeptide [GIP] and glucagon-like peptide-1 (GLP-1); and the glucose modulators insulin and glucagon induce changes in the gastrointestinal motility and elicit haemodynamic effects [169].

Late dumping or post-bariatric hypoglycaemia symptoms occur within 90 min to 3 h after the meal ingestion and are explained by sudden nutrient exposure to the small intestine with insulin and incretin secretion disproportionate to the blood glucose level and with inhibition of glucagon secretion by GLP-1, which further enhances the hypoglycaemia. Additionally, increased sensitivity of pancreatic β-cells to glucose, reduced insulin clearance and insulin-independent glucose uptake may also contribute to hypoglycaemia. Symptoms are related to neuroglycopenia (fatigue, weakness, trouble with concentration, confusion, hunger and syncope) and autonomic/adrenergic reactivity (perspiration, palpitations, tremor and irritability) [169, 170]. Taking a good history is important and scoring systems such as the Sigstad scoring system to grade the dumping symptoms and the Arts's dumping-severity score to grade both early and late dumping symptoms are helpful although not validated for use in bariatric surgery [171, 172] (Tables 6.4 and 6.5). Often, a glucose tolerance test with the ingestion of 50 or 75 g of glucose in solution after an overnight fast is performed with measurements of blood glucose concentrations, haematocrit, pulse rate and blood pressure before and at 30-min intervals up

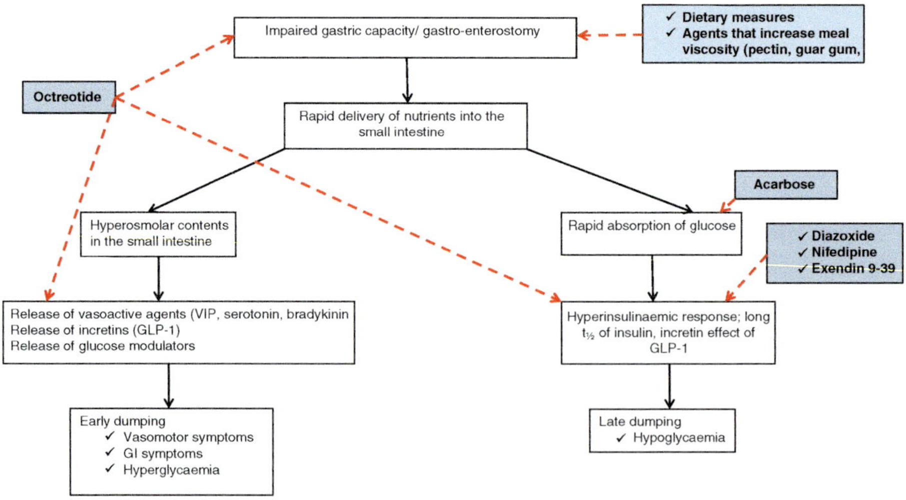

Fig. 6.4 Pathophysiology and points of therapeutic application in the early and late dumping syndrome. Modified and reprinted with permission of MacMillian Publishers Ltd. from Nature Reviews Gastroenterol Hepatol 2009; 6: 583–590, Tack J, Arts J, Caenepeel P, De Wulf D, Bisschops R. Pathophysiology, diagnosis and management of postoperative dumping syndrome

to 180 min after ingestion. The diagnosis of early dumping is positive if in the first 30 min the haematocrit increases by more than 3% or the pulse rate by more than ten beats per minute, the latter being regarded as the most sensitive indicator of early dumping [167, 168]. Late dumping is present when there is initial hyperglycaemia and final hypoglycaemia (<3.33 mmol/L) at 60–180 min post-ingestion. The sensitivity and specificity have been reported as high as 100% and 94%, respectively, but some prefer the mixed-meal tolerance test which is a more physiological representation and more analogous to what is happening in the everyday situation. It should be noted that hypoglycaemia is defined differently with some considering a cut-off of <3.3 mmol/L and others a value of <2.8 mmol/L as indicative of post-bypass hypoglycaemia [169]. Hypoglycaemia which also occurs in the fasting state should raise suspicion for autonomous secretion of insulin by an insulinoma or other hormonal or metabolic disorders.

Table 6.4 Sigstad score for dumping [171]

Symptom	Point(s)
Shock	+5
Loss of consciousness, fainting, syncope	+4
Desire to lie down	+4
Dyspnoea	+3
Weakness, physical fatigue, exhaustion	+3
Sleepiness, apathy	+3
Palpitations	+3
Restlessness, agitation	+2
Dizziness, vertigo	+2
Headache	+1
Warm clammy skin, sweating, pallor	+1
Nausea	+1
Abdominal fullness, distension	+1
Borborygmi	+1
Eructation	−1
Vomiting	−4

Points are given to each symptom, perceived by the patient postprandially [171]. These points are added to give the score. A score >7 suggests dumping, a score <4 suggests another diagnosis. The scoring system is also used to assess the response to therapy and to predict response to therapy. The higher the score the less likely the success of treatment

Table 6.5 Arts score with signs of early and late dumping, each scored on a Likert scale of 4 points with 0 = absent of symptom, 1 = mild, 2 = moderate and 3 = severe intensity of symptoms [172]

Early dumping symptoms	Late dumping symptoms
Sweating	Sweating
Blush	Tachycardia
Tachycardia	Hunger
Abdominal pain	Somnolence
Diarrhoea	Unconsciousness
Swelling	Tremor
Nausea	Irritability

The treatment and level and grading of evidence have been reviewed by van Beek et al. [169] (Fig. 6.4). Dietary modification (level of evidence: III; grade of recommendation: B) includes the consumption of small frequent meals, spaced 3–4 h apart, with a delay of fluid intake until at least 30 min after meals. To prevent late dumping symptoms simple and rapidly absorbable carbohydrates and foods with a high glycaemic index should be eliminated from the diet and low-glycaemic, high-fibre and protein-rich foods should be encouraged [173]. Dieticians often advise to control portions of carbohydrate: 30 g per meal and15 g per snack. In their experience, a 30 g carbohydrate meal may increase glucose ≈5.55 mmol/L (100 mg/dL), and a 15 g carbohydrate snack may increase glucose by ≈2.78 mmol/L (50 mg/dL) [173]. Patients should also eat slowly and chew well. An often forgotten advice is to avoid alcohol. During the metabolism of alcohol by the liver, the endogenous production of glucose by the liver is reduced, increasing the risk for hypoglycaemia [173]. The next step is dietary supplements (level of evidence: III; grade of recommendation: C) such as guar gum, pectin and glucomannan, which increase the viscosity of food and thereby slow the rate of gastric emptying and delay the absorption of glucose [169]. In case of late dumping acarbose (level of evidence: III; grade of recommendation: B) can be advised. Acarbose is an α-glucosidase hydrolase inhibitor. It slows carbohydrate digestion in the small intestine, thereby blunting the postprandial hyperglycaemia and subsequent hypoglycaemia. The last step in the medical treatment is the use of somatostatin analogues (level of evidence: II; grade of recommendation: A) that affects both early and late dumping by its effects of delaying gastric emptying, delaying transit through the small intestine, inhibiting the release of GI hormones, inhibiting insulin secretion, inhibiting the secretion of GLP-1 and inhibiting postprandial vasodilation. Surgical re-intervention (level of evidence: IV; grade of recommendation: C) and continuous enteral feeding, either via a nasojejunal tube, a jejunostomy or a PEG placed in the excluded stomach (level of evidence: V; grade of recommendation: D), are the last steps to be taken in intractable dumping syndrome in desperate patients.

In 2010 two important papers on endoscopic options were published. Reduction of the stoma by argon coagulation, Bard EndoCinch suturing and fibrin glue in six patients with intractable dumping resulted in complete and persistent resolution of the dumping in all and was maintained for 2 years [118]. The goal was to achieve a diameter <10 mm to delay gastric emptying. Before the procedure the pouch length was 5 cm and stoma diameter 23 mm. At least two interrupted stitches were placed and the stoma diameter reduced to 8 mm. One patient bled and had to be treated endoscopically. Leitman et al. treated 42 of 64 patients complaining of severe dumping with the StomaphyX device [128]. Symptom improvement was achieved in all and symptoms resolved in 30 patients (71%). However, a frequently observed side effect was nausea and vomiting which needed often intravenous medication.

6.4.10 Postprandial Hyperinsulinaemic Hypoglycaemia

In a position statement issued by the American Society for Metabolic and Bariatric Surgery (ASMBS) suggestions are given for the management of this rare but invalidating and even life-threatening condition [174]. To this purpose a systematic review of all currently available literature was accomplished. It is characterised by postprandial neuroglycopenic symptoms of weakness, fatigue, light-headedness, dizziness, altered levels of consciousness, confusion, slurred speech and visual disturbances in the presence of documented low blood glucose levels. Autonomic symptoms include anxiety, sweating, tremors and palpitations. The onset is late, between 6 months and even up to 8 years after bariatric surgery. It is a rare condition with an incidence between 0.1 and 0.36% [174].

In the past it was thought to be due to endogenous hyperinsulinaemia from increased β-cell mass and hyperfunctioning islet cells, also called nesidioblastosis, needed to compensate for the insulin resistance associated with morbid obesity. The restoration of insulin sensitivity post-surgery and therefore the decreased need of insulin did not keep abreast with a decrease in β-cell mass and function. Reasoning this way, treatment by partial or total pancreatectomy seemed logic. Most experts now agree that the occurrence of hyperinsulinaemic hypoglycaemia after bariatric surgery is related to alterations in glucose kinetics, changes in multiple glucose regulatory mechanisms and gastrointestinal and pancreatic hormone levels involved in glucose homeostasis, caused by the anatomic changes related to the RYGB. The physiologic counter-regulatory mechanism in response to hypoglycaemia may also be disrupted in post-RYGB hypoglycaemic patients. Two major players in this field are the postprandial increase in GLP-1, thought to be responsible for the major improvement in diabetes after RYGB but probably thereby also contributing to the postprandial hyperinsulinaemic hypoglycaemia, and glucagon, a counter-regulatory hormone against hypoglycaemia. GLP-1 inhibits the secretion of glucagon and α-cells fail to adequately increase the production of glucagon.

To make a definitive diagnosis of postprandial hyperinsulinaemic hypoglycaemia, a patient must have both symptoms and laboratory values that support the diagnosis (plasma glucose level <3.3 or <2.8 mmol/L and serum insulin >450 mU/mL with a corresponding increase in C-peptide). Typically, patients have a spontaneous return to euglycaemia after the hypoglycaemic episode and fasting glucose and insulin levels are normal. The treatments mentioned for the late dumping syndrome are also applicable here. Less well-proven but theoretically sound drugs may be tried in resistant cases such as nifedipine, a calcium channel blocker that reduces insulin secretion; diazoxide, an adenosine-triphosphate-dependent potassium channel agonist of β-cells that reduces insulin release; and exendin 9-39, a GLP-1 receptor antagonist. For the gastroenterologist, it is important to know that placement of a gastrostomy tube into the remnant stomach may provide symptomatic relief as well as nutritional support and should be considered in patients not responding to treatment advices described earlier. Surgery by placing a silastic ring or adjustable band to induce gastrojejunostomy restriction or even reversal of the operation is a major step to be taken when every treatment has failed. Partial pancreatectomy is not recommended [174].

6.4.11 Problems Related to the Bypassed Stomach and Duodenum

The distal stomach and the duodenum are not easily accessible for endoscopy because of the combined length of the oesophagus (25 cm), proximal gastric pouch

(5 cm), Roux limb (75–150 cm), biliopancreatic jejunal limb (35–70 cm), duodenum (20 cm) and excluded stomach (10–15 cm) with a total extension, therefore, in the range of 2–3 m. With specialised equipment the retrograde route can be used through the gastrojejunal anastomosis, Roux limb, enteroenterostomy and duodenopancreatic limb up to the bypassed stomach. The most common reason for failure to enter the bypassed stomach is the acute angulation at the jejunojejunal anastomosis and a too narrow gastrojejunal anastomosis for the passage of the endoscope. Also, a long Roux limb and limited mobility of the mesentery present difficulties. It is occasionally difficult to determine at the jejunojejunostomy which of the two segments is the afferent limb. Some investigators use the presence of bile and foam or bubbles and others the peristaltic movement – moving away from the endoscope suggests the presence in the efferent limb – as an indication of having entered the right limb [175]. Sinar et al. commented that the presence of contractions coming towards the endoscope is a superior afferent limb landmark than bile [176]. It might be wise to tattoo the entrance of the afferent limb at the way back on removal of the endoscope [177]. Retrograde endoscopy of the bypassed segments was first attempted by push enteroscopy, mainly with a paediatric colonoscope, being successful in 65–66%. Later, overtube-assisted enteroscopy came into the field and double-balloon enteroscopy (DBE), single-balloon enteroscopy (SBE) and spiral-overtube-assisted or rotational enteroscopy (SOAE) may be able to reach the excluded stomach in about 75%. When these studies fail to provide a diagnosis or treatment, it may be elected to get access to the stomach via a gastrostomy. Sometimes, surgeons may tag the stomach to the anterior peritoneal wall and place a radiopaque tubing around the gastrostomy during the Roux-en-Y procedure to enable convenient radiologic localisation for future percutaneous access.

6.4.11.1 Findings in the Excluded Stomach

Data on the excluded stomach after RYGB are scarce as the excluded stomach remnant is without the reach of a normal routine endoscopy. Sinar et al. investigated 51 patients 3–24 months after RYGB and successfully intubated the gastric remnant in 65% with a paediatric colonoscope (135 cm, outer diameter (OD) 11 mm) [176]. Failure was mainly due to the acute angulation at the jejunojejunostomy in 15 patients (28%) and in 3 because of a too narrow gastrojejunostomy [176]. They discovered a high incidence of bile-associated gastritis in 97% and intestinal metaplasia in 12%, apparently – and to their surprise – without symptoms. Safatle-Ribeiro et al. performed a double-balloon endoscopy at mean of 78 months after the RYGB procedure and reached the stomach in 35 out of 40 patients [178]. Upon endoscopy 8 patients (22.8%) had a normal bypassed stomach, in 23 (65.7%) a pangastritis was seen and 4 (11.4%) had antrum gastritis. In 2 (5.7%) intestinal metaplasia was seen. It is not yet known whether the finding of intestinal metaplasia has any implication.

6.4.11.2 Abdominal Pain and Anaemia

A need to examine the distal stomach arises, when the patient complains of epigastric or right upper quadrant pain or when anaemia occurs with positive tests of occult blood in the stool. Unexplained anaemia, which cannot be explained by iron, vitamin B_{12} and folic acid deficiencies, which are to be expected in the context of a bypassed duodenum and malabsorption, can also be a reason. It is without saying that first the whole gastrointestinal tract should be investigated by less invasive investigations such as colonoscopy, MRI enteroclysis or video capsule enteroscopy. Upper GI series can be performed by linear echoendoscopy [179]. The defunctionalised stomach after RYGB is often located in close proximity to the gastric pouch. After transgastric puncture with a 22-gauge needle and removal of the stylet, 100 mL of water-soluble contrast followed by 60 mL of air can be instilled to investigate the excluded stomach and duodenum [179].

Keren et al. examined 24 patients with abdominal pain with no previously defined diagnosis [180]. They performed a push enteroscopy with the enteroscope (Olympus SIF-Q140, working length 2500 mm) in 21 and with a paediatric colonoscope in 3. The excluded stomach was successfully accessed in 19 (79%) patients. Mild-to-severe gastritis was present in 13 patients; 4 of them were positive for *H. pylori*. The other six patients had atrophic gastritis. Intestinal metaplasia was found in 3 of 24 patients (12.5%) in the present study similar to the findings of Sinar et al. [176, 180]. Currently, there is only one case series by Skinner et al. focusing on the efficacy of double-balloon enteroscopy (DBE) to successfully identify and treat lesions responsible for obscure GI bleeding in the bypassed stomach [96]. They performed DBE 17 times in 12 patients with altered anatomy, 6 of them having a gastric bypass. Nine cases had overt bleeding and three had occult bleeding. In 10 of the 12 patients, the bleeding site could be identified with DBE. In nine, the bleeding site was at the anastomosis and once in the afferent limb. The stomach was found to be normal in nine of ten patients (90%), including five of six patients with a gastric bypass.

6.4.11.3 Cholelithiasis and Choledocholithiasis

There has been a lot of discussion about the management of gallstones and prophylactic cholecystectomy. Shiffman et al. examined the development of gallstones [181]. Gallstones developed in 36% and sludge in 13% of 81 patients with a normal gallbladder ultrasound at the start; about 40% developed symptoms and 28% were operated [181]. The risk of gallstone formation increases when the weight loss rate exceeds 1.5 kg/week or when the excess weight loss exceeds 24% [181]. Li et al. studied the rate of gallstone development. Preoperative gallbladder disease or cholecystectomy was present in 25.3% of 670 patients undergoing RYGB, 14.9% of 47 patients with LAGB and 30.4% of 79 patients receiving SG [182]. A total of 586 patients had a post-operative follow-up with a mean FU of 25.9 months. The overall rate of gallstone development was 7.8%, 9.5% after RYGB, 2.6% after LAGB and 3.8% after SG, and the mean time for its development was 10.2 months [183]. While Shiffman et al. found symptoms in 40% of cases, this was the case in 24% in Li's study and the incidence of symptomatic gallstones with complications was only 1.9% [181, 182]. To reduce the risk of gallstone formation and its complications, post-operative prophylactic ursodeoxycholic acid (UDCA, ursochol) has been suggested. The prophylactic use of 600 mg ursochol for 6 months following gastric bypass has been shown to reduce the incidence of gallstones to 2% in the treatment group compared to 32% in the placebo group [184]. Six months' daily intake resulted in prolonged absence of gallstone formation as at 24 months the differences were still present [183]. Adams et al. prescribed 300 mg UDCA twice daily for 6 months versus no therapy in controls in SG [185]. In the control group 40% developed gallstones, and in the treatment group only 11% of patients [185]. More importantly, the effectiveness of ursodeoxycholic acid prophylaxis has been confirmed by a meta-analysis of 5 randomised controlled trials involving 521 patients [186]. The rate of gallbladder disease/gallstone formation was significantly lower in patients receiving post-operative UDCA (8.8% vs. 27.7%) [186]. The updated 2013 ASGE/ASMBS/SAGES guidelines state that 300–600 mg UDCA per day significantly reduces gallstone formation and can be used in patients after bariatric surgery without associated cholecystectomy (grade A), but it is unclear why this guideline is not followed by every surgeon [187]. That said, even if it is prescribed the compliance of patients with intake is low and side effects include diarrhoea and skin rash.

Some surgeons remove the gallbladder even if no gallstones are present. Other surgeons believe that this adds the possibility of further complications to the procedure. Warschkow et al. calculated from 13 retrospective and prospective intervention studies that a cholecystectomy in patients without gallstones is not justified and should be exclusively performed in patients with symptomatic biliary disease [188]. The mean incidence for subsequent cholecystectomy was 6.8% with a risk of 3.1% per year. The reason of cholecystectomy was biliary colic or gallbladder dyskinesia in 5.3%, cholecystitis in 1.0%, choledocholithiasis in 0.2% and biliary pancreatitis in 0.2% [189]. The mortality of cholecystectomy was zero and the conversion rate to open surgery was 1.2%. The overall surgery-related complication rate was 1.8%. Patients undergoing RYGB without concomitant cholecystectomy have a risk of 0.1% to suffer from a cholecystectomy-related complication [188]. So, the rate of subsequent cholecystectomy is low, and complications such as choledocholithiasis and biliary pancreatitis are low, the conversion rate is very low and the complication risk is extremely low. Therefore, a concomitant cholecystectomy in patients without gallstones is not justified and should be exclusively performed in patients with symptomatic biliary disease [188]. Worni et al. demonstrated that in a cohort of 70,287 patients included between 2001 and 2008, concomitant cholecystectomies were performed in 9.1% of patients [190]. This proportion declined significantly over the years: from 26.3% in 2001 to 3.7% in 2008. Patients with a laparoscopic RYGB who underwent concomitant cholecystectomy had a higher rate of mortality, higher number of post-operative complications and re-interventions, a longer adjusted hospital stay and less frequent routine discharge [190]. So, given these higher rates, concomitant cholecystectomy should only be considered in symptomatic gallbladder disease.

Melmer et al. followed about a hundred patients over a period of >10 years [189]. Rapid weight loss following the gastric bypass was associated with up to 35% of gallstone formation. The number needed to harm for gallstone formation was seven in the gastric banding group and two cases in the gastric bypass/sleeve gastrectomy group, meaning that seven LAGB and two RYGB/SG patients had to undergo bariatric surgery for one gallstone formation to occur. The number needed to harm for cholecystectomy was 12 and 3 cases in the gastric banding group and the gastric bypass/sleeve gastrectomy group, respectively. Seen their results after a follow-up of 10 years, the a priori application of pharmacological treatment against gallstone formation such as ursochol should be recommended for at least 24 months up to 5 years after surgery. Pineda et al. evaluated the fate of asymptomatic gallbladder disease [191]. Two-hundred and two bariatric surgeries (184 gastric bypass and 18 sleeve gastrectomy) were performed. The global incidence of preoperative gallbladder disease was assessed in 169 patients and was 34.3%, with 14.2% presenting sludge, 20.1% asymptomatic gallstones and 2.3% symptomatic gallstones. The final analysis was based on 146 patients. After 12 months, *de novo* gallbladder disease was observed in 21.2%, sludge in 18.5%, asymptomatic gallstones in 11.3% and symptomatic gallstones in 2%. The overall rate of cholecystectomy because of symptomatic disease after 12 months was 3.4%, 2% developed acute cholecystitis [191]. These data are at variance with the updated 2013 ASGE/ASMBS/SAGES guidelines that suggest that patients undergoing gastric bypass with a positive ultrasound should undergo prophylactic cholecystectomy to prevent gallbladder complications (grade B) [187].

In suspected choledocholithiasis, magnetic resonance cholangiopancreatography (MRCP) is the preferred diagnostic test in patients with RYGB.

An ERCP for therapeutic interventions is an arduous task but can be accomplished by several methods. Before deciding which of the options are best suited, the endoscopist should take the following factors into consideration in a gastric bypass patient: the Roux limb length (short vs. long); the type of anatomic resection, surgical intervention and anastomosis (end-to-side vs. side-to-side); the indication for the ERCP and likelihood of repeat procedures and need for therapeutic manoeuvres; the patient's surgical risk; and very important: the availability of local expertise (deep enteroscopy, endoscopic ultrasound facilities, interventional radiology, surgery). The endoscopist should also have information about previous or concomitantly performed cholecystectomy or a prior papillotomy. In patients with a native papilla the endoscopist should select a technique that allows for the use of a duodenoscope because it increases the chance of successful selective cannulation of the bile duct and pancreatic duct. They should also consider their experience in performing a sphincterotomy. There are specialised papillotomes to overcome the awkward positioning of the ampulla but most endoscopists prefer to insert a biliary stent as a guide for a needle-knife incision. When biliary sphincterotomy is required, balloon dilation of the papilla may be a useful alternative to biliary sphincterotomy [175]. If repeated ERCPs are anticipated access via a gastrostomy tube placed in the gastric remnant may be recommended. If a repeat balloon-assisted enteroscopy is foreseen, the entrance of the afferent limb at the way back can be indicated by a tattoo on removal of the endoscope [177]. All relevant studies such as MRCP, CT scans and surgery reports should be reviewed [192]. In addition, previous endoscopic interventions, such as a previous endoscopic sphincterotomy or stent placement, should be reviewed. It is also important to consider the interval between the surgery and the endoscopic procedure. In the early post-operative period, the risks of instrumentation with regard to anastomotic disruption must be weighed against the potential benefits of ERCP [192].

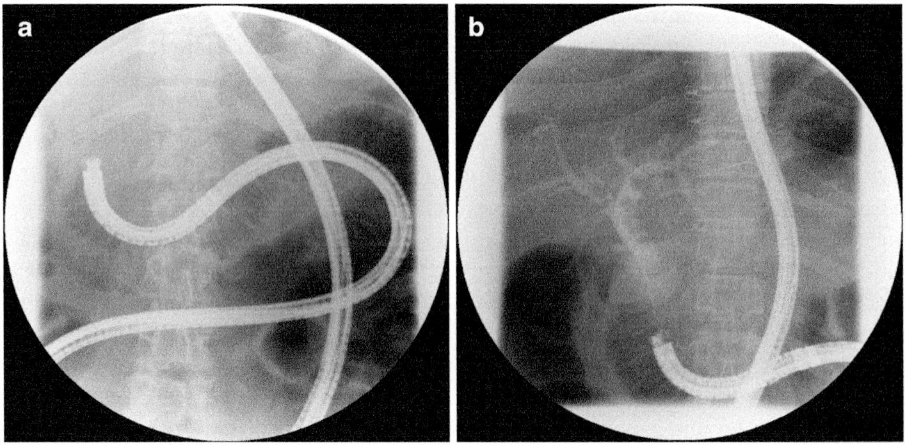

Fig. 6.5 ERCP by push enteroscopy. (**a**) X-ray view of the endoscopic path in the altered anatomy of a gastric bypass, (**b**) opacification of bile duct system loaded with gallstones

Different methods and options are available in accessing the gastric remnant and the papilla of Vater. These can be divided in: A. Retrograde access to the papilla, and B. Antegrade access to the papilla.

Retrograde Access to the Papilla

Retrograde access to the bypassed segments is feasible with a paediatric colonoscope or an enteroscope, the so-called push enteroscopy (Fig. 6.5a, b). A factor that limits deep small-bowel intubation with push enteroscopy is endoscope looping which is counteracted by using the ShapeLock device, and by overtube-assisted enteroscopy such as double-balloon, single-balloon and spiral-overtube enteroscopy, which permit "telescoping" or "pleating" of small-bowel mucosa to bring the target closer to the endoscopist, rather than relying on forward propulsion alone. The disadvantages of this retrograde approach are the forward-viewing perspective with an unfavourable orientation of the native papilla – the ampulla is approached in an oblique orientation not allowing en face viewing of the papilla – the lack of an instrument elevator, the difficult manoeuvrability due to torsion of the scope shaft and loop formation, the limited availability of adequately sized long accessories, and finally the difficult or impossible introduction of accessories through the working channel because of the sharp deflection of the endoscope. Another disadvantage is the 2.8 mm working channel, which limits the size of devices that can be used to less than 8.5 Fr, allowing only biliary stents of 5 and 7 Fr. Therefore, most endoscopists insert at least two stents.

Push Enteroscopy

Using an enteroscope (working length 240 cm) or paediatric colonoscope (working length 164 cm), Elton et al. reported an 84% successful advancement of the endoscope to the level of the papilla, a 94% successful bile duct cannulation (5 of 6 had native papilla) and successful endoscopic treatment in 86% in 18 patients (3 with a RYGB) and a total of 25 attempts [193]. To overcome the above-mentioned disadvantages one can also try to navigate a duodenoscope through the anatomical route over a wire. Once the papilla is reached a guidewire is placed over which the duodenoscope is subsequently advanced. Wright et al. described successful ERCP in 6/11 (55%) patients with a long limb Roux-en-Y gastric bypass and intact papilla by advancing the duodenoscope under fluoroscopic evaluation over a stiff guidewire, previously placed in the bypassed stomach with a forward-viewing endoscope or by pulling up the duodenoscope by means of a wire-guided biliary balloon anchored at the pylorus [194]. The main reason of failure was the inability to pass the endoscope near to the region of the papilla.

A shape-locking guide (ShapeLock endoscopic guide; USGI, San Clemente, CA, USA) was initially developed with the goal of improving colonoscopy and designed to resist loop formation. In the locked state, the ShapeLock guide provides a stable conduit to direct the push forces of the scope without further stretching or looping. Pai et al. inserted the device (100 cm long, OD 16 mm and an inner diameter (ID) of 10.5 mm) over a standard enteroscope in a flexible state before starting [195]. When the tip of the ShapeLock device was positioned across the jejunojejunal anastomosis, the device was locked which made it rigid in the shape of the enteroscope. This allowed the enteroscope to pass the acute angulation of the anastomosis and to move deeply into the pancreatobiliary limb and the excluded stomach. Once the ShapeLock guide is in place and locked, the endoscope can be withdrawn and reinserted multiple times, facilitating procedures that require multiple insertions of the enteroscope or substitution of different endoscopes. Pai et al. were able to reach the gastric remnant in eight of nine patients, without complications [195]. In one patient, the diameter of the gastrojejunal anastomosis prevented passage of the device. There were no complications. Yet, for unknown reasons this study remained the only published one and many more studies are available on the overtube-assisted technology.

Double-balloon enteroscopy, single-balloon enteroscopy and spiral-overtube-assisted enteroscopy can increase the depth of insertion. Balloon enteroscopy was first developed in 2001.

Double-Balloon Enteroscopy

In double-balloon enteroscopy (DBE) both endoscope and overtube are provided with a balloon and a balloon inflation system (EN-450T5, EC-450BI5; Fujifilm USA, Valhalla, NY, USA). The technique is as follows: both enteroscope and overtube are inserted into the stomach. The enteroscope is inserted far into the duodenum and the enteroscope balloon is inflated. Then, the overtube is advanced until the level of the tip of the enteroscope followed by inflation of the balloon of the overtube. Both inflation and deflation are achieved by a balloon pump controller. The enteroscope balloon is deflated and the enteroscope is advanced deeper into the intestines. Again, the enteroscope balloon is inflated and the overtube balloon is deflated and advanced over the enteroscope. This is repeated several times. From time to time, the path has to be straightened by pulling back enteroscope and overtube, both with inflated balloons. There is also a "shorter" DBE system with a 152 cm working length which is compatible with the length of conventional accessories [196]. In 68 patients with Roux-en-Y anatomy (no patient with gastric bypass was included) 103 ERCP procedures were performed. A deep insertion was reported in 100/103, cholangiography in 98/100 and successful therapeutic interventions in 98/98 [197].

Based on data mainly from case reports and a few series on DBE, the papilla can be reached in over 90% of cases and successful selective bile duct cannulation in over 80% of cases. The systematic review by Skinner et al. showed that DBE was able to reach the papilla of Vater or anastomosis in 89% of attempts (range 73–100%) [198]. Cannulation was successful in 93% of attempts (range 85–100%). Overall ERCP success for all attempts was approximately 82% (range 63–95%).

DBE has a few disadvantages: first, attaching the balloon to the tip of the endoscope is troublesome and time consuming; secondly, if the balloon becomes dislodged it may impair the field of view; thirdly, the endoscopist must handle two balloons independently of each other or needs an assistant to do this; fourthly, the cost of DBE equipment is high.

Single-Balloon Enteroscopy

In the single-balloon enteroscopy (SBE) (SIF Q180; Olympus Corporation, Center Valley, PA, USA), a 200 cm long enteroscope with a 2.8 mm working channel is used with a corresponding 13.5 mm OD overtube with a silicone balloon at its tip. The enteroscope and overtube are inserted and the enteroscope is introduced into the small intestine. The overtube is advanced and the balloon is inflated to anchor the small bowel while the enteroscope is advanced as deeply into the small bowel as possible. Once forward motion is no longer possible, the tip of the enteroscope is angulated to create a hook that will help anchor the enteroscope. Once the small bowel is anchored by the tip of the enteroscope the overtube balloon is deflated and advanced until the end of the enteroscope. Then, the balloon is inflated to anchor the small bowel. Also here, from time to time the small bowel has to be reduced and pleated onto the tube by withdrawing both inflated overtube and hooked enteroscope. When the small bowel is sufficiently stretched the procedure is repeated by again advancing the enteroscope.

Success rates ranging from 60 to 80% have been reported. Saleem et al. included 50 patients with Roux-en-Y anatomy who underwent a total of 56 SBEs [177]. Successful ERCP was achieved in 36/56 (70%); therapeutic ERCP was required in 23 cases of which 21 (91%) were successful [177]. Success in patients with Roux-en-Y gastric bypass with native papilla was 7/15 (41%), which was in contrast to the higher success rate in hepaticojejunostomy patients (32/41;78%). SBE-ERCP failed due to not reaching the target site in 14. Failure to identify the afferent limb, failure to enter the afferent limb or marked bowel loop angulation was present each in one case [177].

The systematic review by Skinner showed that when the SBE was used, the papilla of Vater or anastomosis was reached in 82% of attempts (range 75–100%) [198]. Cannulation was successful in 86% of cases (range 76–100%), and overall ERCP success was approximately 68% (range 60–100%). A meta-analysis of 15 trials in 461 patients reported technical, diagnostic and therapeutic success rates of 81%, 69% and 62%, respectively, with large heterogeneity [199]. The largest source of heterogeneity in this meta-analysis is likely the different postsurgical anatomies that were analysed together. So, Abu Dayyeh reanalysed the data for the groups of gastric bypass and other procedures associated with Roux-en-Y anatomy such as Whipple operations [200]. In this reanalysis of gastric bypass surgery, enteroscopy and procedure success rates were 75% (95% CI, 59–87%) and 63% (95% CI, 47–76%) with a low degree of heterogeneity [200]. In patients with successful enteroscopy, the therapeutic success was higher: 78.9% [199]. The results were similar among patients with native papilla and patients with non-native papilla. The adverse event rate was 6.5% (32/489) and major adverse events included pancreatitis (n = 11), bleeding (n = 2), perforation (n = 4) and death from an embolic stroke unrelated to the ERCP (n = 1). Half of the studies (7/15) did not report any adverse event [199].

To accommodate the introduction of a duodenoscope after having performed the enteroscopy, the overtube of the DBE or SBE can be modified to permit the use of a standard endoscope by leaving the overtube in place near the papilla with the balloon inflated to maintain its position [201].

Spiral-Overtube-Assisted or Rotational Enteroscopy

Spiral-overtube-assisted or rotational enteroscopy (SOAE) (Spirus Medical, Stoughton, MA, USA) uses a rotating overtube that pleats the small bowel onto the tube and allows deep advancement of an enteroscope. It has potential advantages over DBE and SBE such as the relative ease of use, better endoscopic control, no need of special pump systems and a shorter learning curve. The systematic review by Skinner et al. included only two studies [198]. So, data about the success of spiral enteroscopy is less robust; however, the ability to reach the papilla of Vater was reported to be as high as 72%, with overall ERCP success reported as 65% [198].

Comparison Between Balloon Methods

Shah et al. compared the results obtained with DBE, SBE and SOAE in 8 centres over 2 years in 129 patients with Roux-en-Y anatomy after surgery (gastric bypass, hepaticojejunostomy, gastrectomy and Whipple procedure) and who had prior attempts in 37/129 (29%) [202]. They underwent a total of 180 ERCPs. The authors noted a 71% successful access to the papilla and a 63% successful cannulation of the common bile duct in the intention-to-treat (ITT) analysis (Table 6.6). When they considered the patient with successful access to the papilla only, the successfully intubated patients had an 88% successful cannulation of the ducts and a 79% successful therapeutic intervention rate. Failures in 48 were due to not reaching the papilla in 23, a too sharp afferent limb angulation in 8 and no identification of the jejunojejunostomy in 6. In 11 the cannulation failed. The results were similar with DBE, SBE and SOAE. The data on 63 patents with gastric bypass could be extracted from the article and are presented for comparison in Table 6.6. In the 73 patients with native papilla, 46 (63%) had a successful ERCP, of whom 9 of 46 (20%) required pre-cut needle-knife papillotomy. In the total group a pre-cut papillotomy

Table 6.6 Data on the comparison of DBE, SBE and SOAE in performing ERCP in the total group ($n = 129$) and in the subgroup of patients with gastric bypass ($n = 63$) in intention-to-treat analysis and in patients with endoscopic success [202]

Enteroscopy	Enteroscopy success $N = 129$	ERCP success $N = 129$	Enteroscopy success $N = 63$	ERCP success $N = 63$
SBE	31/45 (69%)	27/45 (60%)	16/22 (73%)	13/22 (59%)
DBE	20/27 (74%)	17/27 (63%)	13/15 (87%)	10/15 (67%)
Spiral (SOAE)	41/57 (72%)	37/57 (65%)	19/26 (73%)	16/26 (92%)
Overall ITT	92/129 (71%)	81/129 (63%)	48/63 (76%)	29/63 (62%)
ERCP success with achieved access to the papilla	92/129 (71%)	81/92 (88%)	48/63 (76%)	29/48 (60%)

Enteroscopy success was defined as visualising the pancreaticobiliary-enteric anastomosis or native papilla. ERCP success was defined as completing the intended pancreaticobiliary intervention

SBE single-balloon enteroscopy, *DBE* double-balloon enteroscopy, *SOAE* spiral-overtube-assisted enteroscopy, *ITT* intention to treat

was needed in 29, performed freehand in 19, over a pancreatic stent in 2 and over a biliary stent in 8. Complications occurred in 16 patients (12.4%) and included acute pancreatitis in 4 (one severe pancreatitis), mild bleeding in 1, abdominal pain in 4 and throat pain in 5. There were two perforations, one related to needle-knife stricturoplasty, treated conservatively, and one perforation of the afferent limb, treated surgically. There was one death because of an embolic stroke, which may have been related to high intraluminal and/or intraductal air pressures during the procedure, the reason why the authors advise to use CO_2 and water insufflation [202]. Fifteen patients with failed ERCP had a percutaneous transhepatic cholangiography (PTC) and eight patients had a laparoscopically assisted ERCP. So, ERCP was successful in two-thirds of patients in the ITT and in 88% in the per-protocol analysis. The authors also provided two tips to enhance the chances of success: firstly, to use an EMR cap on the tip of the endoscope to minimise enteroscope tip slippage and to provide endoscope tip stabilisation by mucosal suctioning within the EMR cap, and secondly, to change the patient position from the typical semiprone to a left lateral or supine position to improve access to an acutely angled afferent limb or enhance visualisation of the papilla [203].

A systematic review on overtube-assisted enteroscopic ERCPs which included single-balloon, double-balloon and spiral enteroscopy found 23 relevant reports including a total of 945 procedures in 679 patients [1991]. Ten studies reported on gastric bypass patients. Overall ERCP success for all attempts was approximately 74% across all modalities and anatomical configurations. Cannulation is believed to be much more difficult in patients with a native papilla; however, results from successful cannulation attempts in 271 patients with a native papilla (90%) and in 270 with anastomoses (90%) showed less than a 2% difference between the populations. Among 286 patients who underwent Roux-en-Y gastric bypass, endoscopic success was 80% (230/286) and ERCP success was 70% (187/266). Success rates were the lowest in patients with Roux-en-Y gastric bypass, followed by those with pancreaticoduodenectomy and Roux-en-Y hepaticojejunostomy, and they were highest in patients with Billroth II anatomy. There were 32 major complications among the 945 procedures (3.4%), which included cholangitis ($n = 1$), pancreatitis ($n = 11$), bleeding ($n = 3$), perforation ($n = 13$) and death ($n = 1$). Six of the perforations required subsequent surgery [198].

Antegrade Access to the Papilla

In contrast to the previous techniques where the endoscope approaches the papilla from a reverse position, the alternative techniques mentioned here allow direct access to the papilla in a familiar orientation. The first case described by Baron in 1998 was a RYGB patient in whom a Stamm gastrostomy was created during open surgery using a 24 Fr gastrostomy tube. After maturing of the gastrostomy tract for 2 weeks, the tube was removed, the gastrostomy opening was widened by dilation and the insertion of a duodenoscope was permitted.

However, the ideal procedure would be one that can be performed by a single team, without the need of a surgeon or an interventional radiologist, in a single session with a high technical success rate. So, a one-stage and a two-stage procedure can be discerned with the need of a single team or two teams.

One-Stage Procedure

Single team procedures include the endoscopic ultrasound (EUS)-guided antegrade treatment, the EUS-guided gastrogastric antegrade ERCP and the percutaneous-assisted transprosthetic endoscopic therapy (PATENT). Two teams are needed for the laparoscopy-assisted ERCP (LA-ERCP) and the laparoscopic transgastric rendezvous (LATG-RV) procedure. The procedures through a gastrostomy, discussed in the two-stage procedures, can also be performed as one-stage procedure when T-anchors for the apposition of gastric and abdominal walls are used.

One-Stage One-Team Procedure

Endoscopic Ultrasound (EUS)-Guided Antegrade Treatment

Weilert et al. describe their experience in five patients, which involves a stepwise approach after the introduction of a linear echo endoscope into the remnant gastric pouch: (1) EUS-fine-needle aspiration (FNA) puncture into an intrahepatic bile duct, located sonographically; (2) EUS-guided cholangiography and visualisation of the main duct under fluoroscopy; (3) guidewire advancement across the ampulla; (4) dilation of the transhepatic-transgastric access tract; (5) anterograde balloon sphincteroplasty: a through-the-scope, over-the-wire balloon dilator is advanced over the stiff guidewire and across the ampulla and dilation is done under fluoroscopic guidance to obliterate the ampullary waist; and (6) anterograde advancement of stones across the ampulla using a balloon catheter [204]. EUS-guided transhepatic puncture and cholangiography were successful in all and revealed choledocholithiasis in every patient. Tract dilation, antegrade balloon sphincteroplasty and stone extraction were successful in three; in two patients, dilation of the tract was unsuccessful. They then decided to leave the guidewire in place, to remove the echo endoscope and to insert a double-balloon enteroscope. The enteroscope was advanced up to the level of the guidewire which was captured with a snare and pulled through the working channel of the enteroscope. The enteroscope was advanced over the guidewire by a push-and-pull manoeuvre up to the level of the ampulla and retrograde balloon sphinctero-plasty and stone extraction were successful via a rendez-vous procedure. Apart from a subcapsular hepatic haematoma there were no complications. Although bile leaks are a concern during EUS-guided biliary interventions, the transhepatic puncture trajectory may minimise the chance for leakage [204].

Iqbal et al. reviewed the literature on the efficacy and safety of endoscopic ultrasound-guided cholangiopancreatography (EUS-CP) in decompression of biliary and pancreatic ducts and found an overall technical and clinical success rate of about 90% for biliary and 70% for pancreatic duct drainage [203]. The overall EUS-CP complication rate was around 15% and most complications were minor. They also described in detail the access of the bile duct by either an extrahepatic or an intrahepatic approach. In patients with Roux-en-Y anatomy only the intrahepatic, transgastric-transhepatic route seems possible [203]. EUS-CP is, however, a technically challenging procedure and should be performed by an experienced endoscopist skilled in both EUS and ERCP.

Endoscopic Ultrasound (EUS)-Guided Gastrogastric Antegrade ERCP

Kedia et al. described a technique that used a novel, fully silicone-covered, lumen-apposing metal stent with two large end flanges (AXIOS; XLumena, Mountain View, CA, USA) which has been previously applied to form cholecystogastrostomy and gastrojejunostomy fistulas [205]. After the introduction of a linear echo endoscope into the gastric pouch the excluded stomach was located sonographically and punctured with a 19-gauge EUS needle. Injection of contrast to confirm the adequate position within the excluded stomach and injection of 120 mL of water to distend the excluded stomach were followed by advancement of a guidewire through the needle. The gastrogastric connection was dilated with a balloon enabling advancement of the delivery system of the lumen-apposing metal stent into the excluded stomach. The distal flange was deployed in the excluded stomach under fluoroscopic and sonographic guidance. The proximal flange was deployed under endoscopic visualisation in the gastric pouch. To allow for the antegrade passage of a duodenoscope, the lumen of the metal stent was expanded to 18 mm with a dilating balloon. After the ERCP procedure, the gastrogastric lumen-apposing metal stent was removed and the artificially created gastrogastric fistula closed with endoscopic suturing. Also this procedure is a technically challenging and skill-requiring technique.

Percutaneous-Assisted Transprosthetic Endoscopic Therapy (Patent)

In this technique, a double-balloon enteroscopy is used to access the excluded stomach, followed by the creation of a gastrostomy [206]. First, 3T-anchors are placed around the intended site of the gastrostomy. The T-anchors secure the apposition of gastric and abdominal walls and the gastrostomy is created using the Russell introducer method. Within the gastrostomy tract, a fully covered oesophageal self-expandable metal stent (SEMS, 7 cm long and up to 12 cm in length depending on the abdominal wall thickness, 18 mm mid-body diameter, non-foreshortening) is placed with the stent flanges just outside the skin and just within the gastric body. The SEMS is then dilated with a balloon. Antegrade ERCP is performed via the transgastric SEMS using a standard duodenoscope. The double-balloon enteroscope remains within the distal duodenum before and during the ERCP to assist when needed. After the procedure the SEMS can be left in place or otherwise a 26 Fr balloon bumper gastrostomy tube is placed through the SEMS. The SEMS is sectioned longitudinally during removal with a pair of scissors to facilitate removal. Four weeks after the procedure, a period needed to allow for tract maturation, the gastrostomy tube can be removed [206]. A similar device as used for measuring the shaft length of a gastrostomy button can be used to measure the SEMS length: a balloon catheter is introduced through the percutaneous tract. Once the excluded stomach has been entered, the balloon is inflated and retracted. A mark on the catheter indicates the wall thickness in centimetres and an additional 2 cm is added to the measurement to account for the extension of both flanges, and the appropriate skin-level button can be placed. Law et al. reported on the technique and their results in five patients after a gastric bypass, who all had successful biliary sphincterotomy and balloon clearance of the bile duct [206]. There was one perforation caused by sphincterotomy that was treated successfully with a fully covered biliary SEMS.

One-Stage Two-Teams Procedure

Laparoscopy-Assisted ERCP (LA-ERCP)

Laparoscopy-assisted transgastric ERCP has the advantage to perform the laparoscopic cholecystectomy at the same time and also to explore the abdomen for internal hernias, which may develop in as many as 9% of Roux-en-Y gastric bypass patients and which are a frequent cause of recurrent abdominal pain and not easily to be detected by non-invasive diagnostic modalities. In contrast to purely endoscopic approaches it carries the inherent risks of general anaesthesia and surgery. Laparoscopy-assisted ERCP involves the laparoscopic creation of an access port to the gastric remnant or the small bowel (Fig. 6.6a, b). Usually, LA-ERCP is performed through the left upper quadrant port. A locking clamp is placed distally on the biliopancreatic limb to minimise distension of the small bowel from insufflation by the duodenoscope. A 2-0 silk purse-string suture is placed on the antrum or body of the stomach, a gastrotomy is made in the centre of the purse-string suture and a trocar is inserted into the stomach and secured by tightening of the purse-string suture, which also helps to maintain insufflation pressure. The duodenoscope is then placed through the trocar. Some authors reported problems with limited handling of the endoscope because of the distance between trocar and stomach during pneumoperitoneum [207]. Therefore, most prefer to tighten the purse string and to lift the gastric remnant to the anterior abdominal wall, thereby providing a better controlled access [208]. Also, a gastropexy by suturing the stomach against the abdominal wall can be performed. In these techniques, the endoscope is inserted almost directly from the skin into the stomach allowing optimal movements. This strategy also reduces the risks of escape of gastric content or room air during endoscopy. The escape of room

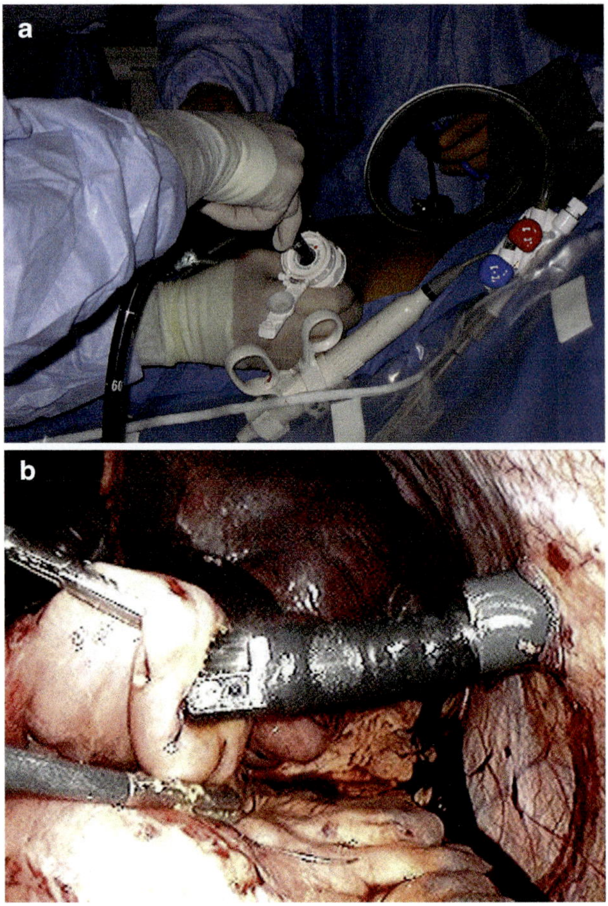

Fig. 6.6 Laparoscopy-assisted ERCP. (**a**) Insertion of sterilised side-viewing duodenoscope by the endoscopist through a 15 mm trocar into the abdomen. (**b**) Visualisation of the insertion of the side-viewing endoscope by the surgeon and surgical help with the insertion of the endoscope into the chosen site of access (biliopancreatic Roux limb), followed by the performance of ERCP in the usual fashion. Reprinted from Gastrointest Endosc 2009; 70: 1254–1259.214, Lopes TL, Clements RH, Mel Wilcox CM. Laparoscopy-assisted ERCP: experience of a high-volume bariatric surgery center (with video), with permission from Elsevier

air in a pneumoperitoneum may cause problems like room-air gas embolism. Also the trocar length may impede controlled movements of the endoscope and a small rigid sigmoidoscope (with the obturator removed) may replace the trocar [209].

A sterilised duodenoscope is then easily advanced through the pylorus into the duodenum. After the procedure the duodenoscope is used to desufflate the stomach and small bowel and after removal the gastrostomy is closed either by suturing or by stapling the defect, whereas others create a gastrostomy when the need of repeated access is foreseen. Also, the place of the gastropexy can be marked by a few clips to facilitate puncture of the stomach, should a repeat procedure be necessary [210].

The success rate reported is high (90–100%) with a relatively low complication rate. In the case of significant adhesions, however, open laparotomy may be required for access to the excluded stomach in 4–13% of patients. Lopes et al. reported successful bile duct cannulation in patients with Roux-en-Y anatomy in 9/10 (90%) and successful pancreatography in 3/3 [211]. Mild pancreatitis was seen in two and one developed a tension pneumothorax. Internal hernias were diagnosed and corrected in four patients [211]. Falcao et al. also reported a successful ERCP and papillotomy without incident in 23 patients [212]. Ten patients underwent simultaneous cholecystectomy. One patient had mild acute pancreatitis that resolved clinically. There was no mortality. Saleem et al. had 100% successful cannulation and sphincterotomy in 15 patients and discovered 3 internal hernias [213]. They had an unusual high rate of pre-cut in 28% which they related to difficulties associated with laparoscopic assisted ERCP such as a lack of the normal endoscope response (lateral rotation and in-and-out movement) and the slightly oblique orientation relative to the papilla, which occasionally needs help of the surgeon to maintain the scope in position. Bertin et al. reported successful gastrostomy placement in all 22 patients, with successful bile duct cannulation in 94% and pancreatic duct cannulation in 89% with one retroperitoneal perforation after a pre-cut papillotomy [210]. Despite these favourable results they found the transgastric ERCP technically challenging for several reasons. The movement of the scope was different than usual and unresponsive to normal manoeuvers. An assistant was needed to maintain torque and this made cannulation much more difficult because the endoscopist could not directly himself/herself control the fine movements needed. The scope engaged the ampulla in a semi-long scope position with the patient supine and the ampulla was further away than normal, making cannulation and cutting less optimal. However, the authors also noted several helpful points summarised here. Steep positioning of the patient is helpful. The gastrostomy should be made as lateral as possible along the greater curvature for good engagement of the pylorus. The assistant can point the trocar towards the pylorus to permit easier entry into the duodenum.

There are also less enthusiastic reports. For instance, Frederiksen et al. noted a high complication rate of 36% despite a 100% successful cannulation of the common bile duct in 29 patients with choledocholithiasis [214]. Perforation of the wall of the gastric remnant occurred in two patients. Eleven procedures (35.5%) demonstrated surgical complications within 30 days. Three haematomas, 3 intra-abdominal abscesses, 1 wound dehiscence and 2 ongoing bleeds were seen. Two patients developed mild post-ERCP pancreatitis. As they performed cholecystectomy and LA-ERCP procedure simultaneously in 12 patients (39% of the LA-ERCP population) they preferred to offer transcystic choledochoscopy and rendez-vous clearance of the choledochus with concomitant cholecystectomy, a modified approach described below.

Laparoscopic Transgastric Rendez-vous (LATG-RV) Procedure

A slightly modified approach is the laparoscopic transgastric rendezvous (LATG-RV) procedure in patients with bile duct stones who also need a cholecystectomy [215]. All the reported series with transgastric ERCP procedure used regular blind ERCP cannulation. Serious ERCP-related complications (retroperitoneal perforation with pre-cut, bleeding, pancreatitis and even tension pneumothorax) have been described. Pre-cut papillotomy was one of the major technical risk factors. Transcystic guided cannulation of the papilla (rendez-vous procedure) has been proposed to increase a selective cannulation and to reduce ERCP complications. At laparoscopy, a general exploration of the Roux-en Y anatomy was performed and internal hernias were ruled out. The cystic duct was identified and clipped proximally and the gallbladder was dissected in its proximal 2/3 out of the liver bed. The cystic duct was partially cut and a transcystic cholangiography was done. If common bile duct stones were identified, a laparoscopic transgastric rendez-vous procedure was performed. The gastrotomy and the introduction of the duodenoscope into the duodenum are similar to the LA-ERCP (Fig. 6.7). When the duodenoscope faces the papilla, the laparoscopic surgeon advances a radiopaque hydrophilic guidewire through the partially opened cystic duct until it appears in the papilla. This guidewire is then retrieved with a Dormia basket through the duodenoscope working channel and extracted by the endoscopist. A sphincterotome is advanced over the guidewire into the duodenal papilla by the endoscopist. The guidewire guides the sphincterotome into the common bile duct (CBD) avoiding a pancreatic duct cannulation. No pre-cut is needed and sphincterotomy and CBD clearance are performed in a regular fashion. Then the gastrotomy is closed, the cystic duct clipped and the cholecystectomy completed. The procedure was performed in four patients and indeed no pancreatitis, which is often due to inadvertent cannulation of the pancreatic duct and repeated trauma to the papilla, and no perforation in the absence of pre-cut papillotomy were observed.

This one-stage two-teams approach requires a great deal of cooperation between endoscopic and surgical teams.

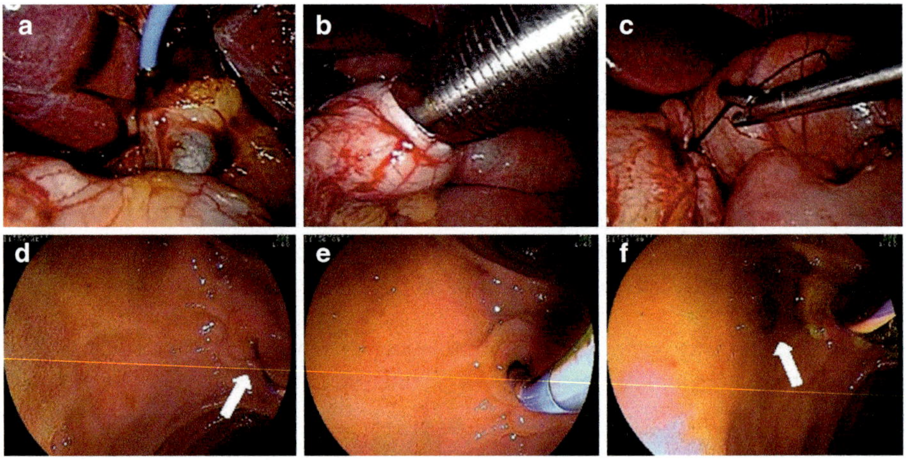

Fig. 6.7 Laparoscopy-assisted transgastric rendezvous. (**a–c**) Laparoscopic phase: (**a**) Cystic duct cannulation and guidewire installation. (**b**) Transgastric 15 mm trocar placement. (**c**) Laparoscopic gastrorrhaphy. (**d–f**) Endoscopic phase: (**d**) Endoscopic view of guidewire inserted by the surgeon through the cystic duct and the papilla (*arrow*). The guidewire is grabbed and extracted through the working channel of the endoscope by the endoscopist. (**e**) Advancement of the sphincterotome over the guidewire into the duodenal papilla for sphincterotomy. (**f**) Endoscopic bile duct clearance of biliary stones (*arrow*). Reprinted from Obes Surg 2016; 26: 2809–2813, Mejía R, Achurra P, Gabrielli M, Briceño E, Rebolledo R, Torres A, et al. Laparoscopy-assisted trans-gastric rendezvous for the treatment of common bile duct stones in patients with prior Roux-en-Y gastric bypass, with permission from Springer

Two-Stage Procedure

The two-stage approach involves first the creation of a gastrostomy and maintenance with a large-calibre catheter, followed by dilation after tract maturation which usually takes 4 weeks and ERCP via the gastrostomy tract. Successful access to the excluded stomach and creation of a gastrostomy have been previously described using various techniques, including surgical, interventional radiologic, and balloon-assisted enteroscopic and endoscopic ultrasound (EUS)-guided procedures. Gastrostomy placement by interventional radiologic methods (except perhaps for CT-guided gastrostomy) and balloon-assisted enteroscopy have the major disadvantage to be not informed about the bowel loops interjacent between gastric remnant and abdominal wall.

Surgical Gastrostomy

In the largest series to date, 28 of 32 patients received a surgical gastrostomy via laparoscopy and in 23 of them an ERCP was performed with a 100% successful cannulation of the common bile duct and pancreatic duct, when indicated [216]. Ten patients were found to have internal hernias which were repaired. One patient developed post-ERCP pancreatitis and in two other patients an intra-abdominal leak required surgical repair [216]. These results were much more favourable than those in the 11 patients who received an open Stamm gastrostomy [217]. Despite a successful ERCP in everyone, these patients developed complications in 5 (45%), including post-ERCP pancreatitis (n = 2), post-sphincterotomy bleeding (n = 1), gastrostomy site bleed (n = 1) and gastric perforation at the site of the endoscopic dilation (n = 1). The authors concluded that the technique enabled therapeutic intervention but that it was associated with significant complications [217].

EUS-Assisted Gastrostomy

Attam et al. reported a successful EUS-assisted placement of a gastrostomy in nine of ten patients (90%) without complications [218]. In one patient with an antegastric Roux limb, the insufflated gastric remnant could not be accessed percutaneously because of an inadequate fluoroscopic window. The echo endoscope is advanced transorally into the gastric pouch and the excluded gastric remnant is identified. The gastric remnant is punctured with a 19-gauge EUS biopsy needle, preflushed with contrast medium, and when adequate positioning is confirmed the gastric remnant is inflated by manually injecting air to a point of maximal distention to push the anterior gastric wall against the anterior abdominal wall. Under fluoroscopic guidance an introducer needle is used to puncture the lumen of the gastric remnant and by radiopaque contrast injection the positioning of the needle tip in the gastric remnant is confirmed. A guidewire is passed into the gastric remnant, the gastric wall is anchored to the abdominal wall with T-anchors (Cope Gastrointestinal Suture Anchor Set, Cook Endoscopy, Winstom-Salem, CA, USA) and a gastrostomy tube of 18 Fr to 20 Fr is placed following the Russell introducer technique in the gastric remnant under fluoroscopic guidance.

Kedia et al. performed an EUS-assisted gastrostomy in the same way, however without using the T-anchors at the placement itself [219]. After a mean of 5.8 days (range, 3–9) a guidewire was placed through the PEG tube, the PEG tube was removed and a small-calibre endoscope was inserted over the wire into the excluded stomach. Subsequently three T-anchors were placed percutaneously under endoscopic and fluoroscopic vision to fix the stomach wall to the abdominal wall. The fistula tract was dilated with dilators over the wire and a fully covered metal oesophageal stent was subsequently deployed over the wire into the stomach with the proximal end outside of the skin. A duodenoscope was inserted through the transcutaneous metal stent over the wire into the second portion of the duodenum, and an ERCP was performed, which was successful in all six patients without complications. After the ERCP, the metal stent was removed over the wire and a 30-Fr Foley catheter inserted over the wire and thereafter the wire was removed. The authors suggest that with the use of T-fasteners a one-stage procedure should be feasible [219].

Comparison of Techniques

Before going into detail into comparative studies the advantages and disadvantages of all mentioned methods should be resumed. Lopes and Wilcox published an excellent table which was modified for this chapter (Table 6.7) [220].

Azeem et al. compared single-balloon enteroscopy ERCP (SB-ERCP) with adult or paediatric colonoscopy ERCP in 90 patients with Roux-en-Y biliary anastomosis [221]. The rates of successful biliary cannulation were similar: 46% for SB-ERCP versus 70% for adult colonoscope ERCP, but SB-ERCP had a higher success rate of biliary cannulation (76% vs. 59%) than when using a paediatric colonoscope. There was no difference between SB-ERCP and adult colonoscopies in therapeutic success rates (71% vs. 66%) but there was a difference compared to paediatric colonoscopy (70% vs. 54%).

Choi et al. compared the indications and technical outcomes of ERCP via a gastrostomy and double-balloon-assisted enteroscopy (DBE-ERCP) for patients with previous Roux-en-Y gastric bypass [222]. They found that ERCP via a gastrostomy accessed the major papilla in 95% (42/44) of cases with cannulation and interventions successful in all 42 cases, whereas in DBE-ERCP the success rates of accessing major papilla, cannulation and therapeutic intervention were 78%, 63% and 56%, respectively [222]. However, the complications were higher with ERCP via a gastrostomy (14.5%) compared with DBE-ERCP (3.1%) ($p = 0.022$)]. There was one (3.1%) post-ERCP pancreatitis in DBE-ERCP. Complications occurred in 11 gastrostomy-ERCP procedures (14.5%), 1 with a mild pancreatitis and 10 related to the gastrostomy. The complications associated with the gastrostomy were as follows: gastrostomy-site infection ($n = 5$), spontaneous dislodgement of the tube ($n = 2$), gastrostomy tract leak ($n = 1$), gastrostomy-site bleeding ($n = 1$) and persistent gastrocutaneous fistula ($n = 1$). Four of the gastrostomy site infections were superficial and resolved with antibiotics. One patient experienced a severe infection at the gastrostomy site, which required hospitalisation and percutaneous drain placement. The authors concluded that ERCP via a gastrostomy is more effective than DBE-ERCP in gaining access to the pancreaticobiliary tree in patients with

Table 6.7 Approaches for ERCP in patients with Roux-en-Y gastric bypass anatomy with advantages and disadvantages and suggestions for best application approaches (modified after Lopes and Wilcox [220], reprinted from Gastroenterol Clin North Am 2010; 39: 99–107, Lopes TL, Wilcox CM. Endoscopic retrograde cholangiopancreatography in patients with Roux-en-Y anatomy with permission from Elsevier)

Technique	Advantages	Disadvantages	Best application
Duodenoscope transorally through anatomic route	• Ideal instrument for cannulation and therapy of native ampulla • Minimally invasive	Frequently unsuccessful due to inability to reach the papilla	Patients with short Roux limb and native papilla
Colonoscope/ enteroscope transorally through anatomic route	• Greater depth of insertion compared to duodenoscope • Minimally invasive	• Frequently unsuccessful in long Roux limb • Forward view • Lack of elevator	Patients with short Roux limb
Overtube-assisted enteroscopic ERCP	Greater reliability in reaching target, even in patients with long limbs	• Forward view • Lack of elevator • Limited availability of accessories	Patients with long Roux limb
Percutaneous assisted transprosthetic endoscopic therapy (PATENT)	• Gastrostomy created by overtube-assisted enteroscopy • Allows use of side-viewing duodenoscope and all standard accessories	More complicated and requires skills	RYGB patients with native papilla
Endoscopic ultrasound (EUS)-assisted antegrade transhepatic-transgastric routing	EUS-guided transhepatic-transgastric route without need of a duodenoscope	Requires fluoroscopy and EUS skills	RYGB patients with native papilla
Endoscopic ultrasound (EUS)-assisted antegrade gastrogastrostomy ERCP	• EUS-guided gastrogastrostomy • Allows use of side-viewing duodenoscope and all standard accessories	Requires EUS skills and suturing skills	RYGB patients with native papilla
Transgastrostomy tract ERCP	• Allows use of side-viewing duodenoscope and all standard accessories • Provides reliable access for repeat procedures	More invasive than purely endoscopic techniques	RYGB patients with native papilla or when repeated procedures are anticipated
Laparoscopy-assisted ERCP	• Allows use of side-viewing duodenoscope and all standard accessories • Ability to diagnose and treat internal hernias • Ability to perform cholecystectomy	• More invasive than purely endoscopic techniques • Requires significant cooperation between surgery and endoscopy teams	RYGB patients with native papilla, particularly when internal hernia is suspected or concomitant cholecystectomy is needed
Percutaneous approach via interventional radiology	Less invasive than surgical approaches	• Morbidity (pain, external drains) • No access to pancreas	Patients with biliary tract pathology who are poor surgical candidates

Roux-en-Y gastric bypass, but the delay by the gastrostomy maturation and the higher morbidity related to the gastrostomy are disadvantageous [222].

Schreiner et al. compared 32 balloon enteroscope-assisted ERCPs (BEA-ERCP) with 24 laparoscopy-assisted ERCP (LA-ERCP) in 56 post-gastric bypass patients [209]. Double-balloon enteroscopy and short double-balloon enteroscopy were used in 26, and single-balloon enteroscopy in 6 patients. LA-ERCP was significantly superior to BEA-ERCP in papilla identification (100% vs. 72%), cannulation rate (100% vs. 59%) and therapeutic success (100% vs. 59%). When restricting the data to those with identified papilla in BEA-ERCP, the successful cannulation rate went up to 83%. There was no difference in post-procedure hospital stay or complication rate between the two groups: both groups had a case of pancreatitis and the LA-ERCP group also had one case of an enterocutaneous fistula. In three of the LA-ERCP patients (13%) the procedure had to be converted from a laparoscopic to an open procedure because of extensive adhesions. In univariate and multivariate analyses, the only predictor associated with therapeutic success was the length of Roux and biliopancreatic (from ligament of Treitz to jejunojejunal anastomosis) limb, being less than 150 cm. The success rate with a limb length <150 cm was 88%, with a limb length of 150–225 cm it was 33%, and with a limb length >225 cm it was 0%. When a limb length of 150 cm or longer is present, LA-ERCP should be the preferred approach. Also, from a cost perspective, starting with BEA-ERCP and continuing with LA-ERCP after a failed BEA-ERCP saved $1015 compared with starting with LA-ERCP. Lo et al. reported that apart from a Roux limb ≥150 cm, also clinical findings that may suggest a long Roux limb such as a large weight loss after RYGB and a body mass index greater than 55 at the start may predict failure when performing a peroral ERCP in post-RYGB patients [223]. These findings were combined in a treatment algorithm by the authors, modified for the purpose of this chapter (Fig. 6.8).

Similar findings were found when spiral-overtube-assisted enteroscopic ERCP (SOAE-ERCP) was compared with LA-ERCP in post-bypass patients. Bile duct cannulation was successful in 57% with SOAE-ERCP compared with 100% with LA-ERCP [224].

Alternative Approaches When ERCP Fails

Besides for diagnostic purposes a percutaneous transhepatic cholangiography with dilation of the track to the bile duct can also establish a route for stone removal, for stent placement in case of bile duct stenosis and for a rendez-vous procedure [192]. Percutaneous transhepatic cholangioscopy may be an option for patients in whom an ERCP cannot be successfully performed. PTC has a reported complication rate of up to 30% [192]. The above-mentioned endoscopic ultrasound-guided cholangiopancreatography (EUS-CP) is a novel approach to achieve ductal access and perform therapies when transpapillary access is unsuccessful. A recent review by Iqbal et al. documented a complication rate of 15% and a 90% success rate with accessing the biliary tree when ERCP fails, although the experience in the setting of altered anatomy is very limited [203]. Finally, laparoscopic common bile duct exploration is a one-stage procedure for cholelithiasis and choledocholithiasis but long-term results to rule out common bile duct strictures are lacking especially in high-risk thin bile ducts [215].

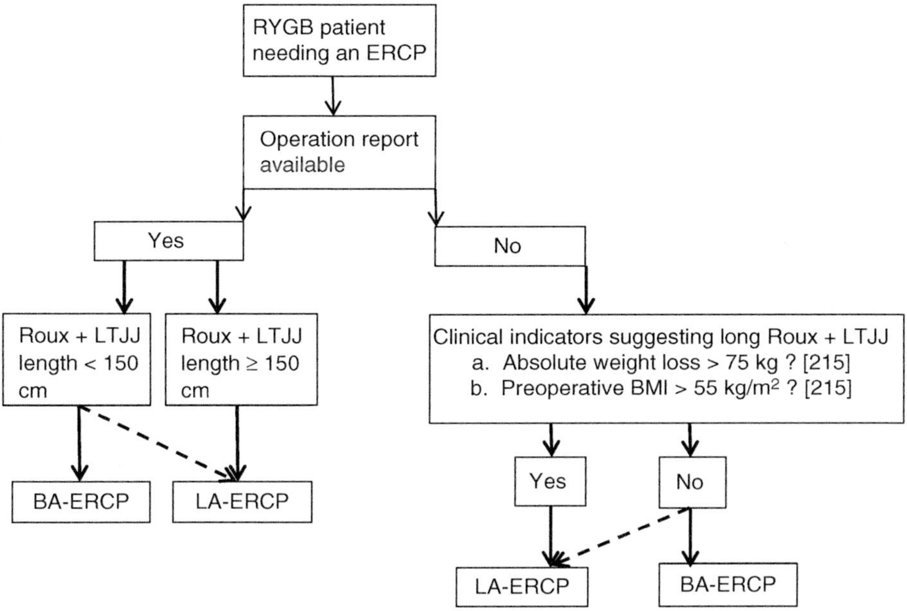

Fig. 6.8 Algorithm to decide the approach to ERCP according to available technology and expertise; the stippled line – – – indicates what to do in case of insufficient experience (modified after Schreiner et al. [201] and Lo et al. [215]). Reprinted from Gastrointest Endosc 2012; 75: 748–756, Schreiner MA, Chang L, Gluck M, Irani S, Gan I, Brandabur JJ, et al. Laparoscopy–assisted versus balloon enteroscopy–assisted ERCP in bariatric post–Roux-en-Y gastric bypass patients, with permission of Elsevier

6.4.12 Gastro-Oesophageal Reflux Disease

The prevalence of gastro-oesophageal reflux disease (GORD) had been reported as high as 45% in morbidly obese subjects, significantly higher than the prevalence of GORD in the general population being in the range of 8–26%. Lifestyle interventions, acid suppression by H_2 receptor antagonists or proton pump inhibitors (PPI), sometimes prokinetic agents and weight loss, are advised. Indeed, Ness-Jensen reported their findings in the HUNT study (HUNT 2 1995–1997 and HUNT 3 2006–2009) with 29,610 patients who provided data on weight loss and GORD symptoms [225]. A reduction of >3.5 BMI units (compared with weight loss <0.5 BMI units) gave an adjusted OR of the loss of having any GORD symptoms of 1.98 (95% confidence interval 1.45/2.72) when using no or less than weekly medication, and an adjusted OR of 3.95 (2.03/7.65) when using at least weekly anti-reflux medication, with a clear dose-response. The OR for loss of severe symptoms was 0.90 (0.32/2.55) and 3.11 (1.13/8.58), respectively. Weight loss was dose-dependently associated with a reduction of GORD symptoms and treatment success with anti-reflux medication in the general population. Obese patients are not as responsive to medical treatments as normal-weight subjects. McDougall et al. found an association between higher BMI and the requirement of longer term H_2 receptor antagonists or antacid therapy [226]. One study suggested that the efficacy of PPIs in obese patients with GORD was not affected by BMI [227], but three studies notified that higher doses of PPIs and even doubling the dosage of pantoprazole in obese or overweight patients provided better control of symptoms [228–230]. Moreover, obese people react less favourably when submitted to anti-reflux surgery: about 31% of obese patients undergoing a laparoscopic Nissen fundoplication or transthoracic Belsey-Mark IV had an operative recurrence compared to an 8% recurrence rate in overweight patients (BMI 25–30 kg/m^2) and 4.5% in normal-weight patients (BMI <25 kg/m^2) [231].

All these data, combined with the favourable, almost reflux-annulling results after RYGB, led surgeons to consider RYGB as both the ideal anti-reflux and weight-loss surgery in obese patients. From a mechanistic standpoint, the good results after RYBG can be predicted: the volume of the new gastric pouch is small, averaging 30 cc, thereby minimising any reservoir capacity to promote regurgitation [232–234]. It relatively lacks parietal cells with a virtually absent basal and stimulated gastric acid secretion, and the reflux of bile is avoided by the Roux-en-Y biliary diversion. The peristaltic activity of the oesophagus is retained and the gastric pouch remains in the abdomen. Also, the excellent weight loss with loss of visceral adipose tissue reduces the intra-abdominal pressure.

Many studies have confirmed the beneficial effects of RYGB on GORD. The Bariatric Outcomes Longitudinal Database (BOLD) graded GORD on a scale of 0 (no GORD); grade 1 (intermittent symptoms, no medication); 2 (intermittent medication); 3 (H_2 blockers or low-dose PPI); 4 (high-dose PPI); and 5 (need for surgery) [235]. Pallati et al. only considered patients with score 2–4 [235]. Almost 32% of 116,136 subjects had evidence of preoperative GORD, severely enough to require medication. Excluding patients undergoing hiatal repair or fundoplication left 22,870 patients with a 6-month follow-up. GORD score before RYGB was 2.80 and post-operatively 1.33. Similarly, LAGB had improvement in GORD score of 2.77 towards 1.63 and SG of 2.82 towards 1.85. GORD score improvement was best in RYGB (56.5% of patients), followed by LAGB (46%) and SG (41%). Worsening of GORD was seen in a small number of patients, mostly in SG (4.6%), followed by RYGB (2.0%) and LAGB (1.2%) [236]. The greater the loss in excess weight the greater the improvement in GORD score. Patients with score 0 or 1 showed worsening and significantly more after SG (9.2%) followed by RYGB (4.6%) and LAGB (2.7%) [235]. There are also limited data on the GORD complication of Barrett's oesophagus and bariatric surgery [236]. Complete regression of cardia-type intestinal metaplasia was observed in 67% of patients; 57% of patients with short-segment Barrett's epithelium and 20% of patients with a long-segment Barrett had complete resolution at repeat endoscopy after gastric bypass [237].

6.5 Sleeve Gastrectomy (SG)

Sleeve gastrectomy (SG) has been considered as technically simple and this fact has contributed to its adoption by a large number of surgeons. Yet, initially there was a heavy combat between believers and non-believers. Those who asked themselves in 2013 "Sleeve gastrectomy: is it always a reasonable surgical option?" mentioned that when complications arise, morbidity numbers are high and referred to their own studies in which 7 of the 22 patients with a leak or stenosis had to undergo a total gastrectomy [236]. But this negative experience from 2013 was more positively addressed by the question in 2016 "Sleeve gastrectomy: have we finally found the holy grail of bariatric surgery?" [238].

Leaks and early staple-line disruption and bleeding are feared acute complications and have been discussed extensively earlier in Chap. 5. Late and more chronic complications are stenosis, fistula and weight regain. Persisting gastro-oesophageal reflux symptoms and *de novo* gastro-oesophageal reflux disease (GORD) will be discussed at length in Chap. 7 and as endoscopy will not only be diagnostic but also therapeutic it will be discussed here as well. The endoscopist should pay attention to the presence of oesophagitis and its staging, to the presence of a hiatal hernia and to staple-line defects and ulcerations. Also, the size of the fundus, which should be small, and any resistance at the gastro-oesophageal junction and midway in the stomach at the incisura angularis, should be reported.

6.5.1 Stenosis and Stricture

Patients with sleeve gastrectomy may have stenosis at the gastro-oesophageal junction, at the incisura angularis in the mid-sleeve, or distally. Stenosis proximally at the level of the oesophagus is the result of chronic inflammation and fibrosis following a leak. Most of the stenoses are located at the incisura angularis for anatomic reasons and their aetiology is functional or mechanical. Functional strictures are transient and derive from oedema or haematoma. Mechanical strictures usually derive from the use of small bougies, stapling too close to the bougie, twisting of the staple line or oversewing of the staple line. Transection too close to the pylorus will result in a distal stenosis. Using a bougie smaller than 32 French could make the sleeve too narrow and too tight and increases the risk of leak and stenosis. Also twisting should be avoided; it can cause distal obstruction and a narrowed sleeve at the incisura angularis. Brethauer et al. showed in their review of studies that included more than 100 patients that 0.6% of sleeve gastrectomy patients required post-operative endoscopic or operative intervention [239]. Later studies reported sleeve stenosis in 0.1–3.9% [240]. Strictures requiring endoscopic dilation or surgical revision occur less than 1% of the time after SG. However, in the presence of a proximal fistula, the downstream obstruction may result in a persistent fistula that does not resolve with conservative management unless dilation is included in the treatment strategy.

Early strictures are symptomatic in the first 6 weeks following surgery; they should be managed by hydration, anti-emetics and upper GI studies. Stable patients can be observed for 24–48 h to allow postsurgical oedema to resolve. However, when patients cannot handle their own secretions a nasogastric tube decompression should be given preferably under fluoroscopic guidance. When no response to conservative managements occurs, a surgical intervention is needed. Laparoscopy will demonstrate the kinking of the gastric sleeve, a tight suture or a haematoma. Sutures used to oversew the staple line should be removed and an intraoperative endoscopy should be performed to confirm the resolution of the stricture.

Chronic strictures often present with mild symptoms and such patients can be initially managed by PPIs. Those who develop severe symptoms, such as persistent dysphagia to solids and liquids with nausea and vomiting, are candidates for further endoscopic or surgical interventions. Endoscopic dilation is a good treatment for short-segment strictures and requires sometimes multiple treatments in 4–6-week intervals [241, 242]. Series such as discussed in the gastric bypass and in Table 6.2 are not available for sleeve gastrectomy. Moreover, different from the gastric bypass, symptomatic stenosis can occur in the presence of a twisted or spiral sleeve. An endoscope can pass through by pushing and twisting in the same direction, and a balloon dilator can be used to open the stenosis. However, the stenosis returns at withdrawal of the endoscope or deflation of the balloon dilator. Also, the stricture has to be defined according to their length into short, i.e. ≤3 cm, and long strictures, and the latter will be resistant to endoscopic dilation.

In treatment-refractory stenosis Zundel et al. used a protocol of pneumatic dilation, first with a CRE TTS balloon at 20 mm Hg for 20 min, followed by achalasia balloons of 30 mm for 20 min with 10–25 psi in the second session, 30 psi in the third session and 35 psi in the fourth session [243]. In the fifth session endoscopic needle cautery cuts are performed in four quadrants including the muscular layer and a 35 mm achalasia balloon at 20 psi for 20 min is used. All nine patients experienced pain for about 2 days. One had a post-procedure bleed and others needed monthly pneumatic dilation. Seven recovered completely and two needed surgery. Parikh et al. treated 8 out of 230 patients (3.5%) who developed symptomatic stenosis with balloon dilation [241]. Endoscopy in these eight patients showed a short-segment stenosis, one near the gastro-oesophageal junction and seven located at the mid-sleeve. Successful dilation was achieved in every patient with median balloon sizes of 15 mm (15–18 mm) in 1.6 (1–2) dilation sessions. Two patients referred from elsewhere had a long-segment stenosis, multiple dilations and endoluminal stenting were to no purpose and although longitudinal seromyotomy was considered it resulted in operative conversion to RYGB in both. Burgos et al. reported a favourable response to 45 Fr Savary-Gilliard bougie dilations in five of six (83%) patients [240]. In a larger series of 26 patients – 1% of the total group of 2500 patients – 9 patients had an early presentation of obstructive symptoms (≤3 months from surgery) and 17 presented late (>3 months) [244]. Dilation was performed with a 30 mm achalasia balloon and inflated to the predetermined diameter under fluoroscopic and endoscopic guidance for 2–5 min. The endoscopic view was needed to avoid unnecessary dilation of the oesophagus or the lower oesophageal sphincter. Fluoroscopy was needed to confirm complete obliteration of the waist of the balloon. With improvement of symptoms, treatment was carried out for an additional 1–2 sessions, 2–4 weeks apart with the same-size balloon. If the patient continued to have symptoms, further dilations were carried out using a 35 mm and, if needed, a 40 mm balloon every 2–4 weeks. A total of 60 sessions was performed in 26 patients. A complete resolution of symptoms was seen in 88.5% of the patients and no adverse events were reported in a mean follow-up of 156 days from the last endoscopic balloon dilation.

Ogra and Kini managed seven long strictures at the incisura level with achalasia balloon as a first-line treatment, of which 71.4% ($n = 5$) were successful and 28.6% ($n = 2$) required subsequent self-expanding metal stents [245].

Although it is difficult to abstract the data on stenting, specifically for the sleeve gastrectomy, from the study by Eubanks et al., it is evident that the use of endoscopic silicone-covered stents to treat strictures was only successful in 83% of the six patients treated and intolerance of the stent with complaints of pain led to the removal of stents after 7 days [92]. Moreover, migration was a frequent finding leading to twice a laparoscopy to remove the stent from the small intestine. A very recent and new approach is the development of ultra-large expandable stents specifically tailored for bariatric surgery leaks [246, 247]. These Megastents (Taewoong Medical, Seoul, South Korea) are fully covered metallic stents with a specific design supposed to minimise migration and to better conform to the anatomy of a gastric sleeve. The wider diameter also provides sufficient radial force to cause dilation of mid-stomach stenosis [246]. Shehab et al. used these stents in 13 patients with a sleeve gastrectomy with post-bariatric surgery leaks (Fig. 6.9) [247].

In the rare case of a banded sleeve gastrectomy, banded with a silastic ring with internal thread, the method by Ferraz et al. may be applied in patients with obstructive symptoms, before deciding to surgically remove the band (Fig. 6.3) [162]. As described in the paragraph on banded gastric bypass, they promoted rupture or stretch of the thread running inside the silastic ring by dilation with a 30 mm Rigiflex balloon. In their study two patients with such a banded sleeve gastrectomy were included.

In case of intractable symptoms not reacting to endoscopic treatment, surgical options are a seromyotomy, stricturoplasty or conversion to a gastric bypass.

6.5.2 Sleeve Dilation and Weight Regain

Surgeons present at the 5th summit reported a conversion rate because of weight loss failure of 4.7% [248]. Several authors related the increase in gastric volume to weight regain and mentioned that the sleeve should measure 75–120 mL at the end of the surgery. The mechanisms mostly involved in sleeve dilation are patients' eating habits, but also surgical aspects such as an incompletely dissected upper posterior gastric pouch or a narrow gastric incisura with consequent gastric upstream dilation of the remnant stomach. Weiner and colleagues reported that a volume of the resected stomach less than 500 mL predicted weight loss failure or weight regain [249]. Himpens et al. showed weight regain in 75% [250]. Reasons for weight gain were a dilation of the gastric tube with increased gastric capacity, an incomplete removal of the gastric fundus thereby retaining too many appetite-stimulating ghrelin-secreting cells, and a too large sleeve due to calibration over a too large orogastric bougie during the operation. Sabbagh and colleagues compared the gastric volume at 2 years after the SG by CT scan and discovered that those with failure of weight loss had larger gastric volumes [251]. Volumes were

>400 mL compared to the mean in the group of 300 mL. Deguines et al. found a mean gastric volume of 255 cc [252]. However, when they compared failures with successful weight losers, success being defined as a >50% excess weight loss, failing patients had volumes of 309 cc versus successful cases one of 225 cc. Weight regain after 5 years was associated in 15.7% with a doubling in gastric volume from 120 to 240 cc [252]. Very recently, Disse et al. performed gastric volumetry

a

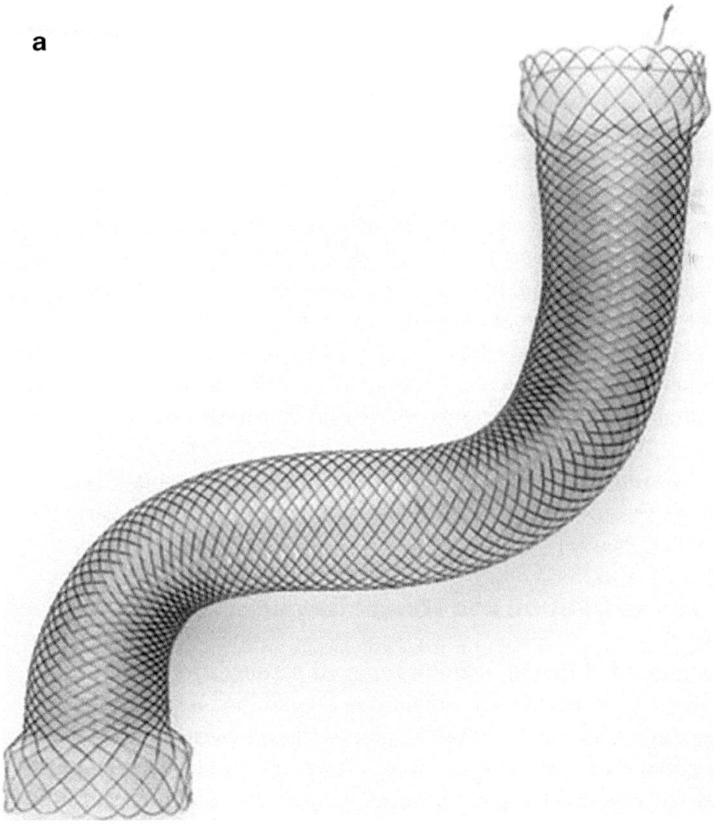

Fig. 6.9 Use of megastent, adapted for use in bariatric surgery, in this case after a gastric bypass. (**a**) The ultra-large stent formed of an s-configuration nitinol mesh fully covered by silicon with significant flexibility despite its large diameter. (**b**) (*a*) A large leak cavity seen at gastro-oesophageal junction leaking into the left subphrenic space. (*b*) Over-the-scope clip (OTSC) loaded on endoscope tip with the deployed tissue anchor device to grasp the tissue and to pull it inside the OTSC cap; red arrow indicates leak into left subphrenic space. (*c*) OTSC deployed (yellow arrow), no contrast is leaking further into left subphrenic space. (*d*) Megastent insertion through gastrojejunal stricture in the same session. (*e* and *f*) Endoscopic and fluoroscopic view after stent removal 6 weeks later with a complete healing of the leak. Reprinted from Obes Surg 2016; 26: 941–948, Shehab HM, Hakky SM, Gawdat KA. An endoscopic strategy combining mega stents and over-the-scope clips for the management of post-bariatric surgery leaks and fistulas (with video), with permission from Springer

b

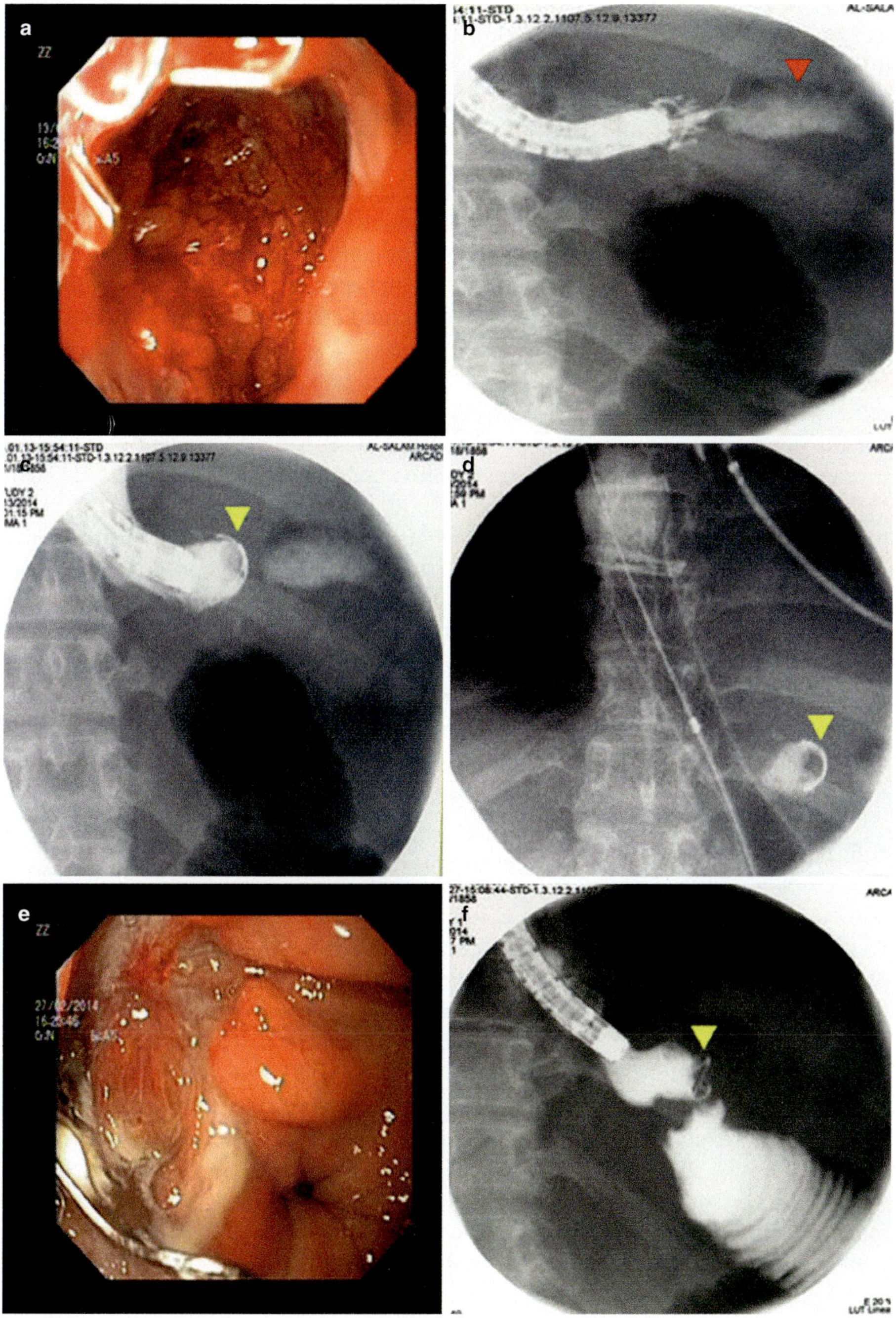

Fig. 6.9 (continued)

using 3D gastric computed tomography with gas expansion [253]. Total gastric volume, volume of the gastric tube and the antrum, and diameter of the gastric tube were assessed after multiplanar reconstructions. An increase of at least 25% of the total gastric volume was considered as a sleeve dilation. Measurements were done at 3 and 12 months post-surgery. Sixty-one per cent of the 54 subjects experienced sleeve dilation 1 year after surgery. The total gastric volume, the volume of the gastric tube and the diameter of the gastric tube were significantly higher in the group with gastric dilation compared to those in the group without gastric dilation, whereas the volume of the antrum was similar between the groups. However, sleeve dilation was not linked to an increase of daily caloric intake and insufficient weight loss during the first 18 months. The authors conclude that sleeve dilation, assessed prospectively in their study, is not a predictive factor of early weight loss failure following SG [253].

Lauti et al. reviewed the literature on weight regain after sleeve gastrectomy and retrieved 21 papers with data on subjects >2 years after surgery [254]. Regain of weight is reported in nine heterogeneous studies as 5.7% at 2 years to 75.6% at 6 years. Only one of these studies reported weight regain rates yearly [255]. Their definition of weight regain was an increase in excess weight loss of ≥25%. They reported regain rates of 0%, 1.0%, 11.6%, 19.2% and 29.5% at 1, 2, 3, 4 and 5 years post-operatively, respectively, confirming the increasing susceptibility to weight regain experienced by patients as time from surgery increases and mainly starting from 18–24 months after surgery [255]. Both surgical-technical factors and patient-related factors are involved in weight regain. Surgical-technical factors are a large sleeve size, the development of a neofundus and a large antral remnant; patient-related factors are incompliance with follow-up visits, maladaptive eating habits and lack of exercise [254, 255].

6.5.3 Fistula

Although fistula by definition is a communication between two epithelialised surfaces, the term fistula is also used in the context of a leak having a single outlet. Many endoscopic treatments such as endoscopic clips, stents and tissue sealants, alone or in different combinations, are available but sometimes repeat endoscopic procedures are necessary: 1–13 procedures in Surache's study, 1–6 in the study by Eisendrath et al. and 2–16 in the study by Bège et al. [93, 256, 257].

Over-the-scope clips (OTSC). Mercky et al. reported that 19 of the 30 patients had a gastric fistula after laparoscopic sleeve gastrectomy and the overall success rate of using the OTSC system was 71% [147]. Surache et al. treated 19 patients with a gastric fistula with OTSC clips to close the fistula, but the data on the 11 patients with a sleeve gastrectomy were reported separately [256]. Among the 11 patients with a gastrectomy, 54.5% were healed with primary efficacy and 36.5% with secondary efficacy requiring a subsequent endoscopic treatment by glue, stents or clips, and treatment failed in 1 patient (9%), thus resulting in an overall 91%

success rate. There was one complication related to the delivery system of the clip because the Ovesco anchor, a device to approximate the edges of the fistula, was blocked within the clip and was therefore unable to be withdrawn immediately. The problem could be resolved by endoscopy a week later.

Multimodal therapy. Bege et al. first assessed the 27 fistulae (2 in gastric bypass and 25 in sleeve gastrectomy patients) before starting treatment [257]. The fistula was simple, defined as having a single outlet in 6, multiple in 9 or complex in 13. A complex fistula corresponded to a cavity with multiple outlets or to a communicating fistula that drained into another organ (e.g. an oesophagobronchial fistula). They had three successive stages in their treatment: first, debridement and drainage of the residual fluid collection with saline lavage, and placement of a nasocystic catheter and double-pigtail stent; the second stage placement of a covered metal stent that remained for 6 weeks; and finally the closure or filling of the hole with endoclips in case of a hole of <1 cm, or, in the case of larger or complex fistulas, a synthetic glue consisting of *N*-butyl-2-cyanoacrylate. All fistulas except two were larger than 10 mm. Debridement was necessary in 19/27 (70%) of cases, a stent was used in 22/27 (81%) of cases and occlusion of the opening was achieved with complementary methods in 18 (70%). Migration of the stent occurred in 13/22 (59%), irrespective of clipping or not. The first procedure was successful in 11 (41%) of cases, and in the others more endoscopic procedures were necessary to achieve a final resolution in all [257]. There were two factors influencing the outcome: the time of referral – when referred early within 390 days a faster healing with fewer sessions was seen – and the origin of the fistula. Fistulas from sleeve gastrectomy may be less likely to heal than the fistulas from gastric bypass, possibly because of exposure to gastric acid but also because of the exposure to high intragastric pressure [257]. In this context therefore, the results reported are very favourable.

Baretta et al. described a novel endoscopic procedure using stricturotomy to treat gastric fistula complicated by stricture after bariatric surgery [258]. All 27 patients studied presented with His angle fistula; 8 patients had anastomotic stricture after RYGB treated with balloon dilation to 20 mm, whereas 9 SG and 4 DS patients had stenosis at the incisura treated with 30 mm achalasia balloon dilation. In every patient a stricturotomy was performed using the Needle Knife (Boston Scientific, Natick, MA, USA) or APC. The mean time to fistula closure was 18 days with a success rate of 100% [259].

6.5.3.1 Gastrocutaneous Fistula

As discussed earlier, Toussaint et al. achieved good results by applying a SurgiSIS plug [156]. Vilallonga et al. tried to treat ten patients with sleeve gastrectomy and a gastrocutaneous fistula, which was visualised by fistulography [260]. First, a catheter was advanced over a guide wire through the fistula until well into the stomach and then *N*-butyl-2-cyanoacrylate was applied from the gastric orifice distally by pulling back the catheter outwards. One patient had the tissue sealing applied before endoscopic stent placement and five after stent placement. Of these six patients, immediate healing occurred only in those five with the sequence of stent followed by *N*-butyl-2-cyanoacrylate (83% healing rate). In the group of patients, who required a Roux limb placement (four patients with chronic gastrocutaneous fistula and the failed patient), the gastrocutaneous fistula healed [259, 260].

6.5.3.2 Gastrobronchial Fistula

In the review by Bezerra Silva et al. the majority (67%) of gastrobronchial fistula occurred after a sleeve gastrectomy [157]. French surgeons reviewed their personal experience and a multicentre experience [159, 261]. Rebibo et al. reported their series of 750 primary sleeve gastrectomies [261]. Eighteen of these patients developed a post-operative gastric fistula (2.4%) and six patients a gastrobronchial fistula. The gastrobronchial fistula was located at the angle of His in all cases. They emphasised the importance of an adequate preoperative nutritional status in the outcome. Guillaud et al. reviewed the data of five French academic bariatric centres and found an incidence of 0.22%, similar to the 0.25% reported by Sakran et al. and 0.37% reported by van de Vrande et al. [159, 259, 262]. In discordance with the study of Campos et al., 9 of their 13 patients (69%) had endoscopic treatment attempts, but it did not permit healing without complementary abdomino-thoracic surgery. Campos et al. treated ten gastric bypass patients and five sleeve gastrectomy patients with a very aggressive scheme of balloon dilation, stricturotomy, septoplasty and stenting (see subchapter of gastrobronchial fistula in gastric bypass) with fistula closure in 93.3%, with only one patient needing surgery [158]. Albanopoulos et al. reported another two cases which occurred late after surgery with an unfavourable outcome of total gastrectomy and one fatality [262]. Almadi et al. discussed a patient with a fatal aorto-oesophageal fistula as a result of a self-expandable metallic stent for the management of a gastric pouch leak after a laparoscopic sleeve gastrectomy [263].

6.5.4 Post-bariatric Hypoglycaemia

Although less common compared with RYGB, there have also been reports of postprandial hypoglycaemia after sleeve gastrectomy between 2 and 4 years after the operation. As with the gastric bypass, laboratory investigations should exclude an insulinoma and fasting hypoglycaemia does not fit in post-bariatric hypoglycaemia. The reader is referred to this subchapter in the gastric bypass section for an extensive discussion.

6.5.5 Gastro-Oesophageal Reflux Disease

The data on gastro-oesophageal reflux disease (GORD) seem less favourable after sleeve gastrectomy. Referring to the earlier discussed BOLD (Bariatric Outcomes Longitudinal Database) data, DuPree et al. retrospectively reviewed the outcomes of patients with GORD symptoms undergoing sleeve gastrectomy or gastric bypass [264]. Pre-existing GORD was present in 44.5% of the 4832 SG and in 50.4% of 33,867 RYGB patients. Resolution of symptoms occurred in 15.9% of

SG patients whereas 84.1% of patients continued to have symptoms, and even 9% had worsening. In RYGB GORD symptoms resolved in most patients, i.e. in 62.8%, 17.6% had stabilisation and 2.2% had worsening of symptoms. In patients without GORD symptoms newly developed symptoms were seen in 8.6% after sleeve gastrectomy. Moreover, when comparing sleeve gastrectomy patients with gastric bypass patients, preoperative GORD symptoms were associated with significantly increased post-operative complications (15.1% vs. 10.6%, respectively, and even 15.1% in those with severe GORD), gastrointestinal adverse events (6.9% vs. 3.6%, respectively, and even 7.5% in those with severe GORD) and increased need for revision operations (0.6% vs. 0.3%, respectively). These revisions were mostly indicated for GORD or weight gain. The presence of GORD had also an adverse effect on weight loss: a >50% excess weight loss was not obtained by 34.0% of sleeve gastrectomy patients with GORD compared with 28.0% of SG patients without GORD [264].

Factors related to a higher chance of gastro-oesophageal reflux after sleeve gastrectomy are the sleeve volume of 100 mL with a loss of distensibility and compliance and thereby increased intraluminal pressure, a disrupted phreno-oesophageal ligament and a smaller antrum delaying gastric emptying [238, 265–267]. According to the law of Newton, the intraluminal pressure correlates inversely with the diameter of the gastric tube and thus a sleeve is a high-pressure condition. As the oesophagus has to empty against a resistance, a disturbed oesophageal clearance of acid may ensue. A narrow sleeve might worsen GORD by resecting/dividing the sling fibres, thereby lowering the LOS pressure, decreasing the LOS length and blunting the angle of His [265]. A narrow sleeve at the angularis and preserving the pylorus might create an obstruction and thus promote reflux [265].

Also, a dilated upper sleeve and intrathoracic migration of the sleeve may result in persistent regurgitation. Himpens et al. reported a biphasic pattern of reflux, with an increase in the first 6 months related to poor patient compliance, and then a decrease in GORD up till 3 years, and between 3 and 6 years GORD symptoms increased to being present in 21% of patients, usually after meals and never at night [250]. The 6-year increase in reflux paralleled the increase in BMI and at 6 years they found fundic regrowth. In the 11-year follow-up on 65 of the 110 patients, none of the 7 preoperatively GORD-positive patients improved; 6 continued PPI intake and 1 required conversion to RYGB primarily because of GORD (remission rate 0%) [268]. Of the 56 preoperatively GORD-negative patients, 14 were re-operated because of weight issues not related to GORD; in the remaining 42 individuals, 9 (21.4%) developed *de novo* GORD, which required conversion to RYGB in 1 [268].

Technical mistakes may further contribute such as a narrowing segment at the junction between the vertical and horizontal parts of the sleeve, twisting of the sleeve and persistence of (a part of) the gastric fundus and/or a hiatal hernia that has not been diagnosed before surgery [266]. One study showed that the prevalence of hiatal hernias increased significantly following sleeve gastrectomy [269]. Another study reported that a significant number of patients had migration of the proximal sleeve above the level of the hiatus on CT scans [270]. An aggressive identification of a hiatal hernia, both before the operation by endoscopy and during surgery, is mandatory and diaphragmatic defects should be closed after the sleeve procedure is completed [271, 272].

However, there are also reasons why the sleeve may reduce gastro-oesophageal reflux: removal of the fundus with less transient LOS relaxations and reduced acid production, accelerated gastric emptying and a decrease in intra-abdominal pressure due to weight loss. Melissas et al. have shown acceleration in gastric emptying up to 2 years after the operation, thought to be due to absence of receptive relaxation of the excised fundus [273].

There are at least four reviews that tried to estimate the effect of sleeve gastrectomy on either *de novo* GORD or GORD by aggravation of pre-existing symptoms [266, 274–276]. All reviews complain about the poor to moderate quality of studies and the high heterogeneity because of the absent standardisation of the technique with many different tube calibration sizes, absence of data on reinforcement of the staple line or when present, done with different materials and methods, non-reporting of hiatal hernia repair, etc. Chiu et al. performed a systematic review and found data to be inconclusive [274]. Of the included studies four showed an increased incidence of GORD post-operatively and seven a decreased incidence. Stenard et al. found 13 studies including 5953 patients which suggested a negative influence of SG on GORD and 12 studies including 1863 patients that reported a favourable impact of SG on GORD [266]. Oor et al. included 33 articles with 8092 obese patients [275]. Of the included studies, 12 report a decrease in the post-operative prevalence of GORD symptoms, whereas 16 studies reported an increase. The relative difference in prevalence of GORD symptoms ranged from a relative decrease of 97% to an increase of 300% following surgery. Eleven studies used validated questionnaires to assess changes in the prevalence of GORD symptoms and found a not-significant pooled difference of 4.3% (95% confidence interval (CI) −9.7/18.4). More relevant as to the debate on the existence of new-onset GORD are the data of seven studies using (standardised) questionnaires. The pooled incidence of new-onset GORD symptoms for these patients was 20% (98/434; with a 95% CI 12.9/27.0; p 0.004) [275]. Very few studies with objective measurements were found. Two studies found an increase in oesophageal acid exposure after sleeve gastrectomy; one study found a decrease with a *de novo* pathological pH measurement in 10% [277–279].

As discussed above, whether or not a hiatal hernia repair was performed simultaneously was not mentioned by every study. The relevance of this is shown by Soricelli et al. [280]. The authors compared the outcomes of SG by differentiating patients with hiatal hernia repair from those who had no hiatal hernia repair and observed a significant decrease in GORD, from 42.1 to 3.1% when hiatal hernia repair was added to the sleeve procedure. Although the follow-up of 12 months was short, the post-operative development of *de novo* reflux symptoms was significantly greater in patients who underwent a SG without a hiatal hernia repair compared to those with a hiatal hernia repair (22.9% vs. 0%, $p = 0.01$). A recent systematic review on simultaneous SG and hiatal hernia surgery by Mahawar et al. included 17 papers with 737 patients [276]. They reported a post-operative GORD of 12.6% at a mean follow-up of 24 months. Sixteen out of 17 papers recommended simultaneous repair of a hiatal hernia during sleeve gastrectomy [276].

GORD should be carefully defined with an exhaustive workup including upper gastrointestinal endoscopy, high-definition manometry and pH impendance-metry. If indicated, volumetric assessment of the gastric sleeve by computerised tomography (CT) scan should be performed as this will assist in the decision of performing a re-sleeve or a gastric bypass when it comes to surgery.

The role of the gastroenterologist is to estimate during endoscopy the grading of oesophagitis, the size of the gastric fundus, the narrowing at the incisura and the presence of a gastric outlet obstruction distally. He/she should review the data of the manometry and pH measurements and, when conservative therapy is indicated, give advices on lifestyle changes, high-dose PPI medication and prokinetics. Because of the gastro-oesophageal motility disturbances, the usual prokinetics may not be effective enough and erythromycin three times daily 250 mg is the best option [281].

When this conservative treatment is tried consciously and does not provide sufficient relief of symptoms, new endoluminal methods may be tried [267, 282]. Four methods are available, although the last three are still investigational: (1) radiofrequency energy delivery to the gastro-oesophageal junction (Stretta procedure); (2) the transoral fundoplication therapy with moulding of the tissue and placement of polypropylene suture material in the region of the gastro-oesophageal junction; (3) the MUSE™ endoscopic stapling system, a technique that creates an endoscopic partial fundoplication; and (4) the anti-reflux mucosectomy (ARMS) with endoscopic mucosal resection and endoscopic submucosal dissection creating a sharp mucosal valve at the gastric cardia [267, 282]. Unfortunately, the StomaphyX equipment that created an endoluminal cuff by stomach plication is no longer available. Leitman et al. treated 64 patients with the StomaphyX method, of whom 18 suffered from severe gastro-oesophageal reflux [128]. After treatment symptoms of gastro-oesophageal reflux improved in 80% and resolved in 20%. In the Stretta procedure (Curon Medical, Sunnyvale, CA, USA) radiofrequency ablation of the submucosa is used to reduce the compliance of the tissue at the gastro-oesophageal junction and to control the transient relaxations of the LOS, helping to prevent GORD [283]. The system utilises temperature-controlled radiofrequency energy, endoscopically delivered by a balloon assembly with needle electrodes that are positioned 1 cm above the gastro-oesophageal junction. Complications include mucosal injury, bleeding and perforation of the oesophagus with a morbidity rate of less than 0.6%. There are no data of its use in sleeve gastrectomy but 10-year follow-up data in non-bariatric patients has shown a 50% decreased use of PPIs in 64% of patients with entire elimination of PPI use in 41% and a significant improvement in quality of life [284]. Pre-existing Barrett's metaplasia regressed in 85% of biopsied patients. However, a systematic review and meta-analysis of trials evaluated the efficacy of Stretta for the management of GORD in non-bariatric patients [285]. The pooled data from 4 trials and 153 analysed patients showed no differences between Stretta and sham or PPI therapy for the outcomes of mean oesophageal acid exposure, lower oesophageal sphincter pressure, ability to stop PPIs or quality of life [285].

6.6 Biliopancreatic Diversion (BPD) with (BPD-DS) or Without Duodenal Switch

In the original version of the biliopancreatic diversion, a large proximal pouch was intentionally made to ensure an adequate intake protein after the disastrous experience with the jejunoileal bypass. This 200–500 mL gastric reservoir in combination with a gastroileostomy makes this operation potentially ulcerogenic. Indeed, the incidence of marginal ulcer after BPD is higher than that after RYGB and reported to occur in 12.5%, but ultimately reduced to 3.2% by changes of surgical techniques and prophylactic medication [286]. As such, the biliopancreatic diversion with duodenal switch is an attempt to reduce the chance of marginal ulceration, to provide gastric restriction and to maintain the regulation of gastric emptying.

Complicated marginal ulcer (with bleeding or perforation), bleeding, small-bowel obstruction due to internal hernia (biliopancreatic limb, alimentary limb, common channel) or incisional hernia, small-bowel or gastric perforation, leak from a staple line or anastomosis, intra-abdominal abscess or anastomotic stenosis are complications to mention, but their discussion and treatment are covered by the previous chapter, Chap. 5, and the subchapters of gastric bypass and sleeve gastrectomy in this chapter. Since 1999 laparoscopic BPD-DS is feasible with quicker recovery time, but bleeding from the gastric staple line was seen more often than with laparotomy [287]. Today, a biliopancreatic diversion with duodenal switch is performed, either as a sole procedure or as a second step after the sleeve gastrectomy procedure. Complications related to the sleeve gastrectomy are discussed above. Specific late complications are mainly nutrition related and include protein malnutrition, Wernicke's encephalopathy, iron deficiency and severe anaemia. Initially, BPD included cholecystectomy, appendectomy and liver biopsy but these procedures are not routinely performed since the introduction of laparoscopy.

6.6.1 Fistula

Papavramidis et al. reported a high-output gastrocutaneous fistula in 6 of 96 patients after a BPD-DS [288]. Four originated from the duodenojejunal anastomosis and two from the gastric pouch. Every patient was treated by total parenteral nutrition (TPN), PPI and somatostatin for at least 7 days after the appearance of the fistula. When the fistula did not close after 7 days, the fibrin sealant (Beriplast P; Behring, Marburg, Germany) was used as a tissue adhesive and sessions were repeated up to complete closure of the fistula at intervals of 2–3 days. This fibrin sealant has, in addition to a mechanical role in occluding the defect, a predominant role in wound healing, including cellular response to wound damage and by forming matrix-building strands which assist neovascularisation and fibroblast proliferation. All patients were treated successfully with conservative treatment, either solely with TPN and somatostatin (3) or with endoscopic fibrin-sealing sessions (3). No evidence of fistula was observed at gastroscopy 3 and 24 months after therapy.

Sometimes many treatments are necessary as demonstrated by Schweitzer et al. in a case report [289]. This patient needed drainage, total parental nutrition and intravenous antibiotics, followed by a stent 2 weeks later. Because of migration a second stent was placed that overlapped the previous stent. Three months later, despite two overlapping stents and retrograde fibrin glue injection, the fistula persisted. A combination of APC denuding and cytology brush abrading of the surrounding tissue and endoscopic suturing by StomaphyX, use of fibrin glue and three endoclips finally resulted in closure of the fistula.

6.6.2 Postprandial Hyperinsulinaemic Hypoglycaemia

Postprandial hyperinsulinaemic hypoglycaemia has been most often associated with RYGB. However, it has been observed after a BPD with duodenal switch, in which nutrients are directly delivered to the mid or distal small intestine. The reader is referred to this subchapter in the gastric bypass section for an extensive discussion.

6.7 Laparoscopic Adjustable Gastric Banding (LAGB)

In the 1990s, when only vertical banded gastroplasty and Roux-en-Y gastric bypass as open bariatric procedures were available, the laparoscopic adjustable gastric banding (LAGB) was introduced as an easy, safe, effective and durable short-stay procedure with a very short learning curve. The intervention was thought to be reversible and safe to be revised in case of problems such as intolerance. Also the adjustment of the inner band, with the possibility of tightening by injecting saline into the reservoir, or loosening by withdrawing saline, made the band a tailor-made instrument attuned to the needs of the patients. To some extent, in retrospect, the introduction of the concept was somewhat premature: the many problems of band slippage, pouch dilation and band erosion reported by the perigastric approach (accessing the right crus perigastrically) were significantly reduced after adoption of the pars flaccida technique (accessing the right crus through the pars flaccida). Furthermore, anterior gastrogastric imbrications and postponement of band fill until 4–6 weeks post-operatively were recommended [290–292]. This also explained the unfavourable results of the two US clinical trials under the FDA protocol starting in 1995 and 1999, compared with the experience in Europe and Australia [293–295]. The FDA-monitored studies used the perigastric method, but the relatively high rates for some complications were also attributed to the relatively few number of procedures performed by each surgeon and their lack of experience with adjustments of the band [293, 294]. In 2001 the FDA approved the Lap-Band (Apollo Endosurgery, Austin, Texas, USA) with a low-volume, high-pressure inflatable band. The Swedish band, available in Europe since 1987, was finally approved in 2007 in the USA as the Realize band (Realize, Ethicon Endo-Surgery Cincinnati, Ohio, USA; Swedish Adjustable Gastric Banding (SAGB), Obtech Medical Sarl, Le

Locle, Switzerland; AMI band, AMI, GmbH, Feldkirch, Austria) with a high-volume, low-pressure balloon design. A meta-analysis of 129 studies (28,980 patients; 4273 patients in 33 Swedish band studies and 24,707 patients in 104 Lap-Band studies) showed a greater absolute weight loss but a similar excessive weight loss and BMI change for the Swedish band [296]. The frequency of late slippage or migration (4.0% and 6.2% for the Swedish and Lap-Band, respectively) and pouch dilation (1.7% and 5.1% for the Swedish and Lap-Band, respectively) were lower for Swedish band. Almost half of the studies with the Lap-Band used the perigastric technique and when the analysis was controlled for the use of the pars flaccida technique, the differences in the complication rates were reduced (from 4.3 to 2.6% for the Swedish and from 6.9 to 3.1% for the Lap-Band). At that time already, it was suggested that probably the low-pressure restriction could have a bearing on the development of long-term complications. Indeed, the most recent version of the Lap-Band (Lap-Band AP) has a fully 360° encircling, high-volume, low-pressure balloon attached to a wide height band [291, 292].

Despite all these improvements the decline in use around the world continued, paralleled by an increase in gastric sleeve procedures. And similar to the sleeve there are surgeons who advocate a "Laparoscopic gastric banding: game over" postulating that the decline in popularity of the band is driven by a lack of long-term efficacy, high revision surgery rates, food intolerance and difficulties with band adjustments [297]. However others from very dedicated teams with good results rebut these arguments and testify that "The band must not be abandoned" [298]. The band adjustments, on the one hand being a unique concept of the band, also resulted in an inability and undesirability of a lifetime commitment to the patient on the other. To facilitate band adjustments, a new type of adjustable gastric band with an innovative adjustment mechanism by a telemetrically activated electric motor (the Easyband (Allergan, Lausanne, Switzerland)) was developed as an alternative to the conventional method of adjustment via an access port and percutaneous injection of a saline solution [299]. Unfortunately, 20.9% of the bands had ≥1 functional test failures, with five technical failures requiring explant of the device, but while engineering solutions were identified the Easyband project was discontinued at the moment of its greatest promise.

Two recent reports on large groups of patients should be mentioned here, because they put the results into perspective. One study compared the effectiveness of bariatrics in the USA. Data from the Bariatric Surgery Center of Excellence Data File was searched from June 2007 to September 2011 for 30-day and 1-year adverse events, 1-year weight loss and comorbidity resolution [1] (Table 6.1). As mentioned earlier, the rates of bleeding at 30 days were 0.1% for LAGB, 0.6% for SG, 1.4% for RYGB and 1.0% for BPD-DS. At 1 year, the bleeding rate was 0.1% for LAGB, and only slightly higher at 0.7% for SG, 1.5% for RYGB and 1.0% for BPD-DS. Leaks were rare after LAGB (0.01%) and increased to 0.1% for SG, 0.4% for RYGB and 0.9% for BPD-DS. Similarly, leak rates were similar at 1 year for LAGB (0.01%), but increased to 0.2% for SG, 0.4% for RYGB and 1.2% for BPD-DS. So, in the short term of 1 year the results with gastric banding are excellent. The more complex the operation the greater the number of adverse and serious adverse events and this has to be weighed against the benefits of a greater weight loss and better comorbidity resolution. In the long term, however, the durability of the LAGB can be questioned.

Altieri et al. tracked all patients in the state of New York over the years 2004–2013 who underwent a gastric band procedure and had their band removed or revised to either Roux-en-Y gastric bypass or sleeve gastrectomy [300]. There were 19,221 records of LAGB placements and 6567 records (34.2%) of revision or removal. From 3158 (16.4%) patients there were follow-up data. Initial revision procedures were coded as band removal in 32.8% ($n = 1035$), band revision in 30.5% ($n = 964$), band removal and replacement in 19.1% ($n = 603$), removal and conversion to SG in 5.6% ($n = 178$), or removal and conversion to RYGB in 12.0% ($n = 378$). From the 3158 patients, 643 (20.4%) required two or more revisions. Albeit being the largest series at present, the major limitation of this study is the inability to determine the reasons for the need of removal or revision, such as device malfunction, band slippage, band obstruction, band erosion or insufficient weight loss.

6.7.1 Band Slippage or Pouch Slippage

Pouch slippage or band slippage is a herniation of a portion of the stomach in a cephalad direction through the band or a caudal movement/slippage of the band. It is difficult to distinguish between these entities and many other names, such as gastric prolapse, slippage of the gastric wall or eccentric pouch dilation, are used to describe the same findings in the end: the post-operative development of an overly large upper gastric pouch which is characterised by food intolerance, dysphagia, epigastric pain and reflux (Fig. 6.10a, b) [290]. A clearly oversized pouch is usually asymmetric. Band slippage or gastric prolapse should be considered when patients who had a normal post-operative period begin to experience changes in their eating ability, e.g. an increase in the sense of restriction or obstruction. It occurs in 2.2–7.8% of the European/Australian studies and between 3.1 and 24% in the US studies [293–295, 301]. Many of the problems such as gastric prolapse and pouch dilation were related to the surgical technique and were more often seen with the perigastric technique (13.3%) than the currently recommended pars flaccida technique (1.8%) with gastrogastric sutures and a 4–6-week postponement of band fill [290–294, 302]. O'Brien and Dixon reported 125 episodes of band slippage (25%) in their first 500 patients using the perigastric approach and only 28 episodes (4.8%) in the last 600 patients after adoption of the pars flaccida technique [303]. In one study with over 1000 consecutive patients a reduction from 20.5 to 1.4% had been described [304]. A meta-analysis of band slippage and band erosion in at least 500 patients and >2-year follow-up resulted in 19 studies with 19,657 patients with a mean follow-up of 6.2 years [302]. Erosion is the process of intragastric band migration. The rates of erosion and slippage were 1.03% (range, 0–3.7) and 1.93% (range, 0.3–12.5), respectively, with a statistically significant overall correlation between erosion and slippage. This correlation was very strong when considering the perigastric technique and not significant in the pars flaccida technique, strongly suggesting that erosion and slippage share a common pathophysiology. Surgical techniques that

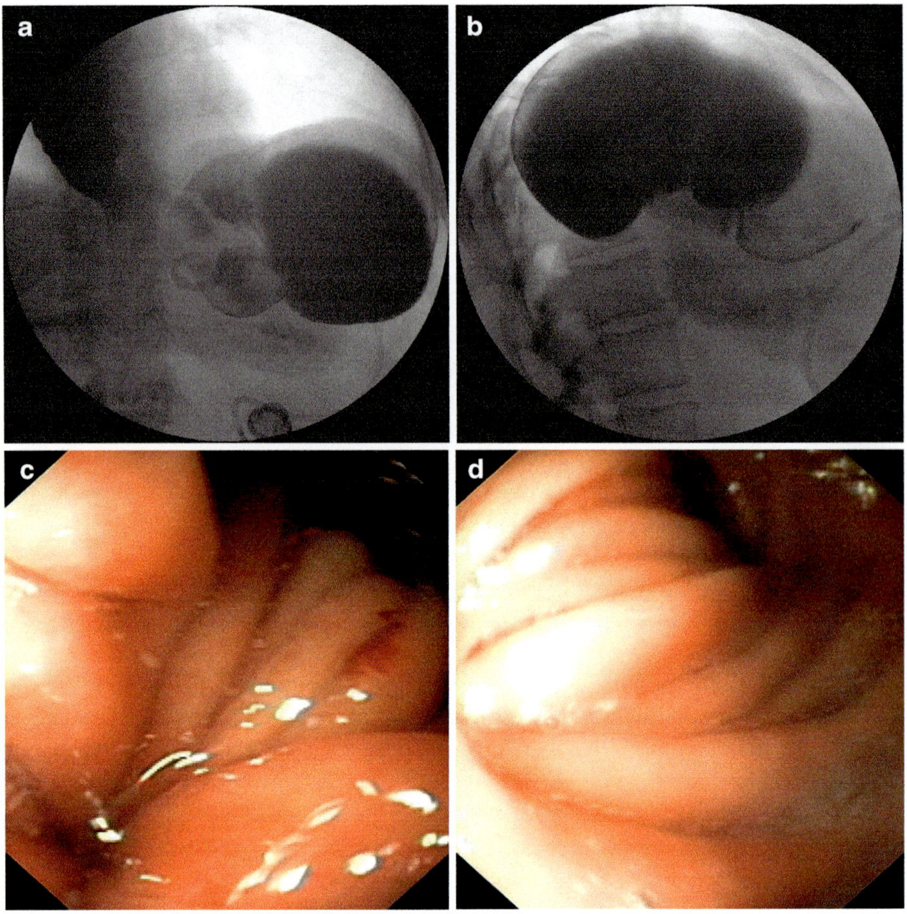

Fig. 6.10 Pouch slippage, band slippage or pouch gastric prolapse. (**a** and **b**) Radiologic appearance of two cases with pouch slippage, the band with its connected tubing and the access port is visible underneath an overly large upper gastric pouch filled with contrast. (**c** and **d**) Endoscopic view of the eccentric pouch dilation with inability or difficulty to enter the distal stomach because of the very eccentric position of the entrance

reduce the slippage should also reduce the rate of erosions and indeed both rates have fallen dramatically following a change from the perigastric to the pars flaccida technique. Another conspicuous finding related to the change in technique was an almost complete annulling of the posterior prolapse and a significant decrease of the anterior prolapse [292].

A change in the band position from baseline radiographic images may suggest gastric prolapse. The most appropriate placement of the band is at an approximately 45° angle towards the left shoulder with the medial aspect of the band juxtaposed to the left pedicle of the vertebra [305]. Based on the portion of herniated stomach, the slippage is divided into anterior or posterior slippage. The herniation of the stomach changes the orientation of the axis of the band; the posterior prolapse (mostly occurring in the perigastric technique) determines a counterclockwise rotation of the band with the axis of the band becoming almost parallel to the vertebral column with a typical O sign of the prolapsed band [292]. In the anterior prolapse (mostly seen with pars flaccida technique), the gastric tissue displaces the band clockwise, resulting in a horizontal appearance of the band [292]. There is no indication for an endoscopy in these cases; endoscopy might even aggravate the situation by air insufflation and by many, often fruitless, attempts to find the path through the band (Fig. 6.10c, d).

Patients usually present with signs of outlet obstruction such as dysphagia, vomiting, regurgitation, food intolerance and abdominal pain. Due to increased tissue mass in the fixed cross-sectional lumen within the band patients may also experience this as feeling the band being too tight [302]. Complications related to band slippage include gastric perforation, necrosis of the slipped stomach, upper gastrointestinal bleeding and aspiration pneumonia. The first action should be to deflate the band, decompress the stomach, give intravenous hydration as needed and determine whether the patient can swallow liquids. If symptoms persist for 3–5 days or if symptoms worsen and tachycardia, raised lactate levels and acidosis complete the picture, this is an emergency as gastric pouch ischaemia and gastric necrosis are imminent. Band removal and occasionally band repositioning are indicated.

6.7.2 Stoma Obstruction

Stoma obstruction is defined as an obstruction to the flow of food from the gastric pouch to the remainder of the stomach. Stoma obstruction in the early post-operative period has a number of causes. Stoma obstruction is usually caused by incorporation of too much tissue inside the band in the perigastric technique or associated with too small bands applied over a thick gastro-oesophageal junction area in the pars flaccida technique [290]. In some cases the band is positioned too distally, causing a large amount of stomach wall to be encompassed by the band. Early stoma obstruction can also be initiated by post-operative oedema of the area incorporated by the band or due to haematoma. The lumen can also be obstructed by insufficiently chewed food, pills or stones; endoscopy is anticipated to remove the offending items. Otherwise, a Gastrografin swallow is indicated. Conservative treatment with intravenous rehydration, deflation of the band and gastric decompression or explorative laparoscopy, when they do not improve, are indicated. Conservative treatment carries a risk of aspiration and ischaemia or necrosis of the occluded tissue in case of an overtight band. Late stoma obstructions are usually related to gastric pouch dilation, gastric prolapse, band slippage or angulation, and band erosion. Deflation of the band, a liquid diet and medical treatment with a PPI can prove salutary [306, 307]. If symptoms of stoma stenosis do not reappear, the band can be inflated step by step. Czeiger et al. tried to relate the intra-band pressure with symptom improvement by band deflation in patients coming to the emergency department with gastric band obstruction [309]. They did not deflate the band entirely but

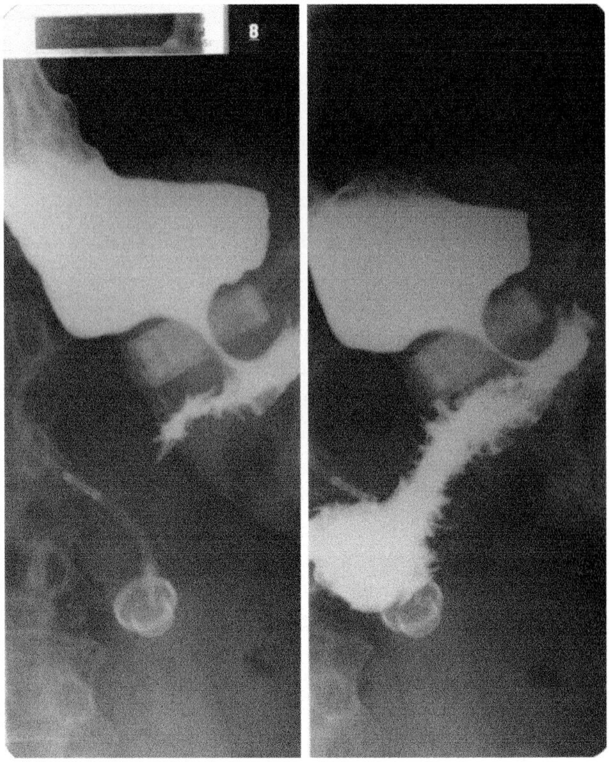

Fig. 6.11 Radiology appearance of a too tight band

discovered that nearly 30% of 48 patients required as little as 0.5 mL of fluid removal, and 60% of them were free of symptoms with removal of 1 mL [308].

One word of caution is adequate here: symptoms may be caused by an excessively tight band, and endoscopy in this setting may lead to perforation (Fig. 6.11). A contrast radiological study should be performed first to assess the degree of constriction and the position of the band. Endoscopy should be performed if symptoms persist after band deflation.

6.7.3 Pouch Dilation and Oesophageal Dilation

Pouch dilation is a common problem, resulting in late functional stenosis and in oesophageal dilation. The endoscopist will find a relatively large pouch with no pouch outlet and during air insufflation the pouch dilation will temporarily increase and occlude the outlet even more. Upper GI barium study reveals the presence of a clearly dilated pouch with "overhanging wall" with regard to the band. One cause of pouch dilation is excessive vomiting. Overeating and ingestion of sparkling drinks may lead to excessive vomiting. However, the most likely cause of gastric pouch dilation is overinflation of the band in patients who do not comply with instructions regarding oral intake [308]. Inappropriate intake can stretch and dilate the gastric pouch and oesophagus which will finally result in an atonic pouch and potentially a dilated atonic oesophagus. Also an underlying oesophageal motility problem may be causal.

Oesophageal dilation is a serious concern seen in 6–10% of patients in the FDA clinical trial and in 0.2% of studies from Europe/Australia [293–295, 301]. The incidence depends on the follow-up with the best data coming from centres that perform a barium swallow each year. Milone et al. performed a 3-year retrospective study on 440 patients and 121 had a follow-up clinic visit and barium swallow performed at 1 year [309]. An oesophagus measuring 35 mm or greater was considered to be dilated. Seventeen patients (14%) were found to have oesophageal dilation with an average diameter of 40.9 mm. GORD symptoms and emesis were more frequent in patients with dilated oesophagus than in those without dilation, but the weight loss was not different. About 29% were asymptomatic. A few years later, Naef et al. reported their data on 167 patients with yearly barium swallow over a follow-up of 12 years [310]. They also considered an oesophageal diameter of 35 mm or greater as being dilated. Oesophageal dilation occurred in 40 patients (25.5%) with a mean oesophageal diameter of 47.3 mm after a follow-up of 73.8 months (range, 36–120 months) compared with 26.2 mm in patients without dilation. Oesophageal dysmotility disorders were found in 108 patients (68.8% of patients followed). They also classified the oesophageal dilation according to Dargent [311]. Stage I was defined by a moderate dilation with delayed emptying; stage II by a hypercontracting oesophagus (nutcracker oesophagus); stage III by a significant dilation with anterior/posterior pouch slipping; and stage IV by major achalasia-like dilation [311]. Of these 40 patients, 34 suffered from stage III dilation (in which band dilation is necessary) and 6 from stage IV (in which band removal is mandatory) [310]. In 29 patients, an upper GI endoscopy was carried out because of heartburn/dysphagia. In 18 patients, the endoscopy was normal; 9 patients suffered from gastro-oesophageal reflux disease, 1 from a stenosis and 1 from a hiatus hernia. One should, however, be aware that stasis and regurgitation of food may mimic symptoms considered to be characteristic for acid reflux.

Already in the past there has been a lively discussion about performing manometry preoperatively, as discussed earlier in Chap. 4, which in itself is not irrelevant with regard to the many abnormal motility patterns associated with obesity, as has been discussed in Chap. 1.

Both Lew et al. and Klaus et al. published their data on oesophageal motility in 2006 [312, 313]. Lew et al. performed preoperative manometry in 77 patients [312]. Fourteen (18.2%) were found to have oesophageal dysmotility. The presence of GORD-like symptoms was evident both in patients with (29%) or without (39%) oesophageal dysmotility. After surgery, in both groups of patients, GORD-like symptoms were improved or completely resolved (100% and 92%, respectively). Klaus et al. described GORD-like symptoms in 164 (27.9%) of 587 patients before gastric banding [313]. In 52 of these patients the symptoms persisted after surgery. These 52 patients were found to have more often disturbed oesophageal motility than those without symptoms post-operatively (20.7% vs. 12%). In the group with oesophageal dysmotility, 18 patients (34.6%) experienced oesophageal dilation after adjustable gastric banding, as did 20 patients (17.9%) in the group without dysmotility. Three of the 18 patients (0.5%) required band removal [313]. In contrast to the recommendations by Klaus et al., the incidence of oesophageal motility disturbances is too low to justify costly routine preoperative testing in everyone [314]. However, in Naef's study 15% of the 40 patients did not recover after band deflation and required removal of the band [310]. Burton et al. tried to get a better understanding of anatomical abnormalities and abnormal oesophageal motility [315–317]. They investigated 143 patients with adverse symptoms or unsatisfactory weight loss after LAGB, with a normal liquid contrast swallow and upper gastrointestinal endoscopy. A stress barium test identified the following appearances: gastric enlargement (n = 57), transhiatal enlargement (n = 44), pan-oesophageal dilation (n = 9) and an anatomically normal situation (n = 33). Twenty-four (72%) of the anatomically normal patients had deficient oesophageal motility. This combination of findings also predicted the outcome: revision LAGB surgery was performed in 56 patients. This was successful in gastric enlargements when oesophageal motility was intact with significant improvement of symptoms and weight loss, but revision surgery for transhiatal enlargements improved symptoms such as dysphagia and reflux but did not improve poor weight loss [317]. From these data they developed the CORE classification which combines anatomical appearance with an assessment of oesophageal motility [317]. Three general anatomical appearances at stress barium test were identified and as mentioned above were a guide in treatment:

1. Gastric enlargements, with subdivision of symmetric gastric enlargement, gastric prolapse and transhiatal gastric enlargement, with mainly reflux as the primary symptom
2. Oesophageal enlargements, with transhiatal oesophageal enlargement, deficient oesophageal motility and pan-oesophageal enlargement, with transhiatal oesophageal enlargement presenting with reflux and dysphagia and pan-oesophageal dilation with loss of satiety
3. Anatomically normal, presenting more commonly with dysphagia complaints, likely a reflection of impaired bolus transit [317]

Treatment comprises complete deflation of the band, gastric decompression, a course of PPIs and a liquid diet for at least 4–6 weeks. Dietary (re)education should be given. If symptoms resolve the band is very prudently inflated step by step and frequent X-ray examinations are performed to follow the pouch volume. A study by Moser and colleagues demonstrated that this conservative approach to pouch enlargement was successful in up to 77% [318]. If pouch dilation reappears, band reposition or removal has to be planned.

6.7.4 Band Erosion

Band erosion is the process of intragastric band migration. Acute erosion is characterised by the free leakage of gastric contents into the peritoneum, similar to

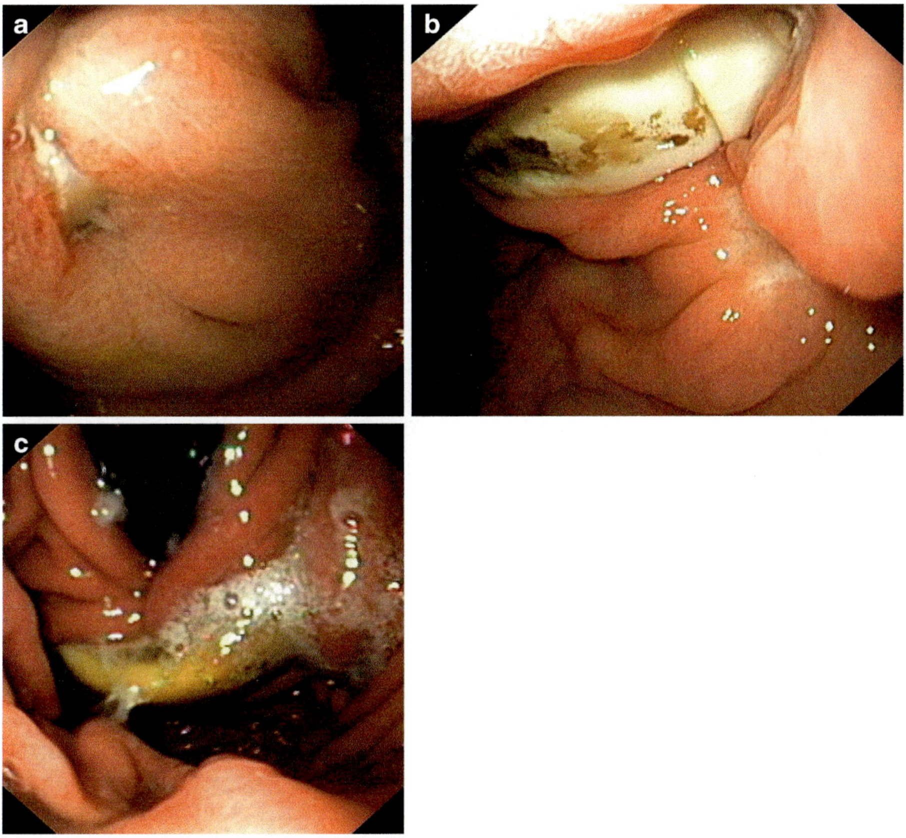

Fig. 6.12 Endoscopic view in retroflexion of an eroded gastric band. (**a**) A very early case of band erosion. (**b**) Erosion of a greater part of the band of recent date with respect to the whitish appearance of the band. (**c**) A longer existing band erosion with yellow colouring of the band due to the contact with bile

the clinical picture of a free gastric perforation with peritonitis, and emergency surgery is indicated [290–292]. In chronic band erosion, the migration process of the band is very slow and the band abrades constantly and slowly against the lumen. It induces significant perigastric localised inflammation and scar tissue formation. At endoscopy the band is visible in the stomach, whitish where it recently penetrated and black discoloured by the long-standing influence of bile (Fig. 6.12a–c). Often, the band erosion is only detected by retroflexion of the endoscope. Many patients are asymptomatic and present only with a non-functioning band with no restriction to the flow of food, they may gain weight and band adjustment has no effect. In many cases, the first indication of possible erosion is infection at the access port by gastric bacteria, ascending along the connecting tubing and reaching the subcutaneous port. Some patients have mild symptoms such as new dysphagia or reflux or more evident obstructive symptoms such as nausea, vomiting and epigastric pain. Also, occasionally referred pain to the shoulder and rarely haematemesis from band erosion into a gastric vessel have been described [319, 320]. In a large Italian survey over the years 1997–2009 intragastric band migrations were seen in 177/6839 (2.8%) which mainly occurred in the first 2 years (41.8%) [321]. It occurred after 24 months in 7.9%, after 36 months in 21.4%, after 48 months in 22.6%, after 60 months in 3.4% and after 72 months in 2.2%. The fate of 165 of the 177 bands was known: 27.7% were removed by laparotomy, 41.8% by laparoscopy and 31.5% by endoscopy [321]. A systematic review of 25 articles in 15,775 patients reported 1.46% erosions (range 0.23–32.7%) [322]. The rate of erosions was predicted by the number of patients and the experience of the surgeon: 4 reports involving less than 100 patients reported an incidence of 10% (27/270) whereas the remaining 21 reports mentioned an incidence of 1.39% (180/12,978) [323]. In a review of 19 studies with 19,657 patients with a mean follow-up of 6.2 years, the rate of erosion was 1.03% (range 0–3.7) [302].

The use of the pars flaccida is associated with a lower erosion rate but there are only a few studies to support this [302]. Boschi et al. reported a drop from 8 to 0.9% [324]. Also in the study by O'Brien et al., who reviewed their data in the three subsequent periods of perigastric technique, pars flaccida technique and the newer band (Lap-Band AP), the erosion rates went down from 8.5 to 2.25%, and 0.8% in the three evolution periods, respectively [292, 295].

The aetiology of band erosion has been attributed to small, undetected operative injuries to the gastric wall, ischaemia from pressure of the gastric band especially when inflated too tightly or due to the inclusion of too much gastric wall at operation, foreign-body reaction against the silicon material, exaggerated stress on the upper gastric pouch by forced endoscopy, excessively large food boluses or excessive vomiting for instance in early pregnancy, and gastric lesions caused by aspirin, NSAIDs, alcohol or smoking [302, 321–323, 325–327]. The erosion site corresponds to the posterior wall where peritoneum coverage is lacking [321].

The band can be removed by laparoscopy or laparotomy. A minimally invasive technique would be the removal by endoscopy. Whatever endoscopic method is used, the port and the maximum length of catheter tubing should first be removed through a cutaneous exploration. Initially, at least a 50% migration into the gastric lumen was required for endoscopic removal by using scissors and diathermy or laser technique, by enhancing migration through increasing the filling volume of the band, or by cutting the small bridge of tissue which held the device to the gastric wall with a needle-knife papillotome, or argon plasma coagulation [325, 328]. This resulted in a gastric fistula in two of the three cases where this was tried in the Italian experience but this complication could be managed by further endoscopies [321]. Blero et al. demonstrated removal of LAGB bands and VBG silastic rings by inducing full band migration by temporary self-expanding plastic stents (SEPS) [329].

Endoscopic removal should only be attempted if the band buckle is visible and >50% of the band is visible. When <50% of the band is eroded, expectant management is advised with evaluation each 2–3 months for serious complications such as haemorrhage, gastrointestinal obstruction, and intra-abdominal or subcutaneous infection. Campos et al. challenged this assertion in a patient with <50% of the band visible [319]. After infiltration with adrenaline they slowly incised the gastric wall covering the LAGB using a endoscopic needle knife with pure coagulation current. To avoid perforation, the incision was limited to the area covering the band near the erosion, under the cardia, and at the anterior wall of the stomach. A second upper endoscopy was performed 7 days later and at this time, after greater penetration of the band, it was possible to visualise its lock. With endoscopic scissors the thread and part of the band lock were cut and once the band was open it was removed orally using a polypectomy snare.

The easiest and almost 100% effective method to cut the band is the tourniquet technique. A metallic thread is passed through the biopsy channel of the endoscope and introduced around the migrated band and retracted out with a forceps to the mouth (Figs. 6.13 and 6.14). Then the two ends of the metallic thread are introduced into an external narrow metal tube or sheath and passed into the tourniquet of the handle of a Gastric Band cutter device (Agency for Medical Innovation (AMI) GmbH, Gotzis, Austria; C.J. Medical, Haddenham, Buckinghamshire, England) or a Soehendra Biliary Mechanical Lithotriptor (Fig. 6.15). The metal tube or sheath containing the cutting wire looped around the intragastric band is passed through the oesophagus to the stomach. By twisting the handle the band is cut under direct vision by strangulation [330, 331].

The largest experience concerns a number of 82 migrated bands; 78 bands (95%) could be transected and removed [332]. In four the bands could be transected but not removed. The band cutter was only used in cases with sufficient erosion, i.e. >50% of the band. Five cases of pneumoperitoneum occurred (6.3% morbidity); three were treated conservatively with nil per mouth, antibiotics and PPIs. One needed laparoscopy and one was treated by abdominal puncture. Some endoscopists recommend CT imaging of the abdominal cavity and band to confirm

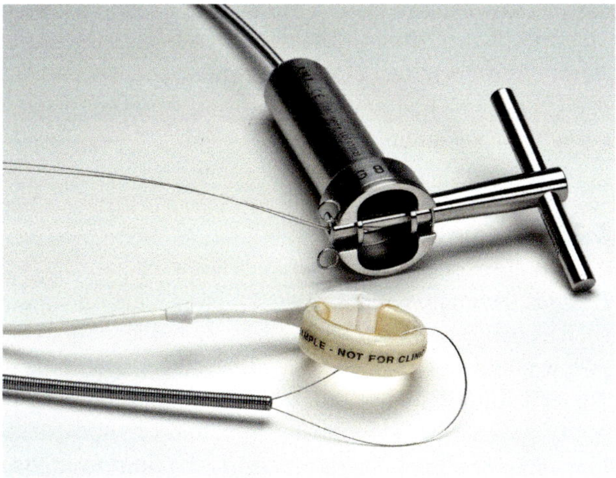

Fig. 6.13 Endoscopic equipment and procedure to cut the band in case of band erosion. The gastric band cutter device with the visible tourniquet, the metallic thread guided around the band with both ends introduced into an external narrow metal tube and into the tourniquet, which by twisting the handle of the tourniquet will cut the band (Agency for Medical Innovation (AMI) GmbH, Gotzis, Austria)

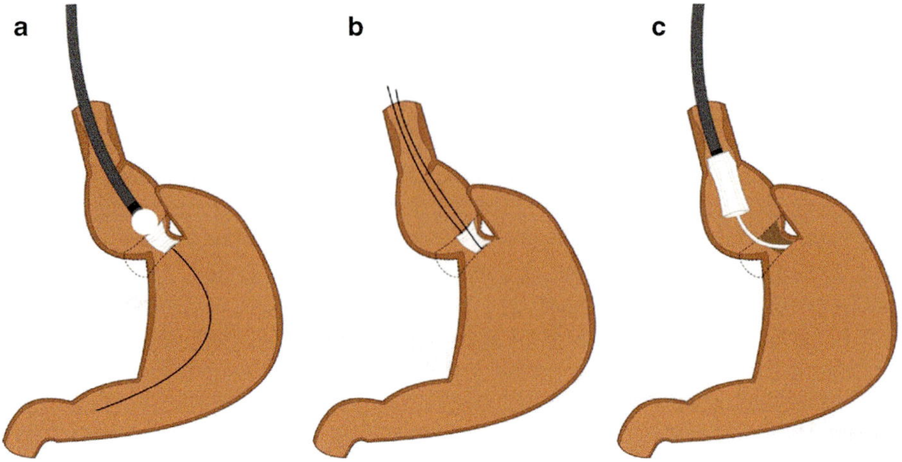

Fig. 6.14 Schematic drawing of the band removal with the gastric band cutter. (**a**) Passage of metallic thread in between eroded band and gastric wall. (**b**) Recovery of thread by endoscope. (**c**) Oral removal of band after cutting it. Reprinted from Surg Obes Relat Dis 2010; 6: 423–427, Galvao Neto MP, Ramos AC, Campos JM, Murakami AH, Falcao M, Moura EH, et al. Endoscopic removal of eroded adjustable gastric band: lessons learned after 5 years and 78 cases, with permission from Elsevier

band encapsulation before attempting endoscopic removal. O'Brien et al. cautioned that due to the low erosion rate of 11 (0.8%) of 1293 patients over a period of 6 years, for most surgeons this would represent ≤2 erosions treated annually and therefore experience, if at all, will come slowly [333]. Although cutting the band was possible in almost every patient, Dogan et al. describe one case where twisting of the cutting wire required conversion from endoscopy to laparotomy [327]. Mozzi et al. reported multiple kinking of the thread due to its thinness above the band and inside the stomach, needing removal of the band and thread by laparoscopy [334]. They propose a different endoscopic wire, the Zebra guidewire (Boston Scientific Corp, Miami, FL, USA), which is thicker and so never coils nor kinks. Also, cutting the band does not guarantee successful removal of the band as the band can be locked in the gastric wall because of severe adhesions and sometimes being fixed by sutures [327, 332, 334].

6.7.5 Weight Regain

Besides the many patient-related factors causing weight regain, band-related causes such as band erosion or disintegration, but also tube- and port-related causes such as port leakage and tube leakage or breakage, should be considered. In these cases the injected fluid does not reach the balloon inside the band and sometimes patients notify pain or swelling during injection of saline. Also, the radiologist or surgeon may recognise the reduction of retrieved fluid from the port as a sign of port leakage or tube fracture or leakage.

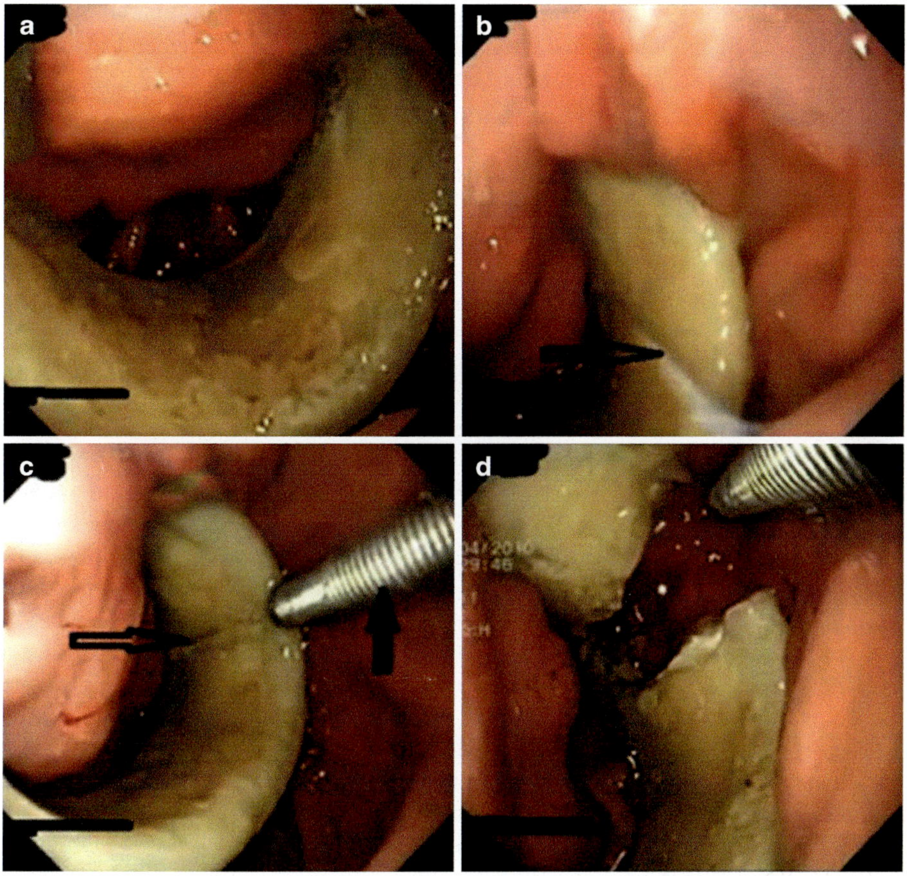

Fig. 6.15 Endoscopic removal of an eroded gastric band by means of a gastric band cutter. (**a**) The gastric band migrated into the stomach. (**b**) The cutting thread of the device (shown by the *open arrow*) is positioned into the stomach through the working channel of the endoscope next to the gastric band and thereafter folded around the band using a snare to retrieve it. (**c**) A metallic tube shown by the solid arrow is inserted into the stomach over both ends of the cutting thread (*open arrow*) and it is pushed against the gastric band under direct endoscopic view. (**d**) The outer edge of the metallic tube is inserted into the tourniquet of the handgrip. By twisting the handle of the device the band is strangulated and cut. Reprinted with permission from Annals of Gastroenterology, Ann Gastroenterol 2016; 29: 249–257, Malli CP, Sioulas AD, Emmanouil T, Dimitriadis GD, Triantafyllou K. Endoscopy after bariatric surgery

6.7.6 Phytobezoar

Four cases of phytobezoars, which are complexes of undigested plant fibres, seeds, skin and peels of fruits and vegetables, have been reported [165]. All four were located in the gastric pouch above the band. Their formation may be due to poor pouch emptying and pouch stasis and because of limited exposure of the high-fibre food to acid, needed to break down the cellulose coatings. The first-line treatment for bezoars after LAGB is deflation of the band. Enzymatic dissolution with papain or endoscopic fragmentation and removal by endoscopy can be tried and advices to prevent phytobezoar formation should be given.

6.7.7 Gastro-Oesophageal Reflux Disease

Within the medical and surgical communities, there is a widely held belief that the LAGB procedure may cause gastro-oesophageal reflux disease (GORD), particularly in patients with weak oesophageal body motility. In this case, a food bolus has to be transported down against a resistance formed by the band, resulting in achalasia-like oesophageal dilation and GORD-like symptoms [313, 314]. Yet, GORD symptoms may have been provoked by overtightening the LAGB system in a patient failing to lose weight. Therefore is it important to study – in a prospective way – patients without symptoms receiving a gastric band as well as patients with GORD complaints who will undergo surgery and will be followed up in time. But the main question is if there is any influence of the gastric band on the normal physiology. De Jong et al. performed a systematic review and found that LAGB has anti-reflux properties, resulting in resolution or improvement of reflux symptoms, normalising pH monitoring, increasing LOS pressure, decreasing transient LOS relaxations and decreasing the risk of oesophagitis in the short term, but in a subset of patients worsening or newly developed symptoms and oesophagitis were found in prolonged follow-up [335]. The anti-reflux effect of the band is likely to be caused by an augmentation of the LOS by creating a longer intra-abdominal pressure zone and by pulling the stomach more into the abdomen in the presence of a hiatal hernia. Probably in the long term, the progressive filling of the band and pouch dilation are responsible for the development of worsened reflux symptoms [310, 336]. Stasis in the pouch and/or oesophagus may also be a factor in increased regurgitation symptoms, and it is well known that symptoms of acid reflux, biliary reflux and food regurgitation in the presence of food stasis converge in the same symptomatology of GORD [337]. Moreover, some surgeons may not conscientiously look for a hiatal hernia at the time of original band placement because of the abundant visceral fat. To do so, the epiphrenic fat pad has to be retracted [301]. With progressive weight loss with loss of visceral fat and diminution of the epiphrenic fat pad, a hiatal hernia may become evident or an existing hiatal hernia may increase, resulting in concentric pouch dilation with GORD symptoms related not so much to the band but to the excessive weight loss [301].

Rebecchi et al. randomly assigned 100 patients to one of the two treatment groups: laparoscopic gastric banding (LAGB) or laparoscopic vertical banded gastroplasty (VBG) [338]. The endpoints of the study were the evaluation of clinical GORD by GORD symptoms and GORD-related quality-of-life questionnaires before the operation and after 3, 12 and 96 months and findings at endoscopy, oesophageal manometry and 24-h pH monitoring before the operation and after 12 and 96 months. At 12 months, GORD had developed in 13 (26%) of the 49 LAGB and 11 (21.6%) of the 51 VBG patients. In the majority of cases, GORD resulted from pouch dilation or poor compliance and required either reoperation (ten after LAGB and three after VBG) or endoscopic dilation (four after VBG). Ten of the LAGB patients had a-peristalsis, all in patients with pouch dilation; six of the VBG patients had a-peristalsis, all in patients with gastric outlet obstruction. A total of 71 patients completed the 96-month follow-up protocol. Three (11.5%) of 26 LASGB patients and 4 (9%) of 45 LVBG patients received PPI therapy for GORD. A-peristalsis was present in one LAGB and two VBG symptomatic GORD patients. This carefully conducted study emphasises the need to measure objectively both patient- and operation-related aspects in order to put symptoms and findings into the right perspective: the increased occurrence of GORD in the early follow-up period of 1 year is often due to a technical defect or poor patient compliance, and during long-term follow-up assessment no significant association between both gastric restrictive procedures and GORD or oesophageal function was found.

Data on GORD in personal series and in large cohorts are available as well: Dixon and O'Brien reported an 89% resolution, 5% improvement and only 2.5% worsening of the symptoms of GORD after LAGB [339]. Data from the Bariatric Surgery Centers of Excellence in the USA compare outcomes of primary bariatric operations in a matched national sample [1]. One of the comorbidities that were taken into consideration was GORD (Table 6.1). GORD was significantly more likely to remit for patients undergoing gastric bypass (OR 1.53, 95% CI: 1.48–1.58) and, although not significant, also for patients undergoing biliopancreatic diversion/duodenal switch (OR 1.20, 95% CI 0.95–1.52) than patients undergoing LAGB, but patients undergoing SG were even less likely to have GORD remit (OR = 0.87, 95% CI: 0.79–0.95).

Very important insights into the relation between GORD and LAGB came from the 5-year prospective APEX study and the 2-year interim analysis of 171 patients (43%) who reported GORD requiring daily medical therapy prior to the LAGB procedure and 224 patients without GORD prior to LAGB surgery (Lap-Band AP) [340]. After 2 years, 122 of the 171 patients (71%) had sufficient data to assess outcomes: 91% of GORD patients experienced resolution and/or improvement of GORD: complete resolution was reported in 98 patients (80%), improvement in 13 (11%), no change in 9 (7%) and worsening in 2 (2%). In the group of 224 patients who completed 2 years of treatment, but did not have GORD symptoms at baseline, 4 patients (1.8%) developed symptoms of GORD, all of whom lost weight. There was no significant correlation between weight loss and reported GORD status after 2 years. Also, device-related adverse events and serious adverse events were similar in patients with GORD and without GORD at baseline, indicating that the Lap-Band AP itself did not increase adverse events in patients with GORD [340]. These data are in contrast to the sleeve data in the BOLD study by DuPree et al., discussed before [264]. Also, revision surgery because of adverse events was necessary in 2.9% of patients (5/171) with GORD at baseline and in 0.45% of patients (1/224) without GORD at baseline after 2 years, a not statistically significant difference. The same was true for pouch dilation which was an uncommon event in 1.2% of patients (2/171) with GORD and 1.8% of patients (4/224) without GORD [340]. The authors provided very strong evidence that the LAGB system does not cause

GORD and suggested that it might even be considered as a therapeutic option in obese patients with the obesity-related GORD comorbidity. The 5-year data are eagerly awaited with this latest Lap-Band AP design [340].

6.8 Vertical Banded Gastroplasty (VBG)

Although vertical banded gastroplasty (VBG) is no longer performed in the USA, due to its popularity in 1980s, many patients still possess this anatomy with its inherent complications [341]. So, endoscopists will very occasionally encounter patients with a vertical banded gastroplasty. The fact that endoscopic solutions for VBG-related problems are still being published up to very recently emphasises the need to remain updated, even for such long-forgotten bariatric interventions.

When patients report problems the endoscopic yield is high [342]. The most commonly reported problems are those of an outlet obstruction, stoma stenosis, band erosion and vertical staple-line disruption. Very important is the surgical report as both silastic rings and mesh materials were used to encircle and enforce the gastric outlet.

6.8.1 Stoma Stenosis

Stenosis of the stoma has to be divided into immediate post-operative, early post-operative (<3 months) and late post-operative (>3 months) stenosis (Fig. 6.16a, b). Oedema or oedema with early scar formation respond well to dilation and the outcome in late scarring is rather poor. Stomal obstruction in the initial post-operative period is often due to oedema and has been simply solved by placement of a nasogastric tube. Stenosis occurring later is believed to result from fibrosis or an inflammatory reaction occurring around the band. In VBG, mainly flexible polyvinyl-tapered bougies (Savary-Gilliard type) have been used. These pass over a previously inserted guidewire; the plastic dilators permit a longer, less traumatic stretching of the stoma. Endoscopic balloons have been used as well. Success rates vary between 46 and 68% for the Savary-Gilliard and 50 and 60% for the fluoroscopic guided balloon dilation [341]. Dilators above 12 mm do not enhance the chance for patient responsiveness but may increase the risk of rupturing the gastric band, thus eliminating weight loss potential. Torsion of the stoma or an angulated channel will predict failure.

A stomal stenosis secondary to tight ring or mesh is traditionally treated with surgical removal of the silastic ring or a complex revision [343]. For the endoscopist, a decompensated pouch after a refractory outlet stoma stenosis without an eroded band after VBG represents another challenge. Blero et al. treated first three patients with an eroded Lap-Band and four patients with an eroded silastic ring and expanded this technique to non-eroded rings that caused outlet stenosis with or without pouch dilation in six patents [329]. The first step involved induction of intragastric migration of the ring or band by the insertion of a plastic self-expandable

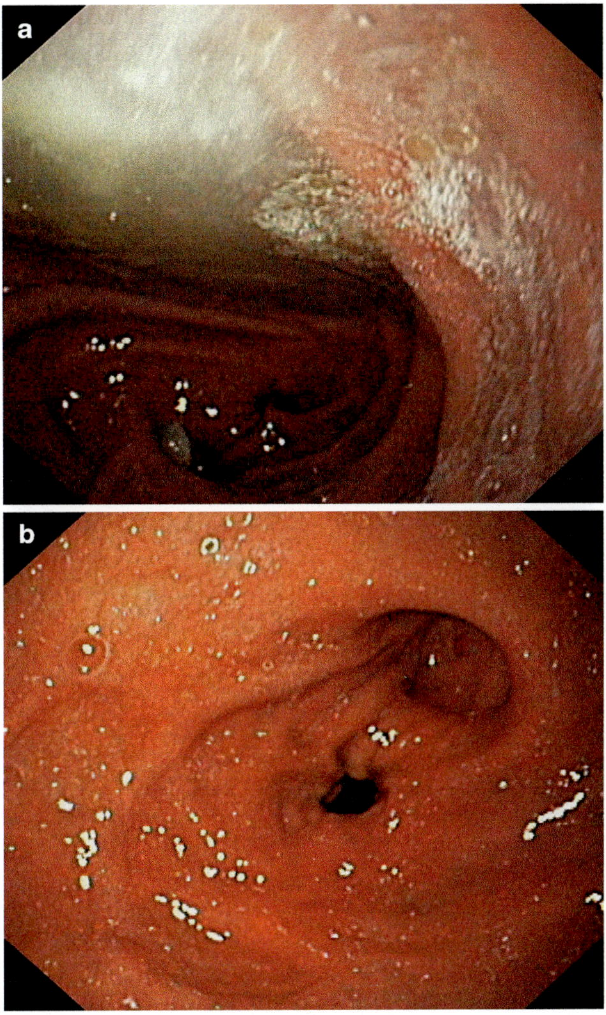

Fig. 6.16 Vertical banded gastroplasty. (**a**) Pouch dilation with stasis of fluid. (**b**) Outlet stenosis as the cause of pouch dilation

stent across the outlet stenosis followed 6–8 weeks later by removal of the stent. The band was cut and the Atkinson extractor was used to remove the band. Lim et al. modified Blero's technique for the removal of the silastic ring but also added a method for the more complicated stenosis caused by mesh material [343].

Aly et al. suggested a minimally invasive technique combining both "transgastric" and "endoscopic" principles for reversal of a VBG stomal stenosis via a single port-site incision [344]. Patients with problematic dysphagia and reflux who just wanted to reverse the stapling without a secondary bariatric procedure were eligible. An endoscope is introduced and negotiated beyond the stoma of the gastric pouch. The stomach is then insufflated via the endoscope and transillumination and indentation is used as is usual in the percutaneous gastrostomy placement to identify a potential point of access through the gastric wall into the antrum of the stomach. From the outside the stomach is punctured to confirm the point of access. A 15 mm incision is made over the chosen point of access and deepened through the rectus fascial layers and peritoneum. Stay sutures are then placed and a gastrotomy is made. A 12 mm blunt-tip balloon self-retaining laparoscopic trocar is then introduced, which secures the gastric wall against the abdominal wall and allows "transgastric" access to a laparoscopic linear cutting stapler. Under direct vision of the endoscopist the stapler is guided across the stoma of VBG. By firing the stapler the stoma of the VBG is cut. The trocar is removed and the gastrotomy is pulled into the wound with the stay sutures and closed. If needed an air leak test can be performed with saline in the wound and air insufflation via the endoscope. The abdominal wound is then closed in layers. They warned that reversal by applying a linear cutting stapler across the stoma is effective and safe, when a polypropylene mesh is used, but that this may not apply to all materials used, such as a silicone ring [344].

Lim et al. treated 14 symptomatic patients with an outlet stenosis at a mean of 14.5 years after the creation of a vertical banded gastroplasty [343]. Two endoscopic methods were developed to remove the band: endoscopic removal of the silastic ring with self-expanding metal stent or endoscopic guided transgastric stapled stricturoplasty. The first method was adapted from Blero et al. and the second was an adaptation of the technique of Aly et al. [329, 344]. The choice of the method depends on whether a silastic ring or a mesh was used to create and enforce the outlet of the VBG and prevent the stretch effect over a period of time in an attempt to improve weight loss. Nine patients who had a silastic ring underwent endoscopic stenting: insertion of a self-expanding stent through the silastic ring. Because of pressure-induced necrosis of the gastric wall interposed between the ring and the stent and migration of the ring inward into the stomach over a period of 4–6 weeks, endoscopic removal of the stent resulted in successful removal of the silastic ring riding on the stent (Figs. 6.17 and 6.18). Two patients in the silastic ring group were not successfully treated (2/9; 22.2%): in one symptoms persisted despite successful removal of the silastic ring due to extensive fibrosis. This patient switched to the second method and was treated successfully. The other suffered from stent migration with obstruction and the need for urgent endoscopic removal, and the ring was removed laparoscopically. Four patients had mesh-induced stenosis and underwent an endoscopic transgastric stapled stricturoplasty. First, a safe area for percutaneous entry as described earlier is chosen. Under endoscopic view the stomach is punctured from outside and a guidewire is introduced into the stomach. Surrounding this puncture site on four locations the stomach is fixed to the anterior abdominal wall as in a gastropexy. Under endoscopic view a 12 mm trocar is introduced and an Endo-GIA stapling device is introduced helped by the endoscopist to provide the best trajectory, and a 30 mm Endo-GIA staple row is fired from the inferior edge of the VBG cephalad, reconnecting the previously excluded fundus with the rest of the stomach. The 12 mm trocar is exchanged for a gastrostomy tube and when access is not any longer needed the tube is removed after 6 weeks. All four were successfully treated with complete symptom resolution.

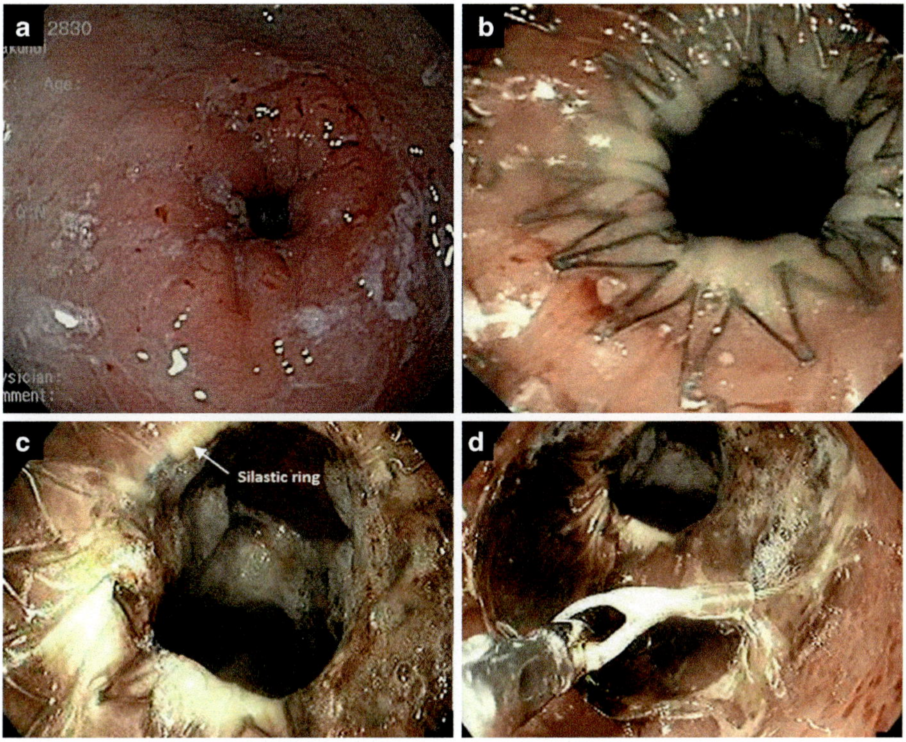

Fig. 6.17 (**a**) Vertical banded gastroplasty stricture. (**b**) Stent placed through the stricture under endoscopic guidance. (**c**) Intragastric migration of the silastic ring due to pressure necrosis of the interjacent tissues towards the stent. (**d**) Stent removal with endoscopic rat tooth grasping forceps. Reprinted from Obes Surg 2016; 26: 2802–2808, Lim CH, Amateau SK, Ikramuddin S, Leslie DB. Endoscopic management of vertical banded gastroplasty stricture: feasibility, safety, and efficacy, with permission of Springer

6.8.2 Band Erosion

Generally, band erosions occur 1–3 years after surgery because of excessively tight bands, infection of the band, and mechanical stress by vomiting or forced endoscopy. Bands of silastic material are easy to remove as they lack the incorporation into surrounding structures or tissues [161]. Bands consisting of Marlex or non-silastic materials are difficult to remove because they integrate in the gastric tissue and surgery is often needed to remove these bands. Surgical removal of the band is complicated by difficulty in locating the band, inability to remove the entire band and damage to surrounding structures with often the need of a gastrotomy. In these cases, removal of eroded bands by endoscopy may pose less risks. Fobi et al. utilised endoscopy to remove an eroded band but they were successful in only 9/14

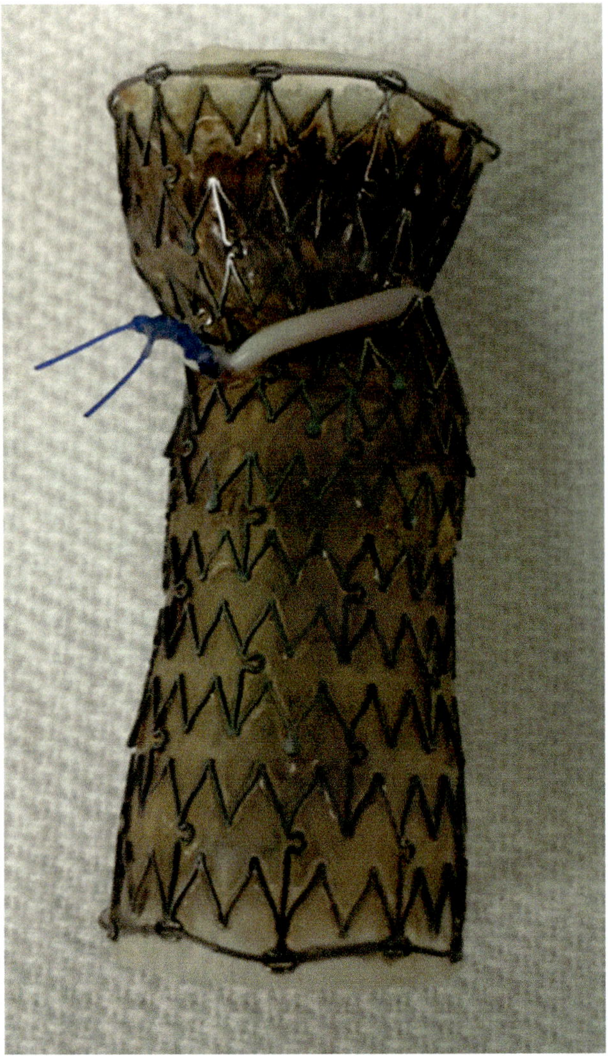

Fig. 6.18 Silastic ring and Prolene suture noted around the stent. Reprinted from Obes Surg 2016; 26: 2802–2808, Lim CH, Amateau SK, Ikramuddin S, Leslie DB. Endoscopic management of vertical banded gastroplasty stricture: feasibility, safety, and efficacy, with permission of Springer

patients [160]. The failures were secondary to inadequate equipment and limitations of the endoscopist. Nd:YAG laser ablation of the band has been reported, but vaporisation of the band was incomplete and required additional techniques to remove the eroded band [345]. Partially eroded Marlex mesh can be transected by argon plasma coagulation at 80 Watts and Meyenberger et al. reported the utilisation of argon plasma coagulation to transect an eroded band [328]. This may work well for conductive material but is not feasible for nonconductive media such as Gore-Tex, silastic or other synthetic materials. On occasion, endoscopic scissor transection is successful in cutting the ring enabling endoscopic removal. Endoscopic scissors were helpful to transect and remove the Gore-Tex band or Marlex mesh [346].

Karmali et al. described their technique of transecting a silastic band [347]. They used a double-channel endoscope, introduced a rat-toothed grasping forceps through the 3.8 mm channel, grasped a segment of the eroded band and pulled it slightly back into the channel to create traction. The straight endoscopic scissors were advanced through the 2.8 mm instrument channel and the band was sequentially transected successfully in all nine patients. Another method was based on Blero's technology of stenting [329]. Forced erosion of the fixed band by endoscopic stenting with self-expandable covered metal stents was successful in 15 cases with in 13 complete band removal and in 2 partial band removal [161]. Initially, to avoid migration, the stent-in-stent procedure was followed, but this caused pain, so that in a later phase covered stents with phalanges were used. Stents remained in place for 3 weeks. The band was cut with endoscopic scissors before extraction. There were five complications: substernal pain in two patients, requiring early stent removal, migration of the stent in one patient, severe nausea and vomiting in one patient and a once a stricture 2 weeks after removal. There was no perforation.

6.8.3 Vertical Staple-Line Disruption

In contrast to the gastric bypass where staple-line disruption will result in weight gain and a marginal ulcer, weight gain and less restriction of food intake are the only symptoms of staple-line disruption in VBG. The endoscopist will see two entrances to the stomach but usually diagnosis is made by barium swallow which will show the gastrogastric fistula.

6.8.4 Weight Regain

Weight regain following VBG may be related to staple-line dehiscence, a gastric outlet obstruction by a too tight band or an eroded band, and pouch dilation. A staple-line breakdown results in a gastrogastric fistula which results in loss of the restrictive benefit of the VBG. Techniques as have been discussed in the subchapter of gastrogastric fistula in gastric bypass may be tried, although data on VBG are not reported. In a gastric outlet obstruction, patients are unable to tolerate solid foods and supplement their diet with high-calorie fluids. In pouch dilation, sometimes accompanied by stoma dilation, a widening of the tube-like structure allows the storage and easy passage of food. Endoluminal therapy might be an option instead of revision surgery. StomaphyX (Endogastric Solutions Inc., Redmond, WA, USA) is an endoluminal plication device that uses H-fasteners to create full-thickness, serosa-to-serosa, endoluminal plications. Manouchehri et al. used the system in 14 patients with regain of at least 15% of the excess body weight lost and an enlarged stoma diameter and enlarged gastric pouch [348]. Eleven patients needed one and three patients needed two separate StomaphyX procedures. Multiple fasteners were fired at each procedure, varying between 23 and 27 fasteners. It was successful in all and resulted in 9.9 kg or 3.6 BMI unit weight loss. There were only minor complications: headache in three patients and back pain in one patient. They discussed the limitations of the procedure in asymmetrical dilation, staple-line dehiscence and band erosion and had the best results in patients with symmetrical dilation of the VBG pouch [348].

6.8.5 Phytobezoar

In the studies that investigated the yield of endoscopy 14% of patients were treated because of food impaction or a bezoar [342]. Bezoars are a rare complication of poor mastication, eating quickly and stasis. These can be dissolved by one-half teaspoon of meat tenderiser (containing the proteolytic enzyme papain) in 250 mL of liquid sipped over 90 min or extracted or fragmented during endoscopy [164, 165, 342]. Metoclopramide to increase motor activity may be of help to prevent the formation in patients with recurrent bezoars.

6.8.6 Gastro-Oesophageal Reflux Disease

Already in 1988, Deitel et al. showed that the vertical banded gastroplasty procedure worked on the same principles as used in the surgical treatment of gastro-oesophageal reflux disease (GORD), such as the repositioning of the gastro-oesophageal junction within the abdomen and constructing an elongated intra-abdominal oesophagus, by converting a part of the lesser curvature into a tube [349]. They observed a reduction in heartburn from 77 to 22% and in regurgitation from 55 to 3% after VBG [349]. Nevertheless, some patients report GORD symptoms after VBG. True reflux from the distal stomach, postprandial oesophageal loading with regurgitation of food, staple-line disruption with a gastrogastric fistula allowing the passage of acid into the pouch and the oesophagus, and large pouches including an increased amount of acid-secreting mucosa may be involved. As has been discussed earlier in the subchapter on GORD in the gastric band procedure, Rebecchi et al. randomised patients to LABG or VBG and studied GORD symptoms, quality of life, findings at endoscopy, manometry and 24-h pH monitoring for up to 96 months [338]. After 12 months GORD was diagnosed in 21.6% (11/51) with a-peristalsis due to gastric outlet obstruction in 6, of whom 4 needed dilation. Three patients underwent a RYGB because of insufficient weight loss. After 96 months 41 patients remained of whom only 4 (9.7%) complained of gastro-oesophageal reflux needing PPIs, with a-peristalsis in 2. So, in the short term mainly technical factors were responsible for symptoms, and indeed when patients present with symptoms also surgical technical factors should be taken into account.

6.9 Guidelines

With all the endoscopic technologies mentioned in the different subchapters it is important to know what guidelines advise. As such the European guideline is rather disappointing [350]. The guideline only discusses early and late dumping with dietary advices and gastrointestinal symptoms with a possible role of endoscopy not discussed at all. In case of failed treatment, further bariatric surgery is advised (evidence level (Oxford) B, C, D) [350].

In contrast, the American Association of Clinical Endocrinologists, The Obesity Society and the American Society for Metabolic and Bariatric Surgery (AACE/TOS/ASMBS) guidelines discuss both diagnosis and treatment with grading of evidence and best evidence levels (BEL) [187]. The diagnosis of post-operative hypoglycaemia is discussed as well as the treatment by diet, medication, gastric restriction and reversal procedures (Grade C, BEL 3). Persistent and severe gastrointestinal symptoms (e.g. nausea, vomiting, abdominal pain, constipation and diarrhoea) warrant evaluation by upper endoscopy (Grade C, BEL 3). In the presence of symptoms suggestive of stricture or foreign body, endoscopy may be the preferred procedure as it can serve at the same time a diagnostic and therapeutic aim (Grade C, BEL 3). Treatment of marginal ulcer should include PPIs, sucralfate and, if *H. pylori* is identified, eradication with triple therapy (Grade C, BEL 3). Patients who underwent RYGB with non-partitioned stomach who develop a gastrogastric fistula with symptoms of weight regain, marginal ulcer, stricture or GORD may benefit from a revision procedure (Grade C, BEL 3). In a detailed discussion, they mention endoscopic plication and suturing but the technology required and endoscopic skills needed to perform these endoluminal procedures are not widely available and are considered investigational at this time (BEL 3). Persistent vomiting, regurgitation or upper gastrointestinal obstruction after LAGB should be treated with immediate removal of fluid from the band (Grade D). However, persistent symptoms of GORD, regurgitation, chronic cough or recurrent aspiration raise the concern of the band being too tight or the development of pouch dilation or oesophageal dilation and should promptly be referred to a bariatric surgeon (Grade D). Prophylactic cholecystectomy may be considered with RYGB to prevent gallbladder complications (Grade B, BEL 2). Oral administration of ursodeoxycholic acid, at least 300 mg/d in divided doses, significantly decreases gallstone formation after RYGB and may be considered for use in patients not having had a cholecystectomy (Grade A, BEL 1) [187].

The Standard Practice Committee of the American Society for Gastrointestinal Endoscopy (ASGE) in conjunction with the Society of Gastrointestinal and Endoscopic Surgeons (SAGES) and the American Society for Metabolic and Bariatric Surgery (ASMBS) searched the literature between January 1980 and December 2013 and issued their recommendations about the role of endoscopy in the bariatric surgery patient [11]. Weaker recommendations were phrased as suggestions and stronger advices as recommendations. The quality of the evidence (QoE) was graded as high, moderate, low and very low. They recommend the following:

1. Endoscopy as a first-line diagnostic study in patients with abdominal pain, nausea or vomiting: In the immediate post-operative period consultation with the surgeon is recommended (moderate QoE). They suggest endoscopic management in fistulas and leaks in consultation with a bariatric surgeon (very low QoE).

2. Endoscopic dilation of symptomatic stomal stenosis up to 15 mm, which should be avoided after LAGB and VBG (moderate QoE).

They suggest the following:

1. Endoscopic removal of suture material from the mature gastrojejunal anastomosis in symptomatic patients (low QoE).
2. An individualised approach to ERCP in patients with RYGB (low QoE).
3. Any attempt to stoma reduction in patients with weight regain be conducted in a multidisciplinary weight management as there are sparse data regarding its effectiveness (low QoE).

Conclusions

Many gastrointestinal symptoms may occur after bariatric surgery, even when the anatomy may remain relatively intact. The timing of symptoms and the type of bariatric surgery are helpful in estimating the chance of finding significant abnormalities when performing endoscopy. Each time, the appropriate diagnostic procedure as well as the sequence should be considered (i.e. radiology or endoscopy). Many of the abnormalities found are treatable, either medically though dietary adjustments, behavioural changes and medication or endoscopically with minimally invasive methods, and eventually surgery. The Natural Orifice Transluminal Endoscopic Surgery (NOTES), aimed at minimisation of abdominal trauma, contributed to the concept of endoscopic addressing of major complications both by its philosophy of reducing the invasiveness of abdominal surgery by choosing other entries and by being conceptual in the development of new instruments. However, it should be realised that some of the endoscopic approaches and solutions for problems require a lot of skills. A good example is the whole spectrum of possibilities to perform an ERCP after a gastric bypass, but this is still within the reach of an experienced endoscopist who is used to perform ERCPs and who can decide which of the methods can be applied in his/her hospital. None of the methods require extravagant equipment. On the contrary, when endoluminal procedures such as plication come into the field, special equipment, often still investigational, is needed and the skills have to be learned. With a rather low frequency of certain complications, the question arises whether enough cases can be treated to get enough skills and experience and to maintain these skills over time. Another implication of the rarity of some complications is that a scientific proof of the efficacy and safety of its treatment will be very hard to obtain.

References

1. Sudan R, Maciejewski ML, Wilk AR, Nguyen NT, Ponce J, Morton JM. Comparative effectiveness of primary bariatric operations in the United States. Surg Obes Relat Dis. 2017;13:826–35.

2. Byrne TK. Complications of surgery for obesity. Surg Clin North Am. 2001;81:1181–93, vii-viii
3. Huang CS, Farraye FA. Endoscopy in the bariatric surgical patient. Gastroenterol Clin North Am. 2005;34:151–66.
4. Ukleja A, Stone RL. Medical and gastroenterologic management of the post-bariatric surgery patient. J Clin Gastroenterol. 2004;38:312–21.
5. Livingston EH. Complications of bariatric surgery. Surg Clin North Am. 2005;85:853–68.
6. Eisenberg D, Duffy AJ, Bell RL. Update on obesity surgery. World J Gastroenterol. 2006;12:3196–203.
7. Mathus-Vliegen EMH. The role of endoscopy in bariatric surgery. Best Pract Res Clin Gastroenterol. 2008;22:839–65.
8. Obstein KL, Thompson CC. Endoscopy after bariatric surgery (with videos). Gastrointest Endosc. 2009;70:1161–6.
9. Levitzky BE, Wassef WY. Endoscopic management in the bariatric surgical patient. Curr Opin Gastroenterol. 2010;26:632–9.
10. Kumar N, Thompson CC. Endoscopic management of complications after gastrointestinal weight loss surgery. Clin Gastroenterol Hepatol. 2013;11:343–53.
11. Evans JA, Muthusamy VR, Acosta RD, Bruining DH, Chandrasekhara V, Chathadi KV, et al. The role of endoscopy in the bariatric surgery patient. Gastrointest Endosc. 2015;81:1063–72.
12. Mathus-Vliegen EMH. The cooperation between endoscopists and surgeons in treating complications of bariatric surgery. Best Pract Res Clin Gastroenterol. 2014;28:703–25.
13. Kalfarentzos F, Kechagias I, Soulikia K, Loukidi A, Mead N. Weight loss following vertical banded gastroplasty: intermediate results of a prospective study. Obes Surg. 2001;11:265–70.
14. Jaffin BW, Knoepflmacher P, Greenstein R. High prevalence of asymptomatic esophageal motility disorders among morbidly obese patients. Obes Surg. 1999;9:390–5.
15. Yu S, Jastrow K, Clapp B, Kao L, Klein C, Scarborough T, et al. Foreign material erosion after laparoscopic Roux-en-Y gastric bypass: findings and treatment. Surg Endosc. 2007;21:1216–20.
16. Ryou M, Mogabgab O, Lautz DB, Thompson CC. Endoscopic foreign body removal for treatment of chronic abdominal pain in patients after Roux-en-Y gastric bypass. Surg Obes Relat Dis. 2010;6:526–31.
17. Nguyen NT, Longoria M, Chalifoux S, Wilson SE. Gastrointestinal hemorrhage after laparoscopic gastric bypass. Obes Surg. 2004;14:1308–12.
18. Karmali S, Brar B, Shi X, Sharma AM, de Gara C, Birch DW. Weight recidivism post-bariatric surgery: a systematic review. Obes Surg. 2013;23:1922–33.
19. Schirmer B, Erenoglu C, Miller A. Flexible endoscopy in the management of patients undergoing Roux-en-Y gastric bypass. Obes Surg. 2002;12:634–8.
20. Huang CS, Forse RA, Jacobson BC, Farraye FA. Endoscopic findings and their clinical correlations in patients with symptoms after gastric bypass surgery. Gastrointest Endosc. 2003;58:859–66.
21. Marano BJ Jr. Endoscopy after Roux-en-Y gastric bypass: a community hospital experience. Obes Surg. 2005;15:342–5.
22. Wilson JA, Romagnuolo J, Byrne TK, Morgan K, Wilson FA. Predictors of endoscopic findings after Roux-en-Y gastric bypass. Am J Gastroenterol. 2006;101:2194–9.
23. Lee JK, Van Dam J, Morton JM, Curet M, Banerjee S. Endoscopy is accurate, safe, and effective in the assessment and management of complications following gastric bypass surgery. Am J Gastroenterol. 2009;104:575–82.
24. Podnos YD, Jimenez JC, Wilson SE, Stevens CM, Nguyen NT. Complications after laparoscopic gastric bypass: a review of 3464 cases. Arch Surg. 2003;138:957–61.
25. Csendes A, Torres J, Burgos AM. Late marginal ulcers after gastric bypass for morbid obesity. Clinical and endoscopic findings and response to treatment. Obes Surg. 2011;21:1319–22.
26. Carr WJR, Mahawar KK, Balupuri S, Small PK. An evidence-based algorithm for the management of marginal ulcers following Roux-en-Y gastric bypass. Obes Surg. 2014;24:1520–7.

27. Coblijn UK, Lagarde SM, de Castro SMM, Kuiken SD, van Wagensveld BA. Symptomatic marginal ulcer disease after Roux-en-Y gastric bypass: incidence, risk factors and management. Obes Surg. 2015;25:805–11.
28. Csendes A, Burgos AM, Burdiles P. Incidence of anastomotic strictures after gastric bypass: a prospective consecutive routine endoscopic study 1 month and 17 months after surgery in 441 patients with morbid obesity. Obes Surg. 2009;19:269–73.
29. Mason EE, Munns JR, Kealey GP, Wangler R, Clarke WR, Cheng HF, et al. Effect of gastric bypass on gastric secretion. 1977. Surg Obes Relat Dis. 2005;1:155–60.
30. MacLean LD, Rhode BM, Nohr C, Katz S, McLean AP. Stomal ulcer after gastric bypass. J Am Coll Surg. 1997;185:1–7.
31. Capella JF, Capella RF. Gastro-gastric fistulas and marginal ulcers in gastric bypass procedures for weight reduction. Obes Surg. 1999;9:22–7.
32. Gilmore MM, Kallies KJ, Mathiason MA, Kothari SN. Varying marginal ulcer rates in patients undergoing laparoscopic Roux-en-Y gastric bypass for morbid obesity versus gastroesophageal reflux disease: is the acid pocket to blame? Surg Obes Relat Dis. 2013;9:862–6.
33. Pope GD, Goodney PP, Burchard KW, Proia RR, Olafsson A, Lacy BE, et al. Peptic ulcer/stricture after gastric bypass: a comparison of technique and acid suppression variables. Obes Surg. 2002;12:30–3.
34. Sacks BC, Mattar SG, Qureshi FG, Eid GM, Collins JL, Barinas-Mitchell EJ, et al. Incidence of marginal ulcers and the use of absorbable anastomotic sutures in laparoscopic Roux-en-Y gastric bypass. Surg Obes Relat Dis. 2006;2:11–6.
35. Rasmussen JJ, Fuller W, Ali MR. Marginal ulceration after laparoscopic gastric bypass: an analysis of predisposing factors in 260 patients. Surg Endosc. 2007;21:1090–4.
36. Csendes A, Smok G, Burgos AM. Prospective sequential endoscopic and histologic studies of the gastric pouch in 130 morbidly obese patients submitted to Roux-en-y gastric bypass. ABCD Arq Bras Cir Dig. 2012;25:245–9.
37. Papasavas PK, Gagné DJ, Donnelly PE, Salgado J, Urbandt JE, Burton KK, et al. Prevalence of Helicobacter pylori infection and value of preoperative testing and treatment in patients undergoing laparoscopic Roux-en-Y gastric bypass. Surg Obes Relat Dis. 2008;4:383–8.
38. Hartin CW Jr, ReMine DS, Lucktong TA. Preoperative bariatric screening and treatment of Helicobacter pylori. Surg Endosc. 2009;23:2531–4.
39. Scheffel O, Daskalakis M, Weiner R. Two important criteria for reducing the risk of postoperative ulcers at the gastrojejunostomy site after gastric bypass: patient compliance and type of gastric bypass. Obes Facts. 2011;4(Suppl 1):39–41.
40. Loewen M, Giovanni J, Barba C. Screening endoscopy before bariatric surgery: a series of 448 patients. Surg Obes Relat Dis. 2008;4:709–14.
41. D'Hondt MA, Pottel H, Devriendt D, van Rooy F, Vansteenkiste F. Can a short course of prophylactic low-dose proton pump inhibitor therapy prevent stomal ulceration after laparoscopic Roux-en-Y gastric bypass? Obes Surg. 2010;20:595–9.
42. Gonzalez R, Lin E, Venkatesh KR, Bowers SP, Smith CD. Gastrojejunostomy during laparoscopic gastric bypass: analysis of 3 techniques. Arch Surg. 2003;138:181–4.
43. Azagury DE, Abu Dayyeh BK, Greenwalt IT, Thompson CC. Marginal ulceration after Roux-en-Y gastric bypass surgery: characteristics, risk factors, treatment, and outcomes. Endoscopy. 2011;43:950–4.
44. Keith JN. Endoscopic management of common bariatric surgical complications. Gastrointest Endosc Clin N Am. 2011;21:275–85.
45. Kaplan LM. Gastrointestinal management of the bariatric surgery patient. Gastroenterol Clin North Am. 2005;34:105–25.
46. Cai JX, Schweitzer MA, Kumbhari V. Endoscopic management of bariatric surgery complications. Surg Laparosc Endosc Percutan Tech. 2016;26:93–101.
47. Garrido AB Jr, Ross M, Lima SE Jr, Brenner AS, Gomes CAR Jr. Early marginal ulcer following Roux-en-Y gastric bypass under proton pump inhibitor treatment – prospective multicentric study. Arq Gastroenterol. 2010;47:130–5.

48. Moon RC, Teixeira AF, Goldbach M, Jawad MA. Management and treatment outcomes of marginal ulcers after Roux-en-Y gastric bypass at a single high volume bariatric center. Surg Obes Relat Dis. 2014;10:229–34.
49. Ying VW, Kim SH, Khan KJ, Farrokhyar F, D'Souza J, Gmora S, et al. Prophylactic PPI help reduce marginal ulcers after gastric bypass surgery: a systematic review and meta-analysis of cohort studies. Surg Endosc. 2014;29:1018–23.
50. Jirapinyo P, Watson RR, Thompson CC. Use of a novel endoscopic suturing device to treat recalcitrant marginal ulceration (with video). Gastrointest Endosc. 2012;73:435–9.
51. Barola S, Magnuson T, Schweitzer M, Chen Y-I, Ngamruengphong S, Khashab MA, et al. Endoscopic suturing for massively bleeding marginal ulcer 10 days post Roux-en-Y gastric bypass. Obes Surg. 2017;27:1394–6.
52. Wetter A. Role of endoscopy after Roux-en-Y gastric bypass surgery. Gastrointest Endosc. 2007;66:253–5.
53. Haddad A, Tapazoglou N, Singh K, Averbach A. Role of intraoperative esophagogastroenteroscopy in minimizing gastrojejunostomy-related morbidity: experience with 2,311 laparoscopic gastric bypasses with linear stapler anastomosis. Obes Surg. 2012;22:1928–33.
54. Al Hadad M, Dehni N, Elamin D, Ibrahim M, Ghabra S, Nimeri A. Intraoperative endoscopy decreases postoperative complications in laparoscopic Roux-en-Y gastric bypass. Obes Surg. 2015;25:1711–5.
55. Go MR, Muscarella P, Needleman BJ, Cook CH, Melvin WS. Endoscopic management of stomal stenosis after Roux-en-Y gastric bypass. Surg Endosc. 2004;18:56–9.
56. Barba CA, Butensky MS, Lorenzo M, Newman R. Endoscopic dilation of gastroesophageal anastomosis stricture after gastric bypass. Surg Endosc. 2003;17:416–20.
57. Ahmad J, Martin J, Ikramuddin S, Schauer P, Slivka A. Endoscopic balloon dilation of gastroenteric anastomotic stricture after laparoscopic gastric bypass. Endoscopy. 2003;35:725–8.
58. Campos MS, Mello FS, Ferraz AAB, Brito JN, Nassif PN, Galvao-Neto MP. Endoscopic dilatation of gastrojejunal anastomosis after gastric bypass. Arq Bras Cir Dig. 2012;25:283–9.
59. Malli CP, Sioulas AD, Emmanouil T, Dimitriadis GD, Triantafyllou K. Endoscopy after bariatric surgery. Ann Gastroenterol. 2016;29:249–57.
60. Escalona A, Devaud N, Boza C, Perez G, Fernandez J, Ibanez L, et al. Gastrojejeunal anastomotic strictures alter Roux-en-Y gastric bypass: ampulatory management with the Savary-Gillard dilator. Surg Endosc. 2007;21:765–8.
61. Fernandez-Esparrach G, Bordas JM, Llach J, Lacy A, Delgado S, Vidal J, et al. Endoscopic dilation with Savary-Gillard bougies of stomal strictures after gastric bypass laparoscopic in morbidity obese patients. Obes Surg. 2008;18:155–61.
62. Costa AF, Almeida FF, Brado JL, Takahashi W. Endoscopic treatment of postoperative complications following Roux-en-Y gastric bypass (RYGB): Results of 73 cases. Gastrointest Endosc. 2009;69:AB200–1.
63. Vance PL, Delange EE, Shaiffer B. Gastric outlet obstruction following surgery for morbid obesity: efficacy of fluoroscopy guided balloon dilatation. Radiology. 2002;222:70–2.
64. Schwartz ML, Drew RL, Roiger RW, Ketover SR, Chazin-Caldie M. Stenosis of the gastroenterostomy after laparoscopic gastric bypass. Obes Surg. 2004;14:484–91.
65. Sanyal AJ, Sugerman HJ, Kellum JM, Engle KM, Wolfe L. Stomal complications of gastric bypass: incidence and outcome of therapy. Am J Gastroenterol. 1992;87:1165–9.
66. Nguyen NT, Stevens CM, Wolfe BM. Incidence and outcome of anastomotic strictures after laparoscopic gastric bypass. J Gastrointest Surg. 2003;7:997–1003.
67. Goitein D, Papasavas PK, Gagne D, Ahmad S, Caushaj PF. Gastrojejunal strictures following laparoscopic Roux-en-Y gastric bypass for morbid obesity. Surg Endosc. 2005;19:628–32.
68. Carrodeguas L, Szomstein S, Zundel N, Lo Menzo E, Rosenthal P. Gastrojejunal anastomotic strictures following laparoscopic Roux-en-Y gastric bypass surgery: analysis of 1291 patients. Surg Obes Relat Dis. 2006;2:92–7.
69. Catalano M, Chua T, Rudig G. Endoscopic balloon dilation of stomal stenosis following gastric bypass. Obes Surg. 2007;17:298–303.

70. Peifer KJ, Shiels AJ, Azar R, Rivera RE, Eagon JC, Jonnalagadda S. Successful endoscopic management of gastrojejunal anastomotic strictures after Roux-en-Y gastric by-pass. Gastrointest Endosc. 2007;66:248–52.
71. Takata MC, Clovica R, Cello JP, Posselt AM, Rogers SJ, Campos GM. Predictors, treatment, and outcomes of gastrojejunostomy stricture after gastric bypass for morbid obesity. Obes Surg. 2007;17:878–84.
72. Caro L, Sanchez C, Rodriguez P, Bosch J. Endoscopic balloon dilation of anastomotic strictures after LRYGB. Dig Dis. 2008;26:314–7.
73. Ukleja A, Afonso BB, Pimentel R, Szomstein S, Rosenthal R. Outcome of endoscopic balloon dilation of strictures after laparoscopic gastric bypass. Surg Endosc. 2008;22:1746–50.
74. Alasfar F, Sabnis AA, Liu RC, Chand B. Stricture rate after laparoscopic Roux-en-Y gastric bypass with a 21-mm circular stapler: the Cleveland Clinic experience. Med Princ Pract. 2009;18:364–7.
75. Dolce CJ, Dunnican WJ, Kushnir L, Bendana E, Ata A, Singh TP. Gastrojejunal strictures alter Roux-en-Y gastric bypass with a 22-mm stapler. JSLJ. 2009;13:306–11.
76. Ryskina KL, Miller KM, Aisenberg J, Herron DM, Kini SU. Routine management of stricture after gastric bypass and predictors of subsequent weight loss. Surg Endosc. 2010;24:554–60.
77. Da Costa M, Mata A, Espinós J, Vila V, Roca JM, Turró J, et al. Endoscopic dilation of gastrojejunal anastomotic strictures after laparoscopic gastric bypass. Predictors of initial failure. Obes Surg. 2011;21:36–41.
78. Espinel J, de-la-Cruz JL, Pinedo E, Canga J, de-la-Cruz F. Stenosis in laparoscopic gastric bypass: management by endoscopic dilation without fluoroscopic guidance. Rev Esp Enferm Dig. 2011;103:508–10.
79. Yimcharoen P, Henegham H, Chand B, Talarico JA, Tariq N, Kroh M, et al. Successful management of gastrojejunal stricture after gastric bypass: is timing important? Surg Obes Relat Dis. 2012;8:151–7.
80. Rossi TR, Dynda DI, Estes NC, Marshall JS. Stricture dilation after laparoscopic Roux-en-Y gastric bypass. Am J Surg. 2005;189:357–60.
81. Mathew A, Veliuona MA, DePalma FJ, Cooney RN. Gastrojejunal strictures after gastric bypass and efficacy of endoscopic intervention. Dig Dis Sci. 2009;54:1971–8.
82. Rosenthal RJ, Szomstein S, Kennedy CI, Soto FC, Zundel N. Laparoscopic surgery for morbid obesity: 1,001 consecutive bariatric operations performed at the Bariatric Institute, Cleveland Clinic Florida. Obes Surg. 2006;16:119–24.
83. Campos GM, Ciovica R, Rogers SJ, Posselt AM, Vittinghoff E, Takata M, et al. Spectrum and risk factors of complications after gastric bypass. Arch Surg. 2007;142:969–75.
84. Carter JT, Tafreshian S, Campos GM, Tiwari U, Herbella F, Cello JP, et al. Routine upper GI series after gastric bypass does not reliably identify anastomotic leaks or predict stricture formation. Surg Endosc. 2007;21:2172–7.
85. Papasavas PK, Caushaj PF, McCormick JT, Quintin RF, Hayetian FD, Maurer J, et al. Laparoscopic management of complications following laparoscopic Roux-en-Y gastric bypass for morbid obesity. Surg Endosc. 2003;17:610–4.
86. Perugini RA, Mason R, Czerniach DR, Novitsky YW, Baker S, Litwin DE, et al. Predictors of complication and suboptimal weight loss after laparoscopic Roux-en-Y gastric bypass: a series of 188 patients. Arch Surg. 2003;138:541–5.
87. Blackstone RP, Rivera LA. Predicting stricture in morbidly obese patients undergoing laparoscopic Roux-en-Y gastric bypass: a logistic regression analysis. J Gastrointest Surg. 2007;11:403–9.
88. Hirdes MMC, van Hooft JE, Koornstra JJ, Timmer R, Leenders M, Weersma RK, et al. Endoscopic corticosteroid injections do not reduce dysphagia after endoscopic dilation therapy in patients with benign esophagogastric anastomotic strictures. Clin Gastroenterol Hepatol. 2013;11:795–801.
89. Yimcharoen P, Heneghan HM, Tariq N, Brethauer SA, Kroh M, Chand B. Endoscopic stent management of leaks and anastomotic strictures after foregut surgery. Surg Obes Relat Dis. 2011;7:628–36.

90. Iqbal A, Miedema B, Ramaswamy A, Fearing N, de la Torre R, Pak Y, et al. Long-term outcome after endoscopic stent therapy for complications after bariatric surgery. Surg Endosc. 2011;25:515–20.
91. Wei W, Ramaswamy A, de la Torre R, Miedema BW. Partially covered esophageal stents cause bowel injury when used to treat complications of bariatric surgery. Surg Endosc. 2013;27:56–60.
92. Eubanks S, Edwards CA, Fearing NM, Ramaswamy A, de la Torre RA, Thaler KJ, et al. Use of endoscopic stents to treat anastomotic complications after bariatric surgery. J Am Coll Surg. 2008;206:935–9.
93. Eisendrath P, Cremer M, Himpens J, Cadiere GB, Le Moine O, Deviere J. Endotherapy including temporary stenting of fistulas of the upper gastrointestinal tract after laparoscopic bariatric surgery. Endoscopy. 2007;39:625–30.
94. Puig CA, Waked TM, Baron TH Sr, Wong Kee Song LM, Sarr MG. The role of endoscopic stents in the management of chronic anastomotic and staple line leaks and chronic strictures after bariatric surgery. Surg Obes Relat Dis. 2014;10:613–7.
95. Schubert D, Kuhn R, Lippert H, Pross M. Endoscopic treatment of benign gastrointestinal anastomotic strictures using argon plasma coagulation in combination with diathermy. Surg Endosc. 2003;17:1579–82.
96. Skinner M, Peter S, Wilcox CM, Mönkemüller K. Diagnostic and therapeutic utility of double-balloon enteroscopy for obscure GI bleeding in patients with surgically altered upper GI anatomy. Gastrointest Endosc. 2014;80:181–6.
97. Issa H, Al-Saif O, Al-Momen S, Bseiso B, Al-Salem A. Bleeding duodenal ulcer after Roux-en-Y gastric bypass surgery: the value of laparoscopic gastroduodenoscopy. Ann Saudi Med. 2010;30:67–9.
98. Magro DO, Geloneze B, Delfini R, Pareja BC, Callejas F, Pareja JC. Long-term weight regain after gastric bypass: a 5-year prospective study. Obes Surg. 2008;18:648–51.
99. Hsu LK, Benotti PN, Dwyer J, Roberts SB, Saltzman E, Shikora S, et al. Nonsurgical factors that influence the outcome of bariatric surgery: a review. Psychosom Med. 1998;60:338–46.
100. Biron S, Hould FS, Lebel S, Marceau S, Lescelleur O, Simard S, et al. Twenty years of biliopancreatic diversion: what is the goal of the surgery? Obes Surg. 2004;14:160–4.
101. Santo MA, Riccioppo D, Pajecki D, Kawamoto F, de Cleva R, Antonangelo L, et al. Weight regain after gastric bypass: influence of gut hormones. Obes Surg. 2016;26:919–25.
102. Abu Dayyeh BK, Jirapinyo P, Thompson CC. Plasma ghrelin levels and weight regain after Roux-en-Y gastric bypass surgery. Obes Surg. 2017;27:1031–6.
103. Abu Dayyeh BK, Lautz DB, Thompson CC. Gastrojejunal stoma diameter predicts weight regain after Roux-en-Y gastric bypass. Clin Gastroenterol Hepatol. 2011;9:228–33.
104. Yimcharoen P, Heneghan HM, Singh M, Brethauer S, Schauer P, Rogula T, et al. Endoscopic findings and outcomes of revisional procedures for patients with weight recidivism after gastric bypass. Surg Endosc. 2011;25:3345–52.
105. Heneghan HM, Yimcharoen P, Brethauer SA, Kroh M, Chand B. Influence of pouch and stoma size on weight loss after gastric bypass. Surg Obes Relat Dis. 2012;8:408–15.
106. Himpens J, Coromina L, Verbrugghe A, Cadière G-B. Outcomes of revisional procedures for insufficient weight loss or weight regain after Roux-En-Y gastric bypass. Obes Surg. 2012;22:1746–54.
107. Dakin GF, Eid G, Mikami D, Pryor A, Chand B. Endoluminal revision of gastric bypass for weight regain—a systematic review. Surg Obes Relat Dis. 2013;9:335–42.
108. Spaulding L. Treatment of dilated gastrojejunostomy with sclerotherapy. Obes Surg. 2003;13:254–7.
109. Catalano FM, Rudic G, Anderson JA, Chua TY. Weight regain after bariatric surgery as a result of a large gastric stoma: Endotherapy with sodium morrhuate may prevent the need for surgical revision. Gastrointest Endosc. 2007;66:240–5.
110. Spaulding L, Osler T, Patlak J. Long-term results of sclerotherapy for dilated gastrojejunostomy after gastric bypass. Surg Obes Relat Dis. 2007;3:623–6.

111. Loewen M, Barba C. Endoscopic sclerotherapy for dilated gastrojejunostomy of failed gastric bypass. Surg Obes Relat Dis. 2008;4:539–42.
112. Madan AK, Martinez JM, Khan KA, Tichansky DS. Endoscopic sclerotherapy for dilated gastrojejunostomy after gastric bypass. J Laparoendosc Adv Surg Tech A. 2010;20:235–7.
113. Abu Dayyeh BK, Jirapinyo P, Weitzner Z, Barker C, Flicker MS, Lautz DB, et al. Endoscopic sclerotherapy for the treatment of weight regain after Roux-en-Y gastric bypass: outcomes, complications, and predictors of response in 575 procedures. Gastrointest Endosc. 2012;76:275–82.
114. Giurgius M, Fearing N, Weir A, Micheas L, Ramaswamy A. Long-term follow-up evaluation of endoscopic sclerotherapy for dilated gastrojejunostomy after gastric bypass. Surg Endosc. 2014;28:1454–9.
115. Schweitzer M. Endoscopic intraluminal suture plication of the gastric pouch and stoma in postoperative Roux-en-Y gastric bypass patients. J Laparoendosc Adv Surg Tech A. 2004;14:223–6.
116. Thompson CC, Slattery J, Bundga EM, Lautz BD. Peroral endoscopic reduction of dilated gastrojejunal anastomosis after Roux-en-Y gastric bypass: a possible new option for patients with weight regain. Surg Endosc. 2006;20:1744–8.
117. Thompson CC, Chand B, Chen YK, Demarco DC, Miller L, Schweitzer M, et al. Endoscopic suturing for transoral outlet reduction increases weight loss after Roux-en-Y gastric bypass surgery. Gastroenterology. 2013;145:129–37.
118. Fernandez-Esparrach G, Lautz DB, Thompson CC. Peroral endoscopic anastomotic reduction improves intractable dumping syndrome in Roux-en-Y gastric bypass patients. Surg Obes Relat Dis. 2010;6:36–40.
119. Kumar N, Thompson CC. Comparison of a superficial suturing device with a full-thickness suturing device for transoral outlet reduction (with videos). Gastrointest Endosc. 2014;79:984–9.
120. Ryou M, Mullady DK, Lautz DB, Thompson CC. Pilot study evaluating technical feasibility and early outcomes of second generation endo-surgical platform for treatment of weight regain after gastric bypass surgery. Surg Obes Relat Dis. 2009;5:450–4.
121. Mullady DK, Lautz DB, Thompson CC. Treatment of weight regain after gastric bypass surgery when using a new endoscopic platform: initial experience and early outcomes (with video). Gastrointest Endosc. 2009;70:440–4.
122. Horgan S, Jacobsen G, Weiss GD, Oldham JS, Denk PM Borao F, et al. Incisionless revision of post-Roux-en-Y bypass stomal and pouch dilation: multicentre registry results. Surg Obes Relat Dis. 2010;6:290–5.
123. Brengman ML, Schroder GL. 12-month outcomes after revision of post Roux-en-Y bypass stomal and pouch dilation with an endoscopic tissue anchoring system: a prospective case series report. Bariatric Times. 2010;7:14–7.
124. Borao F, Gorcey S, Capuano A. Prospective single-site case series utilizing an endolumenal tissue anchoring system for revision of post-RYGB stomal and pouch dilatation. Surg Endosc. 2010;24:2308–13.
125. Raman SR, Holover S, Garber S. Endolumenal revision obesity surgery results in weight loss and closure of gastric-gastric fistula. Surg Obes Relat Dis. 2011;7:304–8.
126. Gallo AS, DuCoin CG, Berducci MA, Nino DF, Almadani M, Sandler BJ, et al. Endoscopic revision of gastric bypass: holy grail or epic fail? Surg Endosc. 2016;30:3922–7.
127. Mikami DJ, Needleman B, Narula V, Durant J, Melvin WS. Natural orifice surgery: initial US experience utilizing the StomaphyX device to reduce gastric pouches after Roux-en-Y gastric bypass. Surg Endosc. 2010;24:223–8.
128. Leitman IM, Virk CS, Avgerinos DV, Patel R, Lavarias V, Surick B, et al. Early results of trans-oral endoscopic plication and revision of the gastric pouch and stoma following Roux-en-Y gastric bypass surgery. JSLS. 2010;14:217–20.
129. Ong'uti SK, Ortega G, Onwugbufor MT, Ivey GD, Fullum TM, Tran DD. Effective weight loss management with endoscopic gastric plication using StomaphyX device: is it achievable? Surg Obes Relat Dis. 2013;9:113–7.

130. Goyal V, Holover S, Garber S. Gastric pouch reduction using StomaphyXTM in post Roux-en-Y gastric bypass patients does not result in sustained weight loss: a retrospective analysis. Surg Endosc. 2013;27:3417–20.
131. Eid GM, McCloskey CA, Eagleton JK, Lee LB, Courcoulas AP. StomaphyX vs a sham procedure for revisional surgery to reduce regained weight in Roux-en-Y gastric bypass patients. A randomized clinical trial. JAMA Surg. 2014;149:372–9.
132. Galvao Neto M, Rodriguez L, Zundel N, Ayala JC, Campos J, Ramos A. Endoscopic revision of Roux-en-Y gastric bypass stomal dilation with a suturing device: preliminary results of a first out-of United States series. Bariatric Times. 2011;8:32–4.
133. Jirapinyo P, Slattery J, Ryan MB, Abu Dayyeh BK, Lautz DB, Thompson CC. Evaluation of an endoscopic suturing device for transoral outlet reduction in patients with weight regain following Roux-en-Y gastric bypass. Endoscopy. 2013;45:532–6.
134. Gitelis M, Ujiki M, Farwell L, Linn J, Wang C, Miller K, et al. Six month outcomes in patients experiencing weight gain after gastric bypass who underwent gastrojejunal revision using an endoluminal suturing device. Surg Endosc. 2015;29:2133–40.
135. Kumar N, Thompson CC. Transoral outlet reduction for weight regain after gastric bypass: long-term follow-up. Gastrointest Endosc. 2016;83:776–9.
136. Thompson CC, Jacobsen GR, Schroder GL, Horgan S. Stoma size critical to 12-month outcomes in endoscopic suturing for gastric bypass repair. Surg Obes Relat Dis. 2012;8:282–7.
137. Heylen AM, Jacobs A, Lybeer M, Prosst RL. The OTSC(R)-clip in revisional endoscopy against weight gain after bariatric gastric bypass surgery. Obes Surg. 2011;21:1629–33.
138. Baretta GA, Alhinho HC, Matias JE, Marchesini JB, de Lima JHF, Empinotti C, et al. Argon plasma coagulation of gastrojejunal anastomosis for weight regain after gastric bypass. Obes Surg. 2015;25:72–9.
139. Kumar N. Weight loss endoscopy: development, applications, and current status. World J Gastroenterol. 2016;22:7069–79.
140. Abidi WM, Aihara H, Thompson CC. Modified endoscopic submucosal dissection techniques before endoscopic revision of a gastric bypass. Gastrointest Endosc. 2016;83:1281–2.
141. Kumar N, Thompson CC. The pursestring technique for endoscopic revision of gastric bypass. Gastrointest Endosc. 2015;82:956.
142. Brethauer SA, Pryor AD, Chand B, Schauer P, Rosenthal R, Richards W, et al. Endoluminal procedures for bariatric patients: expectations among bariatric surgeons. Surg Obes Relat Dis. 2009;5:231–6.
143. Valli PV, Gubler C. Review article including treatment algorithm: endoscopic treatment of luminal complications after bariatric surgery. Clin Obes. 2017;7:115–22.
144. Filho AJ, Kondo W, Nassif LS, Garcia MJ, Tirapelle RA, Dotti CM. Gastrogastric fistula: a possible complication of Roux-en-Y gastric bypass. JSLS. 2006;10:326–31.
145. Bhardwaj A, Cooney RN, Wehrman A, Rogers AM, Mathew A. Endoscopic repair of small symptomatic gastrogastric fistulas after gastric bypass surgery: a single center experience. Obes Surg. 2010;20:1090–5.
146. Griffith PS, Birch DW, Sharma AM, Karmali S. Managing complications associated with laparoscopic Roux-en-Y gastric bypass for morbid obesity. Can J Surg. 2012;55:329–36.
147. Mercky P, Gonzalez JM, Aimore Bonin E, Emungania O, Brunet J, Grimaud J-C, et al. Usefulness of over-the-scope clipping system for closing digestive fistulas. Dig Endosc. 2015;27:18–24.
148. Law R, Wong Kee Song LM, Irani S, Baron TH. Immediate technical and delayed clinical outcome of fistula closure using an over-the-scope clip device. Surg Endosc. 2015;29:1781–6.
149. Winder JS, Kulaylat AN, Schubart JR, Hal HM, Pauli EM. Management of non-acute gastrointestinal defects using the over-the-scope clips (OTSCs): a retrospective single-institution experience. Surg Endosc. 2016;30:2251–8.
150. Haito-Chavez Y, Law JK, Kratt T, Arezzo A, Verra M, Morino M, et al. International multicenter experience with an over-the-scope clipping device for endoscopic management of GI defects (with video). Gastrointest Endosc. 2014;80:610–22.
151. Thompson CC, Carr-Locke DL, Saltzman J, Lautz D, Slattery J, Robinson MK. Peroral endoscopic repair of staple-line dehiscence in Roux-en-Y bypass: a less invasive approach. Gastroenterology. 2004;126(Suppl 2):A810 (abstract).

152. Fernandez-Esparrach G, Lautz DB, Thompson CC. Endoscopic repair of gastrogastric fistula after Roux-en-Y gastric bypass: a less-invasive approach. Surg Obes Relat Dis. 2010;6:282–8.
153. Spaun GO, Martinec DV, Kennedy TJ, Swanström LL. Endoscopic closure of gastrogastric fistulas by using a tissue apposition system (with videos). Gastrointest Endosc. 2010;71:606–11.
154. Flicker MS, Lautz DB, Thompson CC. Endoscopic management of gastrogastric fistulae does not increase complications at bariatric revision surgery. J Gastrointest Surg. 2011;15:1736–42.
155. Maluf-Filho F, Hondo F, Halwan B, de Lima MS, Giordano-Nappi JH, Sakai P. Endoscopic treatment of Roux-en-Y gastric bypass-related gastrocutaneous fistulas using a novel biomaterial. Surg Endosc. 2009;23:1541–5.
156. Toussaint E, Eisendrath P, Kwan V, Dugardeyn S, Devière J, Le Moine O. Endoscopic treatment of postoperative enterocutaneous fistulas after bariatric surgery with the use of a fistula plug: report of five cases. Endoscopy. 2009;41:560–3.
157. Bezerra Silva L, Moon RC, Teixeira AF, Jawad MA, Bandeira Ferraz AA, Galvão Neto M, et al. Gastrobronchial fistula in sleeve gastrectomy and Roux-en-Y gastric bypass—a systematic review. Obes Surg. 2015;25:1959–65.
158. Campos JM, Pereira EF, Evangelista LF, Siqueira L, Galvão Neto M, Dib V, et al. Gastrobronchial fistula after sleeve gastrectomy and gastric bypass: endoscopic management and prevention. Obes Surg. 2011;21:1520–9.
159. Guillaud A, Moszkowicz D, Nedelcu M, Caballero-Caballero A, Rebibo L, Reche F, et al. Gastrobronchial fistula: a serious complication of sleeve gastrectomy. Results of a French multicentric study. Obes Surg. 2015;25:2352–9.
160. Fobi M, Lee H, Igwe D, Felahy B, James E, Stanczyk M, et al. Band erosion: incidence, etiology, management and outcome after banded vertical gastric bypass. Obes Surg. 2001;11:699–707.
161. Wilson TD, Miller N, Brown N, Snyder BE, Wilson EB. Stent induced gastric wall erosion and endoscopic retrieval of nonadjustable gastric band: a new technique. Surg Endosc. 2013;27:1617–21.
162. Ferraz A, Campos J, Dib V, Silva LB, de Paula PS, Gordejuela A, et al. Food intolerance after banded gastric bypass without stenosis: aggressive endoscopic dilation avoids reoperation. Obes Surg. 2013;23:959–64.
163. Swain JM, Scott P, Nesset E, Sarr MG. All strictures are not alike: laparoscopic removal of nonadjustable Silastic bands after banded Roux-en-Y gastric bypass. Surg Obes Relat Dis. 2002;8:190–3.
164. Powers WF, Miles DR. Phytobezoar causing small bowel obstruction seven years after laparoscopic Roux-en-Y gastric bypass. Surg Obes Relat Dis. 2011;7:e3–5.
165. Ben-Porat T, Dagan SS, Goldenshluger A, Yuval JB, Elazary R. Gastrointestinal phytobezoar following bariatric surgery: systematic review. Surg Obes Relat Dis. 2016;12:1747–54.
166. Hewitt AN, Levine MS, Rubesin SE, Laufer I. Gastric bezoars: reassessment of clinical and radiographic findings in 19 patients. Br J Radiol. 2009;82:901–7.
167. da Silva Chaves Y, Destefani AC. Pathophysiology, diagnosis and treatment of dumping syndrome and its relation to bariatric surgery. ABCD Arq Bras Cir Dig. 2016;29(Suppl.1):116–9.
168. Berg P, McCallum R. Dumping syndrome: a review of the current concepts of pathophysiology, diagnosis, and treatment. Dig Dis Sci. 2016;61:11–8.
169. van Beek AP, Emous M, Laville M, Tack J. Dumping syndrome after esophageal, gastric or bariatric surgery: pathophysiology, diagnosis, and management. Obes Rev. 2017;18:68–85.
170. Hammer HF. Medical complications of bariatric surgery: focus on malabsorption and dumping syndrome. Dig Dis. 2012;30:182–6.
171. Sigstad H. A clinical diagnostic index in the diagnosis of the dumping syndrome. Changes in plasma volume and blood sugar after a test meal. Acta Med Scand. 1970;188:479–86.
172. Arts J, Caenepeel P, Bisschops R, Dewulf D, Holvoet L, Piessevaux H, et al. Efficacy of the longacting repeatable formulation of the somatostatin analogue octreotide in postoperative dumping. Clin Gastroenterol Hepatol. 2009;7:432–7.

173. Suhl E, Anderson-Haynes S-E, Mulla C, Patti M-E. Medical nutrition therapy for post-bariatric hypoglycemia: practical insights. Surg Obes Relat Dis. 2017;13:888–96.
174. Eisenberg D, Azagury DE, Ghiassi S, Grover BT, Kim JJ. ASMBS position statement on postprandial hyperinsulinemic hypoglycemia after bariatric surgery. Surg Obes Relat Dis. 2017;13:371–8.
175. Feitoza AB, Baron TH. Endoscopy and ERCP in the setting of previous upper GI tract surgery. Part I: reconstruction without alteration of pancreaticobiliary anatomy. Gastrointest Endosc. 2001;54(2001):743–9.
176. Sinar DR, Flickinger EG, Park HK, Sloss RR. Retrograde endoscopy of the bypassed segment of the stomach after gastric bypass surgery. South Med J. 1985;78:255–8.
177. Saleem A, Baron TH, Gostout CJ, Topazian MD, Levy MJ, Petersen BT, et al. Endoscopic retrograde cholangiopancreatography using a single-balloon enteroscope in patients with altered Roux-en-Y anatomy. Endoscopy. 2010;42:656–60.
178. Safatle-Ribeiro AV, Kuga R, Iriya K, Ribeiro U Jr, Faintuch J, Ishida RK, et al. What to expect in the excluded stomach mucosa after vertical banded Roux-en-Y gastric bypass for morbid obesity. J Gastrointest Surg. 2007;11:133–7.
179. Watson RR, Braver JM, Thompson CC. EUS-guided transgastric upper GI series for the evaluation of the defunctionalized stomach after gastric bypass. Gastrointest Endosc. 2012;76:219–20.
180. Keren D, Madi H, Matter I, Assalia A, Rainis T. Feasibility and importance of enteroscopy after gastric bypass. Obes Surg. 2017;27:1309–15.
181. Shiffman ML, Sugerman HJ, Kellum JM, Brewer WH, Moore EW. Gallstone formation after rapid weight loss: a prospective study in patients undergoing gastric bypass surgery for treatment of morbid obesity. Am J Gastroenterol. 1991;86:1000–5.
182. Li VK, Pulido N, Fajnwaks P, Szomstein S, Rosenthal R, Martinez-Duartez P. Predictors of gallstone formation after bariatric surgery: a multivariate analysis of risk factors comparing gastric bypass, gastric banding, and sleeve gastrectomy. Surg Endosc. 2009;23:1640–4.
183. Miller K, Hell E, Lang B, Lengauer E. Gallstone formation prophylaxis after gastric restrictive procedures for weight loss: a randomized double-blind placebo-controlled trial. Ann Surg. 2003;238:697–702.
184. Sugerman HJ, Brewer WH, Shiffman ML, Brolin RE, Fobi MA, Linner JH, et al. A multicenter, placebo-controlled, randomized, double-blind, prospective trial of prophylactic ursodiol for the prevention of gallstone formation following gastric-bypass-induced rapid weight loss. Am J Surg. 1995;169:91–6.
185. Adams LB, Chang C, Pope J, Kim Y, Liu P, Yates A. Randomized, prospective comparison of ursodeoxycholic acid for the prevention of gallstones after sleeve gastrectomy. Obes Surg. 2016;26:990–4.
186. Uy MC, Talingdan-Te MC, Espinosa WZ, Daez ML, Ong JP. Ursodeoxycholic acid in the prevention of gallstone formation after bariatric surgery: a meta-analysis. Obes Surg. 2008;18:1532–8.
187. Mechanick JI, Youdim A, Jones DB, Garvey WT, Hurley DL, McMahon MM, et al. Clinical practice guidelines for the perioperative nutritional, metabolic, and nonsurgical support of the bariatric surgery patient—2013 update: cosponsored by American Association of Clinical Endocrinologists, the Obesity Society, and American Society for Metabolic & Bariatric Surgery. Obesity. 2013;21:S1–S27.
188. Warschkow R, Tarantino I, Ukegjini K, Beutner U, Guller U, Schmied BM, et al. Concomitant cholecystectomy during laparoscopic Roux-en-Y gastric bypass in obese patients is not justified: a meta-analysis. Obes Surg. 2013;23:397–407.
189. Melmer A, Sturm W, Kuhnert B, Engl-Prosch J, Ress C, Tschoner A, et al. Incidence of gallstone formation and cholecystectomy 10 years after bariatric surgery. Obes Surg. 2015;25:1171–6.
190. Worni M, Guller U, Shah A, Gandhi M, Shah J, Rajgor D, et al. Cholecystectomy concomitant with laparoscopic gastric bypass: a trend analysis of the nationwide inpatient sample from 2001 to 2008. Obes Surg. 2012;22:220–9.

191. Pineda O, Maydón HG, Amado M, Sepúlveda EM, Guilbert L, Espinosa O, et al. A prospective study of the conservative management of asymptomatic preoperative and postoperative gallbladder disease in bariatric surgery. Obes Surg. 2017;27:148–53.
192. Amer S, Horsley-Silva JL, Menias CO, Pannala R. Endoscopic retrograde cholangiopancreatography in patients with surgically altered gastrointestinal anatomy. Abdom Imaging. 2015;40:2921–31.
193. Elton E, Hanson BL, Qaseem T, Howell DA. Diagnostic and therapeutic ERCP using an enteroscope and a pediatric colonoscope in long-limb surgical bypass patients. Gastrointest Endosc. 1998;47:62–7.
194. Wright BE, Cass OW, Freeman ML. ERCP in patients with long-limb Roux-en-Y gastrojejunostomy and intact papilla. Gastrointest Endosc. 2002;56:225–32.
195. Pai RD, Carr-Locke DL, Thompson CC. Endoscopic evaluation of the defunctionalized stomach by using ShapeLock technology (with video). Gastrointest Endosc. 2007;66:578–81.
196. Matsushita M, Shimatani M, Ikeura T, Takaoka M, Okazaki K. ERCP for altered Roux-en-Y anatomy: a single-balloon or short-balloon enteroscope? Endoscopy. 2011;43:169.
197. Shimatani M, Matsushita M, Takaoka M, Koyabu M, Ikeura T, Kato K, et al. Effective "short" double-balloon enteroscope for diagnostic and therapeutic ERCP in patients with altered gastrointestinal anatomy: a large scale series. Endoscopy. 2009;41:849–54.
198. Skinner M, Popa D, Neumann H, Wilcox CM, Mönkemüller K. ERCP with the overtube-assisted enteroscopy technique: a systematic review. Endoscopy. 2014;46:560–72.
199. Inamdar S, Slattery E, Sejpal DV, Miller LS, Pleskow DK, Berzin TM, et al. Systematic review and meta-analysis of single-balloon enteroscopy–assisted ERCP in patients with surgically altered GI anatomy. Gastrointest Endosc. 2015;82:9–19.
200. Abu Dayyeh B. Single-balloon enteroscopy-assisted ERCP in patients with surgically altered GI anatomy: getting there. Gastrointest Endosc. 2015;82:20–3.
201. Mönkemüller K, Toshniwal J, Zabielski M. Therapeutic endoscopic retrograde cholangiography and cholangioscopy (ERCC) combining a single-balloon enteroscope and an ultraslim endoscope in altered gastrointestinal anatomy. Endoscopy. 2012;44:E349–50.
202. Shah RJ, Smolkin M, Yen R, Ross A, Kozarek RA, Howell DA, et al. A multicenter, U.S. experience of single-balloon, double-balloon, and rotational overtube–assisted enteroscopy ERCP in patients with surgically altered pancreaticobiliary anatomy (with video). Gastrointest Endosc. 2013;77:593–600.
203. Iqbal S, Friedel DM, Grendell JH, Stavropoulos SN. Outcomes of endoscopic-ultrasound-guided cholangiopancreatography: a literature review. Gastroenterol Res Pract. 2013;2013:869214.
204. Weilert F, Binmoeller KF, Marson F, Bhat Y, Shah JN. Endoscopic ultrasound-guided anterograde treatment of biliary stones following gastric bypass. Endoscopy. 2011;43:1105–8.
205. Kedia P, Sharaiha RZ, Kumta NA, Kahaleh M. Internal EUS-directed transgastric ERCP (EDGE): game over. Gastroenterology. 2014;147:566–8.
206. Law R, Wong Kee Song LM, Petersen BT, Baron TH. Single-session ERCP in patients with previous Roux-en-Y gastric bypass using percutaneous-assisted transprosthetic endoscopic therapy: a case series. Endoscopy. 2013;45:671–5.
207. Badaoui A, Malherbe V, Rosiere A, De Ronde T. ERCP by laparoscopic transgastric access and cholecystectomy at the same time in a patient with gastric bypass who was seen with choledocholithiasis. Gastrointest Endosc. 2010;71:212–4.
208. Peeters G, Himpens J, Leman G. ERCP by laparoscopic transgastric access and cholecystectomy at the same time in a patient with gastric bypass who was seen with choledocholithiasis. Gastrointest Endosc. 2010;72:1115–6.
209. Schreiner MA, Chang L, Gluck M, Irani S, Gan I, Brandabur JJ, et al. Laparoscopy–assisted versus balloon enteroscopy–assisted ERCP in bariatric post–Roux-en-Y gastric bypass patients. Gastrointest Endosc. 2012;75:748–56.
210. Bertin PM, Singh K, Arregui ME. Laparoscopic transgastric endoscopic retrograde cholangiopancreatography (ERCP) after gastric bypass: case series and a description of technique. Surg Endosc. 2011;25:2592–6.

211. Lopes TL, Clements RH, Mel Wilcox CM. Laparoscopy-assisted ERCP: experience of a high-volume bariatric surgery center (with video). Gastrointest Endosc. 2009;70:1254–9.
212. Falcao M, Campos JM, Galvão Neto M, Ramos A, Secchi T, Alves E, et al. Transgastric endoscopic retrograde cholangiopancreatography for the management of biliary tract disease after Roux-en-Y gastric bypass treatment for obesity. Obes Surg. 2012;22:872–6.
213. Saleem A, Levy MJ, Petersen BT, Que FG, Baron TH. Laparoscopic assisted ERCP in Roux-en-Y gastric bypass (RYGB) surgery patients. J Gastrointest Surg. 2012;16:203–8.
214. Frederiksen NA, Tveskov L, Helgstrand F, Naver L, Floyd A. Treatment of common bile duct stones in gastric bypass patients with laparoscopic transgastric endoscopic retrograde cholangiopancreatography. Obes Surg. 2017;27:1409–13.
215. Mejía R, Achurra P, Gabrielli M, Briceño E, Rebolledo R, Torres A, et al. Laparoscopy-assisted trans-gastric rendez-vous for the treatment of common bile duct stones in patients with prior Roux-en-Y gastric bypass. Obes Surg. 2016;26:2809–13.
216. Gutierrez JM, Lederer H, Krook JC, Kinney TP, Freeman ML, Jensen EH. Surgical gastrostomy for pancreatobiliary and duodenal access following Roux en Y gastric bypass. J Gastrointest Surg. 2009;13:2170–5.
217. Tekola B, Wan AY, Ramanath M, Burnette B, Ellen K, Schirmer BD, et al. Percutaneous gastrostomy tube placement to perform transgastrostomy endoscopic retrograde cholangiopancreaticography in patients with Roux-en-Y anatomy. Dig Dis Sci. 2011;56:3364–9.
218. Attam R, Leslie D, Freeman M, Ikramuddin S, Andrade R. EUS-assisted, fluoroscopically guided gastrostomy tube placement in patients with Roux-en-Y gastric bypass: a novel technique for access to the gastric remnant. Gastrointest Endosc. 2011;74:677–82.
219. Kedia P, Kumta NA, Sharaiha R, Kahaleh M. Bypassing the bypass: EUS-directed transgastric ERCP for Roux-en-Y anatomy. Gastrointest Endosc. 2015;81:223–4.
220. Lopes TL, Wilcox CM. Endoscopic retrograde cholangiopancreatography in patients with Roux-en-Y anatomy. Gastroenterol Clin North Am. 2010;39:99–107.
221. Azeem N, Tabibian JH, Baron TH, Othurhu V, Rosen CB, Petersen BT, et al. Use of single-balloon enteroscope compared with variable-stiffness colonoscopies for endoscopic retrograde cholangiography in liver transplant patients with Roux-en-Y biliary anastomosis. Gastrointest Endosc. 2013;77:568–77.
222. Choi EK, Chiorean MV, Cote GA, El Hajj I, Ballard D, Fogel EL, et al. ERCP via gastrostomy vs. double balloon enteroscopy in patients with prior bariatric Roux-en-Y gastric bypass surgery. Surg Endosc. 2013;27:2894–9.
223. Lo DY, Howell DA, Hallagan LD, Lewis J, Wright E, Bakis G, et al. Accessing the papilla for ERCP in bariatric Roux-en-Y gastric bypass (RNYGB): can clinical features predict success of peroral endoscopy? Gastrointest Endosc. 2011;73:AB346 (abstract).
224. Desai SV, Naveed M, Jazwinski A, Jowell PS, Branch MS. Spiral enteroscopy versus laparoscopic-assisted endoscopy for completion of ERCP in patients with Roux-en-Y gastric bypass surgery. Gastrointest Endosc. 2011;73:AB122 (abstract).
225. Ness-Jensen E, Lindam A, Lagergren J, Hveem K. Weight loss and reduction in gastroesophageal reflux: a prospective population-based cohort study: the HUNT study. Am J Gastroenterol. 2013;108:376–82.
226. McDougall NI, Johnston BT, Collins JS, McFarland RJ, Love AH. Three- to 4.5-year prospective study of prognostic indicators in gastro-oesophageal reflux disease. Scand J Gastroenterol. 1998;33:1016–22.
227. Sharma P, Vakil N, Monyak JT, Silberg DG. Obesity does not affect treatment outcomes with proton pump inhibitors. J Clin Gastroenterol. 2013;47:672–7.
228. Chen WY, Chang WL, Tsai YC, Cheng HC, Lu CC, Sheu BS. Double-dosed pantoprazole accelerates the sustained symptomatic response in overweight and obese patients with reflux esophagitis in Los Angeles grades A and B. Am J Gastroenterol. 2010;105:1046–52.
229. Bruley des Varannes S, Coudsy B, Waechter S, Delemos B, Xiang J, Lococo J, et al. On-demand proton pump inhibitory treatment in overweight/obese patients with gastroesophageal reflux disease: are there pharmacodynamic arguments for using higher doses? Digestion. 2013;88:56–63.

230. Becker V, Grotz S, Schlag C, Nennstiel S, Beitz A, Haller B, et al. Positive predictors for gastroesophageal reflux disease and the therapeutic response to proton-pump inhibitors. World J Gastroenterol. 2014;20:4017–24.
231. Perez AR, Moncure AC, Rattner DW. Obesity adversely affects the outcomes of antireflux operations. Surg Endosc. 2001;15:986–9.
232. Tolone S, Savarino E, Yates RB. The impact of bariatric surgery on esophageal function. Ann N Y Acad Sci. 2016;1381:98–103.
233. Khan A, Kim A, Sanossian C, Francois F. Impact of obesity treatment on gastroesophageal reflux disease. World J Gastroenterol. 2016;22:1627–38.
234. Kindel TL, Oleynikov D. The improvement of gastroesophageal reflux disease and Barrett's after bariatric surgery. Obes Surg. 2016;26:718–20.
235. Pallati PK, Shaligram A, Shostrom VK, Oleynikov D, McBride CL, Goede MR. Improvement in gastroesophageal reflux disease symptoms after various bariatric procedures: review of the bariatric outcomes longitudinal database. Surg Obes Relat Dis. 2014;10:502–7.
236. Moszkowicz D, Arienzo R, Khettab I, Rahmi G, Zinzindohoue F, Berger A, et al. Sleeve gastrectomy severe complications: is it always a reasonable surgical option? Obes Surg. 2013;23:676–86.
237. Csendes A, Burgos AM, Smok G, Burdiles P, Henriquez A. Effect of gastric bypass on Barrett's esophagus and intestinal metaplasia of the cardia in patients with morbid obesity. J Gastrointest Surg. 2006;10:259–64.
238. Kehagias I, Zygomalas A, Karavias D, Karamanakos S. Sleeve gastrectomy: have we finally found the holy grail of bariatric surgery? A review of the literature. Eur Rev Med Pharmacol Sci. 2016;20:4930–42.
239. Brethauer SA, Hammel JP, Schauer PR. Systematic review of sleeve gastrectomy as staging and primary bariatric procedure. Surg Obes Relat Dis. 2009;5:469–75.
240. Burgos AM, Csendes A, Braghetto I. Gastric stenosis after laparoscopic sleeve gastrectomy in morbidly obese patients. Obes Surg. 2013;23:1481–6.
241. Parikh A, Alley JB, Peterson RM, Harnisch MC, Pfluke JM, Tapper DM, et al. Management options for symptomatic stenosis after laparoscopic vertical sleeve gastrectomy in the morbidly obese. Surg Endosc. 2012;26:738–46.
242. Schneider BE, Villegas L, Blackburn GL, Mun EC, Critchlow JF, Jones DB. Laparoscopic gastric bypass surgery: outcomes. J Laparoendosc Adv Surg Tech A. 2003;13:247–55.
243. Zundel N, Hernandez JD, Galvao Neto M, Campos J. Strictures after laparoscopic sleeve gastrectomy. Surg Laparosc Endosc Percutan Tech. 2010;20:154–8.
244. Al Sabah S, Al Haddad E, Siddiqui F. Endoscopic management of post-laparoscopic sleeve gastrectomy stenosis. Surg Endosc. 2017;31:3559–63. https://doi.org/10.1007/s00464-016-5385-9.
245. Ogra R, Kini GP. Evolving endoscopic management options for symptomatic stenosis post-laparoscopic sleeve gastrectomy for morbid obesity: experience at a large bariatric surgery unit in New Zealand. Obes Surg. 2014;25:242–8.
246. Southwell T, Lim TH, Ogra R. Endoscopic therapy for treatment of staple line leaks post-laparoscopic sleeve gastrectomy (LSG): experience from a large bariatric surgery centre in New Zealand. Obes Surg. 2016;26:1155–62.
247. Shehab HM, Hakky SM, Gawdat KA. An endoscopic strategy combining mega stents and over-the-scope clips for the management of post-bariatric surgery leaks and fistulas (with video). Obes Surg. 2016;26:941–8.
248. Gagner M, Hutchinson C, Rosenthal R. Fifth international consensus conference: current status of sleeve gastrectomy. Surg Obes Relat Dis. 2016;12:750–6.
249. Weiner RA, Weiner S, Pomhoff I, Jacobi C, Makarewicz W, Weigand G. Laparoscopic sleeve gastrectomy –influence of sleeve size and resected gastric volume. Obes Surg. 2007;17:1297–305.
250. Himpens J, Dobbeleir J, Peeters G. Long-term results of laparoscopic sleeve gastrectomy for obesity. Ann Surg. 2010;252:319–24.
251. Sabbagh C, Verhaeghe P, Dhahri A, Brehant O, Fuks D, Badaoui R, et al. Two-year results on morbidity, weight loss and quality of life of sleeve gastrectomy as first proce-

dure, sleeve gastrectomy after failure of gastric banding and gastric banding. Obes Surg. 2010;20:679–84.
252. Deguines J-B, Verhaeghe P, Yzet T, Robert B, Cosse C, Regimbeau J-M. Is the residual gastric volume after laparoscopic sleeve gastrectomy an objective criterion for adapting the treatment strategy after failure? Surg Obes Relat Dis. 2013;9:660–6.
253. Disse E, Pasquer A, Pelascini E, Valette J-P, Betry C, Laville M, et al. Dilatation of sleeve gastrectomy: myth or reality? Obes Surg. 2017;27:30–7.
254. Lauti M, Kularatna M, Hill AG, MacCormick AD. Weight regain following sleeve gastrectomy—a systematic review. Obes Surg. 2016;26:1326–34.
255. Liu SYW, Wong SKH, Lam CCH, Yung MY, Kong AP, Ng EK. Long-term results on weight loss and diabetes remission after laparoscopic sleeve gastrectomy for a morbidly obese Chinese population. Obes Surg. 2015;25:1901–8.
256. Surace M, Mercky P, Demarquay J-F, Gonzalez J-M, Dumas R, Ah-Soune P, et al. Endoscopic management of GI fistulae with the over-the-scope clip system (with video). Gastrointest Endosc. 2011;74:1416–9.
257. Bege T, Emungania O, Vitton V, Ah-Soune P, Nocca D, Noel P, et al. An endoscopic strategy for management of anastomotic complications from bariatric surgery: a prospective study. Gastrointest Endosc. 2011;73:238–44.
258. Baretta G, Campos J, Correia S, Alhinho H, Marchesini JB, Lima JH, et al. Bariatric postoperative fistula: a life-saving endoscopic procedure. Surg Endosc. 2015;29:1714–20.
259. van de Vrande S, Himpens J, El Mourad H, Debaerdemaeker R, Leman G. Management of chronic proximal fistulas after sleeve gastrectomy by laparoscopic Roux-limb placement. Surg Obes Relat Dis. 2013;9:856–61.
260. Vilallonga R, Himpens J, Bosch B, van de Vrande S, Bafort J. Role of percutaneous glue treatment after persisting leak after laparoscopic sleeve gastrectomy. Obes Surg. 2016;26:1378–83.
261. Rebibo L, Dhahri A, Berna P, Yzet T, Verhaeghe P, Regimbeau JM. Management of gastrobronchial fistula after laparoscopic sleeve gastrectomy. Surg Obes Relat Dis. 2014;10: 405–10.
262. Albanopoulos K, Tsamis D, Leandros E. Gastrobronchial fistula as a late complication of sleeve gastrectomy. Surg Obes Relat Dis. 2013;9:e97–9.
263. Almadi MA, Bamihriz F, Aljebreen AM. Fatal aortoesophageal fistula bleeding after stenting for a leak post sleeve gastrectomy. World J Gastrointest Surg. 2013;5:337–40.
264. DuPree CE, Blair K, Steele SC, Martin MM. Laparoscopic sleeve gastrectomy in patients with preexisting gastroesophageal reflux disease. A national analysis. JAMA Surg. 2014;149:328–34.
265. Braghetto I, Lanzarini E, Korn O, Valladares H, Molina JC, Henriquez A. Manometric changes of the lower esophageal sphincter after sleeve gastrectomy in obese patients. Obes Surg. 2010;20:357–62.
266. Stenard F, Iannelli A. Laparoscopic sleeve gastrectomy and gastroesophageal reflux. World J Gastroenterol. 2015;21:10348–57.
267. Crawford C, Gibbens K, Lomelin D, Krause C, Simorov A, Oleynikov D. Sleeve gastrectomy and anti-reflux procedures. Surg Endosc. 2017;31:1012–21.
268. Arman GA, Himpens J, Dhaenens J, Ballet T, Vilallonga R, Leman G. Long-term (11+ years) outcomes in weight, patient satisfaction, comorbidities, and gastroesophageal reflux treatment after laparoscopic sleeve gastrectomy. Surg Obes Relat Dis. 2016;12:1778–86.
269. Tai CM, Huang CK, Lee YC, Chang CY, Lee CT, Lin JT. Increase in gastroesophageal reflux disease symptoms and erosive esophagitis 1 year after laparoscopic sleeve gastrectomy among obese adults. Surg Endosc. 2013;27:1260–6.
270. Baumann T, Grueneberger J, Pache G, Kuesters S, Marjanovic G, Kulemann B, et al. Three-dimensional stomach analysis with computed tomography after laparoscopic sleeve gastrectomy: sleeve dilation and thoracic migration. Surg Endosc. 2011;25:2323–9.
271. Rosenthal RJ, Diaz AA, Arvidsson D, Baker RS, Basso N, Bellanger D, et al. International sleeve gastrectomy expert panel consensus statement: best practice guidelines based on experience of >12,000 cases. Surg Obes Relat Dis. 2012;8:8–19.

272. Daes J, Jimenez ME, Said N, Daza JC, Dennis R. Laparoscopic sleeve gastrectomy: symptoms of gastroesophageal reflux can be reduced by changes in surgical technique. Obes Surg. 2012;22:1874–9.
273. Melissas J, Leventi A, Klinaki I, Perisinakis K, Koukouraki S, de Bree E, et al. Alterations of global gastrointestinal motility after sleeve gastrectomy: a prospective study. Ann Surg. 2013;258:976–82.
274. Chiu S, Birch DW, Shi X, Sharma AM, Karmali S. Effect of sleeve gastrectomy on gastroesophageal reflux disease: a systematic review. Surg Obes Relat Dis. 2011;7:510–5.
275. Oor JE, Roks DJ, Ünlü C, Hazebroek EJ. Laparoscopic sleeve gastrectomy and gastroesophageal reflux disease: a systematic review and meta-analysis. Am J Surg. 2016;211:250–67.
276. Mahawar KK, Carr WRJ, Jennings N, Bakpuri S, Small PK. Simultaneous sleeve gastrectomy and hiatus hernia repair: a systematic review. Obes Surg. 2015;25:159–66.
277. Rebecchi F, Allaix ME, Giaccone C, Ugliono E, Scozzari G, Morino M. Gastroesophageal reflux disease and laparoscopic sleeve gastrectomy: a physiopathologic evaluation. Ann Surg. 2014;260:909–15.
278. Burgerhart JS, Schotborgh CA, Schoon EJ, Smulders JF, van de Meeberg PC, Siersema PD, et al. Effect of sleeve gastrectomy on gastroesophageal reflux. Obes Surg. 2014;24:1436–41.
279. Gorodner V, Buxhoeveden R, Clemente G, Sole L, Caro L, Grigaites A. Does laparoscopic sleeve gastrectomy have any influence on gastroesophageal reflux disease? Preliminary results. Surg Endosc. 2015;29:1760–8.
280. Soricelli E, Iossa A, Casella G, Abbatini F, Cali B, Basso N. Sleeve gastrectomy and crural repair in obese patients with gastroesophageal reflux disease and/or hiatal hernia. Surg Obes Relat Dis. 2013;9:356–61.
281. Keidar A, Appelbaum L, Schweiger C, Elazary R, Baltasar A. Dilated upper sleeve can be associated with severe postoperative gastroesophageal dysmotility and reflux. Obes Surg. 2010;20:140–7.
282. Triadafilopoulos G. Endoscopic options for gastroesophageal reflux: where are we now and what does the future hold? Curr Gastroenterol Rep. 2016;18:47.
283. Triadafilopoulos G, DiBaise JK, Nostrant TT, Stollman NH, Anderson PK, Wolfe MM, et al. The Stretta procedure for the treatment of GERD: 6 and 12 month follow-up of the U.S. open label trial. Gastrointest Endosc. 2002;55:149–56.
284. Noar M, Squires P, Noar E, Lee M. Long-term maintenance effect of radiofrequency energy delivery for refractory GERD: a decade later. Surg Endosc. 2014;28:2323–33.
285. Lipka S, Kumar A, Richter JE. No evidence for efficacy of radiofrequency ablation for treatment of gastroesophageal reflux disease: a systematic review and meta-analysis. Clin Gastroenterol Hepatol. 2015;13:1058–67.
286. Scopinaro N, Marinari G, Camerini G, Papadia F. Biliopancreatic diversion for obesity: state of the art. Surg Obes Relat Dis. 2005;1:317–28.
287. Sekhar N, Gagner M. Complications of laparoscopic biliopancreatic diversion with duodenal switch. Curr Surg. 2003;60:279–80.
288. Papavramidis TS, Kotzampassi K, Kotidis E, Eleftheriadis EE, Papavramidis ST. Endoscopic fibrin sealing of gastrocutaneous fistulas after sleeve gastrectomy and biliopancreatic diversion with duodenal switch. J Gastroenterol Hepatol. 2008;23:1802–5.
289. Schweitzer M, Steele K, Mitchell M, Okolo P. Transoral endoscopic closure of gastric fistula. Surg Obes Relat Dis. 2009;5:283–4.
290. Spivak H, Favretti F. Avoiding postoperative complications with the LAP-BAND system. Am J Surg. 2002;184(Suppl 2):31S–7S.
291. Richardson J, Smith B. Laparoscopic gastric banding. Minerva Chir. 2012;67:1–12.
292. Lo Menzo E, Szomstein S, Rosenthal P. Update on treatment of morbid obesity with adjustable gastric banding. Surg Clin North Am. 2016;96:795–813.
293. Rubenstein RB. Laparoscopic adjustable gastric banding at a U.S. center with up to 3-year follow-up. Obes Surg. 2002;12:380–4.
294. DeMaria EJ, Jamal MK. Laparoscopic adjustable gastric banding: evolving clinical experience. Surg Clin North Am. 2005;85:773–87.

295. O'Brien PE, MacDonald L, Anderson M, Brennan L, Brown WA. Long-term outcomes after bariatric surgery: fifteen-year follow-up of adjustable gastric banding and a systematic review of the bariatric surgical literature. Ann Surg. 2013;257:87–94.
296. Cunneen SA, Phillips E, Fielding F, Banel B, Estok R, Fahrbach K, et al. Studies of Swedish adjustable gastric band and lap-band: systematic review and meta-analysis. Surg Obes Relat Dis. 2008;4:174–85.
297. Dargent J. Laparoscopic gastric banding: game over? Obes Surg. 2017;27:1914–6.
298. Brown WA, O'Brien PE. The band must not be abandoned. Obes Surg. 2017;27:1911–3.
299. Handgraaf HJM, Ashton D, Favretti F, Segato G, van Ramshorst B, Meesters B, et al. The gastric band that is not to be. Efficacy, safety and performance of the Easyband™: a multicenter experience. Obes Surg. 2015;25:2239–44.
300. Altieri MS, Yang J, Telem DA, Meng Z, Frenkel C, Halbert C, et al. Lap band outcomes from 19,221 patients across centers and over a decade within the state of New York. Surg Endosc. 2016;30:1725–32.
301. Parikh MS, Fielding GA, Ren CJ. U.S. experience with 749 laparoscopic adjustable gastric bands. Intermediate outcomes. Surg Endosc. 2005;19:1631–5.
302. Singhal R, Bryant C, Kitchen M, Khan KS, Deeks J, Guo B, et al. Band slippage and erosion after laparoscopic gastric banding: a meta-analysis. Surg Endosc. 2010;24:2980–6.
303. O'Brien PE, Dixon JB. Weight loss and early and late complications—the international experience. Am J Surg. 2002;184:42S–5S.
304. Ponce J, Paynter S, Fromm R. Laparoscopic adjustable gastric banding: 1,013 consecutive cases. J Am Coll Surg. 2005;201:529–35.
305. Eid I, Birch DW, Sharma AM, Sherman V, Karmali S. Complications associated with adjustable gastric banding for morbid obesity: a surgeon's guide. Can J Surg. 2011;54:61–5.
306. Busetto L, Segato G, De Luca M, De Marchi F, Foletto M, Vianello M, et al. Weight loss and postoperative complications in morbidly obese patients with binge eating disorder treated by laparoscopic adjustable gastric banding. Obes Surg. 2005;15:195–201.
307. Busetto L, Segato G, De Marchi F, Foletto M, De Luca M, Caniato D, et al. Outcome predictors in morbidly obese recipients of an adjustable gastric band. Obes Surg. 2002;12: 83–92.
308. Czeiger D, Abu-Swis S, Shaked G, Ovnat A, Sebbag G. Management of gastric obstruction caused by adjustable gastric band. Obes Surg. 2016;26:2931–5.
309. Milone L, Daud A, Durak E, Olivero-Rivera L, Schrope B, Inabnet WB, et al. Esophageal dilation after laparoscopic adjustable gastric banding. Surg Endosc. 2008;22:1482–6.
310. Naef M, Mouton WG, Naef U, van der Weg B, Maddern GJ, Wagner HE. Esophageal dysmotility disorders after laparoscopic gastric banding—an underestimated complication. Ann Surg. 2011;253:285–90.
311. Dargent J. Esophageal dilatation after laparoscopic gastric banding: definition and strategy. Obes Surg. 2005;15:843–8.
312. Lew JI, Daud A, DiGorgi MF, Olivero-Rivera L, Davis DG, Bessler M. Preoperative esophageal manometry and outcome of laparoscopic adjustable silicone gastric banding. Surg Endosc. 2006;20:1242–7.
313. Klaus A, Gruber I, Wetscher G, Nehoda H, Aigner F, Peer R, et al. Prevalent esophageal body motility disorders underlie aggravation of GERD symptoms in morbidly obese patients following adjustable gastric banding. Arch Surg. 2006;141:247–51.
314. Klaus A, Weiss H. Is preoperative manometry in restrictive bariatric procedures necessary? Obes Surg. 2008;18:1039–42.
315. Burton PR, Brown WA, Laurie C, Korin A, Yap K, Richards M, et al. Pathophysiology of laparoscopic adjustable gastric bands: analysis and classification using high-resolution video manometry and a stress barium protocol. Obes Surg. 2010;20:19–29.
316. Burton PR, Brown WA, Laurie C, Hebbard G, O'Brien PE. Criteria for assessing esophageal motility in laparoscopic adjustable gastric band patients: the importance of the lower esophageal contractile segment. Obes Surg. 2010;20:316–25.
317. Burton PR, Brown WA, Laurie C, Hebbard G, O'Brien PE. Predicting outcomes of intermediate term complications and revisional surgery following laparoscopic adjustable gastric

banding: utility of the CORE classification and Melbourne motility criteria. Obes Surg. 2010;20:1516–23.
318. Moser F, Gorodner MV, Galvani CA, Baptista M, Cretien C, Horgan S. Pouch enlargement and band slippage: two different entities. Surg Endosc. 2006;20:1021–9.
319. Campos JM, Evangelista LF, Galvao Neto MP, Ramos AC, Martins JPC, dos Santos MC Jr, et al. Small erosion of adjustable gastric band: endoscopic removal through incision in gastric wall. Surg Laparosc Endosc Percutan Tech. 2010;20:e215–7.
320. Cappell MS, Mogrovejo E, Desai T. Case report of patient presenting in shock from band penetration into stomach after LAGB surgery: diagnosis by emergency EGD after misdiagnosis by abdominal CT. Dig Dis Sci. 2016;61:3366–8.
321. Di Lorenzo N, Lorenzo M, Furbetta F, Favretti F, Giardiello C, Boschi S, et al. Intragastric gastric band migration: erosion: an analysis of multicenter experience on 177 patients. Surg Endosc. 2013;27:1151–7.
322. Egberts K, Brown WA, O'Brien PE. Systematic review of erosion after laparoscopic adjustable gastric banding. Obes Surg. 2011;21:1272–9.
323. Meir E, Van Baden M. Adjustable silicone gastric banding and band erosion: personal experience and hypotheses. Obes Surg. 1999;9:191–3.
324. Boschi S, Fogli L, Berta RD, Patrizi P, Di Dominico M, Vetere F, et al. Avoiding complications after laparoscopic esophago-gastric banding: experience with 400 consecutive patients. Obes Surg. 2006;16:1166–70.
325. De Palma GD, Formato A, Pilone V, Rega M, Giuliano ME, Simeoli I, et al. Endoscopic management of intragastric penetrated adjustable gastric band for morbid obesity. World J Gastroenterol. 2006;12:4098–100.
326. Forestieri P, Pilone V, TramontanoS FA, Monda A, Esposito E. Laparoscopic gastric band migration: role of environmental factors in the experience of a single team in three operating rooms. Obes Surg. 2010;20:1333–9.
327. Dogan UB, Dal MB. An 8-year experience with endoscopic management of eroded gastric bands. Surg Laparosc Endosc Percutan Tech. 2015;25:e140–4.
328. Meyenberger C, Gubler C, Hengstler PM. Endoscopic management of a penetrated gastric band. Gastrointest Endosc. 2004;60:480–1.
329. Blero D, Eisendrath P, Vandermeeren A, Closset J, Mehdi A, Le Moine O, et al. Endoscopic removal of dysfunctioning bands or rings after restrictive bariatric procedures. Gastrointest Endosc. 2010;71:468–74.
330. Regusci L, Groebli Y, Meyer JL, Walder J, Margalith D, Schneider R. Gastroscopic removal of an adjustable gastric band after partial intragastric migration. Obes Surg. 2003;13:281–4.
331. Sakai P, Hondo FY, Almeida Artifon EL, Kuga R, Ishioka S. Symptomatic pneumoperitoneum after endoscopic removal of adjustable gastric band. Obes Surg. 2005;15:893–6.
332. Galvao Neto MP, Ramos AC, Campos JM, Murakami AH, Falcao M, Moura EH, et al. Endoscopic removal of eroded adjustable gastric band: lessons learned after 5 years and 78 cases. Surg Obes Relat Dis. 2010;6:423–7.
333. O'Brien P. Comment on: endoscopic removal of eroded adjustable gastric band: lessons learned after 5 years and 78 cases. Surg Obes Relat Dis. 2010;6:427–8.
334. Mozzi E, Lattuada E, Zappa MA, Granelli P, De Ruberto F, Armocida A, et al. Treatment of band erosion: feasibility and safety of endoscopic band removal. Surg Endosc. 2011;25:3918–22.
335. de Jong JR, Besselink MG, van Ramshorst B, Gooszen HG, Smout AJ. Effects of adjustable gastric banding on gastroesophageal reflux and esophageal motility: a systematic review. Obes Rev. 2010;11:297–305.
336. de Jong JR, van Ramshorst B, Timmer R, Gooszen HG, Smout AJ. The influence of laparoscopic adjustable gastric banding on gastroesophageal reflux. Obes Surg. 2004;14:399–406.
337. Klaus A, Weiss H. Esophageal dilation after laparoscopic adjustable gastric banding. Surg Endosc. 2009;23:909–10.

338. Rebecchi F, Rocchietto S, Giaccone C, Talha A, Morino M. Gastroesophageal reflux disease and esophageal motility in morbidly obese patients submitted to laparoscopic adjustable silicone gastric banding or laparoscopic vertical banded gastroplasty. Surg Endosc. 2011;25:795–803.
339. Dixon JB, O'Brien PE. Gastroesophageal reflux in obesity: the effect of lap-band placement. Obes Surg. 1999;9:396–8.
340. Woodman G, Cywes R, Billy H, Montgomery K, Cornell C, Okerson T. Effect of adjustable gastric banding on changes in gastroesophageal reflux disease (GERD) and quality of life. Curr Med Res Opin. 2012;28:581–9.
341. Sataloff DM, Lieber CP, Seinige UL. Strictures following gastric stapling for morbid obesity. Results of endoscopic dilatation. Am Surg. 1990;56:167–74.
342. Deitel M, Bendago M. Endoscopy of vertical banded gastroplasty. Am Surg. 1989;55:287–90.
343. Lim CH, Amateau SK, Ikramuddin S, Leslie DB. Endoscopic management of vertical banded gastroplasty stricture: feasibility, safety, and efficacy. Obes Surg. 2016;26:2802–8.
344. Aly A, Sweeney T, Michell I, Lim K. Single port trans-gastric reversal of high gastric reduction. Obes Surg. 2014;24:483–6.
345. Lunde OC. Endoscopic laser therapy for band penetration of the gastric wall after gastric banding for morbid obesity. Endoscopy. 1991;23:100–1.
346. Evans JA, Williams NN, Chan EP, Kochman ML. Endoscopic removal of eroded bands in vertical banded gastroplasty: a novel use of endoscopic scissors (with video). Gastrointest Endosc. 2006;64:801–4.
347. Karmali S, Snyder S, Wilson EB, Timberlake MD, Sherman V. Endoscopic management of eroded prosthesis in vertical banded gastroplasty patients. Surg Endosc. 2010;24:98–102.
348. Manouchehri N, Birch DW, Menzes C, Shi X, Karmali S. Natural orifice surgery: endoluminal pouch reduction following failed vertical banded gastroplasty. Obes Surg. 2011;21:1787–91.
349. Deitel M, Khanna RK, Hagen J, Ilves R. Vertical banded gastroplasty as an antireflux procedure. Am J Surg. 1988;155:512–6.
350. Fried M, Yumuk V, Oppert J-M, Scopinaro N, Torres AJ, Weiner R, et al. Interdisciplinary European guidelines on metabolic and bariatric surgery. Obes Facts. 2013;6:449–68.
351. Sakran N, Assalia A, Keidar A, Goitein D. Gastrobronchial fistula as a complication of bariatric surgery: a series of 6 cases. Obes Facts. 2012;5:538–45.

Perioperative and Postoperative Guidance of the Bariatric Patient

7

Contents

E. M. H. Mathus-Vliegen, J. Dargent, *Bariatric Therapy*,
https://doi.org/10.1007/978-3-319-90074-2_7

Abbreviations

AACE	American Association of Clinical Endocrinologists
ASA	American Society of Anaesthesiologists
ASMBS	American Society for Metabolic and Bariatric Surgery
BAROS	Bariatric Analysis and Reporting Outcomes System
BCS	Biopharmaceutics Classification System
BMI	Body mass index
BIA	Bioelectrical impedance analysis
BMD	Bone mineral density
BPD	Biliopancreatic diversion
BPD-DS	BPD-duodenal switch
CBT	Cognitive-behavioural therapy
DR	Discharge readiness
DVT	Deep venous thrombosis
DXA	Dual-energy X-ray absorptiometry
EASO	European Association for the Study of Obesity
EBW	Excess body weight
ERAS	Enhanced recovery after surgery
FDA	Food and Drug Administration
FFM	Fat-free mass
GI	Gastrointestinal
GP	General practitioner
IFSO	International Federation for the Surgery of Obesity
IU	International units
IV	Intravenous
IWQOL	Impact of weight on quality of life
LAGB	Laparoscopic adjustable gastric banding
LBM	Lean body mass
LSG	Laparoscopic sleeve gastrectomy
NHS	National Health Service
NICE	National Institute for Health and Clinical Excellence
NIV	Non-invasive ventilation
NBSR	National Bariatric Surgery Registry
NPD	Normal protein diet
PED	Protein-enriched diet
PPI	Proton pump inhibitors
PCP	Primary care physician
PTH	Parathyroid hormone
QOL	Quality of life
RCT	Randomised controlled trials
RMR	Resting metabolic rate
RYGB	Roux-en-Y gastric bypass
SG	Sleeve gastrectomy
T2DM	Type 2 diabetes mellitus

TA	Time to ambulate
TOS	The Obesity Society
TWL	Total weight loss

7.1 Introduction

A detailed follow-up scheme is of utmost importance to ensure long-term acceptable results after any kind of bariatric treatment. There should be no major differences in the principles of this guidance, whether the technique has been surgical or endoscopic. The only difference is probably the duration of action that is expected to be part of a given technique, i.e. more prolonged guidance after malabsorptive techniques. On the other hand, obesity will never be cured by whatever intervention and as such obesity is a lifelong disease that requires lifelong guidance and/or treatment irrespective of the treatment given. Lessons can be learned from the recent past: some surgical techniques have a rather short duration of efficacy (gastric banding for instance), or others, as argued in Chap. 9 of this book, have an on-off effect (e.g. gastric banding, neuromodulation), not much different from a gastric balloon for example. The FDA therefore has recently approved in the USA three different balloons and the gastric aspiration only when imbedded in a 12-month intensive lifestyle programme. This may seem rather short, but it is for the first time that this requirement had been so explicitly stated. On the other hand, some endoscopic techniques may have an average longer duration of efficacy, or can be repeated, although much about this is unknown at the present time. Gastric aspiration, repeated swallowing of balloons and endoscopic plication may claim a longer effect, beyond 18 months in selected cases, either on its own or because of the possibility of repeating the therapy. The bottom line is that whatever the technique, post-operative guidance has very similar objectives; the intensity and quality of the programme depend on the quality of the follow-up team. Yet, the ASMBS [1], AACE/TOS [2] and the European EASO/IFSO [3] issued guidelines about the minimum requirements of follow-up, which concentrated mainly on laboratory-technical and dietary/supplemental items and not so much on fitness, quality of life and psychological, social and societal issues. A great deal of these issues has also been taken by the EASO accreditation of Centres of Excellence [3].

The post-operative guidance has several goals that will be examined in detail:

- The detection of surgical or medical complications
- The coaching and guidance as to diet counselling, physical exercise, and weight loss support and weight loss maintenance
- The avoidance of nutritional and vitamin deficiencies
- The quality-of-life issues
- The medical follow-up of comorbidities
- The choice of the moment and the specific features in case of a redo intervention
- The desirability, timing and coaching of pregnancy

7.2 Preoperative and Perioperative Guidance

7.2.1 Preoperative Guidance

In a sense, the guidance starts already at/before baseline, when a patient is screened and deemed eligible for a bariatric intervention and should be prepared and tested for the perioperative and post-operative compliance. It starts as soon as the patient is enrolled and begins to line up in prevision of a surgical procedure. The preoperative assessment aims at testing the willingness and commitment to a lifelong monitoring [4], with patient-centred education programmes.

Hesitations and misunderstandings regarding the choice of being operated or not are a common experience for patients being on the waiting list for surgery, or simply being referred for surgery. They often do not realise that surgery is only a part of the whole treatment armamentarium and that it is not a quick fix, and thus it is understandable that a significant number of patients withdraw themselves. For instance, only 36% of the patients referred to the Toronto bariatric programme starting in 2011 underwent surgery, out of 1237 referred patients [5]. Variations exist depending on the health systems in place, and in this study half of the Canadian patients who withdrew did so because of insurance denial. Nevertheless, there will always be a significant number of patients that will drop out from a given programme including surgical options, whatever the endeavour of the professionals committed to the programme will be.

Preoperative weight loss has been debated and has also been discussed exhaustively in Chap. 4, and in Chap. 2 in the preoperative balloon application and "BIB" test. Most authors concur in recommending weight loss preoperatively because it will facilitate the surgical procedure in very obese patients, e.g. with BMI above 60 kg/m^2, and will decrease the size of massive livers with liver steatosis (which often hinders accessibility to the lesser gastric curve/gastro-oesophageal junction). The rate of immediate surgical and medical complications could be decreased, whereas there is no such evidence regarding an effect on 1-year weight loss and beyond.

Correlation between weight loss before bariatric surgery and post-operative success has been discussed and investigated. The fact that one can lose weight before the operation has been a requirement for some surgeons and insurance companies, especially in the USA. A study was performed at a community teaching hospital in Michigan, with 204 patients who underwent LSG between 2011 and 2015 [6]. The study demonstrated that the group who lost >5% of their excess body weight (EBW) before surgery had initially (<6 months) a statistically significant greater weight loss than those who lost <5%, but the difference faded away with a similar post-operative weight loss at 1 year. However, for Alami et al., in a prospective randomised trial, there was no real benefit of preoperative weight loss in RYGB patients [7]. Likewise, for Carlin et al., preoperative weight loss is not a predictor of post-operative weight loss after laparoscopic Roux-en-Y gastric bypass [8].

On the other hand, the preoperative period also serves to adequately inform patients about the ins and outs of the operation and realistic expectations from the operation. The surgeon or obesity nurse can communicate the results obtained in their own hospital and take advantage of all their knowledge to deal with this kind of patients which are usually not a cross section of the normal population. Good information plays an utmost important role. As commonly shown, one cannot truly rely on information that is available "out there" on the Internet, for instance very few smartphone applications dealing with obesity surgery having been proven relevant [9]. We can only recommend exhaustive and fair information from the multidisciplinary team, as a necessity in accompanying any bariatric patient prior to a given procedure.

So, it remains difficult to infer the final results from the preoperative workup, and even if formal criteria emerged they would not be sufficient reason for ruling out every patient who falls into a least favourable category. This emphasises once again the importance of the decision-taking in a team that is well informed about their results and that has discussed a particular patient in depth and thus may even consider patients with a high initial BMI, older age, presence of T2DM and all factors that have been correlated to a less favourable outcome and a less important weight loss [10]. However, there is also no consensus on how to incorporate these unfavourable characteristics of patients, emerging from univariate and multivariate analyses from the literature, into guidelines. Likewise, self-reported behavioural changes before bariatric surgery have not been found to be reliable. Moreover, supposed changes in dietary habits may be less predictive of further weight loss than reported changes in physical activity [11].

A comprehensive preoperative evaluation and estimation of the commitment of the patient are mainly based on years of experience and as such the ideal tool to operate. Also, definite criteria for a specific procedure have not been established, although many attempts have been made to define patients into eating categories such as carbohydrate cravers, sugar addicts, sweat eaters, gorgers, snackers and grazers and to correlate this eating pattern to outcomes after certain operations. It even resulted in a sweat-eater questionnaire, although this questionnaire has never been studied prospectively [12]. One can very commonly read or hear that a certain technique "works if patient selection has been rigorous," which is depreciative to others who apparently with less good results were said not to select their patients well. It does not also make much sense: on a normal basis, each bariatric procedure should follow the same path and as yet we are far from an algorithm where characteristics of a patient can be put in in the beginning and the most ideal bariatric surgery figures out in the end.

The basics of preoperative workup are summarised in Table 7.1:

In case of redo surgery, there is no reason why the preoperative assessment should be shorter or less rigorous than in primary cases. Many patients are seeking a simple alternative solution to a technical failure without acknowledging the underlying behaviour that hampered the continuation of weight loss or simply weight maintenance. Yet, most often and whatever the duration of the in-between surgeries' interval, it is the duty of a dedicated team to start all over again with the basics of preoperative evaluation. This is also the case when sequential therapies involve different sets of options, e.g. when a bariatric surgery is performed some years after a

Table 7.1 Preoperative workup before bariatric surgery

General assessment	History of obesity/medical records Possible surgical and bariatric records Obvious contraindications to bariatric surgery
Risk assessment (anaesthesiology)	Pulmonary function (obstructive sleep apnoea/hypoventilation syndrome/pulmonary hypertension/airway assessment) ASA score Vascular access
Gastrointestinal change assessment	GI evaluation/upper GI endoscopy
Nutritional and metabolic workup	Endocrinology/potential deficiencies
Psychological evaluation	Detection of formal or temporary contraindications/additional preparation
Multidisciplinary assessment	Review of team evaluation
Choice of an operation	Patient selection for a specific intervention (?) implementation of algorithm (?)
Preparation to surgery	Information sessions and support groups/informed consent

balloon implantation, or the other way around, when a gastric endoscopic plication is performed in case of pouch enlargement after a gastric bypass.

7.3 Enhanced Recovery After Bariatric Surgery

The enhanced recovery after surgery (ERAS) protocol is well established in many surgical disciplines and leads to a decrease in the length of hospital stay and morbidity. Multimodal protocols have also been introduced into bariatric surgery and guidelines established [13], which could benefit probably more than other categories from ERAS, but it seems that the ERAS protocol leads only to a reduction of the length of hospital stay while having barely or no influence on morbidity. One may object that ERAS is just a new way to name a tendency that exists for years, but it seems that the focus on establishing standardised protocols has been worth the efforts of the surgical community, in conjunction with anaesthesiologists.

In a very recent systematic review in 2017, Małczak et al. evaluated the current literature on ERAS in obesity surgery. The primary outcome was the length of hospital stay; the secondary outcomes included overall morbidity, specific complications, mortality, readmissions and costs [14]: 11 papers were analysed, but only 2 were RCTs. The meta-analysis of the length of stay presented a significant reduction in hospital stay with a standard mean difference of 2.4 days (2.8 vs. 4.6, significant). Overall morbidity, mortality, specific complications and Clavien-Dindo classification, readmissions and costs were not significantly different between ERAS and non-ERAS groups. Also, Singh et al. analysed the efficiency and safety of the application of ERAS protocols in bariatric surgery with also the primary outcome of length of hospital stay [15]. According to their criteria only five studies were included that all had a high degree of heterogeneity. They found a 1.56 days' shorter length of stay in the ERAS group, without any benefit of ERAS in overall complications, readmissions and anastomotic leaks. The length of stay as a primary outcome has been criticised in general surgery but in contrast to general surgery is characterised by clearly defined discharge criteria in bariatric surgery.

From the anaesthesiologist point of view, similar conclusions can be drawn [16]. Sinha et al. performed a retrospective analysis of prospectively collected data of 823 patients who underwent laparoscopic bariatric surgery, and assessed the effects of BMI in 4 categories (severely obese, morbidly obese, super-morbidly obese and super-super-morbidly obese) on recovery and anaesthetic outcome parameters. The main focus was prehabilitation, including aggressive preoperative optimisation of medical comorbidities, familiarising with perioperative protocols, thromboprophylaxis and opioid-free multimodal analgesia. This would allow early ambulation, time to ambulate (TA) being the primary outcome, and early discharge as a positive correlate. Requirement for non-invasive ventilation (NIV) was the only significant predictor of TA and discharge readiness (DR); the DR was further affected by functional capacity and presence of chest pain. The analysis indicated that each unit increase in BMI (kg/m^2) contributed to increase TA by 1.24 min and a prolonged discharge readiness by 0.5 h. For instance, whereas a morbidly obese subject had a time to ambulate of 155 min and a discharge readiness of 27.4 h, these figures in the super-super-morbidly obese (BMI > 60 kg/m^2) were 191.6 min and 43.3 h, respectively. The authors concluded that prehabilitation before surgery with the many different items in each phase of preoperative optimisation and preparation has a significant impact on anaesthesiology and the herewith associated outcomes such as ambulation and discharge.

7.4 Prevention of Thromboembolic Complications

Risk of thrombosis and thromboembolic prophylaxis is an important part of obesity surgery and requires specific measures, including low extremity compression, pharmacologic prophylaxis or both. But the optimal use is still unclear, because of evaluation to a limited extent only (strategies of adjusted-dose heparins, post-discharge anticoagulant therapies, role of vena cava filters), as pointed out by Bartlett et al. [17]. These risks were analysed based on the data from the German Bariatric Surgery Registry by Stroh et al. [18]. Using antithrombotic prophylaxis, the risk of deep venous thrombosis (DVT) and its complications have to be balanced with the increased bleeding risk. A total of 31,668 primary bariatric procedures were performed between 2005 and 2013 (3999 LAGB, 13,722 RYGB, 11,840 SG). Gender, surgical procedure or administration of thromboembolic prophylaxis had no statistical impact on the DVT incidence. By contrast, BMI and duration of thromboembolic prophylaxis did impact the frequency of onset of DVT. Age, BMI, male gender and a previous history of DVT were the most important risk factors. The drug of choice is heparin. Low-molecular-weight heparin should be preferred over unfractionated heparins due to their improved pharmacological properties, i.e. better bioavailability and longer half-life as well as ease of use. Stroh et al. concluded that prospective randomised studies are needed to determine the optimal thrombosis prophylaxis [18].

7.5 Post-operative Guidance

7.5.1 Follow-Up: Guidelines to Follow

Both the ASMBS and the EASO-IFSO European chapter and the American Heart Association have developed guidelines, stating the frequency of follow-up and the frequency of blood sampling with different schemes according to the operations. O'Kane et al. reviewed the guidelines and graded the level of evidence [19]. Bariatric surgery has a profound impact on nutrition; patients need access to follow-up and aftercare. NICE guidelines emphasised the importance of a minimum of 2-year follow-up in the bariatric surgical service and recommended an annual monitoring as part of a shared care model of chronic disease management. NHS England Obesity Clinical Reference Group commissioned a multi-professional subgroup, which included patient representatives, to develop bariatric surgery follow-up guidelines concerning the annual review, ability of a general practitioner (GP) to refer back to specialist centre and submission of follow-up data to the national database to the National Bariatric Surgery Registry (NBSR).

7.5.2 Follow-Up Quality: How Strict Should We Be?

In terms of general experience, what happens when a given patient skips regular appointments, or even does not come back? Most often and dealing with restrictive operations, not much, except that it means that the patient is disappointed, dissatisfied or ashamed for not having achieved what he/she was supposed to! Should he/she actively be traced? The answer should be yes, because the physician has been committed himself/herself for a lifelong guidance and the patient himself/herself will not undertake any action because of his/her sense of shame. However, time and resources will mostly thwart any action. This is very different with malabsorptive operations, where loss of follow-up in addition to disappointing weight loss results may have significant consequences with respect to nutritional deficiencies. For both kind of operations, the rule is that initial weight loss predicts further weight loss, and that the less support a patient gets over the long term, the more likely he/she is going to fail. "Being strict" does not ensure efficacy in times of self-empowerment, best exemplified by expressions like "therapeutic alliance" or "therapeutic education" that are supposed to express the co-partnership that exists between patient and caregivers, a bond that is more meaningful than the one resulting from "guidance," connected with "authority." Nevertheless, it is not obvious to organise long-term surveillance and gradually the recognition that also the general practitioner has a role to play or even obesity health workers or obesity nurses can be involved as is the case with an as great problem as diabetes, which may facilitate a better long-term follow-up. It is obvious that the surgeon who performed the operation cannot do this on his/her own but the analogue of diabetes nurse and diabetes dietician, under the supervision of the GP and specialist, can be picked up in obesity management. The confidence of the patient that he/she is always welcome to come back and also the consultations via e-mail contact are helpful. Mehaffey et al. studied the way to go after a gastric bypass, when nutrient deficiency is a potential threat, and they asked the very relevant question: Who is responsible? [20] They compared nutrient supplementation and time since last visit when surgeon or primary care physician (PCP) followed their patients. The group of patients was divided into patients with short-term versus long-term follow-up [20]. All patients undergoing LRYGB at a single institution in 2004 (long-term group, $n = 281$) or in 2012–2013 (short-term group, $n = 149$) were evaluated. Complete follow-up was available in 172 (61%) of the long-term and 107 (72%) of the short-term patients. There was a significant difference ($p < 0.0001$) in time since last surgeon follow-up (13.3 months for the short-term vs. 86.9 months for the long-term group) with no difference in PCP follow-up (3.1 vs. 3.7 months). Nutrient supplementation was higher in the short-term group, including multivitamin (70.3% vs. 58.9%, $p < 0.05$), iron (84.2% vs. 67.1%, $p = 0.02$), folate (14.2% vs. 4.5%, p 0.01) and calcium (49.5% vs. 32.9%, $p = 0.01$), whereas according to the guidelines blood sampling should follow a certain scheme. In the group operated 2 years ago, a complete blood count was performed 12 months before; in the 10-year post-surgery group this was 33 months, so almost 3 years before. However, nothing is mentioned about more detailed blood samples for vitamins, minerals, PTH, and liver and kidney function. After adjusting for interval since surgery, %EBMI (excess BMI) loss and current comorbidities, logistic regression demonstrated that a shorter time since last surgeon visit was independently predictive of multivitamin use ($p = 0.001$). While patients preferred to be followed up by their PCP, it seems that the PCP should be educated on the recognition of malnutrition and on the need of nutrient supplementation.

7.6 Detection of Surgical or Medical Complications

Complications related to surgery have been explained in Chaps. 5 and 6; they may occur even in the long term and should be referred to the multidisciplinary team, or any team dedicated to bariatric surgery with full equipment, without further delay. One dreads for instance late post-operative small-bowel obstruction due to internal hernia, late gastric ulcer, stenosis, etc. Medical complications may include post-bariatric hypoglycaemia, protein malnutrition, vitamin deficiencies, dumping syndrome and fear of osteopenia/osteoporosis (see also Chap. 6). Most must be dealt with on a multidisciplinary basis, including endoscopy, radiology, endocrinology and other medical fields.

7.7 Coaching and Physical Exercise, Weight Loss Support and Maintenance, Diet Counselling

A recent systematic review article reviewed the patient education practices in weight loss surgery [4]. Twenty-four publications were included with 16 studies dealing with preoperative and 8 studies dealing with post-operative patient guidance. Evidence levels were high, i.e. I–III in 5 studies, and moderate to low (IV–VII) in 17 studies. The education programmes varied substantially in composition, teaching methods and education, and in depth. Factors commonly discussed were the surgical procedure, nutrition, activity and psychosocial behaviours. Whereas preoperative education was mostly provided in small groups, individual sessions were used post-operatively. Many healthcare experts from multiple disciplines were involved in both phases and commonly used passive learning methods with little active involvement of patients. Written or Web-based aides supported the education in both phases and can be used to more actively involve patients. For those who want to set up this education, the article gives an extensive overview of what has been tried in the different centres [4].

It is commonly assumed that physical activities play a positive role if started while a given patient is getting prepared for bariatric surgery, provided that functional limitations are not extensive, which is called functional rehabilitation [4, 19, 21]. More accurate data are available, from a study by Marcon et al., who compared exercise, exercise and group therapy with cognitive-behavioural therapy (CBT), or conventional waiting list patients before bariatric surgery [22]. This RCT investigated the effect of a 4-month low-intensity exercise programme (two-weekly sessions of 25 min each) on 66 morbidly obese individuals. The weight change was −7.4 kg, −4.2 kg and + 2.9 kg for the groups of exercise, exercise + CBT and waiting list controls, respectively. Changes were significant when compared to the control group ($p < 0.001$), but there were no differences between the two intervention arms. Functional capacity and cardiometabolic parameters significantly improved in both intervention arms and worsened in the control group. The adherence to the exercise programme in both groups was above 78%.

Insistence on post-operative exercise is even more important, owing to a mutual benefit: weight loss enhances physical capacity, and exercise contributes to sustained weight loss, with a relative sparing of the breakdown of muscles and maintenance of muscular capacities. Functional capacity, balance and mobility are increased as early as 6 months post-operatively, such as shown in the study by Gallart-Arago et al. [23]. However, muscle and/or protein deficiencies may alter some of these capacities, which therefore should be evaluated more in detail, as shown in a pilot that randomised patients to an exercise programme specifically adapted for post-bariatric patients [24]. Fifty-one post-bariatric patients, 6–24 months post-surgery, were randomly assigned to usual care control ($n = 25$) or the exercise intervention ($n = 26$). The intervention included twice-weekly 60-min group exercise classes with functional strength, flexibility and aerobic activities; at least 3 days per week of self-directed exercise; daily pedometer; recording of steps and activities; and weekly telephone counselling. There was also a 6-month maintenance period. Patients were 49 years old, 84% female, with a BMI of 32.9 kg/m^2, and per cent excess BMI loss since surgery of 56%. Patients were 14 months post-surgery. A total of 44 patients (86%) completed both phases of the programme and all assessments. The following measures improved significantly in patients in the intervention group with no changes in control participants: the number of yards walked in 6 min, number of seconds for 8-foot up-and-go, number of arm curls and distance in inches for chair sit-and-reach. The change brought about by the intervention remained over the 6-month maintenance period.

A valuable adjunction to exercise could be represented by wearable technologies or Internet on things, which is also an interesting tracking tool. Yet, the assumption that weight loss, enhanced by the use of technology, would automatically result in greater or more sustained weight loss could be presumptuous, as shown in a recent study in non-surgical patients over a period of 24 months [25]. A total of 471 adults (BMI 25–40 kg/m^2) seeking weight loss were randomised to a standard lifestyle intervention group ($N = 234$) or a group with a wearable device + Web interface ($N = 237$) to monitor diet and physical activity. The primary end point was the change in weight between the two groups. The second group achieved no better results in terms of weight loss. Such studies are not available in surgical patients yet, but we may infer similar results.

Supportive therapy through lifestyle modifications represents of course the bigger picture, requesting the participation of the whole bariatric team, dedicated to weight loss and well-being of the obese patients. Likewise, support groups and meetings are encouraged on a regular basis. There is no need to emphasise this, and it has been widely endorsed. Diet prescription post-operatively does not fundamentally differ from the advice given to the general population, except immediate post-operative diets (liquid and semi-liquid diets for a few weeks for any kind of procedures, with between-meals if necessary). The guidelines emphasise an adequate protein consumption, especially after RYGB and the more malabsorptive procedures [1]. Special requirements exist on a case-to-case basis, e.g. in the presence of an ulcer or a dumping. Although supplements are routinely prescribed, one may advise food with more balanced nutrients and micronutrients. More generally, a focus on food preferences is worthwhile, owing to changes that are very common after RYGB or LSG for instance, new tastes and aversions coming up, such as for red meat or poultry or intolerances such as for milk and milk products. There is consensus on not recommending a low-calorie diet post-operatively, except occasionally in case of weight regain, and not insisting on nutrient exclusion, while low-lipid diets are generally advised in case of diarrhoea following bypass surgeries, and low-carbohydrate (and/or dairy) diets in case of dumping syndrome. Dietary adjustments in case of dumping are discussed in Chap. 6. Dealing with endoscopic techniques, with usually less ambitious weight loss goals, a low-calorie diet can be recommended.

7.8 Quality of Life

The appreciation of the quality of life (QOL) is a key issue in bariatric surgery, since weight loss per se may induce problems of its own, and create others that had not been anticipated. QOL in general is significantly improved by bariatric surgery, whatever the questionnaire used. Various questionnaires exist, among which are the BAROS (Bariatric Analysis and Reporting Outcomes System) and the IWQOL (31-item questionnaire, assessing the Impact of Weight on Quality Of Life), both disease-specific questionnaires for obesity, and the more general RAND-36 (general health-related QOL questionnaire with 36 questions and 9 scales) [26].

Other criteria are also important, that may impact the QOL, such as the digestive side effects of an intervention. A specific gastrointestinal QOL questionnaire (GIQLI, 36 items with response ranging from 0 to 4) has been developed and showed improvements both after sleeve gastrectomy and bypass, despite digestive side effects such as GORD or potential complications/side effects (irritable bowel, diarrhoea, dumping syndrome, pouch inflammation, ulcer, stenosis, etc.) [27].

7.9 Medical Follow-Up of Comorbidities

The comorbidities that have been described in Chap. 1 entail surveillance and monitoring over the time. A favourable outcome is to be expected in most of them, although improvements occur at different paces depending on each patient's profile and characteristics, and on the surgical procedure, with bypass interventions having in general more rapid and stronger effects.

7.10 Short-Term and Long-Term Nutritional Support and Supplementation

Numerous guidelines are available regarding general requirements and more specific detailed needs according to different operations [1–3]. The multidisciplinary team may either follow one of the international guidelines or the local national guidelines or set up a list of required number of visits per year and laboratory measures and eventually more specialised examinations such as DEXA for bone status, which will be more exhaustive the greater the impact of surgery on the normal anatomy. Although all types of operation entail supplements at least in the beginning, they are strictly requested only with the operations with a significant malabsorptive component, RYGB, BPD-DS, etc. Blood tests are recommended every year [1–3]. Nutrient deficiencies may be due to changes in intake, complaints leading to avoid some foods, and changes in taste and hedonic responses to food but these are easy to cover with temporary supplements and dietary advices in patients after a LSG or LAGB. This is different in patients with a RYGB or BPD with or without duodenal switch, who have an added problem of maldigestion and malabsorption, which will be discussed when indicated.

7.11 Macronutrients

7.11.1 Proteins

A very significant part of the absorption takes place in the proximal part of the small intestine, and the remainder in the distal small intestine. Mankind cannot make essential amino acids himself, so these should be provided by daily nutrition with proteins of high biological value. The rate-limiting step in protein synthesis is the smallest available amount of the essential amino acid. There are many factors that may contribute to protein malnutrition after bariatric surgery: decreased intake by poor tolerance for animal protein (e.g. red meat) or dumping of protein-rich milk products, increased losses as with chronic diarrhoea and intractable vomiting, and decreased absorption due to loss of pepsinogen, gastric acid and pancreatic enzymes. Also, bacterial overgrowth with protein consumption and protein breakdown may attribute. Protein shortness is most of the time not revealed by blood tests (very exceptionally hypoalbuminaemia is seen) but symptoms should alert the physician: muscle loss and weakness, dermatitis, wound-healing problems, alopecia, bone loss, oedema indicating the need for at least temporary IV nutrition, and possibly reversal of the malabsorptive part of the operation. Although protein supplements are usually recommended for a few months in all kinds of bariatric technique, it is only mandatory in case of RYGB, and BPD-DS (or other malabsorptive procedures). After RYGB, the rate of hypoalbuminaemia can be up to 1.3% after 2 years. Two systematic reviews looked at the influence of dietary protein and its amino acid composition either on post-operative outcomes [28] or on protein status and lean body mass (LBM) post-surgery [29].

Van den Broek et al. investigated the relationship between intake of dietary protein or supplementation with amino acids and post-operative outcomes after gastric bypass surgery in 23 studies [28]. They discovered that convincing evidence of an effect of dietary protein intake on weight loss or other beneficial effects after gastric bypass is lacking. This is in contrast to the finding in non-bariatric patients where higher protein diets were found to be a successful strategy for weight reduction. In the reviewed studies on gastric bypass, three randomised trials did not find an effect of protein intake on weight loss parameters, but two non-randomised studies did. Findings in three other studies suggested that protein intake might be associated with a greater decline in weight or BMI, although these results were not statistically significant. Part of the discrepancy can be explained by the duration of follow-up with positive results being present in the studies with a post-operative follow-up of 12 months, in contrast to the follow-up of only 6–8 weeks or 6 months of the studies with a less positive outcome. Another important fact that has to be taken into consideration is the preservation of lean body mass which consists of more water and thus is heavier than fat mass. So when weight is lost, a distinction between fat loss and lean body weight loss, the latter being less favourable, should be made. The authors, being surprised that in view of the popularity of bariatric surgery, the quality and quantity of protein in the diet did not receive sufficient and science-worth attention, strongly recommend future studies describing the exact quantity and composition of the protein or amino acids in the diet or supplement.

Ito et al. did a systematic review to evaluate the amount of protein intake and its association with lean mass and serum proteins during at least 6 months following Roux-en-Y gastric bypass or sleeve gastrectomy [29]. Twelve studies ($n = 739$) showed that in most patients a protein intake below 60 g/day and significant lean mass loss were observed; changes in body composition were measured by bioelectrical impedance analysis (BIA) or dual-energy X-ray absorptiometry (DXA). Out of the four studies that measured the association between protein intake and lean mass retention, only two supported the hypothesis of this correlation. There is insufficient evidence of the effect of dietary protein on serum protein levels. It may be that certain components of the protein such as amino acids, e.g. branched-chain amino acids or leucine, are clinically more relevant than the total amount of protein. Further studies are needed to better estimate the minimal protein intake needed that supports a healthy nutritional status in the bariatric population.

Schiavo et al. demonstrated in sleeve gastrectomy patients the well-known positive impact of a protein-enriched diet (PED) versus a normal protein diet (NPD) on total weight loss (TWL), fat mass (FM), fat-free mass (FFM) and resting metabolic rate (RMR) [30]. Sixty male patients after LSG received either a NPD ($N = 30$) with protein intake 1.0 g/kg of ideal body weight or a PED ($N = 30$) with protein intake 2.0 g/kg of ideal body weight [30]. Despite a non-significant variation in total body weight (TBW), FM decreased more significantly ($p < 0.01$) with PED compared to NPD. In addition, the PED group showed a significantly ($p < 0.01$) lower decrease in FFM and RMR when compared with the NPD group. Both groups showed a high compliance in following the prescribed diets, without a negative impact on renal function.

7.11.2 Carbohydrates and Lipids

The capacity for storage of these nutrients being extensive, the likelihood of a deficiency is very low. Yet the lack of essential fatty acids can have adverse consequences. Carbohydrate digestion has a large capacity as salivary amylase and pancreatic amylase are responsible for the breakdown in oligosaccharides and disaccharides and the brush border enzymes that further digest the carbohydrate are usually not affected. The only problem occurs when too much small bowel is bypassed, but again this does not result in deficiencies as the liver can make glucose via the gluconeogenesis, but patients may suffer from bacterial degradation of carbohydrates in the colon and suffer from diarrhoea, bloating, flatulence, etc. As to the lipids, lingual lipase and pancreatic lipase and emulsification by the stomach are needed to enable adequate digestion. Bile acids are needed as well for the absorption. So, in the case of fat, maldigestion and malabsorption occur together, the latter being due to the loss of bile salts and their presence below the critical micellar level. This signifies that also fat-soluble vitamins are malabsorbed.

7.11.3 Micronutrients

This issue is more important than previously thought, even in non-bypass surgeries, which can partly be explained by the fact that obese patients, despite having an intake that is far beyond a normal intake, do not eat the right foods and thus often have deficiencies before the operation which should be evaluated at the screening consultation. According to Roust et al. [31], micronutrient deficiencies are common and multiple in obese individuals preoperatively, without an identified profile of deficiency. They concern mostly vitamin D, folate, vitamin B12 and iron. An early supplementation before surgery should be recommended. Gillon et al. examined the vitamin and mineral status in patients up to 5 years after LSG and explored changes that occurred from preoperatively to 1, 2 and 5 years after surgery [32]. Data reviewed included age, sex, weight and body mass index (BMI), micronutrient supplements consumed and blood levels of 25 hydroxyvitamin D (25 (OH) D), parathyroid hormone (PTH), ferritin, haemoglobin, folate and vitamin B12, prior to and post-LSG. There were 336 patients with values preoperatively and 1 year after surgery; 272 had values up to 2 years, and 116 had values up to 5 years after surgery. At 5 years, only 54% (58/107) of patients reported taking daily multivitamin supplements. While most patients had values within the reference range for haemoglobin, vitamin B12, folate and vitamin D 5 years after LSG, 36% (34/94) of the patients had serum ferritin below the reference value. Gudzune et al. followed >21,000 patients over 3 years and could divide their population in patients with restrictive, RYGB and malabsorptive operations (84%) [33]. They demonstrated that the latter had the highest frequency of deficiency in the first 12 months post-operatively: vitamin D (12%), vitamin B12 (60%), folate (47%) and iron (49%) [33]. James et al. discussed the adherence of 287 patients in taking supplements [34], and found that patients' adherence was sustained in 92%, with acceptable rates of deficiencies 6–36 months post-operatively: vitamin A (4.9%), E (0%), B12 (3.7%), D (16.2%), iron (6% in females) and anaemia (12.2% in females). On the other hand, most often composite supplements are used for their ease and safety and one could question whether such supplements suffice for all and can prevent deficiencies [35], although the deficiency rates for iron and vitamin A, B12 and D were significantly lower in compliant patients than in non-compliant patients.

7.11.4 Water-Soluble Vitamins

Thiamin (vitamin B1) deficiency can lead to Wernicke-Korsakoff syndrome and beriberi. It is absorbed in the duodenum and jejunum, which is out of circulation after RYGB. Very dangerous is the combination of frequent vomiting and insufficient intake. Because of dehydration patients receive intravenous fluid administration and when glucose is given without 100 mg vitamin B1 intramuscularly or intravenously they can become very acidotic (lactic acidosis) with adverse consequences and even death. The daily requirements are 1.1–1.3 mg, but there is no toxicity, so when in doubt give 100 mg vitamin B1.

Vitamin B9 (folic acid) should be provided as well, 400 µg/day. The problem of folic acid is that it needs first the removal of the terminal glutamic acid by gastric acid before it can be absorbed in the duodenum. Both the digestion and the absorption are absent in RYGB. Moreover, in the case of bacterial overgrowth, the bacteria may provide and synthesise folic acid. This is very important for infertile obese female patients who will conceive more readily after weight loss after bariatric surgery.

Vitamin B12 (cyanocobalamin) is absorbed in the ileum, together with the intrinsic factor, produced by gastric parietal cells. Due to absence of gastric acid and pepsin it is not cleaved and freed from the protein binding in meat and liver and therefore not available for binding to the intrinsic factor, which is also absent after RYGB (not after a sleeve or BPD-DS), explaining why some malabsorptive surgery can lead to severe symptoms: macroblastic anaemia and polyneuropathy. Also, bacterial overgrowth can decrease vitamin B12 due to bacterial consumption. Supplementation of 2.4–3 µg/day is recommended, usually intramuscularly as a 1000 mcg hydroxycobalamin, but high doses of crystalline B12, 1 mg per day, may also suffice. Different supplementation regimes are available and critically reviewed by Smelt et al. [36]. Based on ten studies, they concluded that a daily oral intake of 350 µg was the appropriate dose.

Vitamin B2, B3, B5, B6 and C and biotin are not to be neglected. The daily recommended doses are as follows: riboflavin (B2): 1.2–1.15 mg; niacin (B3): 13–17 mg; pantothenic acid (B5): 6 mg; pyridoxine (B6): 1.2–1.5 mg; biotin: 30–60 µg; and ascorbic acid (C): 100–150 mg.

7.11.5 Fat-Soluble Vitamins

As discussed earlier, due to the mechanisms leading to fat malabsorption also fat-soluble vitamins may be affected.

Vitamin A: Vitamin A deficiency may cause night blindness, dry skin and respiratory infections. Vitamin A supplementation should be done carefully in pregnancy due to possible teratogenicity.

Vitamin D (calciferol): Vitamin D deficiency is common in obese patients already before surgery, with many causes (inadequate dietary intake, limited sun exposure, decreased bioavailability owing to its retention in adipose tissue). It is possible that the persistence of this deficiency is correlated to the existence of a metabolic syndrome [37]. The vitamin D status and supplementation before and after surgery have been reviewed by Peterson et al. [38]: optimal serum concentrations should be >30 ng/mL; preoperative and post-operative deficiency rate is as high as 98%; a daily intake of 1000–5000 IU is necessary, or even a 50,000 IU weekly + daily supplement. Guidelines on vitamin D replacements were reviewed by Chakhtoura et al. [39], who argued that a daily intake of 1000–2000 IU was necessary in children, adolescents and pregnant women in the Middle East and North Africa. A systematic review by Switzer et al. [40] demonstrated a long-term, 5-year persistence of hyperparathyroidism despite the intake of calcium and vitamin D supplements: from a 5.69 pmol/L level at baseline, average parathyroid hormone levels raised to 8.29 > 5 years, while at that time vitamin D level was low at 20.79 ng/mL.

Vitamin E: Vitamin E is important for reproduction; a major deficiency would result in ataxia, but is rarely observed.

Vitamin K: Vitamin K deficiency seems common, and can translate into increased coagulation time, with usually minimal consequences.

7.11.6 Electrolytes and Trace Elements

Calcium, iron and zinc have the same problems of digestion and absorption after RYGB. They are bound to protein-rich foods such as milk products, meat and fish, and split off from their protein binding by pepsin secreted in the stomach and activated by gastric acid from pepsinogen. Moreover, trivalent iron has to be reduced to bivalent iron for uptake and usually this is done in the presence of gastric acid or by supplementing vitamin C to vegetables. Calcium, iron and zinc when freed are preferentially absorbed in the duodenum, which is out of the circulation in RYGB. As all three are bivalent ions, they can also bind to fatty acids to produce fat soaps and due to the fat malabsorption in RYGB this increases the loss of the bivalent ions in the stool. So, maldigestion, malabsorption and increased losses are instrumental in their deficiency. Magnesium can also bind to the fatty acids and be lost with the stools.

Calcium: Calcium supplementation, together with vitamin D, should start early after bariatric surgery.

Magnesium, zinc, iodine and copper: Supplementation is necessary when symptoms of a deficiency exist (including hair loss). Copper deficiency is rare after RYGB and reviewed by Kumar et al. who advised an annual monitoring, and treatment in case of haematological or neurological disorders [41].

Potassium: Potassium is a problem in case of acute vomiting with dehydration.

Iron: Iron deficiency is the most frequent occurring deficiency and the main reason for post-operative anaemia [42]. It results from several factors post-operatively: insufficient dietary intake; reduction of acid secretion in the stomach whereby there is no reduction of Fe^{3+} to Fe^{2+}, which is the only form that can be absorbed; reduction of absorption in the (absent/bypassed) duodenum and proximal intestine; and losses via marginal ulcer bleeding or menstrual blood loss.

7.12 General Issues in Follow-Up

7.12.1 Medical Follow-Up of Associated Comorbidities and Potential Negative Side Effects of Bariatric Surgery

It is not required for a bariatric surgeon and/or endoscopist to transform himself/herself into an internist, but he/she must be prepared to call for any specialist when associated diseases require fine-tuned adjustments, or sometimes major updates, e.g. when it comes to the rapid and favourable evolution of T2DM or high blood pressure.

7.12.2 Neurological Problems

Mainly due to vitamin B deficiencies several problems may occur which have been summarised by Juhasz-Pocsine et al. [43]: acute complications, including encephalopathy or polyradiculoneuropathy, can occur in the early stage or decades later. Although one would not expect problems with restrictive operations, Wernicke encephalopathy has also been described after a sleeve gastrectomy [44, 45].

7.12.3 Bone Mineral Density

The decreased calcium and vitamin D absorption and the resultant hyperparathyroidism are important side effects of bariatric operations which are predominantly performed in women and mostly at young ages. The commonly prescribed proton pump inhibitors (PPI) are an unfavourable combination with bypass surgery and risk of bone fracture and/or osteoporosis, such as emphasised by Deitel et al. [46]. Raoof et al. examined the bone mineral density (BMD) in 32 patients, and found that in 5-year follow-up 8 developed osteopenia and 1 osteoporosis [47]. A systematic review and a meta-analysis reviewed the relationship between bariatric surgery and BMD [48]: BMD was decreased at the femoral neck, but not at the lumbar spine. Interestingly, the British Medical Journal published two articles on this item, one by Lalmchamed who examined the risk for fractures [49], and the other recently by Rousseau et al. [50]. Lalmchamed et al. used data from the records of the United Kingdom General Practice Research Database, today known as the Clinical Practice Research [49]. Patients with a body mass index of at least 30 kg/m^2 were included and each bariatric surgery patient was matched to up to six controls by age, sex, practice, year and BMI, resulting in 2079 bariatric surgery patients and 10,442 matched controls. In a mean follow-up time of 2.2 years, there was no significantly increased risk of fracture in patients who underwent bariatric surgery. The risk was 8.8 per 1000 person-years compared with 8.2 per 1000 person-years in controls with an adjusted relative risk of 0.89 (95% confidence interval 0.60 to 1.33). Bariatric surgery also did not affect the risk of osteoporotic and non-osteoporotic fractures. The follow-up time was relatively short and although not significant a trend towards an increased fracture risk was seen both after a prolonged observation period of 3–5 years following surgery and in patients who had a greater decrease in BMI after surgery. Rousseau et al. more recently compared 12,676 bariatric surgery patients with 38,028 obese and 126,760 non-obese controls, who were matched by age and sex [50]. Before surgery, fractures were more often seen in patients undergoing bariatric surgery (1326; 10.5%) than in obese (3065; 8.1%) or non-obese (8329; 6.6%) controls. After a mean of 4.4 years after surgery, bariatric patients were more susceptible to fracture (514; 4.1%) than were obese (1013; 2.7%) and non-obese (3008; 2.4%) controls. Adjusted relative risks of bariatric patients were 1.38 (95% confidence interval 1.23 to 1.55) versus obese subjects and 1.44 (95% confidence interval 1.29 to 1.59) versus non-obese controls. Whereas before surgery the risk of distal lower limb fracture was higher, after surgery the risk of upper limb, spine, pelvis, hip or femur fractures increased. When looking at the different bariatric surgeries, the increase in risk of fracture reached significance only for biliopancreatic diversion. So, patients referred to and undergoing bariatric surgery are at increased risk of fractures, which seemed to be site specific, with a change from a fracture pattern being associated with obesity (lower limb fractures) to a pattern associated with osteoporosis after bariatric surgery. But also here the follow-up is relatively short and bariatric patients are mainly young females, who are by themselves at increased risk.

7.12.4 The Problem of Alcohol, Substance Abuse, Depression and Suicide Attempt

The ASMBS made a position paper on alcohol use after bariatric surgery issuing a warning as increasing reports were released on the subject [51]. Ostlund et al. followed 11,115 patients after restrictive surgery for 8.6 years and compared preoperative incidence with post-operative incidence of depression, substance abuse, suicide attempt and alcohol abuse and this separately for men and women [52]. They concluded that in a mean FU time of 8.6 years, there was a twofold increase of inpatient care for alcohol abuse in bypass patients versus restrictive surgery patients. Substance use after bariatric surgery has been reviewed by Li and Wu [53]: in 40 studies, preoperative history of substance use was a reliable correlate of post-operative substance use. No significant change in cigarette smoking from pre- to post-operative period was observed, and the new onset of substance users among bariatric patients ranged from 34 to 89%! Also the question whether alcohol use was amended after bariatric surgery was negatively answered by Gregorio et al. [54].

7.12.5 The Fear of the Return of Diabetes

The exact prevalence of diabetes relapse after initial remission is unknown because of attrition problems and lack of data on the long-term after surgery. The mechanisms of relapse are not fully elucidated, whether in conjunction or not with weight regain, as pointed out by Shad and Laferrère [55].

7.12.6 Drug Treatments

Adaptation of drug prescription concerns all patients who have medication, while potential benefits of weight loss should be translated into new prescriptions, along with improvements of comorbidities. RYGB poses a problem of drug disposition, which can turn into a sensitive issue regarding anticoagulant or contraceptive medication. A review of all pharmacokinetic studies involving at least four subjects who underwent RYGB has been performed [56]. Twenty-five publications were selected and, overall, 25 drugs were studied. Drug solubility and permeability parameters for each drug were defined using different parameters or classifications. Increased rates of oral drug absorption were predominantly observed. Conversely, drug exposure differed from one drug to another. Both the galenic formulation and the Biopharmaceutics Classification System (BCS) class may help predict the outcome of oral drug intake after a RYGB. A strategy aiming to guide prescription and drug monitoring in patients with RYGB is suggested, but further research is clearly needed due to the unique characteristics of the bariatric population. Azran et al. reviewed the literature of oral drug treatment after bariatric surgery and provided an extensive list of publications on the most common drugs with recommendations [57]. They pointed out that patients may be discharged with insufficient instructions regarding post-operative medication therapy [57]. Bland et al. considered the long-term pharmacotherapy after bariatric surgery and discussed the most prominent groups of medications [58]. They argued to assign an important role to the pharmacists [58].

7.13 Weight Regain

Weight regain is one of the most important issues in bariatric surgery, one that puts the whole field at jeopardy, since long-term improvements of related comorbidities are strongly correlated with the long-term weight maintenance. How dedicated the bariatric team may be, it does not prevent the occurrence of technical and surgical problems like gastric band dislodgement, widening of the gastric pouch and gastro-jejunostomy diameter or volume increase of the sleeve gastrectomy, but the team should try to minimise the propensity to weight regain. Among others, the choice of a redo intervention and the choice of the timing of this intervention are difficult decisions to make, whereas intentions of the bariatric team may oppose patient's preferences. This has been explained in Chap. 3. When it comes to the "end-of-the-line operations" such as after a gastric bypass of biliopancreatic diversion, choices are even more difficult. Monaco-Ferreira et al. have investigated weight regain and the associated variables 10 years after RYGB in 166 patients [59]. At 24 months, 50% of the patients ($N = 83$) regained a mean weight of 3.98 kg, and 25.3% a mean weight of 14.6 kg at 120 months ($N = 42$). Excess weight, preoperative BMI, gender, age, nutritional monitoring and iron deficiency did not explain weight regain. Younger patients had regained significantly more weight 96 and 120 months after surgery than older patients.

7.14 Aesthetic Follow-Up

Even relatively "milder" operations, such as those achieved by endoscopic means, may end up with a very significant weight loss and aesthetic aftermaths. Reconstructive and plastic surgery is an important topic of concern for patients, for which information should be delivered from the start, including insurance coverage (which can be denied), sequences for repair and intervals of time in between, and post-operative specific complications (bleeding, scar dehiscence, unsatisfactory results and necessity of surgical adjustments).

In a comprehensive survey, French use of plastic reconstructive surgery has been analysed (unpublished data): from 2007 to 2013, 190,000 bariatric procedures have been performed in 183,000 patients; in the same population, 23,400 plastic surgery procedures have been performed in 18,300 patients. The operations consisted in 62% of abdominoplasties, in 25% of upper or lower limb plasties and in 14% of breast reconstructions. Twenty-one per cent of the bariatric-operated patients had a further plastic surgery at 7 years, yet this percentage was highly variable, depending on regional location, from 2 to 50%!

A study has examined the utilisation of two common procedures, abdominoplasty and panniculectomy, following bariatric surgery in New York State, with 37,806 patients between 2004 and 2010 [60]. Procedures included LSG, RYGB and LAGB. Only 5.58% (n = 2,112) of these patients subsequently had a body-contouring procedure, with 143 of them (6.8%) having ≥1 plastic surgery. The average time to plastic surgery after bariatric surgery was 1134, 984 and 903 days, for LSG, RYGB and LAGB, respectively. Insurance and income issues in this US context have contributed to the fact that plastic surgery was completed by a low number of patients following bariatric procedures.

7.14.1 Pregnancy

Eighty-five per cent of obese patients undergoing bariatric surgery are females, most of them being fertile, so pregnancy is a very important issue before implementing surgery, and during the follow-up.

Because of nutritional complications for the growing child patients are often dissuaded to become pregnant in the first to second years after bariatric surgery. Although pregnancy after bariatric surgery is associated with decreased risk for the mother and the foetus, nutritional complications may occur and apart from the increased requirements may be due to the increased occurrence of vomiting. The focus on deficiencies becomes a very important issue and special attention should be given to vitamin B12 and iron and other micronutrients should be considered such as vitamin A (important in reproduction, and cell differentiation, but in high doses also leading to teratogenicity), folic acid (risk of foetal neural tube defect), zinc (abnormal foetus development) and magnesium (foetal growth retardation).

The usual recommendations are to wait around 18 months after any bariatric procedure before being pregnant, and 24 months after RYGB. There is indeed a risk of low birth weight and micronutrient deficiencies in neonates from mothers after bypass, even if this postponement by 1–2 years has been taken into consideration. Gascoin et al. screened newborns for micronutrient deficiencies: they compared 56 newborns of mothers with RYGB, and 56 newborns of non-obese healthy mothers (controls) after a normal pregnancy [61]. Cord blood micronutrient concentrations from controls were used for establishing normative data. After RYGB, the pregnant women took daily micronutrient supplements; they lost 18.1 units in BMI in the

11–69 months between surgery and onset of pregnancy (% EWL of 79%), reaching a BMI of 30.1 kg/m^2 compared with the BMI of 22.3 kg/m^2 in the normal-weight controls ($P < 0.05$). Neonates born to RYGB mothers were small for gestational age in 23% of cases versus 3.6% in the control group ($P < 0.01$). A higher percentage of RYGB neonates had cord blood concentrations below the 2.5 percentile for calcium (19% vs. 2%), zinc (13% vs. 3%), iron (19% vs. 2%) and vitamin A (13% vs. 3%), and over the 97.5 percentile for magnesium (13% vs. 3%), vitamin E (16% vs. 3%), 25-hydroxyvitamin D (13% vs. 2%) and vitamin B12 (14% vs. 2%) ($P < 0.05$ for all comparisons). The conclusion was that neonates born from RYGB mothers had more blood micronutrient deficiencies than those born from healthy mothers, results from those born from morbidly obese mothers being unknown.

Gimenes et al. evaluated nutritional and biochemical indicators of women who became pregnant after RYGB [62]. The study included 25 patients (35.7 years), who became pregnant 31.3 months after RYGB. Weight loss until the beginning of pregnancy was 32.4%, and the gestational weight gain was 3.8 kg. Total cholesterol (180.9 vs. 148.5 mg/dL), LDL cholesterol (103.5 vs. 85.8 mg/dL), HDL cholesterol (56.4 vs. 46.9 mg/dL) and latent iron-binding capacity (337.6 vs. 277.8 μg/dL) were higher during pregnancy compared to just before pregnancy, while haemoglobin values (11.2 vs. 12.3 g/dL) and sodium (138.8 vs. 141 mmol/L) were lower. No differences of food intake were found when comparing post-RYGB and pregnancy times. There was no difference on gestational weight gain between women who became pregnant before or after the first year. During pregnancy, there was an expected weight gain and maintenance of the lipid profile within the normal range; however, there was a reduction of haemoglobin levels. These findings show the need for individualised follow-up with adequate nutritional intervention in the event of deficiencies.

On a wider scale, pregnancy after bariatric surgery has been reported in the National Survey of Obstetrician's Comfort, Knowledge, and Practice Patterns (USA) [63]. It showed that while most obstetricians are aware of perinatal risks after bariatric surgery, a substantial percentage of obstetricians are unaware of recommended practices regarding nutrition and nutritional monitoring.

Acknowledgments The author wants to acknowledge Lisbeth Mathus-Vliegen for her help with this chapter.

References

1. Mechanick J, Youdim A, Jones DB, Garvey T, Hurley DL, McMahon M, et al. Clinical Practice Guidelines for the Perioperative Nutritional, Metabolic, and Nonsurgical Support of the Bariatric Surgery Patient—2013 Update: Cosponsored by American Association of Clinical Endocrinologists, the Obesity Society, and American Society for Metabolic & Bariatric Surgery. Obesity (Silver Spring). 2013;21(0 1):S1–27.
2. Garvey WT, Mechanick JI, Brett EM, Garber AJ, Hurley DL, Jastreboff AM, et al. American Association of Clinical Endocrinologists and American College of Endocrinology comprehensive clinical practical guidelines for medical care of patients with obesity. American Endocr Pract. 2016;22(Suppl 3):1–203.

3. Fried M, Yumuk V, Oppert JM, Scopinaro N, Torres A, Weiner R, et al. International Federation for Surgery of Obesity and Metabolic Disorders-European Chapter (IFSO-EC); European Association for the Study of Obesity (EASO); European Association for the Study of Obesity, Obesity Management Task Force (EASO OMTF). Interdisciplinary European guidelines on metabolic and bariatric surgery. Obes Surg. 2014;24(1):42–55.
4. Groller KD. Systematic review of patient education practices in weight loss surgery. Surg Obes Relat Dis. 2017;13(6):1072–85.
5. Pitzul KB, Jackson T, Crawford S, Chi Hin Kwong J, Sockalingam S, Hawa R, et al. Understanding disposition after referral for bariatric surgery: when and why patients referred do not undergo surgery. Obes Surg. 2014;24(1):134–40.
6. Steinbeisser M, McCracken J, Kharbutli B. Laparoscopic sleeve gastrectomy: preoperative weight loss and other factors as predictors of postoperative success. Obes Surg. 2017;27(6):1508–13.
7. Alami RS, Morton JM, Schuster R, Lie J, Sanchez BR, Peters A, et al. Is there a benefit to preoperative weight loss in gastric bypass patients? A prospective randomized trial. Surg Obes Relat Dis. 2007;3(2):141–5.
8. Carlin AM, O'Connor EA, Genaw JA, Kawar S. Preoperative weight loss is not a predictor of postoperative weight loss after laparoscopic Roux-en-Y gastric bypass. Surg Obes Relat Dis. 2008;4(4):481–5.
9. Stevens DJ, Jackson JA, Howes N. Obesity surgery smartphone apps: a review. Obes Surg. 2014;24:32–6.
10. Al-Khyatt W, Ryall R, Leeder P, Ahmed J, Awas S. Predictors of inadequate weight loss after laparoscopic gastric bypass for morbid obesity. Obes Surg. 2017;27(6):1446–52.
11. Ledoux S, Sami O, Breuil MC, Delapierre M, Calabrese D, Msika S, et al. Relevance of self-reported behavorial changes before bariatric surgery to predict success after surgery. Obes Surg. 2017;27(6):1453–9.
12. van den Heuvel M, Hörchner R, Wijtsma A, Bourhim N, Willemsen D, Mathus-Vliegen EMH. Sweet eating: a definition and the development of the Dutch sweet eating questionnaire. Obes Surg. 2011;21:714–21.
13. Thorell A, Mac Cormick AD, Awad S, Reynolds N, Roulin D, Demartines N, et al. Guidelines for perioperative care in bariatric surgery: Enhanced Recovery after Surgery Society (ERAS) recommendations. World J Surg. 2016;40(9):2065–83.
14. Małczak P, Pisarska M, Piotr M, Wyzocki M, Budzinsky A, Pedziwiatr M. Enhanced recovery after bariatric surgery: systematic review and meta-analysis. Obes Surg. 2017;27(1):226–35.
15. Singh PM, Panwar R, Borle A, Goudra B, Trikha A, van Wagensveld BA, et al. Efficiency and safety effects of applying eras protocols to bariatric surgery: a systematic review with meta-analysis and trial sequential analysis of evidence. Obes Surg. 2017;27:489–501.
16. Sinha A, Jayaraman L, Punhani D, Chowbey P. Enhanced recovery after bariatric surgery in the severely obese, morbidly obese, super-morbidly obese and super-super morbidly obese using evidence-based clinical pathways: a comparative study. Obes Surg. 2017;27(3):560–8.
17. Bartlett MA, Mauck KF, Daniels PP. Prevention of venous thromboembolism in patients undergoing bariatric surgery. Vasc Health Risk Manag. 2015;11:461–77.
18. Stroh C, Michel N, Luderer D, Wolff S, Lange V, Köckerling F, et al. Risk of thrombosis and thromboembolic prophylaxis in obesity surgery: data analysis from the German Bariatric Surgery Registry. Obes Surg. 2016;26(11):2562–71.
19. O'Kane M, Parretti HM, Hughes CA, Sharma M, Woodcock S, Puplampu T, et al. Guidelines for the follow-up of patients undergoing bariatric surgery. Clin Obes. 2016;6(3):210–24.
20. Mehaffey JH, Mehaffey RL, Mullen MG, Turrentine FE, Malin SK, Schirmer B, et al. Nutrient deficiency 10 years following Roux-en-Y gastric bypass: Who's responsible? Obes Surg. 2017;27(5):1131–6.
21. Colles SL, Dixon JB, O'Brien PE. Hunger control and regular physical activity facilitate weight loss after laparoscopic adjustable gastric banding. Obes Surg. 2008;18(7):833–40.

22. Marcon ER, Baglioni S, Bittencourt L, Lopes CL, Neumann CR, Trindade MR. What is the best treatment before bariatric surgery? Exercise, exercise and group therapy, or conventional waiting: a randomized controlled trial. Obes Surg. 2017;27(3):763–73.
23. Gallart-Arago T, Fernandez-Lao C, Castro-Martin E, Canterero-Villanueva I, Cozar-Ibanez A, Arroyo-Morales M. Health-related fitness improvements in morbid obese patients after laparoscopic sleeve gastrectomy: a cohort study. Obes Surg. 2017;27(5):1182–8.
24. Coleman KJ, Caparosa SL, Nichols JF, Fujioka K, Koebnick C, McCloskey KN, et al. Understanding the capacity for exercise in post-bariatric patients. Obes Surg. 2017;27(1):51–8.
25. Jakicic JM, Davis KK, Rogers RJ, King WC, Marcus MD, Helsel D, et al. Effect of wearable technology combined with a lifestyle intervention on long term weight loss: the IDEA randomized clinical trial. JAMA. 2016;316(11):1161–71.
26. Monpellier VM, Antoniou EE, Aerts EO, Janssen IMC, Jansen ATM. Improvement of health-related quality of life after Roux-en-Y gastric bypass related to weight loss. Obes Surg. 2017;27(5):1168–73.
27. Nickel F, Schmidt L, Bruckner T, Billeter AT, Kenngott HG, Müller-Stich BP, et al. Gastrointestinal quality of life improves significantly after sleeve and Roux-en-Y gastric bypass – a prospective cross-sectional study within a 2-year follow up. Obes Surg. 2017;27(5):1292–7.
28. van den Broek M, de Heide LJ, Veeger NJ, van der Wal-Oost AM, van Beek AP. Influence of dietary protein and its amino acid composition on postoperative outcomes after gastric bypass surgery: a systematic review. Nutr Rev. 2016;74(12):749–73.
29. Ito MK, Gonçalves VSS, Faria SLCM, Moizé V, Porporatti AL, Guerra ENS, et al. Effect of protein intake on the protein status and lean mass of post-bariatric surgery patients: a systematic review. Obes Surg. 2017;27(2):502–12.
30. Schiavo L, Scalera G, Pilone V, De Sena G, Quagliariello V, Iannelli A, et al. A comparative study examining the impact of a protein-enriched Vs normal protein postoperative diet on body composition and resting metabolic rate in obese patients after sleeve gastrectomy. Obes Surg. 2017;27(4):881–8.
31. Roust LR, DiBaise JK. Nutrient deficiencies prior to bariatric surgery. Curr Opin Clin Nutr Metab Care. 2017;20(2):138–44.
32. Gillon S, Jeanes YM, Andersen JR, Våge V. Micronutrient status in morbidly obese Patients prior to laparoscopic sleeve gastrectomy and micronutrient changes 5 years post-surgery. Obes Surg. 2017;27(3):606–12.
33. Gudzune KA, Huizinga MM, Chang HY, Asamoah V, Gadgil M, Clark JM. Screening and diagnosis of micronutrient deficiencies before and after bariatric surgery. Obes Surg. 2013;23(10):1581–9.
34. James H, Lorentz P, Collazo Clavell ML. Patient reported adherence to empiric vitamin/mineral supplementation and related deficiencies after Roux-en-Y gastric bypass. Obes Surg. 2016;26(11):2661–6.
35. Boyce SG, Goriparthi R, Clark L, Cameron K, Rostin MS. Can composite nutritional supplement based on the current guidelines prevent vitamin and mineral deficiency after weight loss surgery? Obes Surg. 2016;26(5):966–71.
36. Smelt HJ, Pouwels S, Smulders JF. Different supplementation regimes to treat perioperative vitamin B12 deficiencies in bariatric surgery: a systematic review. Obes Surg. 2017;27(11):254–62.
37. Obispo Entrenas A, Legupin Tubio D, Lucena Navarro F, Matin Carvajal F, Gandara Adan N, Redondo Bautista M, et al. Relationship between Vitamin D deficiency and the components of metabolic syndrome in patients with morbid obesity, before and 1 year after laparoscopic Roux-en-Y gastric bypass or sleeve gastrectomy. Obes Surg. 2017;27(5):1222–8.
38. Peterson LA, Zeng X, Canfield-Noll CP, Schweitzer MA, Magnuson TH, Stelle KE. Vitamin D status and supplementation before and after bariatric surgery: a comprehensive literature review. Surg Obes Relat Dis. 2016;12(3):693–702.
39. Chakhtoura L, El Ghandour S, Shawak K, Akl EA, Arabi A, Mahfoud Z, et al. Vitamin D replacement in children, adolescents and pregnant women in the Middle-East and North

Africa: a systematic review and meta-analysis of randomized control trials. Metabolism. 2016;70:160–76.
40. Switzer NJ, Marcil G, Prasad S, Debur E, Church N, Mitchell P, et al. Long-term hypovitaminosis D and secondary hyperparathyroidism outcomes of the Roux-en-Y gastric bypass: a systematic review. Obes Rev. 2017;18(5):560–6.
41. Kumar P, Hamza N, Madhok B, De Alwis N, Sharma M, Miras AD, et al. Copper deficiency after gastric bypass for morbid obesity: a systematic review. Obes Surg. 2016;26(6):1335–42.
42. Kheniser KG, Kashyap SR, Schauer PR, Lam ETC, Kullman ES. Prevalence of anemia in subjects randomized into Roux-en-Y gastric bypass or sleeve gastrectomy. Obes Surg. 2017;27(5):1381–6.
43. Juhasz-Pocsine K, Rudnicki SA, Archer RL, Harik SI. Neurologic complications of gastric bypass surgery for, morbid obesity. Neurology. 2007;68(21):1843–50.
44. Kröll D, Laimer M, Bortbély YM, Laederach K, Caudinas D, Nett PC. Wernicke encephalopathy: a future problem even after sleeve gastrectomy. A systematic literature review. Obes Surg. 2016;26(1):205–12.
45. Tabbara M, Carandina S, Bossi M, Polliand C, Genser L, Barrat C. Rare neurological complications after sleeve gastrectomy. Obes Surg. 2016;26(12):2843–8.
46. Deitel M. Bariatric surgery, proton pump-inhibitors, and possibility of osteoporosis. Surg Obes Relat Dis. 2010;6(4):4161–462.
47. Raoof M, Näslund J, Rask E, Szabo E. Effects of gastric bypass on bone mineral density, parathyroid hormone and vitamine D: 5 years follow-up. Obes Surg. 2016;26(5):1141–5.
48. Ko BJ, Myung SK, Cho KH, Park YG, Kim SG, Kim do H, et al. Relationship between bariatric surgery and bone mineral densituy: a meta-analysis. Obes Surg. 2016;26(7):1414–21.
49. Lalmchamed A, de Vries F, Bazelier MT, Cooper A, van Staa TP, Cooper C, et al. Risk of fracture after bariatric surgery in the United Kingdom based population, retrospective cohort study. BMJ. 2012;345:e5085.
50. Rousseau C, Jean S, Gamache P, Lebel S, Mac-Way F, Biertho L, et al. Change in fracture risk and fracture pattern after bariatric surgery: nested case-control study. BMJ. 2016;354:i3794.
51. Parikh M, Johnson JM, Ballem N. American Society for Metabolic and Bariatric Surgery clinical issues committee. AMSBS position statement on alcohol use before and after bariatric surgery. Surg Obes Relat Dis. 2016;12(2):225–30.
52. Ostlund MP, Backman O, Marsk R, Stockeld D, Lagergren J, Rasmussen F, Näslund E. Increased admission for alcohol dependence after gastric bypass surgery compared with restrictive bariatric surgery. JAMA Surg. 2013;148(4):374–7.
53. Li L, Wu LT. Substance abuse after bariatric surgery: a review. J Psychiatr Res. 2016;76:16–29.
54. Gregorio UD, Lucchese R, Vera I, Silva GC, Silva A, Moraes RC. The alcohol consumption is amended after bariatric surgery? An integrative review. Arg Bras Cir Dige. 2016;29Suppl 1(Suppl 1):111–5.
55. Shah A, Laferrère B. Diabetes after bariatric surgery. Can J Diabetes. 2017;41(4):401–6.
56. Hachon L, Declèves X, Faucher P, Carette C, Lloret-Linares C. RYGB and drug disposition: How to do better? Analysis of pharmacokinetic studies and recommendations for clinical practice. Obes Surg. 2017;27(4):1076–90.
57. Azran C, Wolk O, Zur M, Fine-Shamir N, Shaked G, Czeiger D, et al. Oral drug therapy following bariatric surgery: an overview of fundamentals, literature and clinical recommendations. Obes Rev. 2016;17(11):1050–6.
58. Bland CM, Quidley AM, Love BL, Yaeger C, Mc Michael B, Bookstaver PB. Long-term pharmacotherapy considerations in the bariatric patient. Am J Health Syst Pharm. 2016;73(16):1230–42.
59. Monaco-Ferreira DV, Leandro-Merhi VA. Weight regain 10 years after Roux-en-Y gastric bypass. Obes Surg. 2017;27(5):1137–44.
60. Altieri MS, Yang J, Park J, Novikov D, Kang L, Spaniolas K, et al. Utilization of body contouring procedures following weight loss surgery: a study of 37806 Patients. Obes Surg. 2017;27(11):2981–7. https://doi.org/10.1007/s11695-017-2732-4.

61. Gascoin G, Gerard M, Sallé A, Becouarn G, Rouleau S, Sentilhes L, et al. Risk of low birth weight and micronutrient deficiencies in neonates from mothers after gastric bypass: a case control study. Surg Obes Relat Dis. 2017;13(8):1384–91.
62. Gimenes JC, Nicoletti CF, de Souza Pinhel MA, de Oliveira BAP, Salgado Júnior W, Marchini JS, et al. Pregnancy after Roux en Y gastric bypass: nutritional and biochemical aspects. Obes Surg. 2017;27(7):1815–21.
63. Smid MC, Dotters-Katz SK, Mcelwain CA, Volckmann ET, Schulkin J, Stuebe AM. Pregnancy after bariatric surgery: National survey of obstetrician's comfort, knowledge, and practice patterns. Obes Surg. 2017;27(9):2354–9.

8 When the Endoscopist Needs the Surgeon

Contents

Abbreviations

BEA-ERCP	Balloon enteroscopy-assisted ERCP
DJBS	Duodenojejunal bypass sleeve
ERCP	Endoscopic retrograde cholangiopancreaticography
IMAS	Incisionless magnetic anastomotic system
IOP	Incisionless Operating Platform
LA-ERCP	Laparoscopy-assisted ERCP
LAGB	Laparoscopic adjustable gastric banding
LATG-RV	Laparoscopic assisted transgastric rendez-vous
POSE	Primary Obesity Surgery Endoluminal
RYGB	Roux-en-Y gastric bypass
SG	Sleeve gastrectomy
TERIS	Transoral endoscopic restrictive implant system

Both in endoscopic bariatric therapy and in post-bariatric complications where the endoscopist is consulted and called up for help, the endoscopist may request earnestly the assistance of a surgeon, a true cross-pollination between two specialisms and specialists.

Although intragastric balloons date back to the 1980s, endoscopic bariatric therapy is a relatively new sprout on the tree of knowledge of how to treat obesity and lags far behind the surgical experience in this field. Endoscopic techniques to treat

E. M. H. Mathus-Vliegen, J. Dargent, *Bariatric Therapy*,
https://doi.org/10.1007/978-3-319-90074-2_8

obesity stand in between medical treatment and surgical interventions and, as long as they have not proven to serve as an independent, efficacious and long-standing approach, they should always consider – in their aggressiveness on the stomach – the feasibility of bariatric surgery in the future. Modern endoscopic bariatric operations are in a constant state of development, evolution and technical upgrading. This will create several kinds of post-endoscopic issues that should be handled in combination with bariatric surgeons. In the first place, there are immediate or early but also later, more postponed complications that may be managed conservatively or need the help of a surgeon. Even when conservative management is considered, it is always wise to inform the surgeon. Examples where the endoscopist needs the assistance of a surgeon are perforations of the stomach either during placement of an intragastric balloon or later, when the balloon itself causes a gastric perforation. Surgery is then required and to reduce the duration of the operation and the injury to the gastric wall surgeons in their turn often ask endoscopists to remove the balloon by endoscopy in the same setting [1]. Abou Hussein et al. described this approach in 3 cases and reviewed the literature where in total 18 cases were found with 3 deaths [1]. Such a high mortality rate raises doubts about recommendations by Bekheit et al., who managed a gastric perforation secondary to intragastric balloon insertion successfully by conservative means and concluded that such perforations can be treated conservatively in highly selected patients [2]. The balloon can be removed through the perforation itself if large enough by the surgeon. An oesophageal perforation arising during balloon removal may be treated conservatively, depending on the size of the tear, either by a suction tube at the level of the tear, antibiotics and nil per mouth or by placing a stent [3, 4]. This perforation is different from a perforation occurring during dilation of a stenosis. While patients in both cases are fasting, the balloon is often covered with unmeshed food, which may enter and contaminate the area of perforation. So, in case of stent placement one should be prepared for the development of an abscess. When a balloon deflates and cannot be retrieved from the stomach by the endoscopist, the patient should be observed for clinical signs of small-bowel obstruction, and the endoscopist should be deliberate with the surgeon if and when surgical intervention is needed. Sometimes, transabdominal puncture to deflate the balloon by ultrasound is possible as was possible in two of the three balloons that obstructed the small intestine, thus bypassing the need of surgery [5]. Bleeding upon balloon placement or balloon removal may be due to a Mallory-Weiss lesion and is usually treated conservatively or by endoscopic clipping [3, 5]. However, bleeding from an ulcer induced by pressure necrosis or by damage to the wall may be more difficult as the balloon has to be removed first, followed by endoscopic haemostasis techniques [4, 5]. Because of a change in the design of the ReShape Duo intragastric balloon, the ulcer rate went down from 39.6 to 10.3%, and only one of the initial ulcers that were also larger in size bled and needed intervention [4]. In the pivotal US study with the swallowable Obalon balloon only one haemorrhage occurred that was treated conservatively [6]. In the presence of a fulminant bleeding that cannot be controlled by endoscopic measures, there are two choices: that of radiologic embolisation or surgical intervention.

The duodenojejunal bypass sleeve (DJBS) has certain complications such as device migration (4.9%), gastrointestinal bleeding (3.9%) and liver abscess (0.13%) during their stay and complications due to mechanical trauma upon removal such as oesophageal perforation (0.13%) [7, 8]. As is the case with balloon removal, the possibility of a mucosal tear and oesophageal perforation exists by the sharp barbs that hold the DJBS in place and that should be encapsulated within the protective plastic foreign-body retrieval hood mounted on the endoscope to avoid trauma to the stomach or oesophagus. An uncovered barb caused an oesophageal perforation upon withdrawal of the sleeve [7]. A very exceptional case among 21 DJBS cases has been described [9]. This patient suffered from an acute cholecystitis and duodenal fistula due to bulbar transmural penetration and gallbladder impaction by one of the anchors/barbs of the DJBS 1 month after the implant [9]. DJBS migration can mostly be treated by endoscopy but also once a surgical intervention was needed. Gastrointestinal bleeding can be a major complication when the DJBS corrodes the posterior duodenal artery, which can be so massive to not allowing to remove the sleeve and to re-endoscope the patient. Moreover, the positioning at the rear of the duodenal bulb may thwart a favourable approach for endoscopic haemostasis. In these cases radiologic embolisation is the preferred method and surgery is the second choice. Fortunately, however, the eight bleedings reported by Tarnoff et al. and Gershin et al., although impressive by their demonstration of haematemesis, occurred at the proximal anchor point in the oesophagus and did not need major interventions such as embolisation or surgery [10, 11]. Liver abscesses, reported in only 0.13% in Abu Dayyeh's analysis, but being the main reason of interruption of the US pivotal study because of their occurrence in 3.5%, seldom need a surgical approach as these can be drained by the radiologist [7, 12].

All these complications can be treated by a general of a gastrointestinal surgeon, who should, however, be experienced with laparoscopy and should have knowledge of the special obesity-related problems of less visibility due to the large liver and a fatty and large mesentery, and less manoeuvrability of instruments due to the thick abdominal wall (all of this being nowadays part of the basic training in laparoscopic digestive surgery). This may be different for the more invasive techniques such as gastric suturing or stapling where a bariatric surgeon might be preferred. Both in the Primary Obesity Surgery Endoluminal (POSE) with the Incisionless Operating Platform and in the OverStitch studies intraluminal and extraluminal bleedings have been reported. The intraluminal bleedings emanated from the stitches and sutures and could be treated by the endoscopist. Intraluminal bleeding occurred in 2 of the 20 patients in Lopez-Nava's study using the OverStitch [13]. Two endoscopically treated bleedings in 34 patients and minor bleedings in 147 patients of whom 1 needed hospitalisation were found in two POSE studies [14, 15]. In a multicentre survey of the OverStitch one splenic laceration with a bleeding (0.4%) occurred and in the US pivotal study, the ESSENTIAL study concerning the POSE, one extraluminal gastric bleeding (0.4%) was seen which needed surgical intervention [16, 17]. True symptomatic gastric perforations both after suturing and after gastric plication always needed surgery, whereas pneumoperitoneum was asymptomatic and left untreated or managed conservatively [18, 19]; a case of pneumothorax and pneumoperitoneum needed a chest tube [16]. Two perigastric fluid collections adjacent to the fundus were drained locally [16]. A rare case of incarceration of the gallbladder with endoscopic stitches has been reported that was explained by the lateral position of the patient during the OverStitch procedure.

From these data it is obvious that although conservative treatment may suffice in many cases, the trust in readily accessible surgical help is mandatory. For some endoscopic bariatric therapies, the endoscopist relies on laparoscopic assistance, but this may change in the near future. To avoid a faulty suturing for fixation of the upper part of the ValenTx oesophagogastroduodenal bypass sleeve and to avoid interjacent bowel loops between the two magnets of the incisionless magnetic anastomotic system (IMAS) to create a jejunoileal bypass, these endoscopic procedures are performed under laparoscopic control [20, 21].

As mentioned earlier, the endoscopist should realise that sutures, plications or staples but also sequelae from the duodenal bypass sleeve or intragastric balloons may hamper a bariatric procedure later in life. So, it is important that in their follow-up reports they report which patients needed bariatric surgery in a later stage and to what extent surgeons were troubled by the endoscopic procedure. Presumed or observed thickening of the gastric wall after intragastric balloon treatment is a reason for some surgeons to postpone bariatric surgery for 2 weeks [22]. However, others have not seen any problems and many reports are available of removal of the balloon and bariatric surgery in the same session [23, 24]. Notwithstanding the major intra-abdominal changes observed at the outside of the stomach in animal studies after DJBS, those changes were not seen in the study by Gershin et al. where patients, after a period of DJBS treatment, underwent LAGB and RYGB uneventfully [11]. Yet, three studies reported local inflammation and pseudopolyp formation at the inside, during device removal and up to 2–4 weeks after device removal [10, 25, 26]. Also, gastric plication after a Transoral Endoscopic Restrictive Implant System (TERIS) did not interfere with subsequent RYGB surgery. Much less experience with subsequent surgery is available for the POSE and OverStitch procedures. Besides the materials that have been left in place and often cannot be removed, as they are deep rooted in the tissues, also adhesions as a result of the endoscopic bariatric surgery or resulting from a complication may hinder the bariatric surgeon. Perigastric collections near the fundus may be such an example.

The complication in itself but also the consequences of previous endoscopic bariatric therapy as discussed before should be discussed by both endoscopist and surgeon, not only to decide what to do but also to see to what extent these changes are a technical barrier for the surgeon, such as stapling within or across plicated folds and thicker tissue, but also to discuss sequential strategies that might follow after this complicated endoscopic bariatric treatment. The specifics of surgery become different: for example, during a sleeve gastrectomy, the stapler cartridges might run through the plicated stomach with potential anchors situated on the greater curve, while when performing a bypass the lesser curve should be preserved. Under these circumstances, careful pre-surgical endoscopy is the key element to a roadmap for the surgeon. Moreover, in the discussion of a surgical procedure one should evaluate the response to the preceding endoscopic procedure, whereby algorithms that have been suggested by Ajuha and Nimgaonkar might be useful [27].

It is not possible to foresee all kind of complications that may occur during a given endoscopic procedure and that should be treated by a general of gastrointestinal surgeon. Albeit bariatric knowledge is recommended when dealing with such complications, surgeons with a general surgery background may often be in charge when such complications occur, which, to be fair, is nowadays occasionally also the case with post-bariatric surgery complications. This is certainly not the ideal situation but is not a particular threat when dealing with basic complications such as bleeding and sepsis with or without perforation.

Eventually, we should consider the possibility of "third-stage complication," i.e. first a surgical complication that is treated by the endoscopist, which may then be followed by a potential complication of the endoscopy that should be treated by surgery and/or sometimes by radiology with a surgical backup. Examples thereof are stent migration, perforation after endoscopic dilation of a surgical stenosis, an intractable stenosis after many endoscopic dilations that need surgery again for seromyotomy or a revision, secondary abscesses after endoscopic drainage that cannot be approached by radiology, a persistent fistula despite all endoscopic measures, etc. Moreover, as has been discussed extensively in Chaps. 5 and 6, surgeons asked the help of an endoscopist in certain complications, who for being successful, on his/her turn, needs the assistance of the surgeon, as for instance in the access to the excluded stomach and the biliary tree. These two teams of surgeons and endoscopists are needed for the laparoscopy-assisted ERCP (LA-ERCP) and the laparoscopic transgastric rendez-vous (LATG-RV) procedure, performed in cases where also a cholecystectomy is indicated [28–30]. Both success rate and costs have to be taken into account: Schreiner et al. demonstrated a higher success rate with the LA-ERCP when compared with balloon enteroscopy-assisted ERCP (BEA-ERCP), but cost-effectiveness calculations suggested to start with a BEA-ERCP [31]. However, when balloon enteroscopy is not available, the choice for a LA-ERCP is evident. The ERCP procedures through a gastrostomy, usually two-stage procedures, can also be performed as one-stage procedures when T-anchors for the apposition of gastric and abdominal walls are used. The two-stage approach involves first the creation of a gastrostomy and maintenance with a large-calibre catheter, followed by dilation after tract maturation which usually takes 4 weeks and ERCP via the gastrostomy tract. Successful access to the excluded stomach and creation of a gastrostomy have been previously described using various techniques, including a surgical gastrostomy [32, 33]. In contrast to other techniques such as radiology or gastrostomy, which need the maturation of the gastrostomy tract, a surgical gastrostomy allows an ERCP in the same session.

In conclusion, these examples emphasise the need for a true alliance and cooperation between endoscopists and surgeons. Future techniques, whether surgical or endoscopic, as well as unforeseen complications of the existing ones, make this reality even more obvious.

References

1. Abou Hussein BM, Khammas AA, Al Ani AM, Swaleh AH, Al Awadhi SA, El Tayyeb YH, et al. Gastric perforation following intragastric balloon insertion: combined endoscopic and laparoscopic approach for management: case series and review of literature. Obes Surg. 2016;26:1127–32.
2. Mohamed Bekheit M, Abdelsalam WN, Sgromo B, Catheline J-M, Katri K. Is conservative management for gastric perforation secondary to intragastric balloon possible? Case report and review of literature. Obes Surg. 2014;24:968–70.
3. Mathus-Vliegen EMH. Is endoscopy really necessary for placing intragastric balloons? Obes Surg. 2018;28(1):169–75. https://doi.org/10.1007/s11695-017-2812-5.
4. Ponce J, Woodman G, Swain J, Wilson E, English W, REDUCE Pivotal Trial Investigators, et al. The REDUCE pivotal trial: a prospective, randomized controlled pivotal trial of a dual intragastric balloon for the treatment of obesity. Surg Obes Relat Dis. 2015;11:874–81.
5. Mathus-Vliegen EMH, Tytgat GNJ. Intragastric balloons for morbid obesity: results, patient tolerance, and balloon life span. Br J Surg. 1990;77:76–9.
6. Sullivan S, Swain JM, Woodman G, Edmundowicz S, Hassanein TI, Shayani V, et al. 812d The Obalon swallowable 6-month balloon system is more effective than moderate intensity lifestyle therapy alone: results from a 6-month randomized sham controlled trial. Gastroenterology. 2016;150:S1267.
7. ASGE Bariatric Endoscopy Task Force and ASGE Technology Committee, Abu Dayyeh BK, Kumar N, Edmundowicz SA, Jonnalagadda S, Larsen M, et al. ASGE Bariatric Endoscopy Task Force systematic review and meta-analysis assessing the ASGE PIVI thresholds for adopting endoscopic bariatric therapies. Gastrointest Endosc. 2015;82:425–38.
8. Brethauer SA, Chang J, GalvaoNeto M, Greve JW. Gastrointestinal devices for the treatment of type 2 diabetes. Surg Obes Relat Dis. 2016;12:1256–61.
9. Vilarrasa N, Ruiz de Gordejuela AG, Casajoana A, Duran X, Toro S, Espinet E, et al. Endobarrier® in grade I obese patients with long-standing type 2 diabetes: role of gastrointestinal hormones in glucose metabolism. Obes Surg. 2017;27:569–77.
10. Tarnoff M, Rodriguez L, Escalona A, Ramos A, Neto M, Alamo M, et al. Open label, prospective, randomized controlled trial of an endoscopic duodenal-jejunal bypass sleeve versus low calorie diet for pre-operative weight loss in bariatric surgery. Surg Endosc. 2009;23:650–6.
11. Gersin KS, Rothstein RI, Rosenthal RJ, Stefanidis D, Deal SE, Kuwada TS, et al. Open-label, sham-controlled trial of an endoscopic duodenojejunal bypass liner for preoperative weight loss in bariatric surgery candidates. Gastrointest Endosc. 2010;71:976–82.
12. Kaplan LM, Buse JB, Mullin C, Edmundo-Wicz S, Bass E, Visintainer P, et al. EndoBarrier therapy is associated with glycemic improvement, weight loss and safety issues in patients with obesity and type 2 diabetes on oral antihyperglycemic agents. Diabetes. 2016;65(suppl):A326–LB.
13. Lopez-Nava G, Galvão MP, da Bautista-Castaño I, Jimenez A, De Grado T, Fernandez-Corbelle JP. Endoscopic sleeve gastroplasty for the treatment of obesity. Endoscopy. 2015;47:449–52.
14. López-Nava G, Bautista-Castaño I, Jimenez A, de Grado T, Fernandez-Corbelle JP. The Primary Obesity Surgery Endolumenal (POSE) procedure: one-year patient weight loss and safety outcomes. Surg Obes Relat Dis. 2015;11:861–5.
15. Miller K, Turró R, Greve JW, Bakker CM, Buchwald JN, Espinós JC. MILEPOST multicenter randomized controlled trial: 12-month weight loss and satiety outcomes after posesm vs. medical therapy. Obes Surg. 2017;27:310–22.
16. Lopez-Nava G, Sharaiha RZ, Galvao Neto M, Kumta NA, Topazian M, Shukla A, et al. Endoscopic sleeve gastroplasty for obesity: a multicenter study of 242 patients with 18 months follow-up. Gastroenterology. 2016;150:S26.
17. Sullivan S, Swain JM, Woodman G, Antonetti M, De La Cruz-Munoz N, Jonnalagadda SS, et al. Randomized sham-controlled trial evaluating efficacy and safety of endoscopic gastric plication for primary obesity: the ESSENTIAL trial. Obesity. 2017;25:294–301.

18. Familiari P, Costamagna G, Blero D, Le Moine O, Perri V, Boskoski I, et al. Transoral gastroplasty for morbid obesity: a multicenter trial with a 1-year outcome. Gastrointest Endosc. 2011;74:1248–58.
19. de Jong K, Mathus-Vliegen EM, Veldhuyzen EA, Eshuis JH, Fockens P. Short-term safety and efficacy of the trans-oral endoscopic restrictive implant system for the treatment of obesity. Gastrointest Endosc. 2010;72:497–504.
20. Sandler BJ, Rumbaut R, Swain CP, Torres G, Morales L, Gonzales L, et al. One-year human experience with a novel endoluminal, endoscopic gastric bypass sleeve for morbid obesity. Surg Endosc. 2015;29:3298–303.
21. Machytka E, Bužga M, Zonca P, Lautz DB, Ryou M, Simonson DC, et al. Partial jejunal diversion using an incisionless magnetic anastomosis system: 1-year interim results in subjects with obesity and diabetes. Gastrointest Endosc. 2017;86(5):904–12. https://doi.org/10.1016/j.gie.2017.07.009.
22. Jones M, Healey AJ, Efthimiou E. Early use of self-expanding metallic stents to relieve sleeve gastrectomy stenosis after intragastric balloon removal. Surg Obes Relat Dis. 2011;7:e16–7.
23. de Goederen-van der Meij S, Pierik RG, Oudkerk PM, Gouma DJ, Mathus-Vliegen LM. Six months of balloon treatment does not predict the success of gastric banding. Obes Surg. 2007;17:88–94.
24. Khan O, Irukulla S, Sanmugalingam N, Vasilikostas G, Reddy M, Wan A. Simultaneous intra-gastric balloon removal and laparoscopic sleeve gastrectomy for the super-super obese patients — a prospective feasibility study. Obes Surg. 2013;23:585–7.
25. Rodriguez-Grunert L, Galvao Neto MP, Alamo M, Ramos AC, Baez PB, Tarnoff M. First human experience with endoscopically delivered and retrieved duodenal-jejunal bypass sleeve. Surg Obes Relat Dis. 2008;4:55–9.
26. Schouten R, Rijs CS, Bouvy ND, Hameeteman W, Koek GH, Janssen IM, et al. A multicenter, randomized efficacy study of the EndoBarrier Gastrointestinal Liner for presurgical weight loss prior to bariatric surgery. Ann Surg. 2010;251:236–43.
27. Ahuja NK, Nimgaonkar A. Precision Bariatrics: toward a new paradigm of personalized devices in obesity therapeutics. Obes Surg. 2016;26:1642–5.
28. Badaoui A, Malherbe V, Rosiere A, De Ronde T. ERCP by laparoscopic transgastric access and cholecystectomy at the same time in a patient with gastric bypass who was seen with choledocholithiasis. Gastrointest Endosc. 2010;71:212–4.
29. Bertin PM, Singh K, Arregui ME. Laparoscopic transgastric endoscopic retrograde cholangiopancreatography (ERCP) after gastric bypass: case series and a description of technique. Surg Endosc. 2011;25:2592–6.
30. Mejía R, Achurra P, Gabrielli M, Briceño E, Rebolledo R, Torres A, et al. Laparoscopy-assisted trans-gastric rendez-vous for the treatment of common bile duct stones in patients with prior Roux-en-Y gastric bypass. Obes Surg. 2016;26:2809–13.
31. Schreiner MA, Chang L, Gluck M, Irani S, Gan I, Brandabur JJ, et al. Laparoscopy–assisted versus balloon enteroscopy–assisted ERCP in bariatric post–Roux-en-Y gastric bypass patients. Gastrointest Endosc. 2012;75:748–56.
32. Gutierrez JM, Lederer H, Krook JC, Kinney TP, Freeman ML, Jensen EH. Surgical gastrostomy for pancreatobiliary and duodenal access following Roux-en-Y gastric bypass. J Gastrointest Surg. 2009;13:2170–5.
33. Tekola B, Wan AY, Ramanath M, Burnette B, Ellen K, Schirmer BD, et al. Percutaneous gastrostomy tube placement to perform transgastrostomy endoscopic retrograde cholangiopancreaticography in patients with Roux-en-Y anatomy. Dig Dis Sci. 2011;56:3364–9.

Input of New Ways of Reasoning

9

Contents

Abbreviations

AUC	Area under the curve
BMI	Body mass index
DALYs	Disease-adjusted life years
EBT	Endoscopic bariatric therapy
IFSO	International Federation for the Surgery of Obesity
PIVI	Preservation and Incorporation of Valuable endoscopic Innovations
QUALY	Quality-Adjusted Life Years
TBWL	Total body weight loss

E. M. H. Mathus-Vliegen, J. Dargent, *Bariatric Therapy*,
https://doi.org/10.1007/978-3-319-90074-2_9

9.1 Introduction

New technologies, particularly endoscopic techniques, have elicited a momentum in the bariatric field [1]. It appears that weight loss per se has a different profile when it comes to operations that have a shorter duration than common bariatric surgeries, and that these profiles are worth a separate analysis.[1] Cut-offs for classes

[1] The BMI question entails three discussions, with further consequences

1. Percentage of weight-loss

- Surgeons often use EWL which will be high in less obese patients and low in super-morbidly obese patients with a similar weight loss in kilogram. Therefore this EWL measure should be abandoned. Indeed total weight loss in % is what counts. An obese patient, whatever his/her initial BMI, should lose 5–10% in order to improve his/her morbidities (real or potential), and his/her QOL. The assumption that a patient with a higher BMI needs to lose a higher % is essentially true, but may be discussed: lower BMI suffer from comorbidities too and need in this respect an intensive weight loss whereas those who do not have obvious comorbidities (whatever the BMI) may have hidden comorbidities (see also Chap. 1 on the discussion of the non-existence of a healthy obese). It has never been investigated if the absolute remaining BMI after weight loss or the relative reduction and speed of reduction will determine the life expectancy and fate of a person. Some allusion may be provided by the data of the SOS study where the life expectancy increased by weight loss but only after 10 years and mainly because of cancer-related mortality and that any role of the degree of weight loss by different operations and speed of weight loss could not be discerned (but probably due to insufficient numbers). In other words, and for many searchers/clinicians, there is no such thing as a "healthy obese patient." Moreover, obesity per se is often presented as a morbidity by itself (although others argue that obesity is not necessarily a medical condition).
- Nevertheless, let us take for granted that for patients with BMI > 40 or more, 25% TBWL is a sound objective (for the purpose of comorbidities' improvement), and that this objective can be reasonably achieved only by surgical means. And further, endoscopic techniques have a shorter duration of efficient life, hence less expectations in terms of weight maintenance.

2. Atypical observations

- Short-term and possibly repeated weight loss episodes represent nowadays the privilege of endoscopic techniques: this is not necessarily detrimental since weight cycling per se (if unrelated to medical conditions, such as cancer) has been proven mostly harmless, although this is a complex issue. Likewise, weight cycling does not prevent further weight loss, as shown in other studies.
- When examining the way patients behave once a given technique has stopped to be active (the "on-off" effect), we observe erratic patterns of weight loss, and erratic trajectories. These trajectories may also be present with surgical methods (e.g. banding or neurostimulation), but to a lesser extent. It is important to go into the details of these trajectories, in terms of prevalence and consequences; for example, there is a centre effect, differing with commitments, as it seems very obvious that results are different in dedicated centres with all endoscopic and surgical modalities being available compared to centres where for instance endoscopic solutions are only a part of the options. Moreover, as patient-shared decision is a new paradigm, obesity centres should provide much of the conservative medical, endoscopic and surgical methods as possible.

3. Efficacy and cost/efficacy

We may oppose the reasoning: "If a technique has few side-effects and risks, it may be less efficient or less cost/efficient, and less durable," for two reasons:

of BMI are artificial and fixed by consensus, they are based on risks of comorbidity and mortality and their artificiality is demonstrated by the recent knowledge of different cut-offs in different populations as for instance in Asia, and even here BMI cut-offs for Indian, Chinese and Philippine people within one world continent are different (see for a more detailed discussion Chap. 1) [2]. Moreover, BMI is known to be an imperfect predictor of metabolic risks [3]. Some individuals with a normal BMI have a metabolic pattern characteristic of those with overweight or obesity. Some with high BMI appear to have a healthy metabolic pattern, the so-called healthy obese, suggesting that the disease risks associated with obesity may not be uniform and that apparently a subgroup of obese patients are resistant to the development of obesity-associated diseases [4]. So, there is a continuum over the class I, II and III obesity, which is reflected by the fact that both endoscopic and surgical techniques may address each of these categories, although with nuances: for instance, endoscopic bariatric therapy (EBT) may concern patients who are not eligible for surgery, who are not (yet) fit to undergo surgery or who refuse surgery. The way of analysing these weight and weight loss trajectories is of great importance, and this can be reinforced by the input of new ways of reasoning.

This means a reset of the way of reasoning with the evaluation of new leads, and appreciation of influences stemming from the environment of patients. The focus will be on new leads such as weight loss trajectories, personalised medicine or adaptive trial designs. The environmental issue is more complex to apprehend and is beyond the purpose of this book. Just to briefly mention two of its current components that may play an important role in the future:

- Syndemics is a new approach that evaluates the natural and post-treatment evolution of a given disease in the context of socio-economical trends, culture and recent history, for instance regarding migrant populations [5]. It has not been applied to weight loss so far.
- The quantitative assessment of weight loss has an economical counterpart that needs to be analysed. Cost/benefit and benefit/risk ratios of a given intervention, e.g. EBT or bariatric surgery, are instrumental herein. Disease-adjusted life years or DALYs (which can be conceived of as years of healthy life) give an economical horizon to public health strategies: calculating the difference between baseline DALYs and post-intervention DALYs gives the number of DALYs saved by each intervention. Each disability-adjusted life year (DALY) is connected to

---

- Bariatric methods are weight loss methods that entail an intervention, more or less mediated by a device or several devices, with a risk/benefit ratio, a cost, etc. They belong to a sole armamentarium, regardless the way they are implemented, e.g. open surgery, laparoscopic surgery and endoscopic surgery (which could be similar for instance to a prostatectomy). Within this group, they compete, and represent alternative options that change over the time; sometimes a technique wins it all, and conquers 90% of the market: this is the case with the sleeve gastrectomy for the time being, and OverStitch might hypothetically be a major player in the next few years. This is why we can never be sure that a technique should or should not have less side effects or shortcomings than another one just because it belongs to a different category.
- One never knows for sure especially not at the start which device is the least harmful.

costs and for this a quality-adjusted life year is an economic value of the costs per gained year of life.[2] Importantly, BMI changes can be translated into DALYs saved [6] but also the QUALY (Quality-Adjusted Life Years).

9.1.1 Weight Loss Trajectories

There has been a lot of discussion on the benefits and risks of repeated attempts of less intensive weight loss therapies with a low risk profile and not compromising future strategies such as surgery. The "weight cycling" or "yo-yo dieting," a pattern of alternating phases of dieting and relapse, has been the subject of several studies suggesting that increased risks of morbidity and mortality may be associated with fluctuations in weight, although contested by many others (see Chap. 2). Weight loss curves are worth an analysis for themselves: different trajectories reflect different weight loss patterns.

One must first address "spontaneous" weight loss, and then actual patterns according to different weight loss interventions.

9.1.1.1 Is there a Natural Evolution of Weight?

A study by Fildes et al. [7] dealt with the probability of an obese person to attain normal body weight over the time, through various methods except bariatric surgery. While demonstrating that attaining normal weight was unlikely – and also never the primary aim of weight loss strategies as it departs from the wrong statement that obesity is a curable disease – it provided an overview of the natural evolution of weight in large cohorts of population. It showed that weight stability and, more importantly, weight cycling most commonly occur in 30% and 40%, respectively, over 10 years, both in the general population and in obese population (Figs. 9.1 and 9.2). Weight loss was uncommon in 15%, and also weight gain uncommon in 12%.

9.1.1.2 Does Weight Cycling Have Adverse Consequences?

When seeking weight loss, most overweight or obese patients commonly have experienced weight cycling, pertaining to what we may call a "natural history of obesity." In a study already dating back to the 1990s, Colditz et al. demonstrated that weight cycling is common, with a stronger tendency to weight gain over the time in the general population [8].

---

[2] To give a pregnant example: in the Netherlands there has been a discussion about the reimbursement of medication for very rare diseases such as Pompe and Fabry and in the past it was decided that 1 QUALY may cost a maximum of 80,000 euros. As 1 QUALY with Fabry's disease costs 0.3–0.9 million euro and 1 QUALY of Pompe's disease 3.3 million, it was decided not to reimburse their treatment. This evoked a lot of discussion and to set the discussions into medical perspective: 1 QUALY by breast cancer screening costs 4200 euro, by the national child vaccination programme 18,000 euro and by heart transplantation 38,000 euro, all well accepted by the Council of Health. In that same report, they also contrasted the healthcare costs for 1 QUALY against societal measures: 1 QUALY gained by the obligatory check-up of cars costs 80,000 euro, and 1 QUALY gained by the DELTA works to protect against floods costs two million and when the incomes from the DELTA works are subtracted it still costs 300,000 euro.

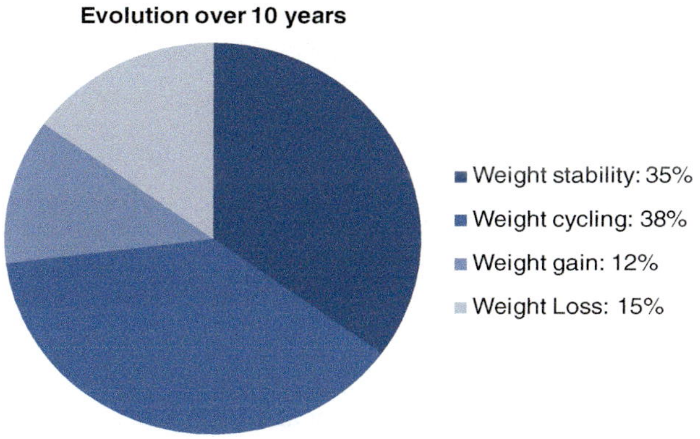

Fig. 9.1 Weight in the general female population (2004–2014): 149,788 pts. (Fildes et al.) [7]

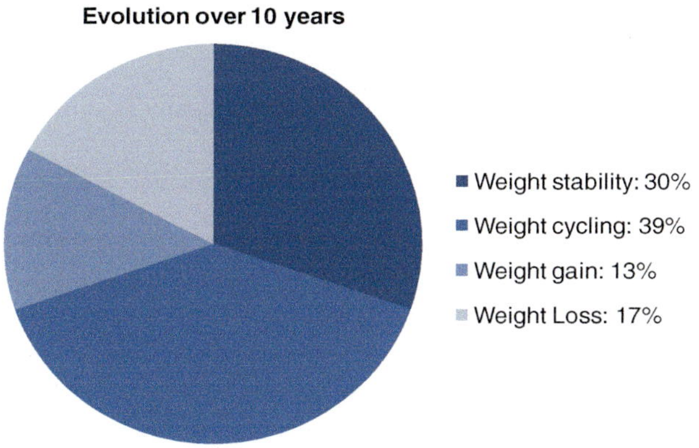

Fig. 9.2 Weight in the female population, BMI 30–35 (2004–2014): 27,251 pts. (Fildes et al.) [7]

Does this strong tendency to weight cycling (regardless the weight status) have adverse consequences? Although Sorensen et al. found that in overweight subjects without comorbidities the intention to lose weight could be related to excessive mortality [9], Mehta et al. have shown that despite the fact that over the last two decades weight cycling has been thought to be associated with many morbid health conditions and increased mortality, the evidence for an adverse effect of weight cycling appears very thin [10]. Yet, weight regain following successful weight loss remains the most challenging aspect of long-term body weight regulation, and the uncritical reiteration of weight cycling being detrimental to health is put aside as a myth, once confounding factors have been taken out of the equation [11].

Furthermore, the majority of clinical studies in humans, investigated by Muls et al. up to 1995, do not support the hypothesis that weight cycling per se influences the amount and velocity of subsequent weight loss [12]. Both natural and experimental weight cycling studies have failed to demonstrate permanent alterations of body composition or body fat distribution, as well as resting energy expenditure, at least in obese subjects. Kajioka et al. demonstrated the devastating effects of yo-yo

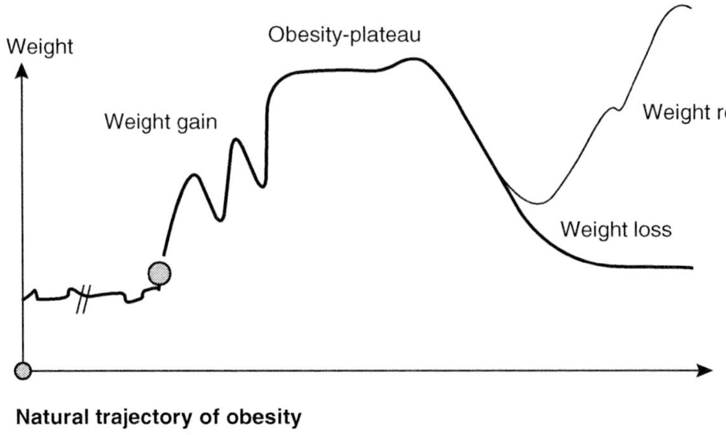

Fig. 9.3 Constitution and evolution of weight gain

dieting in non-obese women with decreased lean body mass, increased blood pressure, increased serum triglycerides and decreased thyroid function as a result [13]. A history of weight cycling is not related to alterations in fat mobilisation or in cardiovascular risk factors [12]. Likewise, weight cycling does not impede future weight loss and its related benefits in postmenopausal women [14].

A careful conclusion may be (1) that repeated short-term weight loss through whatever technique, including EBT, is not necessarily detrimental as such, provided that safety is ensured along the way, and (2) that, instead of focusing solely on the causes of weight gain, weight loss or weight regain, the curves of weight loss after any kind of intervention should be analysed as such. A more comprehensive approach of different categories of weight trajectories might lead to a more unified vision on weight evolution.

9.1.1.3 Is it Important to List Weight Loss Patterns?

The typical weight trajectories are well known: the yo-yo ascending curve on the one hand (Fig. 9.3) and the rather steep weight loss curve followed by a slight or important weight regain in the longer term on the other. Indeed, this is what the literature always mentions, and for instance the SOS-type curves after bariatric surgery are compelling [15] (Fig.9.4).

Weight loss trajectories after medical intervention alone are well documented, and their short-term effectiveness is pointed out (Fig. 9.5).[3]

[3] A critical note should be made here: most programmes are of short duration, not taking back patients who relapse and only addressing the short-term benefits, while it is a generally recognised fact that weight maintenance is even more difficult than losing weight and that weight maintenance requires a different approach than weight loss. Losing weight, but even more so maintenance of that reduced weight, is something that is almost incompatible with normal physiology. Moreover, there are only a few studies (not included in the graphs of Fig. 9.5) that give the optimal intensive lifestyle modification of supervised diet, exercise and behavioural therapy, the latter including coping and relapse prevention.

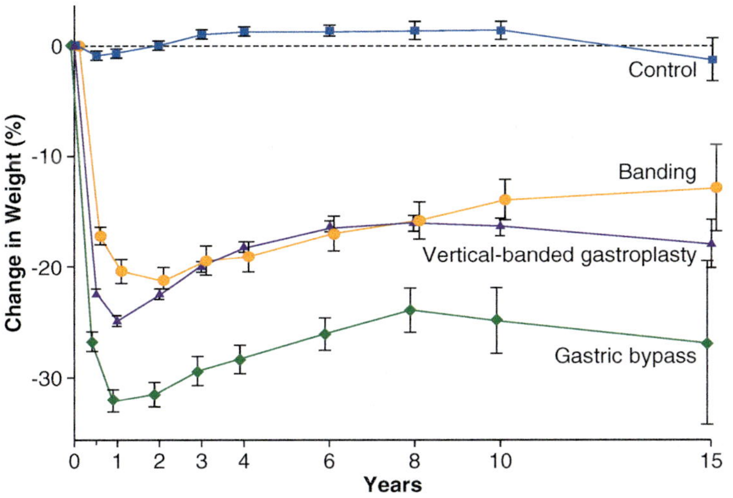

No. Examined

Control	2037	1768	1660	1553	1490	1281	982	886	190
Banding	376	363	357	328	333	298	267	237	52
Vertical-banded gastroplasty	1369	1298	1244	1121	1086	1004	899	746	108
Gastric bypass	265	245	245	211	209	166	92	58	10

Fig. 9.4 Typical post-bariatric surgery evolution, the SOS Study

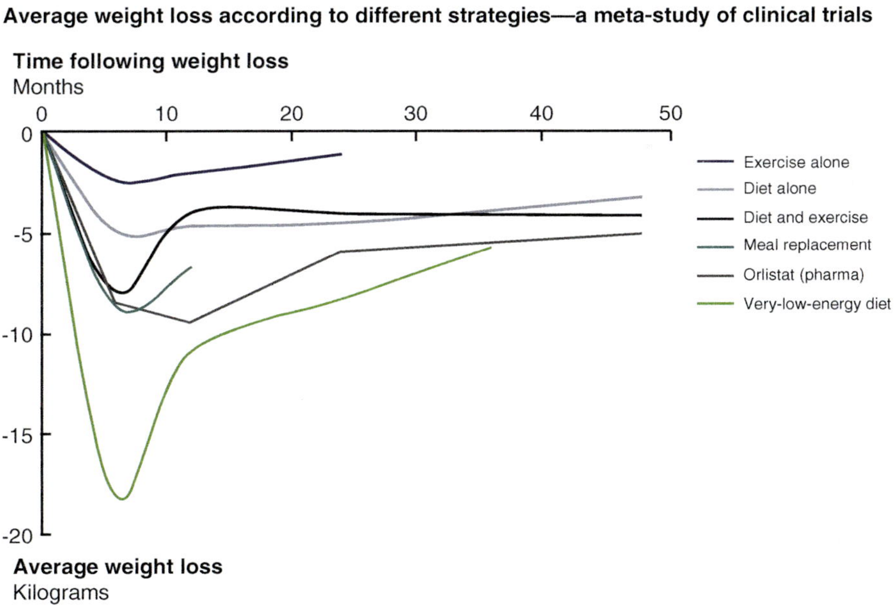

Fig. 9.5 Post-medical intervention weight evolution

Table 9.1 Patterns of weight loss according to various surgical/endoscopic procedures

Patterns	Typical	Others
Incremental	Gastric plication	Lap-banding
One shot[a]	Gastric balloon	Endoscopic techniques
Long-standing	Gastric bypass	Sleeve gastrectomy
Very long-standing	Biliopancreatic bypass and duodenal switch	Jejunoileal bypass
On-off	Neurostimulation	Lap-banding

[a]One-shot techniques can be repeated, e.g. balloon or endo-plication

For the time being, most of the current techniques that fit into EBTs have the disadvantage of short duration of maximally 1 year and thus have rather short-term effects, which are strongly influenced by external factors, in a much more important way than "regular" bariatric surgeries are. On the other hand, as emphasised by the FDA approval, EBTs should be accompanied by a 12 months' intensive lifestyle programme. The appearance of such new technologies makes it necessary to reframe the list of options for patients and to redefine the access of patients to different techniques according to different weight loss patterns, which would capture more data than just the magnitude of weight loss. Each operation may have a specific signature in terms of weight loss trajectory that may evolve over the time. These curves are worth an analysis for themselves. While some of these trajectories remain to be described along with the experience that should be collected in the future, a start has been made with the most established current operations in bariatric surgery and some EBTs which suggest some basic patterns of weight loss in Table 9.1.

Attempting to refine post-operative trajectories, de Hollanda et al. have identified different patterns [16] after sleeve gastrectomy and gastric bypass (Fig. 9.6), but the variations that they have described are limited to three: steady weight loss followed by stability, primary poor weight loss, or secondary poor weight loss following a period of steady weight loss. They did not describe another pattern of successful weight loss followed by weight regain, but this might be related to the rather short and probably incomplete follow-up in a decreasing number of patients.

Atypical trajectories may be observed when comparing cross-sectional with a longitudinal observation of weight loss per subject (Fig. 9.7). This discrepancy can be attenuated when considering other statistical models, e.g. multivariate mixed-effects model analysis, such as published by Dallal et al. [17] (Fig. 9.8).

Lessons could also be drawn from another atypical trajectory, which is the preoperative weight loss, that is asked by some insurance companies and that many surgeons advise – probably sometimes under the pressure of those who have to reimburse the costs of the operation – as a sound measure before surgery, to facilitate the procedure and improve the outcome (Fig. 9.9). The sense and nonsense of preoperative weight loss has been discussed in Chap. 4. As being discussed there, the outcome is very different when looking at the six meta-analyses or at large cohorts. Summarising the six meta-analyses and reviews there is little strong evidence to support or refute the recommendation for preoperative weight loss management. The uncertainty is due

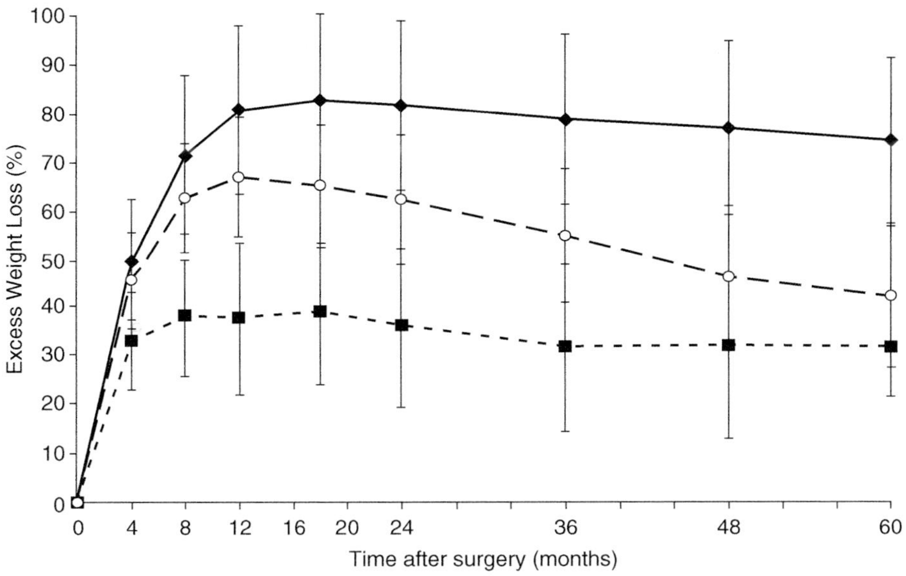

Fig. 9.6 Post-surgery evolution, regular patterns [16]

to lack of consensus on how to implement and how to standardise preoperative weight loss programmes and also due to methodological concerns with previous studies on this subject. The goal of preoperative weight management should be better defined and may be that the focus should be more on nutrition, psychoeducation, physical activity and behaviour modification rather than on the current measure of preoperative weight loss. The cohort data strongly suggest that weight loss prior to bariatric surgery is associated with marked reduction in the risk of post-operative complications and increased chances of ongoing and higher post-operative weight loss. There was a positive dose-response relationship between pre- and post-operative weight loss and preoperative weight loss and complications, the most pronounced in the highest BMI region, signifying that especially patients in the higher range of BMI are likely to benefit most from preoperative weight loss measures.

9.1.1.4 Micro-Trajectories

Current EBTs, like gastric balloon or endoscopic plication, have a limited time of application by definition and as in the case of balloons by FDA approval, hence a shorter time for being efficacious, than typical surgical techniques, like gastric bypass or sleeve gastrectomy, which are permanent and enable sustainable weight loss by most patients. Whereas 1- to 5-year results are reported for bariatric surgeries, with a 10–15-year horizon, in EBTs much shorter periods are commonly analysed with a horizon rarely beyond 18 months. These micro-trajectories are more likely to be erratic.

These atypical trajectories during short intervals (i.e. micro-trajectories) were shown in a study comparing three groups of patients: those being treated with a

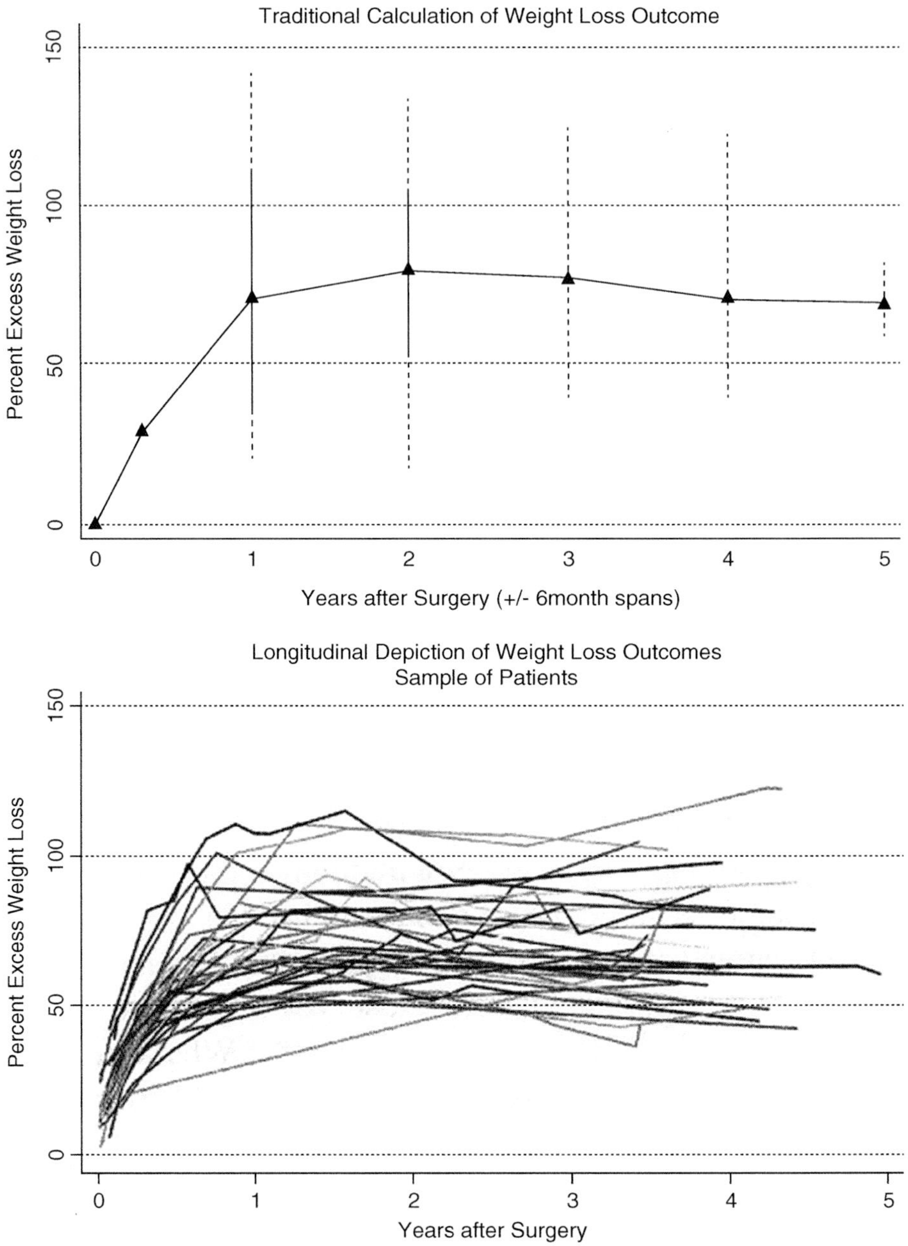

Fig. 9.7 Weight cycling within weight loss curves. Cross-sectional depiction of weight loss: average % of WL each year, computed over all patients versus individual depiction of weight loss (plots for each patient)

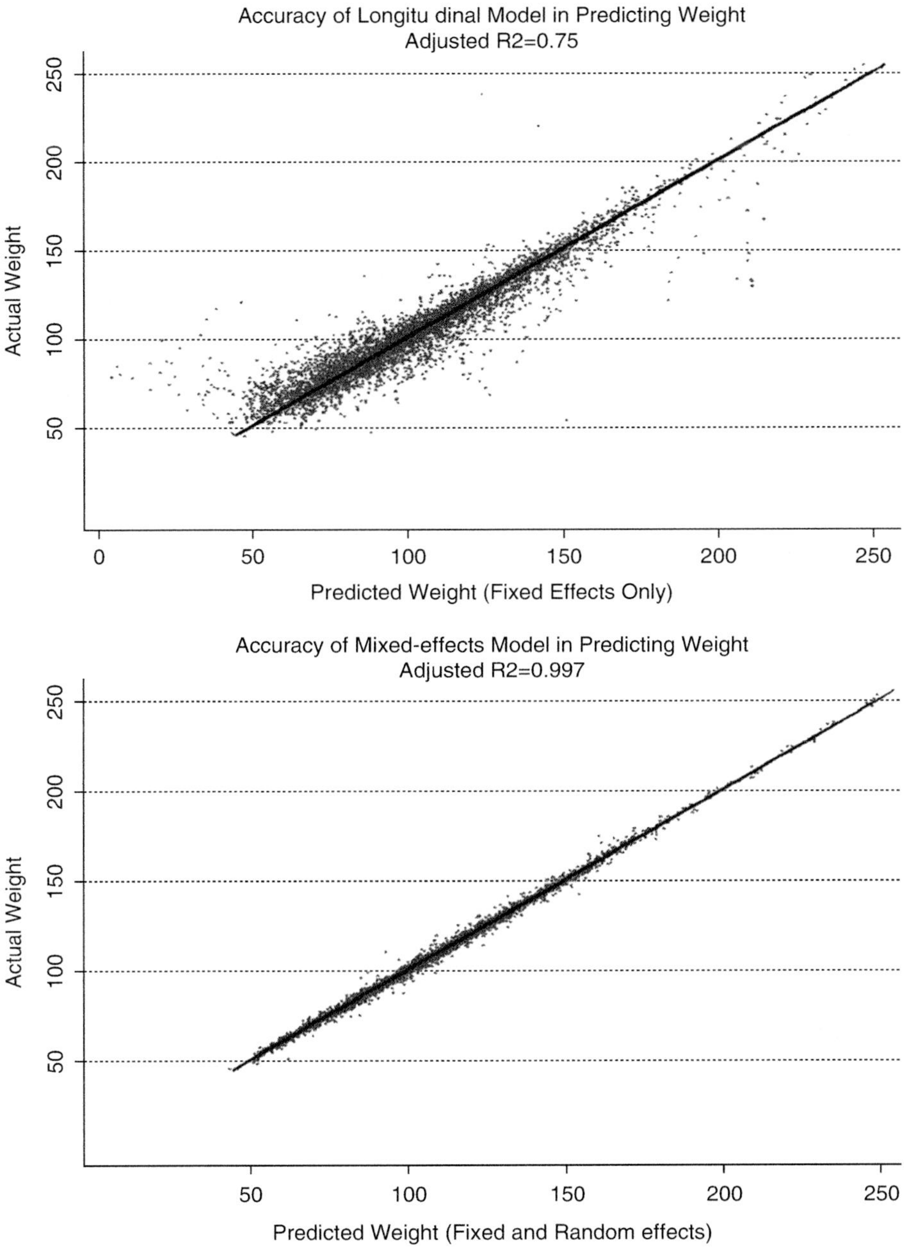

Fig. 9.8 Linear modelling. Multivariate model considering only the fixed effects (observed predictor variables) versus mixed-effects model that combines the within-patient and between-patient regression coefficients into a single one [17]

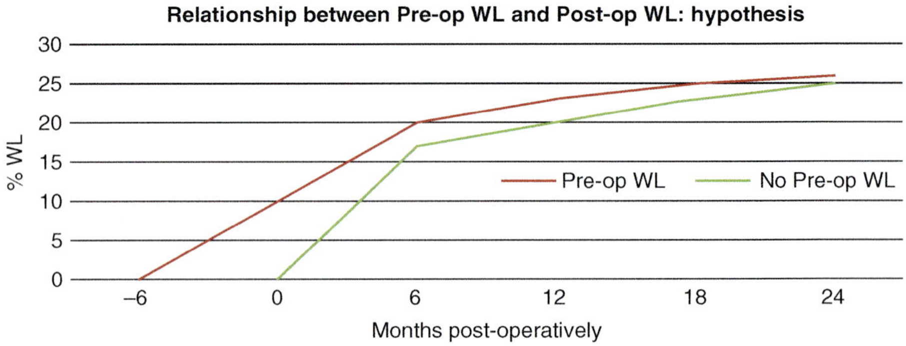

Fig. 9.9 Pre-op weight loss versus no pre-op WL: less post-operative risks

balloon only, those who first received hyaluronic acid injections followed by a balloon or the reverse: those that first received a balloon followed by the hyaluronic acid injections [18]: Figs. 9.10 and 9.11.

Many patient-related factors have been investigated over time and as far as they are known they are reported in Chap. 2 with each EBT. There are also other factors that may account for weight loss profiles such as the following:

- Differences among physicians in terms of experience, training and learning curve; differences among settings (e.g. centres of excellence, insistence on lifestyle modifications).
- Differences in the setting of a study environment or academic setting or the usual everyday practice (see Chap. 2).
- Differences over the time: modifications and improvements of a given technique such as EBTs and the ways some operations evolve, when confronted with other – more successful – operations. For example, the acceptance of gastric banding has changed once sleeve gastrectomy had been proven successful, also explaining a tendency to suggest a revision more often when a band seemed to fail and to cause a less successful weight loss trajectory. Typically, when an operation is less favoured, surgeons stop to include it in their armamentarium and its overall efficacy collapses rapidly, certainly in the case of a band where a constant liability to band adjustments had to be present.

There are many questions left. Can we create a model for analysing weight loss curves in minimally invasive techniques? Is repeated short-term weight loss such as achieved by these techniques productive or not? Do micro-trajectories reflect or influence typical bariatric surgery trajectories?

9.1.1.5 On-off Patterns

The existence of an "on-off" pattern renders weight loss curves more complex to analyse. It consists of alternative periods of time when a given device or operation is supposed to be active or not. Such an effect can be observed in typical surgical

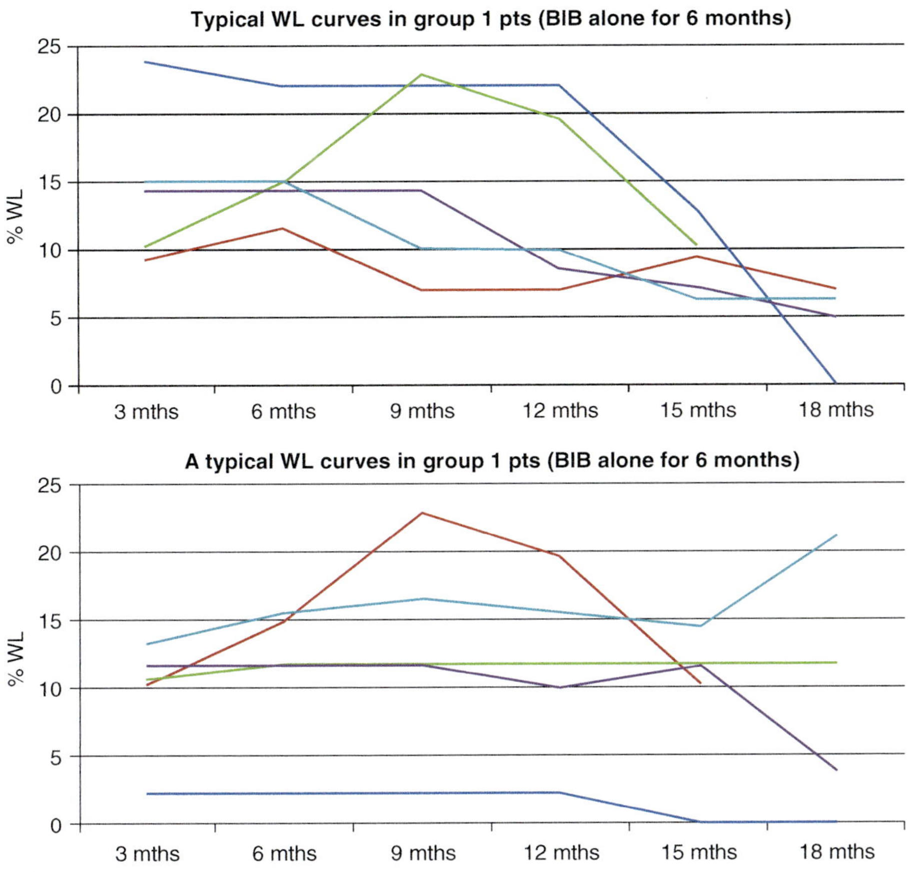

Fig. 9.10 and 9.11 Micro-trajectories. In the typical patient, weight loss occurs up to the moment of balloon removal after 6 months as shown in Fig. 9.10. Variations occur, till complete or incomplete weight regain at 18 months for some patients, while others still achieve 5–10% TBWL. Some patients had an atypical, erratic weight evolution as shown in Fig. 9.11, with some starting to lose weight effectively after the balloon had been removed

procedures like gastric banding (band inflation or deflation) or gastric neurostimulation (equipment in the on or off stand), but probably also new technologies may reveal complex weight loss trajectories. The knowledge of weight loss trajectories may have a valuable input into the whole bariatric field. In the study just mentioned, some patients only started to lose weight when the given device, an intragastric balloon, was removed and was no longer active [18].

It would have been interesting to have patient's characteristics beforehand and to see whether a previous pattern of weight cycling would have predicted this erratic outcome. Also, one should realise that some patients wrongly ascribe the movement of the balloon in their stomach to having hunger and being unable to ingest large amounts of solid food, they escape to energy-rich drinks, and by stopping that behaviour after balloon removal they would then lose weight.

9.1.2 GI and Other Traits as a Predictor and Personalised Medicine (Systems Biomedicine)

New approaches may benefit from the study of weight loss trajectories combined with the adjunction of weight loss-predicting factors which can be found by accruing data and new ways of designing studies.

Systems biomedicine is the application of systems biology to the understanding and modulation of developmental and pathological processes; its purpose consists of gathering comprehensive data to determine optimised therapeutic outcomes. For example, it may be that individual factors pertaining to gastrointestinal anatomy and physiology could be exploited as significant predictors of weight loss related to various techniques. Acosta et al. cite satiation and gastric emptying measurements that could be turned into "actionable phenotypes" [19], thus leading to a selection of procedures and/or drugs such as liraglutide or phentermine-topiramate, according to various patterns. For instance, having low satiety levels would lead to gastric neurostimulation, and rapid emptying at the start could indicate a preference for balloon treatments or an endoscopic plication, as has been demonstrated by Gomez [20] et al., and Abu Dayyeh et al. [21].

9.1.2.1 Individual Predictive Factors should Be Balanced by Larger Predictive Factors

Exploring patient characteristics is a valid approach, but might in itself be insufficient if other factors are not acknowledged. There are many reasons why the characteristics of an operation per se are at least as important. Many themes should pass under review:

- Preferences: Patient preferences in general apply in a specific context (country, area, local guidelines, Internet recommendations, chat sites, etc.). They may change according to the existence of more attractive operations. More generally speaking, the attractiveness of a procedure (e.g. incisionless) will change over time. Provider preferences are important as well (or team preferences, academic schools, countries, mindsets, promoters of a given technique). Lobbying or pre-emptive action from different corporations can interfere, such as emphasised by the IFSO statement on class I obesity [22], claiming further territory for obesity surgery.
- Evolution: A procedure evolves owing to modifications whether they are in the light of competing operations or owing to technical upgrades. While introducing new techniques some questions become obsolete as soon as they have been raised, as for instance now the question of laparoscopy versus laparotomy. The choice of a bariatric technique is today not an easy task because the field moves rapidly, and current gold standards may appear obsolete a few years ahead. More importantly, choices and preferences most often result from the power of an intervention regarding weight loss.
- Complexity: This includes the simplicity of a procedure, its availability, the learning curve that is necessary, the potential for side effects, or severe adverse events. Costs and reimbursement process are considered as well.

- Commercial considerations: The capacity of a company making a new device to hold its ground, finance delays, implement additional trials, participate in training, etc.
- Post-operative follow-up: This depends on the patient's adherence, stimulated by the intensive lifestyle intervention that accompanies the EBT programme. It has been demonstrated many times that the number of contacts with the multidisciplinary team is essential for ensuring weight loss maintenance, not only for EBT but even for less invasive diet treatments [23, 24]. In this context, the gastric banding was thought to enhance the compliance as patients had to return for adjustment of their band. Yet, most of these contacts can be remote, as shown in a recent study on diet follow-up [25].
- Physical exercise is an important part of the maintenance of weight loss. The American Heart Association, the American College of Cardiologists and The Obesity Society have advised ≥150 min per week of moderate intensity for weight loss and more exercise is needed for weight loss maintenance: 200–300 min per week of moderate-intensity exercise [26]. Daily life activities have been stressed in terms of obesity prevention [27], but having seen the above-mentioned recommendations such an approach is insufficient as an alternative to exercise after bariatric surgery.

9.1.3 Adaptive Trial Designs and the Future Role of Big Data: A Changing Paradigm?

This new way of designing clinical trials could be of value to bariatric treatments. The principle is to adjust study populations and treatment at predefined interval points during a prospective investigation [28]. It allows re-combinations of sequential therapeutic arms in any kind of RCT in a less rigid way than commonly recommended. Statistics will become much more complicated and not anymore easy to perform for physicians or to explain in manuscripts. As pointed out by Ahuja and Nimgaonkar, it is worth combining this kind of study to specific obesity subtypes [29], i.e. combining systems biomedicine and adaptive clinical design. These authors suggest a methodology characterising obesity phenotypes based on integrating a systems biology approach into an adaptive clinical trial design. "Phenotype assay" at each stage of the trial allows to reroute further randomisation with or without a crossover between groups within the study.

The way new trials can be designed highlights the "on-off" pattern (and subsequently weight cycling), since "on" or "off" periods entail different possibilities in terms of algorithm design.[4]

---

[4]When one implements a technique that has an "on-off effect," such as a gastric balloon, a gastric band with or without inflation, and a digestive neurostimulation with the device on or off, one assumes that when it is off, one may restart with whatever other technique without the interference of the previous one, at least theoretically. One may implement a new algorithm that is more or less influenced by the results of the previous one. This is influenced by the results because of the

9.1.4 Redistribution of Bariatric Indications

The various new ways of reasoning that we have listed may greatly affect the way we consider bariatric techniques and the role dedicated for each procedure. Repeated and less intensive weight loss therapies may be instrumental, provided that they keep a low-risk profile and do not compromise future surgical strategies. It is difficult to foresee these evolutions, owing to shifts that often go unnoticed. Hence it is even more difficult to make a choice that ought to be theoretically simple (EBT versus bariatric surgery):

- Bariatric surgery claims new territory (IFSO Statement on class I obesity with comorbidities), while endoscopy can be used in class II–III obese patients that are unwilling to undergo a surgical procedure, are not eligible or are too fragile for invasive methods.
- Overlapping techniques are submitted to scrutiny and debates. For instance, gastric plication can be performed with traditional laparoscopic tools, or with a purely endoscopic device, with discussions regarding indications, outcomes, complications and acceptances.
- Evolutions and upgrades can produce unexpected results, or rejuvenate older techniques that would seem abandoned for a long time, e.g. the jejunoileal bypass that may have a second life if performed endoscopically, although it is not entirely comparable with the older abandoned technique.
- Public and physicians' preferences/expectations are unknown at this stage. For example, swallowable balloons (which do not require endoscopy for placement and sometimes also not for removal and do not require anaesthesia) could represent a breakthrough or not. Costs also play a role as long as bariatric surgery is often reimbursed and EBTs not at all or exceptionally.
- Thresholds are to be defined. We may be alerted by, for instance, the American Society for Gastrointestinal Endoscopy [30] document on Preservation and Incorporation of Valuable endoscopic Innovations (PIVI), which states the following goals: for primary treatment the excess weight loss (EWL) should be $\geq 25\%$, and a significantly 15% EWL greater than the control group in subjects with a BMI $\geq$ 35 kg/m^2. For non-primary treatment a total body weight loss (TBWL) >5% should be demonstrated with efficacy of the device over the whole range of BMIs. For primary treatment in a less heavy group with a BMI 30–35 kg/m^2, an adverse event rate of <5% should be present and a significant change in one or more comorbidities. Likewise, caution is recommended when evaluating the benefits of a given technique, and its safety profile, and when designing the methods of randomised control trials in obesity treatment. These points have been outlined in an IFSO Statement on New Technologies [31].

---

necessities of the trial (failure vs. success, etc.), but not in the sense that the previous technique had remnant effects.

Conclusion

The input of several new ways of reasoning may have an immediate consequence: we should no longer consider "separate blocks" of obesity range (namely class I–III obesity class) but see them as a continuum and we should take into consideration the dynamics of weight loss. A unified and in-continuity model seems more appropriate, and weight loss curves could benefit from renewed biostatistical approaches, such as calculation of the area under the curve (AUC) in different weight loss trajectories, with multi-compartmental models, similarly to pharmacokinetics models.

Acknowledgments The authors acknowledge the contribution of Lisbeth Mathus-Vliegen to this chapter.

References

1. Kumar N. Endoscopic therapy for weight loss: Gastroplasty, duodenal sleeve, intragastric balloons, and aspiration. World J Endosc. 2015;7:847–59.
2. Expert consultation WHO. Appropriate body-mass index for Asian populations and its implications for policy and intervention strategies. Lancet. 2004;363:157–63.
3. Heymsfield SB, Cefalu WT. Does body mass index adequately convey a patient's mortality risk? JAMA. 2013;309:87–8.
4. Wildman RP, Muntner P, Reynolds K, McGinn AP, Rajpathak S, Wylie-Rosett J, et al. The obese without cardiometabolic risk factor clustering and the normal weight with cardiometabolic risk factor clustering. Arch Intern Med. 2008;168:1617–24.
5. Editorial. Syndemics: health in context Lancet 2017; 389, March 4. www.mckinsey.com.
6. Overcoming obesity, an initial economic analysis. Mc Kinsey Global Institute, discussion paper, 2014.
7. Fildes A, Charlton J, Rudisill C, Littlejohns P, Prevost AT, Gulliford MC, et al. Probability of an obese person attaining normal body weight: cohort study using electronic health records. Am J Public Health. 2015;105(9):e54–9.
8. Colditz GA, Willet WC, Stampfer MJ, London SJ, Segal MR, Speizer FE. Patterns of weight change and their relation to diet in a cohort of healthy women. Am J Clin Nutr. 1990;51:1100–5.
9. Sorensen TI, Rissanen A, Korkeila M, Kapri J. Intention to lose weight, weight changes, and 18-y mortality in overweight individuals without co-morbidities. PLoS Med. 2005;2(6):e171.
10. Mehta T, Smith DL, Muhammad J, Casazza K. Impact of weight cycling on risk of morbidity and mortality. Obes Rev. 2014;15(11):870–81.
11. Casazza K, Pate R, Allison DB. Myths, presumptions, and facts about obesity. N Engl J Med. 2013;368(5):446–54.
12. Muls E, Kempen K, Vansant G, Saris W. Is weight cycling detrimental to health? A review of the literature in humans. Int J Obes Relat Metab Disord. 1995, Sep;19(Suppl 3):546–50.
13. Kajioka T, Tsuzuku S, Shimokata H, Sato Y. Effects of intentional weight cycling on non-obese young women. Metabolism. 2002;51:149–54.
14. Mason C, Foster-Schubert KE, Imayama I, Xiao L, Kong A, Campbell KL, et al. History of weight cycling does not impede future weight loss or metabolic improvements in postmenopausal women. Metabolism. 2013;62(1):127–36.
15. Sjöström L, Lindroos AK, Peltonen M, Torgerson J, Bouchard C, Carlsson B, et al. Swedish Obese Subjects Study Scientific Group. Lifestyle, diabetes, and cardiovascular risk factors 10 years after bariatric surgery. N Engl J Med. 2004;351(26):2683–93.

16. De Hollanda A, Ruiz T, Jimenez A, Flores A, Lacy A, Vidal J. Patterns of weight loss response following gastric bypass and sleeve gastrectomy. Obes Surg. 2015;25(7):1177–83.
17. Dallal RM, Quebbemann BB, Hunt LH, Braitman LE. Analysis of weight loss after bariatric using mixed-effects linear modeling. Obes Surg. 2009;19(6):732–7.
18. Dargent J, Mion F, Costil V, Ecochard P, Pontette F, Mion V, et al. Multicenter randomized study of obesity treatment with minimally invasive injection of hyaluronic acid versus and combined with intragastric balloon. Obes Surg. 2015;25(10):1842–7.
19. Acosta A, Camilleri M, Shin A, Vasquez-Roque MI, Iturrino J, Burton D, et al. Quantitative gastrointestinal and psychological traits associated with obesity and response to weight-loss therapy. Gastroenterology. 2015;148(3):258–62.
20. Gomez V, Woodman G, Abu Dayyeh BK. Delayed gastric emptying as a proposed mechanism of action during intragastric balloon therapy: results of a prospective study. Obesity. 2016;24:1849–53.
21. Abu Dayyeh BK, Acosta A, Camilleri M, Mundi MS, Rajan E, Topazian MD, et al. Endoscopic sleeve gastroplasty alters gastric physiology and induces loss of body weight in obese individuals. Clin Gastroenterol Hepatol. 2017;15:37–43.
22. Busetto L, Dixon J, De Luca M, Shikora S, Pories W, Angrisani L. Bariatric surgery in class I obesity. A position statement from the International federation for the Surgery of Obesity and Metabolic Disorders (IFSO). Obes Surg. 2014;24(4):487–519.
23. Lopez Nava G, Galvao M, Bautista-Castano I, Fernandez-Corbelle JP, Trell M. Endoscopic sleeve gastroplasty with 1-year follow-up: factors predictive of success. Endosc Int Open. 2016;4(2):E222–7.
24. Sacks FM, Bray GA, Carey VJ, Smith SR, Ryan DH, Anton SD, et al. Comparison of weight-loss diets with different compositions of fat, protein, and carbohydrates. N Engl J Med. 2009;360:859–73.
25. Little P, Stuart B, Hobbs FR, Kelly J, Smith ER, Bradbury EJ, et al. An internet-based intervention with brief nurse support to manage obesity in primary care (POWeR+): a pragmatic, parallel-group, randomised controlled trial. Lancet Diabetes Endocrinol. 2016;4:821–8.
26. Jensen MD, Ryan DH, Apovian CM, Ard JD, Comuzzie AG, Donato KA, et al. 2013 AHA/ACC/TOS guideline for the management of overweight and obesity in adults: a report of the American College of Cardiology/American Heart Association Task Force on Practice Guidelines and the Obesity Society. J Am Coll Cardiol. 2014;63:2985–3023.
27. Mensah K, Maire A, Oppert JM, Dugas J, Charreire H, Weber C, et al. Assessment of sedentary behaviors and transport-related activities by questionnaire: a validation study. BMC Public Health. 2016;16:753.
28. Chow SC. Adaptative clinical trial design. Annu Rev Med. 2014;65:405–15.
29. Ahuja NK, Nimgaonkar A. Precision Bariatrics: toward a new paradigm of personalized devices in obesity therapeutics. Obes Surg. 2016;26(7):1642–5.
30. ASGE Bariatric Endoscopy Task Force, Sullivan S, Kumar N, Edmundowicz SA, Abu Dayyeh BK, Jonnalagadda SS, et al. ASGE Bariatric Endoscopy Task Force systematic review and meta-analysis assessing the ASGE PIVI thresholds for adopting endoscopic bariatric therapies. Gastrointest Endosc. 2015;82(3):425–38.
31. Dargent J, Vilallonga R, Katz L, Portenier D, Wilson E, Escalona A, et al. IFSO position statement on new technologies in bariatric surgery. Obes Surg. 2017;27(9):2456–9.

When Surgeons and Endoscopists Should or Could "Act as One" Regardless of Their Conflicts of Interest

10

Contents

Abbreviations

ASGE	American Society for Gastrointestinal Endoscopy
ASMBS	American Society for Metabolic and Bariatric Surgery
DJBS	Duodenal-Jejunal bypass sleeve
DMR	Duodenal mucosal resurfacing
EBT	Endoscopic bariatric techniques
EDNOS	Eating disorders non otherwise specified
ESG	Endoscopic sleeve gastroplasty
EUS	Endoscopic ultrasound
EWL	Excess weight loss
GORD	Gastro-oesophageal reflux disease
IGB	Intra gastric balloon
LOS	Lower oesophageal sphincter
PIVI	Preservation and incorporation of valuable endoscopic innovations
POSE	Primary obesity surgery endolumenal

E. M. H. Mathus-Vliegen, J. Dargent, *Bariatric Therapy*,
https://doi.org/10.1007/978-3-319-90074-2_10

RYGB	Roux-en-Y gastric bypass
SAGS	Society of gastrointestinal and endoscopic surgeons
TBWL	Total body weight loss
IMAS	Incisionless magnetic anastomosis system

Some physicians are eager to jump into new developments, and some are reluctant to perform anything that is unusual and/or that has not been scrutinised and peer reviewed. New technologies require acceptance before being launched on a larger scale.

10.1 Outlook Upon Endoscopic and Surgical Bariatric Techniques by Gastroenterologists, Surgeons and Their Associations

There is a useful contribution to the debate that, although 8 years old and dates back to 2009, is still valid. Brethauer et al. on behalf of the American Society for Metabolic and Bariatric Surgery (ASMBS) Emerging Technologies Committee developed a questionnaire that was distributed to the members of the ASMBS with the aim to assess the expectations and concerns among bariatric surgeons regarding the use, risks and outcome of primary and revision bariatric endoluminal procedures [1]. Risk tolerance was assessed in comparison to commonly performed endoscopic and bariatric procedures. The percentage of excess weight loss (EWL) ranges was provided to assess the expectations of the results 1 year after the procedure. A total of 214 responses were turned back. The respondents believed that the level of success (i.e., % EWL) should be proportionate to the risk of the intervention. An endoluminal intervention that effects 10–20% EWL should carry no more risk than a therapeutic endoscopy, and 81% of respondents agreed herewith for a primary and 76% for a revision endoscopic procedure. An intervention that effects 30–40% EWL should have an equivalent risk to that of standard laparoscopic adjustable gastric banding and this was assented by 45% and 35%, respectively, for a primary or a revision endoscopic procedure. The acceptable level of risk to achieve 30–40% EWL after primary and revision procedures was equivalent to that after laparoscopic Roux-en-Y gastric bypass for only 8% and 22% of the respondents, respectively. In addition, 62% of respondents responded that 10–30% EWL would be acceptable for revision procedures, and 35% responded that 10–30% EWL would be acceptable after a primary procedure. The main concern was unproven efficacy, followed by durability, poor weight loss, availability of equipment, and procedural risk. Risk tolerance and weight loss expectations among bariatric surgeons are different for primary and revision endoscopic procedures, they are less tolerant for primary procedures and 58% of surgeons are unwilling to consider endoluminal procedures for their patients until the efficacy has been proven.

A paper jointly published by the ASGE and ASMBS in 2011 as a White Paper recommends that endoscopic bariatric therapies be evaluated on multiple end points, including weight loss, safety profile, efficacy, durability and impact on anatomy [2]. The systematic review by the ASMBS Emerging Technology Committee by Dakin et al. on the endoluminal revision of a gastric bypass for weight regain in 2013 was endorsed by the executive committee [3]. This committee concluded that there was insufficient data to support the updating of the ASMBS's position statement on this topic of 2009, as the principles of safe and responsible use of any emerging technology outlined in the original statement did not change [4, 5]. A beautiful summary as far as the use of endoscopic modalities in the revision of weight regain after Roux-en-Y gastric bypass (RYGB) are modified after Dakin et al. and given in Table 10.1 [3].

In 2015, the ASGE Bariatric Endoscopy Task Force and ASGE Technology Committee reviewed the endoscopic bariatric therapies and in that same year a joint task force convened by the ASGE and the ASMBS published the thresholds in a Preservation and Incorporation of Valuable endoscopic Innovations (PIVI) document [6, 7]. The PIVI criteria were as follows [7]:

- Endoscopic bariatric therapy (EBT) intended as a primary obesity intervention in class II/III obese individuals (body mass index [BMI] >35 kg/m^2) should achieve a mean minimum threshold of 25% excess weight loss (% EWL) measured at 12 months. Primary obesity interventions are stand-alone interventions in combination with lifestyle modification and/or behavioural therapy to induce weight loss and improvement in obesity-associated medical comorbidities.
- In addition to the above-mentioned absolute threshold of weight loss, the mean % EWL difference between a "primary" EBT and control groups should be a minimum of 15% EWL and be statistically significant.
- Five percent of the total body weight loss (5% TBWL) should represent the absolute minimum threshold for any non-primary EBT (e.g., early intervention, bridge to surgery or metabolic therapy). Patients with a BMI >50 kg/m^2 present greater technical challenges and surgical risk than less obese, healthier patients; therefore, EBTs used for this indication should perform well also in higher BMI groups.
- The risk associated with EBT should equate to a ≤5% incidence of serious adverse events.
- If a low-risk EBT proves to have a significant impact on one or more obesity-related comorbidities, the threshold for intervention may extend to class I obese individuals (BMI 30–35 kg/m^2).

The committees reviewed the different EBTs against these PIVI criteria and found an adequate number of studies for a meta-analysis on the Orbera intragastric balloon and the EndoBarrier duodenojejunal bypass sleeve, which have been discussed in Chap. 2. None of the newer modalities such as the different balloons, aspiration therapy and endoscopic gastroplasty techniques had sufficient data to include in a meta-analysis. Very recently, the ASMBS has written a position statement more specifically focused on intragastric balloons and assigned a level I evidence as to their efficacy and safety [8].

Table 10.1 Different endoscopic therapies used as a revision procedure in case of weight regain after Roux-en-Y gastric bypass (modified after Dakin et al. [2])

Therapy	Weight loss	Safety	Technical feasibility	Repeatability	Efficacy	Durability	General availability	Costs
Sclerotherapy	ND	+++	+++	+++	ND	ND	+	+++
EndoCinch	ND	++	+	++	ND	ND	NA	+
StomaphyX	ND	++	+	++	ND	ND	NA	+
IOP	ND	++	+	++	ND	ND	NA	+
OTSC	ND	+++	++	++	ND	ND	+	++
OverStitch	ND	++	++	++	ND	ND	+	++

ND insufficient data, *NA* not available

Safety: +Moderate risk. ++Modest risk. +++Minimal risk

Technical feasibility +++Simple procedure with no special equipment. ++Moderately complex. +Significantly complex

Repeatability +Not repeatable. ++Repeatable a limited number of times. +++Can repeat treatment on an ongoing basis

Costs +++Equivalent to colonoscopy. ++Equivalent to ERCP with sphincterotomy. +Equivalent to adjustable gastric band

10.2 Conflicting Interests and Suggestions on How to Deal with These Diverging Views

Some of the highly diverging views are related to a possible impediment of future bariatric surgery by endoscopic bariatric therapy, but also to the choice of an appropriate operation in case of GORD and finally the management of patients that failed after their first endoscopic bariatric therapy.

10.2.1 Impairment of Future Bariatric Surgery by Endoscopic Bariatric Therapy

Any kind of endoscopic procedure has consequences in terms of feasibility when a further bariatric surgery is considered. This is especially true for EBT that leads to an altered anatomy and foreign material left in place with or without long-term consequences and possibly detrimental effects. Surgeons have the merit of dealing with sequelae of any previous intervention in the abdomen, and for instance simple adhesions resulting from a pelvic surgery can be an important impediment to the performance of a gastrojejunal bypass; there are reasons to stay more optimistic when it comes to procedures that stay within the digestive lumen, causing limited damage exteriorly to the gastric or intestinal wall, and as a consequence few adhesions that could hinder access to the digestive tract.

Let us cite some current examples of real or anticipated inconvenience:

- Intragastric balloons do not leave any imprint within the gastric wall, at least not after a few weeks of balloon extraction. Nevertheless, it is a common observation, although not reported in the literature except by Jones et al., that when performing a laparoscopic sleeve gastrectomy in a patient having had a balloon a few years back, the gastric fundus is somehow stretched, with usually more cartridges necessary when stapling the greater gastric curve along a calibration tube placed in the gastric lumen intraoperatively [9–11].
- Gastric endoscopic plication, e.g., with the Apollo OverStitch and the USGI-POSE, leaves stitches inside the gastric lumen that go transmurally and appose serosa to serosa with material devoted for cinching (for example "snowshoe anchors"). These materials may become imbedded in the gastric mucosa and may or may not be retrieved prior to a surgical procedure like bypass or sleeve. If not, this may lead to a broken cartridge and a possible staple-line leak.
- Likewise, endoscopic plication leads at least in the short term to an increased thickness of the gastric wall, not necessarily easy to assess through typical means such as preoperative or intraoperative endoscopy, or 3D imaging. To what extent the endoscopic ultrasound (EUS) may assist herewith has not yet been reported. Even during laparoscopy, an accurate assessment of this wall thickness can be hazardous, and one assumes that thicker cartridges than in regular cases will be necessary.

- Non-apparent damages may occur whatever the type of innovative device placed inside the digestive tract. The causes and mechanisms of intra-hepatic abscesses after the insertion of the duodenojejunal bypass sleeve are still unexplained. On the other hand, the gastric wall abnormalities observed in animals were not confirmed in the subjects that after the DJBS underwent a gastric banding of a gastric bypass [12]. Other promising devices, yet very experimental, aim at destroying the duodenal mucosa that in diabetes subjects is hypertrophied with endocrine hyperplasia and thought to contribute as a "sick" mucosa to the origin of diabetes. By duodenal mucosal resurfacing (DMR) or the Revita procedure (Fractyl Laboratories, Cambridge, MA, USA) the mucosa is lifted from the submucosa over a distance starting 2 cm down from the papilla, over 10–15 cm up to the ligament of Treitz, and then burned away by hydroablation, assuming that the following duodenal mucosa rejuvenation will result in a more normal duodenal mucosa. The fact that three stenoses occurred due to overlapping of the heat or to insufficient lifting may suggest that sometimes deeper layers can be involved, which by changes in the technique have been eliminated [13, 14]. SatiSphere, which aligns several intra-duodenal meshes, may irritate the duodenal wall. One can imagine unexpected side effects of these devices [15].
- The incisionless magnetic anastomosis system (IMAS) creates a side-to-side jejunoileal anastomosis through purely endoscopic ways by magnets inserted by jejunoscopy and ileocolonoscopy. Although these magnets are, for the time being, only inserted under laparoscopic guidance with a report on the location of placement and are not likely to create intra-abdominal adhesions, this kind of short circuit may cause partial or total occlusion of the small bowel, with potential intraoperative difficulties to sort out the different intestinal limbs [16].
- We feel compelled to add another delicate item: "rescuing a rescue endoscopic procedure"! Endoscopic stents (more often than internal endoscopic drains or clips) used to seal a surgical leak can cause surgical complications of their own. Displacement and migration are the most frequent complications, but a secondary abscess, bleeding, perforation or necrosis may be seen as well.

10.2.2 Gastro-Oesophageal Reflux Disease: Impact of Endoscopic Bariatric Therapy and Choice of the Operation

Gastro-oesophageal disease has been touched in different chapters of this book and the aggravation or *de novo* occurrence after endoscopic bariatric therapy and bariatric surgery is a hot topic at present.

Reflux is a consequence of some bariatric techniques, or at least should be taken into consideration. Choosing an anti-reflux procedure, surgical or endoscopic, is a difficult issue in an obese patient. In morbidly obese patients, or at least class II obese patients, RYGB comes as the procedure of choice. On the other hand, any kind of anti-reflux intervention, whether surgical or endoscopic, is a likely impediment to a further procedure, again surgical or endoscopic. The choice of a bariatric procedure in a patient who underwent a Nissen fundoplication is a common conundrum, dissection of the angle of His being a difficult part of any bariatric procedure in this case.

The background of endoscopic techniques dedicated to GORD is instrumental. While many of these techniques have evolved and/or have been discarded, most of them have been reproduced and served as a model for bariatric endoscopic procedures, endoscopic plication being the most relevant current example. Techniques that created an internal separation at the level of the gastro-oesophageal junction and that were meant for GORD have an endoscopic aspect that at first glance is comparable to the more modern bariatric techniques meant for weight loss, e.g., gastric plication.

10.2.2.1 Is it Possible that a Given Endoscopic Bariatric Procedure Aggravates GORD Or Creates De Novo GORD?

The group of Mathus-Vliegen demonstrated that an intragastric balloon may provoke GORD and they ascribed the increased gastro-oesophageal reflux and oesophagitis to increased rates of LOS relaxations by the presence of a balloon with a potential involvement of cholecystokinin A receptors in their triggering [17–20]. They also showed a relationship with the rate of weight loss: the weight loss (58.4 kg in 8 months) of those remaining or becoming acid refluxers was significantly different ($P < 0.01$) from those with normal or normalising pH measurements (36.9 kg in 8 months) [21]. Rossi et al. demonstrated an increase in gastro-oesophageal reflux and therefore recommended the use of PPIs during balloon positioning. Apart from balloons, gastro-oesophageal reflux has not been studied with respect to the other EBT devices [22].

10.2.2.2 The Choice of the Appropriate Bariatric Surgery

For the gastroenterologist the choice of the surgical technique is a difficult subject.

In 2015, the American Society for Gastrointestinal Endoscopy (ASGE) in conjunction with the Society of Gastrointestinal and Endoscopic Surgeons (SAGS) and the American Society for Metabolic and Bariatric Surgery (ASMBS) suggested that the decision to perform preoperative endoscopy should be individualised in patients scheduled to undergo bariatric surgery after a thorough discussion with the surgeon, taking into consideration the type of the procedure (low-quality evidence) [23]. Patients with symptoms of GORD or who use chronically H2 blockers or PPIs should have an upper GI endoscopic evaluation. This guideline did not take into consideration that patients with a Barrett's oesophagus may not have gastro-oesophageal reflux symptoms because their oesophagus is adapted to the acid. Also, the fact that an improvement in symptoms might not always correspond with a cure in GORD but may be related to the development of a Barrett's oesophagus with a decrease in complaints was not mentioned. Even more difficulties are encountered in the decision of a sleeve gastrectomy, which potentially carries an increased risk of developing *de novo* GORD symptoms and/or worsening reflux symptoms and oesophageal mucosa injury.

The International Sleeve Gastrectomy Expert Panel Consensus Meeting in 2012 defined severe oesophagitis or Barrett's oesophagus as a contraindication to perform sleeve gastrectomy and Roux-en-Y gastric bypass (RYGB) should be considered instead [24]. At the fifth international Consensus Conference in 2016 the majority of experts tended to agree that Barrett's oesophagus precluded sleeve gastrectomy [25]. This means that most surgeons should propose a preoperative gastroscopy on all their patients. However, this was only done in 1.3%. Moreover 50% of experts in 2012 agreed that all patients should have 24-h pH measurement and manometry before laparoscopic sleeve gastrectomy (SG) if they complained of reflux; this agreement declined to 32.8% in 2016 [24, 25].

So, which would be the appropriate operation in case of GORD is difficult to answer. Even the discussion about *de novo* GORD after a sleeve gastrectomy is hampered by a total lack of prospective studies of significant size that mapped out their population at the start with high-resolution manometry and impedance pH-metry, questionnaires and quality-of-life assessments, and followed them up with the same investigations over years. One should always remember that often a decision of bariatric surgery is taken in the third or fourth decade of life and that a pathologic reflux, when induced or aggravated by the intervention, will exercise its detrimental influence for years. The patient with symptoms is fortunate because he/she will be followed over time, but the difficulty here is the asymptomatic patient or the patient with already a Barrett's oesophagus at the start who will go undetected. Both surgeons and gastroenterologists have to realise that when an oesophagus resection is necessary the normal pull up of the stomach is not feasible and a colon interposition may be the ultimate choice.

10.2.3 The Management of Patients that Failed After Their First Endoscopic Bariatric Therapy

Insufficient weight loss after an endoscopic bariatric method is an option that ought to be considered from the start, possibly taking into consideration that algorithms are being formulated where some gastrointestinal characteristics may be decisive in the EBT procedure to follow, such as gastric emptying or a standardised nutrient drink test.

Abu Dayyeh et al. studied gastric emptying after endoscopic sleeve gastroplasty and Gomez et al. studied the gastric emptying after an intragastric balloon [26, 27]. Although changes in gastric emptying predicted the weight loss, i.e., those with the greatest delay in gastric emptying and with the greatest gastric retention lost the most in body weight, pre-insertion characteristics which might help in the decision which EBT to apply were not available [26]. Yet, the amount of gastric retention correlated with weight loss, not only at balloon removal but also in the period after balloon removal, suggesting that some of the physiologic changes, which resulted in delayed gastric emptying during intragastric balloon treatment, continue to exert some effects even after the device is removed [26]. Abu Dayyeh et al. studied gastric emptying in four subjects after endoscopic sleeve gastroplasty and found a delay in gastric emptying and an increased satiety, measured with the standardised nutrient drink test [27]. This earlier and enhanced satiety was also found by Espinos et al. and Miller et al. after the POSE procedure [28, 29]. But again, this does not help in the decision which EBT for which patient. In a larger multicentre study, published in abstract form [30] and for some parts in articles [26, 27], 118 subjects had paired scintigraphic gastric emptying studies before and after endoscopic bariatric therapy (EBT) including 15 undergoing a sham endoscopic procedure, 14 lifestyle modification only, 45 gastric injections of botulinum toxin A (BTA), 15 saline-filled intragastric balloon (IGB) [26], 25 duodenal-jejunal bypass sleeve (DJBS) and 4 endoscopic sleeve gastroplasty (ESG) [30]. Interestingly, rapid baseline gastric emptying and degree of slowing in gastric emptying after EBTs were associated with % TBWL at 6 months on univariate and multivariate analyses after adjusting for age, sex, BMI, diabetes and intervention [30]. Subjects in the EBT group in the highest gastric emptying quantile lost four times more weight than non-EBT-treated controls. Both baseline gastric emptying and change in gastric emptying after EBT significantly predicted achieving ≥15% TBWL at 6 months [30]. One may conclude from this study that in tailoring the EBT method to the characteristics of the patient, pretreatment measurement of gastric emptying might be of help to assign an IGB to patients with rapid gastric emptying at the start.

In the current context, it is likely that patient's choice will remain the primary incentive, since some of them, although eligible for a surgical "strong" procedure, prefer a technique implemented through natural orifices.

Hence, in patients with an indication for surgery and having failed after EBT it comes naturally in mind to suggest surgery, and if they refuse, other options exist with a sequential endoscopic technique, preferably not identical to the one that proved not to be successful. May be that in the near future predictive tests as mentioned before can be included in an algorithm helping to design the best treatment for a particular patient.

On the other hand, patients might have been successful during endoscopic bariatric therapy but due to the time limitation of most endoscopic methods they may slice back into inappropriate behaviours and in these patients the "balloon-after-balloon" strategy may be an option (see also Chap. 2 for a more detailed discussion). The open studies performed are divergent in their advocacy of such a strategy, but two randomised studies, one in normal subjects and another on subjects with eating disorders otherwise non-specified EDNOS), were truly in favour of using a second balloon after a balloon-free 1-month period [31–34]. An exceptional case of replication with the OverStitch and with the POSE has been reported and appeared to be feasible; however, no data about the outcome and sense of such a repeat procedure are available. Moreover, the kinetics of weight loss and weight regain, or weight cycling, referred to in Chap. 2 and more extensively discussed in Chap. 9 makes it possible to consider alternative and sequential endoscopic options soon.

10.3 Four-Hands and Two-Minds Procedures

Cooperation between bariatric surgeons and endoscopists goes without saying most of the time: endoscopists assess bariatric patients, preoperatively and postoperatively; they fix some of the complications, in the short term and in the long term. More recently, it occurs that some of the primary interventions useful for the treatment of obesity can be performed through endoscopic ways, preferably in class I and II obesity, such as the gastric balloons which have been approved by the FDA for BMI 30–40 kg/m^2, but also the AspireAssist method, which consists of the percutaneous endoscopic gastrostomy that can be connected to a device that aspires the gastric content into the lavatory, are allowed for patients with a BMI between 35 and 55 kg/m^2.

The question very relevant in this topic remains: Who is the most apt to perform both the primary endoscopic bariatric therapies and the secondary surgery-salving procedures? Bariatric surgeons may not have the necessary skills and/or time to perform these procedures on their own, but the same holds true for the average endoscopist, who is either not trained or when trained not able to acquire enough volume of procedures to keep up with expertise and skills. So, everything depends on the circumstances, training and level of mutual understanding in each team or hospital.

The issue of endoscopic bariatric techniques in regard with surgeon's capabilities may be mitigated by a close cooperation between surgeon and endoscopist, a compromise that should equate both specialties. Many bariatric techniques, always on a pace of constant evolution, find their way through the upper gastrointestinal endoscopic channel. With respect to the considerations given above, where the endoscopist could possibly jeopardise a further bariatric intervention, it is relevant that bariatric surgeons become involved in the choice and – although not in every country allowed – in the implementation of such operations. Again, working in a dedicated environment of an obesity department facilitates such an approach and inspires the people involved.

Our experience in Lyon, France, seems original, but could be reproduced in many if not most centres. Complications of surgery that should be dealt with by endoscopic methods are the part of dedicated endoscopists, e.g., dilation of a stenosis of a gastrojejunal anastomosis after gastric bypass and placement of a pigtail drain or a stent after a gastric leak. On the other hand, we have chosen to perform selected primary or secondary bariatric endoscopic interventions with "four hands", combining both endoscopic and surgical skills. One could object that the endoscopist is only holding the camera, the way an assistant would do in a typical laparoscopic procedure, and/or the surgeon is only reproducing manoeuvres, the way a mere assistant would do. Yet, if both agree on using their own skills for the greater good and dedicate time enough to implement such combined procedures, it seemed to us that this strategy was mutually beneficial. From January 2015 to July 2017, we performed 46 endoplication operations with the Apollo OverStitch system in this "four-hands two-minds" approach.

RYGB failures are a real challenge in bariatric surgery nowadays, because they represent the failure of the "ultimate operation" (if we admit leaving BPD or BPD-DS out of the picture for primary patients). Therefore, various solutions have been suggested over the time. The surgical options are the following: lengthening of the alimentary limb and/or the biliopancreatic limb, recalibrating the pouch by placing a band (adjustable or not) around the pouch or at the gastro-oesophageal junction, or resizing the pouch. The endoscopic options, extensively discussed in

Chap. 6, are mostly plicating the pouch and/or the gastrojejunal anastomosis. Injections with sclerosants have been suggested but usually do not suffice and the sclerosant used in the studies is not commercially available anymore. In parallel with the reported experience in the literature, in Lyon, OverStitch was first applied in secondary cases: 13 secondary cases and 33 primary cases. The FDA approved both the POSE and the OverStitch for use in post-bariatric complications as an apposition method and is now considering its use for primary therapy, with the ESSENTIAL trial in POSE which has just been finished, and the PROMISE trial in the OverStitch. Both in Lyon and elsewhere in France, gastric bypass failure (insufficient weight loss or weight regain) was treated according to a government-funded, multicentre and randomised protocol initiated in Montpellier (lifestyle intervention group vs. OverStitch group, unpublished results). We were assisted during the initial ten cases by an assistant of the company, well trained with the specifics of the technique. Mean operative time dropped from 90 min during the initial 20 cases to 60 min during the last 15 ones. There were seven serious adverse events: one postoperative bleeding at day 32 without finding a source by subsequent endoscopy, and 6 cases of pain for more than 12 h, requiring 2 days of hospitalisation. EWL at 6 months has been 25% ($n = 34$) and 22% at 1 year ($n = 20$).

In conclusion, there are many opportunities to be confronted with each other but such a confrontation should be fruitful and productive when each of the specialists involved knows the objections and criticisms of the other, and this should inspire both to follow the same way in the right direction: the best choice of the procedure the best fitting with the characteristics and desires of the patient, carried out by the most experienced person in a fully mutual understanding of both specialisms involved, i.e., gastroenterology and bariatric surgery.

References

1. Brethauer SA, Pryor AD, Chand B, Schauer P, Rosenthal R, Richards W, et al. Endoluminal procedures for bariatric patients: expectations among bariatric surgeons. Surg Obes Relat Dis. 2009;5:231–6.
2. ASGE/ASMBS Task Force on Endoscopic Bariatric Therapy, Ginsberg GG, Chand B, Cote GA, Dallal RM, Edmundowicz SA, et al. White paper: a pathway to endoscopic bariatric therapies. Surg Obes Relat Dis. 2011;7:672–82.
3. Dakin GF, Eid G, Mikami D, Pryor A, Chand B. Endoluminal revision of gastric bypass for weight regain—a systematic review. Surg Obes Relat Dis. 2013;9:335–42.
4. Society of American Gastrointestinal and Endoscopic Surgeons. Position Statement on Endolumenal Therapies for Gastrointestinal Diseases. 2009. http://www.sages.org/publications/guidelines/position-statement-on-endolumenal-therapies-for-gastrointestinal-diseases/. Accessed 16 August 2017.
5. Emerging Technologies and Clinical Issues Committees of the ASMBS. American Society of Metabolic and Bariatric Surgery Position Statement on emerging endosurgical interventions for the treatment of obesity. Surg Obes Relat Dis. 2009;5:197–298.
6. ASGE Bariatric Endoscopy Task Force and ASGE Technology Committee, Abu Dayyeh BK, Edmundowicz SA, Jonnalagadda S, Kumar N, Larsen M, et al. Endoscopic bariatric therapies. Gastrointest Endosc. 2015;81:1073–86.

7. ASGE Bariatric Endoscopy Task Force and ASGE Technology Committee, Abu Dayyeh BK, Kumar N, Edmundowicz SA, Jonnalagadda S, Larsen M, et al. ASGE Bariatric Endoscopy Task Force systematic review and meta-analysis assessing the ASGE PIVI thresholds for adopting endoscopic bariatric therapies. Gastrointest Endosc. 2015;82:425–38.
8. Ali MR, Moustarah F, Kim JJ, on behalf of the American Society for Metabolic and Bariatric Surgery Clinical Issues Committee. American Society for Metabolic and Bariatric Surgery position statement on intragastric balloon therapy endorsed by the Society of American Gastrointestinal and Endoscopic Surgeons. Surg Obes Relat Dis. 2016;12:462–7.
9. Jones M, Healey AJ, Efthimiou E. Early use of self-expanding metallic stents to relieve sleeve gastrectomy stenosis after intragastric balloon removal. Surg Obes Relat Dis. 2011;7:e16–e17.
10. de Goederen-van der Meij S, Pierik RG, Oudkerk PM, Gouma DJ, Mathus-Vliegen LM. Six months of balloon treatment does not predict the success of gastric banding. Obes Surg. 2007;17:88–94.
11. Khan O, Irukulla S, Sanmugalingam N, Vasilikostas G, Reddy M, Wan A. Simultaneous intra-gastric balloon removal and laparoscopic sleeve gastrectomy for the super-super obese patients—a prospective feasibility study. Obes Surg. 2013;23:585–7.
12. Gersin KS, Rothstein RI, Rosenthal RJ, Stefanidis D, Deal SE, Kuwada TS, et al. Open-label, sham-controlled trial of an endoscopic duodenojejunal bypass liner for preoperative weight loss in bariatric surgery candidates. Gastrointest Endosc. 2010;71:976–82.
13. Rajagopalan H, Cherrington AD, Thompson CC, Kaplan LM, Rubino F, Mingrone G, et al. Endoscopic duodenal mucosal resurfacing for the treatment of type 2 diabetes: 6-month interim analysis from the first-in-human proof-of-concept study. Diabetes Care. 2016;39:2254–61.
14. Baar AV, Deviere J, Costamagna G, Galvao Neto M, Rodriguez L, Haidry R, et al. Early experience of duodenal mucosal resurfacing treatment for type 2 diabetes when expanding from single to multiple sites. Gastroenterology. 2016;150:S232.
15. Sauer N, Rosch T, Pezold J, Reining F, Anders M, Groth S, et al. A new endoscopically implantable device (SatiSphere) for treatment of obesity–efficacy, safety, and metabolic effects on glucose, insulin, and GLP-1 levels. Obes Surg. 2013;23:1727–33.
16. Machytka E, Bužga M, Zonca P, Lautz DB, Ryou M, Simonson DC, et al. Partial jejunal diversion using an incisionless magnetic anastomosis system: 1-year interim results in subjects with obesity and diabetes. Gastrointest Endosc. 2017;86(5):904–12. https://doi.org/10.1016/j.gie.2017.07.009.
17. Mathus-Vliegen EM, Tygat GN. Gastro-esophageal reflux in obese subjects: influence of overweight, weight loss and chronic gastric balloon distention. Scand J Gastroenterol. 2002;37:1246–52.
18. Mathus-Vliegen EM, van Weeren M, van Eerten PV. LOS function and obesity: the impact of untreated obesity, weight loss, and chronic gastric balloon distention. Digestion. 2003;68:161–8.
19. Hirsch DP, Mathus-Vliegen EM, Holloway RH, Fakhry N, D'Amato M, Boeckxstaens GE. Role of CCK(A) receptors in postprandial lower esophageal sphincter function in morbidly obese subjects. Dig Dis Sci. 2002;47:2531–7.
20. Hirsch DP, Mathus-Vliegen EM, Dagli U, Tytgat GN, Boeckxstaens GE. Effect of prolonged gastric distention on lower esophageal sphincter function and gastroesophageal reflux. Am J Gastroenterol. 2003;98:1696–704.
21. Mathus-Vliegen LM, Tytgat GN. Twenty-four-hour pH measurements in morbid obesity: effects of massive overweight, weight loss and gastric distension. Eur J Gastroenterol Hepatol. 1996;8:635–40.
22. Rossi A, Bersani G, Ricci G, Petrini C, DeFabritiis G, Alvisi V. Intragastric balloon insertion increases the frequency of erosive esophagitis in obese patients. Obes Surg. 2007;17:1346–9.
23. Evans JA, Muthusamy VR, Acosta RD, Bruining DH, Chandrasekhara V, Chathadi KV, et al. The role of endoscopy in the bariatric surgery patient. Gastrointest Endosc. 2015;81:1063–72.
24. Rosenthal RJ, for the International Sleeve Gastrectomy Expert Panel. International sleeve Gastrectomy expert panel consensus statement: best practice guidelines based on experience of 12,000 cases. Surg Obes Relat Dis. 2012;8:8–19.

25. Gagner M, Hutchinson C, Rosenthal R. Fifth international consensus conference: current status of sleeve gastrectomy. Surg Obes Relat Dis. 2016;12:750–6.
26. Gomez V, Woodman G, Abu Dayyeh BK. Delayed gastric emptying as a proposed mechanism of action during intragastric balloon therapy: results of a prospective study. Obesity. 2016;24:1849–53.
27. Abu Dayyeh BK, Acosta A, Camilleri M, Mundi MS, Rajan E, Topazian MD, et al. Endoscopic sleeve gastroplasty alters gastric physiology and induces loss of body weight in obese individuals. Clin Gastroenterol Hepatol. 2017;15:37–43.
28. Espinós JC, Turró R, Moragas G, Bronstone A, Buchwald JN, Mearin F, et al. Gastrointestinal physiological changes and their relationship to weight loss following the POSE procedure. Obes Surg. 2016;26:1081–9.
29. Miller K, Turró R, Greve JW, Bakker CM, Buchwald JN, Espinós JC. MILEPOST multicenter randomized controlled trial: 12-month weight loss and satiety outcomes after posesm vs. medical therapy. Obes Surg. 2017;27:310–22.
30. Abu Dayyeh BK, Woodman G, Acosta A, Lopes GS, Gostout C, De Moura E, et al. Baseline gastric emptying and its change in response to diverse endoscopic bariatric therapies predict weight change after intervention. Gastroenterology. 2016;150:S86.
31. Dumonceau JM, Francois E, Hittelet A, Mehdi AI, Barea M, Deviere J. Single vs repeated treatment with the intragastric balloon: a 5-year weight loss study. Obes Surg. 2010;20:692–7.
32. Lopez-Nava G, Rubio MA, Prados S, Pastor G, Cruz MR, Companioni E, et al. BioEnterics® Intragastric Balloon (BIB®): single ambulatory center Spanish experience with 714 consecutive patients treated with one or two consecutive balloons. Obes Surg. 2011;21:5–9.
33. Genco A, Cipriano M, Bacci V, Maselli R, Paone E, Lorenzo M, et al. Intragastric balloon followed by diet vs intragastric balloon followed by another balloon: a prospective study on 100 patients. Obes Surg. 2010;20:1496–500.
34. Genco A, Maselli R, Frangella F, Cipriano M, Paone E, Meuti V, et al. Effect of consecutive intragastric balloon (BIB(R)) plus diet versus single BIB(R) plus diet on eating disorders not otherwise specified (EDNOS) in obese patients. Obes Surg. 2013;23:2075–9.

When Surgeons and Endoscopists Are Possible Opponents

11

Contents

Abbreviations

ACE	Articulating circular endoscopic
ARMS	Anti-reflux mucosectomy
ASGE	American Society for Gastrointestinal Endoscopy
ASMBS	American Society of Metabolic Bariatric Surgery
BMI	Body mass index
DJBL	Duodenojejunal bypass liner
DJBS	Duodenojejunal bypass sleeve
EBT	Endoscopic bariatric therapy
EMA	European Medicines Agency
ESG	Endoscopic sleeve gastroplasty
EWL	Excess weight loss
FDA	Food and Drug Administration
FU	Follow-up

E. M. H. Mathus-Vliegen and J. Dargent contributed equally to this work.

E. M. H. Mathus-Vliegen, J. Dargent, *Bariatric Therapy*,
https://doi.org/10.1007/978-3-319-90074-2_11

GI	Gastrointestinal
GLP-1	Glucagon-like peptide-1
GORD	Gastro-oesophageal reflux disease
IFSO	International Federation for the Surgery of Obesity
LAGB	Laparoscopic adjustable gastric banding
LGCP	Laparoscopic greater curve plication
PIVI	Preservation and Incorporation of Valuable endoscopic Innovations
POSE	Primary Obesity Surgery Endolumenal
PPI	Proton pump inhibitor
PYY	Peptide YY
RCT	Randomised clinical trial
RYGB	Roux-en-Y gastric bypass
SG	Sleeve gastrectomy
T2DM	Type 2 diabetes mellitus
TBWL	Total body weight loss
TERIS	Transoral restrictive implant system

11.1 Introduction

Competition between endoscopy and surgery in the bariatric field is not very relevant today but may become so as future surgical developments include devices that are or will become shortly applicable for upper GI endoscopy. When figuring procedures or concepts that are applicable to both endoscopy and laparoscopic surgery, three of them come into mind for the time being: (1) stapling, (2) plication and (3) bypass or any kind of "metabolic procedure". Despite having had a very effective endoscopic stapling device that could suck the tissue into the device, squeeze and fire staples at a pressure of 6 bar and form serosa-to-serosa plications, the further development is on hold after the acquisition of Barosense by Boston Scientific [1]. The endoscopic gastric plication may be a benchmark for surgical gastric plication and vice versa, and the metabolic effect resulting from bypassing biliopancreatic secretions may be compared between the duodenojejunal bypass sleeve (DJBS; EndoBarrier) or even more the oesophagogastroduodenal bypass (ValenTx) and the "true" gastric bypass. These are two emblematic cases of a fair competition between concepts that have been applied to both endoscopy and surgery. While representing novel approaches, many questions can be asked about the relevance and results of endoscopic plication and DJBS in the context of similar and typical surgical approaches. As a matter of fact, the surgical approaches are often questioned as well: gastric bypass is a well-known operation with much dedicated scientific research data but still having underlying mechanisms that are not yet fully understood, and laparoscopic greater curve plication (LGCP) is under scrutiny. Roux-en-Y gastric bypass (RYGB) is still the gold standard of bariatric surgery; it is the oldest and the most effective operation with sufficient background and level of evidence. LGCP represents an alternative to sleeve gastrectomy (SG); while supposedly saving resources (there is no stapling), and complications linked to this stapling, the weight loss it provides is not impressive.

We shall also examine the more complex issue of gastro-oesophageal reflux disease (GORD) and the connections between surgery and endoscopy in this respect.

11.2 Class I Obesity with Associated Comorbidities

Numerous observational studies and RCTs have shown that obesity surgery is effective in patients with a BMI 30–35 kg/m^2 as has been shown in observational studies but also RCTs (Table 11.1). Yet, except for the study of O'Brien et al. [2] and Lee et al. [4], none of the studies has mentioned the proportion of patients in this category and, when looking at the mean, the mean suggests that most patients belonged to a higher BMI category.

Therefore, the International Federation for the Surgery in Obesity (IFSO) has claimed in 2011 that obesity surgery should not be denied for patients with a lower BMI and suffering from comorbidities who are willing to undergo such procedures [7]. Of course, this new frontier may elicit and has already elicited many discussions. While claiming further territory, surgery faces competition from bariatric endoscopic techniques, which have different definitions for success, which is not that strange as authorities, institutions and guidelines have demonstrated that in patients with a BMI between 30 and 40 kg/m^2 significant health benefits can be gained by a 5–10% weight loss, and that for cure of some diseases such as diabetes and sleep apnoea a larger weight loss varying around 15% is required (see Chap. 2) [8–11]. For instance, the American Society for Gastrointestinal Endoscopy (ASGE) together with and endorsed by the American Society of Metabolic Bariatric Surgery (ASMBS) [12] has issued a document on Preservation and Incorporation of Valuable endoscopic Innovations (PIVI), which formulated goals for primary and non-primary endoscopic bariatric therapy (EBT). For primary treatment in subjects with a BMI ≥35 kg/m^2 the intervention has to show an excess weight loss (EWL) ≥25%, and a statistically significant 15% greater EWL more than the control group. For non-primary treatment (i.e. bridge to surgery) a total body weight loss (TBWL) ≥5% is required. The EBT is only allowed for subjects with a lower BMI (BMI 30–35 kg/m^2) when the risk of adverse events is low, i.e. ≤5%, and an impact on at

Table 11.1 Randomised controlled trials documenting the efficacy of bariatric surgery in class I obesity patients

Authors	Patients number	BMI and characteristics	Arms	FU length	FU rate (%)
O'Brien et al. (2006) [2]	80	30–35	LAGB vs. medical	2 year	97
Dixon et al. (2008) [3]	60	30–40 + T2DM	LAGB vs. medical	2 year	92
Lee et al. (2011) [4]	60	25–35 + T2DM	RYGB vs. SG	1 year	100
Schauer et al. (2012) [5]	150	27–43 + T2DM	RYGB vs. SG vs. medical	1 year	93
Ikramuddin et al. (2013) [6]	120	30–40 + T2D	RYGB vs. medical	1 year	95

least one comorbidity can be proven. Abu Dayyeh et al. performed a meta-analysis of 82 studies on the Orbera balloons and 11 studies on the DJBL/EndoBarrier [12]. They compared these findings of the meta-analysis with the PIVI thresholds, and concluded that the Orbera balloon fulfilled the requirements for primary and non-primary therapy in subjects with a BMI ≥35 kg/m^2 and that the DJBS/EndoBarrier did not fulfill the PIVI criteria for whatever group. Unfortunately, they did not formulate a standpoint as regard to EBT for the obesity BMI class I and when looking at the data of complications that have to remain equal of below 5% the balloons should have had that recommendation. Similar rules are also operative in pharmacotherapy trials (pharmacotherapy being indicated for subjects with a BMI ≥30 kg/m^2 or ≥ 27 kg/m^2 in the presence of one or more comorbidities) where the US Food and Drug Administration (FDA) requires a 5% greater weight loss and a significant larger percentage of people attaining a 5–10% weight loss compared with controls, and the European Medicines Agency (EMA) requires an absolute 10% TBWL [13].

The usual surgical definition of success is a ≥ 50% EWL, which should be sustained for 5 years. This does not create a conflict since the claims for EBT are in force irrespective of who applies this method; so they are operative both for surgeons and for gastroenterologist. The rigorous surgical criteria of a ≥50% EWL for 5 years are required for true surgical and invasive interventions such as RYGB or sleeve gastrectomy. In contrast to endoscopic therapies, surgery requires general anaesthesia and certainly entails more risks, while endoscopy rightly claims that the benefit/risk ratio could be superior if the procedures are kept minimally invasive. However, until now, the limited durability of EBT is certainly a disadvantage as long-term benefits are essential when evaluating any kind of bariatric technique or even more so, when evaluating whatsoever treatment of obesity. Confusion might arise by the fact that candidates for surgery are not willing to undergo it and often require an endoscopic therapy, while occasionally less severely obese patients are seeking surgery. To some extent this is discouraged by the FDA approval of three balloons only for patients with a BMI between 30 and 40 kg/m^2 and aspiration therapy for patients with a BMI between 35 and 55 kg/m^2.

It is difficult to predict what will happen in the near future. At the same time, both surgeons and endoscopists have their hands full, given the rapid expansion of the obesity epidemic, while resources that can be dedicated to the bariatric field are not infinite, and always request data in terms of benefit/risk ratio. Nevertheless, if surgeons and endoscopists willingly extend their cooperation, there will not be a matter of dispute!

11.3 Laparoscopic Greater Curve Plication and Endoscopic Plication

Laparoscopic greater curve plication (LGCP) stands as a competitor to laparoscopic sleeve gastrectomy (SG). Although available results are encouraging, it is too early to claim that it represents a match to SG. Long-term weight loss results are not available and the rate of complications is likely to be close to SG. LGCP could also be a valuable tool for reoperation. Usual surgical restrictive procedures involved the use of foreign material, stapling devices or partial gastric resection, while LGCP only involves a shape modification of the stomach to achieve restriction by folding the greater curvature of the stomach inward with suture materials, thus reducing gastric capacity. LGCP is a competitor of SG, although no one knows if it is likely to replace it. In this respect, the term "sleeve-killer" seems exaggerated. On the other hand, LGCP could be matched by endoscopic gastric plication, if a long trajectory of the stomach can be plicated through the endoscopic approach, or at least LCGP may serve as a benchmark for endoscopic plication techniques. The surgical technique includes division of the gastric vessels at 2 cm distance from the gastric wall, the plication concerning specifically the greater curve of the stomach. One or two nonabsorbable running sutures are recommended, with a distance and a depth from 1.5 to 2.5 cm. A calibration with a gastric tube, like the one used for a SG, can be replaced in the beginning of the experience by intraoperative endoscopy. The plication starts 2 cm away from the angle of His, preserves a couple of short gastric vessels and ends at 8–11 cm from the pylorus.

The technique was invented in Iran with long-term results that seemed interesting but have not been repeated [14]. Both animal work and clinical experimentation have demonstrated that vertical plication along the greater curve was the way to go [15, 16]. Series have shown good results [17], but, as explained in Chap. 3, evidence-based medicine is not in favour of LGCP when compared to SG: reoperations are common after LGCP and not easy because of the thickness of gastric wall [18], and mid- or long-term results are inferior to those of SG [19] (Table 11.2). However, LGCP could be a useful benchmark to minimally invasive plication techniques, and other restrictive endoscopic techniques, which have been extensively discussed in Chap. 2.

Among these techniques, procedures with endoluminal plication, either by separated folds with shoe anchors (POSE) or by separated running sutures with a Z-like pattern (OverStitch, also called endoscopic sleeve gastroplasty (ESG)), are already successful for managing mild to moderately obese patients [25].

Initially, the main objective was the downsizing of a gastric pouch and/or anastomosis that had been enlarged a few years after RYGB [26]. The FDA approved both methods for tissue apposition after bariatric surgery. Later, endoscopists deemed it feasible for the primary treatment of patients and obtained safe and

Table 11.2 Twelve-month results of LGCP compared to SG in published series, with 12-month weight loss expressed as %excess weight loss (EWL) and within brackets the number of patients

Authors	SG: 12-month mean % EWL (N patients)	LGCP: 12-month mean % EWL (N patients)
Shen et al. (2013) [20]	80 (20)	58.8 (19)
Chouillard et al. (2016) [21]	61.2 (40)	51.9 (40)
Sharma et al. (2015) [22]	53.8 (15)	42.1 (15)
Abdelbaki et al. (2014) [23]	68.1 (78)	52.1 (62)
Grubnik et al. (2016) [24]	59.5 (27)	45.8 (25)

reproducible results [27]. For instance, Lopez-Nava et al. reviewed the data of three centres who performed an ESG in 248 patients between 2013 and 2015 [28]. Their baseline BMI was 37.8 kg/m^2. At 6 and 24 months, 33 and 35 patients were lost to follow-up, respectively. At 6 and 24 months, % TBWL was 15.2% and 18.6%, respectively. Weight losses were similar in the three centres after 6 and 24 months. At 6 and 24 months, the percentage of patients achieving ≥10% TBWL was 84.2% and 53%, respectively. On multivariable linear regression analysis, only % TBWL at 6 months significantly predicted % TBWL at 24 months. The odds of achieving ≥10% TBWL at 24 months if a patient achieved <10% TBWL at 6 months is 0.18 (95% Confidence interval 0.034–0.84). Five (2%) serious adverse events occurred, of which four were related to the procedure itself: a pneumothorax and pneumoperitoneum that required a chest tube, one splenic laceration causing a haemorrhage and two perigastric collections at the level of the fundus. Especially the latter two have been discussed in the previous Chap. 10 as a possible difficulty in eventual future bariatric surgery. Endoscopists who perform these gastric plications should report their cases that subsequently underwent surgery as both the surgical and endoscopic world should learn lessons from these cases.

11.4 Duodenojejunal Bypass Sleeve (DJBS)

The duodenal-jejunal bypass sleeve (DJBS), or EndoBarrier Gastrointestinal Liner, is supposed to mimic a duodenal-jejunal bypass (see also Chap. 2). It has an anchor to reversibly affix the device to the wall of the duodenum and an impermeable fluoropolymer sleeve extending 60 cm into the small bowel. The impact on type 2 diabetes mellitus (T2DM) is thought to act via exclusion of the foregut from foods, the so-called foregut hypothesis. It is assumed that in the duodenum, when exposed to nutrients, an unknown anti-incretin factor is secreted in patients with T2DM. Excluding the proximal intestine from nutrients by malabsorptive bariatric surgical techniques improves T2DM within days [29]. Moreover, due to the increased exposure of lower bowel loops to nutrients, gut peptides like glucagon-like peptide-1 (GLP-1), an incretin hormone, and peptide YY (PYY) with a major role in motility are secreted and play a role (hindgut hypothesis).

Given its mechanisms of action, this procedure is meant to match the metabolic effects of a genuine gastric bypass (with a Roux-en-Y limb). Provided that side effects can be handled (anchor fixation, lumen obstruction, bleeding, liver abscesses, etc.), it might be promising, although there are two negative and only one positive meta-analyses [30–32]. The DJBS did not pass the above-mentioned PIVI criteria [12]. The studies that looked into the hormonal effects of the DJBS and the explanation for the improvement in diabetes have been discussed in Chap. 2 and unfortunately are not consistent. The beautiful results by de Jonge et al. with data that fitted perfectly in the foregut and hindgut hypothesis have not been replicated by others [33]. Also, the study by Vilarrasa et al. which evaluated the efficacy and safety of the DJBS in 21 grade 1 obese (BMI 30–35 kg/m^2) T2DM patients with poor metabolic control could only partly explain the effects on glucose metabolism [34]. These patients with a diabetes duration of 14.8 years and HbA1c value of 9.1 under insulin therapy lost 14.9 kg of their total body weight over the 12 months of the study. HbA1c decreased 1.3% in the first month, but at the end of the study the reduction was only 0.6%. A HbA1c ≤7% was achieved by 26.3% of patients. No differences in GLP-1 AUC values were found before and after implant. Fasting plasma ghrelin and PYY concentrations increased from months 1 to 12. Conversely, fasting plasma glucagon concentrations decreased at month 1 but increased thereafter. Weight and HbA1c decreases at month 1 were the only variables that predicted the HbA1c values at 12 months. Minor adverse events occurred in 14% of patients and major events in 9.5%.

Apart from bypassing the duodenum the RYGB and the DJBS differ with respect to the fundus with ghrelin secretion. Ghrelin is an orexigen but also has anti-insulin properties. The fundus is excluded from food passage only by the oesophagogastroduodenojejunal bypass (ValenTx) which is thus more similar to the RYGB. However, data on hormones are not yet available. Also, other effects of the RYGB on bile acid metabolism and on microbiota have not yet been investigated with these bypass liners, and very recently van der Wielen et al. investigated the effects of the ACE stapling which largely mimics the effect after POSE (downsizing of the fundus and antral plications to retard gastric emptying), on microbiome and gene expression, and found a downregulation of the secretion of ghrelin and a significant reduction of inflammatory tone in the upper gastrointestinal tract [35]. They could not answer the question whether this might be a consequence of an improved metabolic health status and weight loss or alternatively caused by the procedure itself.

As initially the DJBS did not really provide a marked weight loss, the DJBS was positioned in the market as a metabolic treatment for obese patients with T2DM. It is as yet unclear whether the beneficial metabolic effects will sustain in the long term, suggesting that probably the bypass effect is not long-standing in the absence of significant initial weight loss. More data are needed to sort out the various components of the procedures that bypass the duodenum.

Another, relatively new player in the field also focuses on the role of the duodenal mucosa, which is hypertrophied and shows endocrine hyperplasia in T2DM. Duodenal mucosa resurfacing or Revita is a technique of mucosal ablation of the duodenum mucosa distal from the papilla up to the ligament of Treitz with restoration and rejuvenation of the duodenum mucosa as a result and thereby improving or curing diabetes (see Chap. 2) [36]. Maybe this method may be added to the armamentarium of duodenal exclusion as is done with the DJBS for which safety issues have first to be solved.

11.5 GORD Treatment as a Field of Competition?

11.5.1 Basic Principles

Restriction of the upper part of the stomach may be achieved via endoscopy as was shown with the Transoral Restrictive Implant System (TERIS), an endoscopic bariatric treatment that mimics the laparoscopic gastric banding which is not in vogue anymore (see Chaps. 2 and 3). When performing endoscopy after the TERIS procedure as well as in patients after the positioning of a gastric band a small portion of stomach beneath the Z line and above the band acts as an effective pouch. This forms a cone-like area that can be identified endoscopically as a high-pressure area above the narrowed outlet. The anatomical features of the junction between the longitudinal fibres of the oesophagus and the circular fibres of the stomach may explain why some degree of GORD and/or oesophageal dilation is likely to occur in the long term after a gastric band has been placed, even when it is correctly placed and without the complications of gastric prolapse and band slippage. Similar to the band, also in the sleeve gastrectomy the stomach is a high-pressure zone that is incompliant when being filled and thereby increasing the pressure which may be instrumental in increasing reflux of acid or food.

11.5.2 Treating GORD Endoscopically in Obese Patients?

Many would object dealing endoscopically with GORD in an obese patient who would be eligible for bariatric surgery, which should preferably be a gastric bypass. Yet, patients may be unwilling to undergo a rather aggressive approach, particularly if they are moderately obese.

When intensification of conservative treatment is tried consciously and does not provide sufficient relief of symptoms, new endoluminal methods may be tried [37, 38] (see also Chap. 6). Four methods are available, although the last three are still investigational: (1) radiofrequency energy delivery to the gastro-oesophageal junction (Stretta procedure); (2) the transoral fundoplication therapy with moulding of the tissue and placement of polypropylene suture material in the region of the gastro-oesophageal junction; (3) MUSE™ endoscopic stapling system, a technique that creates an endoscopic partial fundoplication; and 4. anti-reflux mucosectomy (ARMS) with endoscopic mucosal resection and endoscopic submucosal dissection creating a sharp mucosal valve at the gastric cardia [37, 38].

In a fairly old study dating back to 2009, White et al. evaluated the outcomes using two commercially available endoluminal therapies in 22 consecutive obese patients (BMI > 30 kg/m^2) with GORD (DeMeester > 14.5) undergoing either Plicator (NDO Surgical, Mansfield, MA, USA) or Stretta (Stretta System, Curon Medical, Sunnyvale, CA, USA) [39]. The Plicator technique consisted of placing several plication-stitches with pledgets at the gastro-oesophageal junction, under retroflexed view; the Stretta method consisted of applying a radiofrequency catheter endoluminally at the gastro-oesophageal junction, under direct vision. Outcomes assessed were (1) the failure rate, defined as absolutely no symptomatic improvement after the procedure and/or need for subsequent anti-reflux surgery; (2) change in post-treatment vs. pretreatment symptoms (heartburn, chest pain, regurgitation, dysphagia, cough, hoarseness and asthma) scores; and (3) proton pump inhibitor (PPI) medication use. Twenty-two patients underwent an endoluminal therapy (10 Plicator patients and 12 Stretta patients) with a mean follow-up of 1.5 years. There were no treatment-associated complications. Mean BMI was not different between Plicator and Stretta groups (39.6 kg/m^2 vs. 38.6 kg/m^2, respectively). The failure rate for the entire cohort was 28%; 10% of Plicator patients versus 42% of Stretta patients failed ($p = 0.11$). The proportion of patients reporting moderate/severe symptoms post-treatment was significantly less than the proportion of patients reporting these symptoms pretreatment. Chest pain decreased from 13 to 9%; cough from 36 to 22%; voice changes from 36 to 9% and dysphagia from 32 to 9%. The proportion of patients remaining on PPI medications was also less (45% vs. 81%). They concluded that endoluminal treatment can provide a safe means of improving GORD symptoms for some obese patients, though many will continue to require medication.

However, a systematic review and meta-analysis of trials evaluated the efficacy of Stretta for the management of GORD in *non-bariatric* patients [40]. The pooled data from four trials and 153 analysed patients showed no differences between Stretta and sham or PPI therapy for the outcomes of mean oesophageal acid exposure, lower oesophageal sphincter pressure, ability to stop PPIs, or quality of life [40].

11.5.3 Learning from GORD Endoscopic Procedures

Pharmacological treatment and endoscopic therapy for GORD has been a leading research project for more than 15 years and has been shown to partly replace anti-reflux surgery and hiatal hernia repair. However, at that time only surgical procedures via laparotomy were feasible and things might have changed by the current approach by laparoscopic surgery. Various techniques have been described that reinforce the gastro-oesophageal junction. Two of these techniques, i.e. the radiofrequency method (Stretta) and non-circular injection of polymers should probably be discarded in the combination of obesity and GORD. Two others may have potential effects in the bariatric field: circular injection of an absorbable or nonabsorbable polymer that solidifies after injection [41], and full-thickness gastric plication [42], from which the devices and procedures described in the section "plication" are derived. For instance, the first suturing method in endoscopic bariatric therapy was an extension of the EndoCinch, a method used to treat GORD (see Chap. 2). These devices involve strictly the oesophagogastric junction and have no effect on food intake, except for a mild and transient dysphagia in less than 10% of the cases, which has also been observed in anti-reflux surgery. Unfortunately, the StomaphyX equipment that created an endoluminal cuff by stomach plication is no longer available. Leitman et al. treated 64 patients, of whom 18 suffered from severe gastro-oesophageal reflux [43]. After treatment symptoms of gastro-oesophageal reflux improved in 80% and resolved in 20%. Dargent et al. investigated the use of hyaluronic acid to produce such an internal gastric restriction, alone or in combination with an intragastric balloon, but they were disappointed in the end [44] (see Chap. 6).

It is likely that minimally invasive bariatric procedures (via natural orifices) will be performed more frequently in the future. Some surgeons consider that most, if not all, current endoscopic methods are not readily available with unproven cost efficiency, and that long-term outcomes are largely unknown. A more complete understanding of the physiology of the gastro-oesophageal junction after RYGB and sleeve gastrectomy may be highly useful when new types of operations through endoscopic channels are implemented aiming both at obesity and GORD. Creating a gastric restriction without durably impairing the normal gastro-oesophageal anatomy and function will be a key challenge when designing such procedures.

Conclusion

The International Federation for the Surgery of Obesity (IFSO) issued a position statement in 2017, which was intended to provide a framework for examining novel technologies and procedures in the bariatric field [45]. The goal is to keep an open mind about these new upcoming options for obese patients, balancing the ethical challenges that may develop based on the current available outcome data. The bullet points of that position paper are the following:

- Rapid changes in technology require the physician to be flexible, yet there must always remain a balance between the necessities of innovation and a comprehensive evaluation of the safety and merit of such endeavours. Ideally, the new technology should represent a less invasive approach compared to the currently accepted methods, be clinically effective and most importantly provide equally good results with decreased risk of complications.
- While traditional metabolic and bariatric surgery is an accepted option for a broad range of patients (see IFSO statement on class I obesity [7]), endoscopic bariatric techniques may fill a crucial void for the patients deemed not eligible or simply not interested in the traditional surgical interventions.
- Traditionally, individual medical and surgical societies would release their own consensus statements. The modern approach to this dilemma is that the multitude of societies should refer to the available body of work and evidence-based literature that has been published by similarly oriented societies. By issuing a joint consensus statement, it will be possible to establish algorithms that are based on solid fundamentals for the development of new technologies.
- Some of the newer less invasive technologies have not demonstrated the ability to achieve long-standing goals of effective weight loss and comorbidity resolution and could subsequently result in increased use of revision surgical interventions to ameliorate the results of the originally performed technology.
- Bariatric and metabolic surgery has been available for more than five decades and yet it still remains in evolution. It is difficult to fully imagine and foresee which future techniques and devices are going to be available to the bariatric and endoscopic surgeon/gastroenterologist and endoscopists. While the treatment modalities continue to advance, certain basic principles such as respect for evidence, ethical commitment, use of accepted methodology for data analysis and inclusion of patients in proper protocols remain a fundamental requirement. IFSO is engaged in implementing the vision for developing new technologies according to these standards.

References

1. Verlaan T, Paulus GF, Mathus-Vliegen EMH, Veldhuyzen EAML, Conchillo JM, Bouvy ND, et al. Endoscopic gastric volume reduction with a novel articulating plication device is safe and effective in the treatment of obesity. Gastrointest Endosc. 2015;81:312–20.
2. O'Brien PE, Dixon JB, Laurie C, Skinner S, Proietto J, McNeil J, et al. Treatment of mild to moderate obesity with laparoscopic adjustable gastric banding or an intensive medical program: a randomized trial. Ann Intern Med. 2006;144(9):625–33.
3. Dixon JB, O'Brien PE, Playfair J, Chapman L, Schachter LM, Skinner S, et al. Adjustable gastric banding and conventional therapy for type 2 diabetes: a randomized controlled trial. JAMA. 2008;299(3):316–23.
4. Lee WJ, Chong K, Ser KH, Lee YC, Chen SC, Chen JC, et al. Gastric bypass vs sleeve gastrectomy for type 2 diabetes mellitus: a randomized controlled trial. Arch Surg. 2011;146(2):143–8.
5. Schauer PR, Kashyap SR, Wolski K, Brethauer SA, Kirwan JP, Pothier CE, et al. Bariatric surgery versus intensive medical therapy in obese patients with diabetes. N Engl J Med. 2012;366(17):1567–76.
6. Ikramuddin S, Korner J, Lee WJ, Connett JE, Inabnet WB, Billington CJ, et al. Roux-en-Y gastric bypass vs intensive medical management for the control of type 2 diabetes, hypertension, and hyperlipidemia: the Diabetes Surgery Study randomized clinical trial. JAMA. 2013;309(21):2240–9.
7. Busetto L, Dixon J, De Luca M, Shikora S, Pories W, Angrisani L. Bariatric surgery in class I obesity. A position statement from the International Federation for the Surgery of Obesity and Metabolic Disorders (IFSO). Obes Surg. 2014;24(4):487–519.
8. World Health Organization. Obesity: preventing and managing the global epidemic. Report of a WHO Consultation on Obesity, Geneva, 3–5 June 1997. Report 1998 No.: WHO/NUT/NCD/98.1.
9. National Institutes of Health, National Heart, Lung and Blood Institute. Clinical Guidelines on the Identification. Evaluation, and treatment of overweight and obesity in adults- the evidence report. Obes Res. 1998;6(Suppl. 2):1S–209S.
10. National Institute for Health and Care Excellence. Obesity: guidance on the prevention, identification, assessment and management of overweight and obesity in adults and children. London, United Kingdom: National Institute for Health and Care Excellence; 2006. www.NICE.org.uk
11. Jensen MD, Ryan DH, Apovian CM, Ard JD, Comuzzie AG, Donato KA, et al. 2013 AHA/ACC/TOS guideline for the management of overweight and obesity in adults: a report of the American College of Cardiology/American Heart Association Task Force On Practice Guidelines and the Obesity Society. J Am Coll Cardiol. 2014;63:2985–3023.
12. ASGE Bariatric Endoscopy Task Force and ASGE Technology Committee, Abu Dayyeh BK, Kumar N, Edmundowicz SA, Jonnalagadda S, Larsen M, et al. ASGE Bariatric Endoscopy Task Force systematic review and meta-analysis assessing the ASGE PIVI thresholds for adopting endoscopic bariatric therapies. Gastrointest Endosc. 2015;82:425–38.
13. Apovian CM, Aronne LJ, Bessesen DH, McDonnell ME, Murad MH, Pagotto U, et al. Pharmacological management of obesity: an Endocrine Society clinical practice guideline. J Clin Endocrinol Metab. 2015;100:342–62.
14. Talebpour M, Amoli BS. Laparoscopic total gastric vertical plication in morbid obesity. J Laparoendosc Adv Surg Tech A. 2007;17:793–8.
15. Kirk RM. An experimental trial of gastric plication as a means of weight reduction in the rat. Br J Surg. 1969;56:930–3.
16. Brethauer SA, Harris JL, Kroh M, Schauer P. Laparoscopic gastric plication for treatment of severe obesity. Surg Obes Relat Dis. 2010;7(1):15–22.
17. Fried M, Dolezavola K, Buchwald JN, McGlennon TW, Stramkova P, Ribaric G, et al. Laparoscopic greater curve plication (LGCP) for treatment of morbid obesity in a series of 224 patients. Obes Surg. 2012;22(8):1298–307.

18. Zerrweck C, Rodríguez JG, Aramburo E, Viscara R, Rodriguez JL, Solorzano A, et al. Revisional surgery following laparoscopic gastric plication. Obes Surg. 2017;27(1):38–43.
19. Ye Q, Chen Y, Zhan X, Wang Y, Zhu J. Comparison of laparoscopic sleeve gastrectomy and laparoscopic greater curvature plication regarding efficacy and safety: a meta-analysis. Obes Surg. 2017;27:1358–64.
20. Shen D, Ye H, Wang Y, Ji Y, Zhan X, Zhu J, et al. Comparison of short-term outcomes between laparoscopic greater curvature plication and laparoscopic sleeve gastrectomy. Surg Endosc. 2013;27(8):2768–74.
21. Chouillard E, Schoucair N, Alsabah S, Alkandari B, Montana L, Dejonghe B, et al. Laparoscopic Gastric Plication (LGP) as an alternative to Laparoscopic Sleeve Gastrectomy (LSG) in patients with morbid obesity: A Preliminary, Short-Term, Case-Control Study. Obes Surg. 2016;26(6):1167–72.
22. Sharma S, Narwaria M, Cottam DR, Cottam S. Randomized double-blinded trial of laparoscopic gastric imbrication v laparoscopic sleeve gastrectomy at a single Indian institution. Obes Surg. 2015 May;25(5):800–4.
23. Abdelbaki TN, Sharaan M, Abdel-Baki NA, Katri K. Laparoscopic gastric greater curvature plication versus laparoscopic sleeve gastrectomy: early outcome in 140 patients. Surg Obes Relat Dis. 2014;10(6):1141–6.
24. Grubnik VV, Ospanov OB, Namaeva KA, Medvedev OV, Kresyun MS. Randomized controlled trial comparing laparoscopic greater curvature plication versus laparoscopic sleeve gastrectomy. Surg Endosc. 2016;30(6):2186–91.
25. Kumar N. Endoscopic therapy for weight loss: Gastroplasty, duodenal sleeve, intragastric balloons, and aspiration. World J Endosc. 2015;7(9):847–59.
26. Horgan S, Jacobsen G, Weiss GD, Oldham JS Jr, Denk PM, Borao F, et al. Incisionless revision of post-roux-en-Y bypass stomal and pouch dilatation: multicenter registry results. Surg Obes Relat Dis. 2010;6(3):290–5.
27. Espinos JC, Turro R, Mata A, Cruz M, da Costa M, Villa V, et al. Early experience with the incisionless operating platformTM (IOP) for the treatment of obesity. Obes Surg. 2013;23(9):1375–83.
28. Lopez-Nava G, Sharaiha RZ, Vargas EJ, Bazerbachi F, Manoel GN, Bautista-Castaño I, et al. Endoscopic Sleeve Gastroplasty for obesity: a Multicenter Study of 248 patients with 24 months follow-up. Obes Surg. 2017;27(10):2649–55.
29. Rubino F, Zizzari P, Tomasetto C, Bluet-Pajot MT, Forgione A, Vix M, et al. The role of the small bowel in the regulation of circulating ghrelin levels and food intake in the obese Zucker rat. Endocrinology. 2005;146(4):1745–51.
30. Patel SR, Hakim D, Mason J, Hakim N. The duodenal-jejunal bypass sleeve (EndoBarrier gastrointestinal liner) for weight loss and treatment of type 2 diabetes. Surg Obes Relat Dis. 2013;9:482–4.
31. Zechmeister-Koss I, Huic M, Fischer S. The duodenal-jejunal bypass liner for the treatment of type 2 diabetes mellitus and/or obesity: a systematic review. Obes Surg. 2014;24:310–23.
32. Rohde U, Hedbäck N, Gluud LL, Visboll T, Knop FK. Effect of the EndoBarrier gastrointestinal liner on obesity and type 2 diabetes: a systematic review and meta-analysis. Diabetes Obes Metab. 2016;18:300–5.
33. de Jonge C, Rensen SS, Verdam FJ, Vincent RP, Bloom SR, Buurman WA, et al. Endoscopic duodenal-jejunal bypass liner rapidly improves type 2 diabetes. Obes Surg. 2013;23:1354–60.
34. Vilarrasa N, de Gordejuela AG, Casajoana A, Duran X, Toro S, Espinet E, et al. Endobarrier in Grade I obese patients with long-standing Type 2 diabetes: role of gastrointestinal hormones in glucose metabolism. Obes Surg. 2017;27(3):569–77.
35. van der Wielen N, Paulus G, van Avesaat M, Masclee A, Meijerink J, Bouvy N. Effect of endoscopic gastroplication on the genome-wide transcriptome in the upper gastrointestinal tract. Obes Surg. 2017;27:740–8.
36. Rajagopalan H, Cherrington AD, Thompson CC, Kaplan LM, Rubino F, Mingrone G, et al. Endoscopic duodenal mucosal resurfacing for the treatment of type 2 diabetes: 6-month interim analysis from the first-in-human proof-of-concept study. Diab Care. 2016;39:2254–61.

37. Crawford C, Gibbens K, Lomelin D, Krause C, Simorov A, Oleynikov D. Sleeve gastrectomy and anti-reflux procedures. Surg Endosc. 2017;31:1012–21.
38. Triadafilopoulos G. Endoscopic options for gastroesophageal reflux: where are we now and what does the future hold? Curr Gastroenterol Rep. 2016;18:47.
39. White B, Jeansonne LO, Cook M, Chavarriaga LF, Goldenberg EA, Davis SS, et al. Use of endoluminal antireflux therapies for obese patients with GERD. Obes Surg. 2009;19(6):783–7.
40. Lipka S, Kumar A, Richter JE. No evidence for efficacy of radiofrequency ablation for treatment of gastroesophageal reflux disease: a systematic review and meta-analysis. Clin Gastroenterol Hepatol. 2015;13:1058–67.
41. Johnson DA, Ganz R, Aisenberg J, Cohen LB, Deviere J, Foley TR, et al. Endoscopic implantation of enteryx for treatment of GERD: 12-month results of a prospective, multicenter trial. Am J Gastroenterol. 2003;98(9):1921–30.
42. Pleskow D, Rothstein R, Lo S, Hawes R, Kozarek R, Haber G, et al. Endoscopic full-thickness plication for the treatment of GERD: a multicenter trial. Gastrointest Endosc. 2004;59(2):163–71.
43. Leitman IM, Virk CS, Avgerinos DV, Patel R, Lavarias V, Surick B, et al. Early results of trans-oral endoscopic plication and revision of the gastric pouch and stoma following Roux-en-Y gastric bypass surgery. JSLS. 2010;14:217–20.
44. Dargent J, Mion F, Costil V, Pontette F, Ecochard D, Mion M. Multicenter randomized study of obesity treatment with minimally invasive injection of hyaluronic acid versus and combined with intragastric balloon. Obes Surg. 2015;25(10):1842–7.
45. Dargent J, Vilallonga R, Katz L, Portenier D, Wilson E, Escalona A, et al. IFSO position statement on new technologies in bariatric surgery. Obes Surg. 2017;27(9):2456–9.

Printed by Printforce, the Netherlands